Blood Conservation in Cardiac Surgery

Springer
New York
Berlin
Heidelberg
Barcelona
Budapest
Hong Kong
London
Milan
Paris
Santa Clara
Singapore
Tokyo

Editors

Karl H. Krieger, M.D.

Professor and Vice Chairman, Department of Cardiothoracic Surgery, The New York Hospital-Cornell Medical Center, New York, New York

O. Wayne Isom, M.D.

Professor and Chairman, Department of Cardiothoracic Surgery, The New York Hospital-Cornell Medical Center, New York, New York

Blood Conservation in Cardiac Surgery

With 83 Figures

Springer

Karl H. Krieger, M.D.
O. Wayne Isom, M.D.
Department of Cardiothoracic Surgery
The New York Hospital–Cornell Medical Center
New York, NY 10021
USA

Library of Congress Cataloging-in-Publication Data
Blood conservation in cardiac surgery / [edited by]
Karl H. Krieger, O. Wayne Isom.
p. cm.
Includes bibliographical references and index.
ISBN 978-1-4612-7447-6 (hrdcvr : alk. paper)
1. Heart–Surgery. 2. Hemostasis, Surgical. 3. Blood–Transfusion. 4. Blood–Collection and preservation.
I. Krieger, Karl H. II. Isom, O. Wayne.
[DNLM: 1. Heart Surgery. 2. Blood Preservation. 3. Blood Transfusion. WG 169 B652 1997]
RD598.B577 1998
617.4'12059–dc21 96-45492

Printed on acid-free paper.

ISBN-13: 978-1-4612-7447-6 e-ISBN-13: 978-1-4612-2180-7
DOI:10.1007/978-1-4612-2180-7

Softcover reprint of the hardcover 1st edition 1998

Production coordinated by Chernow Editorial Services, Inc., and managed by Lesley Poliner; manufacturing supervised by Jeffrey Taub.
Typeset by TechType, Inc., Ramsey, NJ.

9 8 7 6 5 4 3 2 1

ISBN-13: 978-1-4612-7447-6 Springer-Verlag New York Berlin Heidelberg SPIN 10552889

Preface

Blood conservation has become a primary goal of medical practitioners at both academic and nonacademic medical centers. The term *blood transfusion* was once synonymous with the term *cardiac surgery*, but not blood and blood products are utilized in fewer than half of the cases performed in the United States. In preparation for open heart surgery, most centers type and cross four units of packed red blood cells, where as 15 years ago eight units were routinely prepared.

The impetus to conserve blood has come from multiple sources. In 1985 the general population was startled to learn of contamination of the nation's blood supply by the HIV virus and they became hesitant to undergo cardiac surgery, not because of the risks of surgery itself, but because of the risk of contracting the acquired immunodeficiency syndrome (AIDS) from a blood transfusion. Religious groups that refuse blood transfusions, such as Jehovah's Witnesses, wanted cardiac surgery to become more available to their members. Hospital and blood bank administrators totaled the cost of blood components used in their cardiac surgery programs and asked that transfusion practices be reexamined. Finally, cardiac surgeons and cardiologists became aware that the disadvantages associated with aggressive transfusion policies often outweighed the advantages.

Over the last decade, most hospitals and cardiac surgery centers have instituted a "blood conservation" program and some hospitals promote themselves as "bloodless surgical centers." Yet the meaning of these terms is not well defined. "Blood conservation" at one hospital may mean that cell-saving devices are used in the operating room. At another center "blood conservation" may imply that transfusion triggers have been standardized. On the other hand, some centers, such as the Cleveland Clinic, have used a wide range of physiologic, pharmacologic, and operative innovations to ensure a more broad-based program of blood rationing.

At the New York Hospital–Cornell University Medical Center, we have developed a new, comprehensive, and at times radical approach to blood conservation. We have examined each facet of our cardiac surgery program to devise unique strategies to decrease blood and blood factor utilization.

We believe we have left no stones unturned in attempting to devise original and safe technology that salvages blood and blood products. Working closely with physicians from the departments of hematology, pathology (blood bank), cardiology, and anesthesiology, we have developed a comprehensive program that sets a unique standard in an age of blood rationing. An algorithm has been developed that is safe, understandable, and user friendly, and it can be incorporated into most cardiac surgery guidelines.

This book describes the development of this algorithm. The text is divided into four parts that mirror the clinical course of a cardiac surgical patient. Part I describes the preoperative period, in which issues related to a patient's preparation for cardiac surgery are examined. Part II describes the decision-making experience in the operating room, where procedural and operative techniques often define who will require transfusions. Part III describes the postoperative experience, in which transfusion decisions may no longer rest solely in the hands of the cardiac surgeon. Part IV concludes with an algorithm that summarizes each component of the blood conservation program.

Using the guidelines outlined in the text, we have recently completed 100 consecutive coronary artery bypass operations without a single donor exposure (no red blood cells, no blood factors). We will also describe our large experience with Jehovah's Witness patients, in which complex reoperative procedures were undertaken.

At a time when politicians, patient advocate groups, and managed care programs are scrutinizing every aspect of the medical community for cost-effectiveness and quality guidelines, it behooves all individuals involved in medical care to provide the best possible care at the lowest possible price. Blood conservation in cardiac surgery takes a critical step toward achieving this goal.

The editors would like to thank Jeannette Torres for her help and enthusiasm in the preparation of this text.

Karl H. Krieger, M.D.
Professor and Vice Chairman
Department of Cardiothoracic Surgery
The New York Hospital–Cornell Medical Center
New York, New York

O. Wayne Isom, M.D.
Professor and Chairman
Department of Cardiothoracic Surgery
The New York Hospital–Cornell Medical Center
New York, New York

Contents

III. Postoperative Bleeding and Management

IV. Algorithm for Bloodless Surgery at The New York Hospital–Cornell Medical Center

Contributors

Gabriel S. Aldea, M.D., Associate Professor, Department of Cardiothoracic Surgery, Boston University Medical Center, Boston, MA 02118, USA

Nasser K. Altorki, M.D., Associate Profesor, Department of Cardiothoracic Surgery, The New York Hospital–Cornell Medical Center, New York, NY 10021, USA

Adam S. Asch, M.D., Associate Professor, Department of Medicine, The New York Hospital–Cornell Medical Center, New York, NY 10021, USA

Su-Pen Bobby Chang, Assistant Professor, Department of Anesthesiology, The New York Hospital–Cornell Medical Center, New York, NY 10021, USA

Joseph A. Dearani, Mayo Clinic, Rochester, MN 55905, USA

William DeBois, C.C.P., The New York Hospital–Cornell Medical Center, Room F-10 New York, NY 10021, USA

Nabeel G. El-Amir, M.D., Chief Resident, Department of Cardiothoracic Surgery, Columbia-Presbyterian Medical Center, New York, NY 10032, USA

Jeffrey P. Gold, M.D., Professor and Chairman, Unified Department of Cardiothoracic Surgery, Montefiore Medical Center, Bronx, NY 10467, USA

Maureen E. Gomez, R.N., M.P.H., C.C.R.N., The New York Hospital–-Cornell Medical Center, New York, NY 10021, USA

Robert E. Helm, M.D., Clinical Research Fellow, Department of Cardiothoracic Surgery, The New York Hospital–Cornell Medical Center, New York, NY 10021, USA

O. Wayne Isom, M.D., Professor and Chairman, Department of Cardiothoracic Surgery, The New York Hospital–Cornell Medical Center, New York, NY 10021, USA

Justin S. Kang, M.D., Chief Resident, Department of Cardiothoracic Surgery, Columbia-Presbyterian Medical Center, New York, NY 10032, USA

John D. Klemperer, M.D., Research Fellow, Department of Cardiothoracic Surgery, The New York Hospital–Cornell Medical Center, New York, NY 10021, USA

Karl H. Krieger, M.D., Professor and Vice Chairman, Department of Cardiothoracic Surgery, The New York Hospital–Cornell Medical Center, New York, NY 10021, USA

Stephen J. Lahey, M.D., Assistant Professor, Department of Surgery, Harvard Medical School–New England Deaconess Hospital, Boston, MA 02215, USA

Samuel J. Lang, M.D., Professor, Department of Cardiothoracic Surgery, The New York Hospital–Cornell Medical Center, New York, NY 10021, USA

Kathleen A. Leonard, M.D., Assistant Professor, Department of Pathology, Assistant Director, Blood and Transfusion Services, The New York Hospital–Cornell Medical Center, New York, NY 10021, USA

David C. Mair, M.D., Departments of Pathology and Internal Medicine, University of Virginia Health Sciences Center, Charlottesville, VA 22908, USA

John P. Miller, M.D., Departments of Pathology and Internal Medicine, University of Virginia Health Sciences Center, Charlottesville, VA 22908, USA

Paul D. Mintz, M.D., Professor, Department of Pathology and Internal Medicine, University of Virginia Health Sciences Center, Charlottesville, VA 22908, USA

Thomas W. Nash, The New York Hospital–Cornell Medical Center, New York, NY 10021, USA

Todd K. Rosengart, M.D., Assistant Professor, Department of Cardiothoracic Surgery, The New York Hospital–Cornell Medical Center, New York, NY 10021, USA

Hartzell V. Schaff, Professor, Division of Thoracic and Cardiovascular Surgery, Mayo Clinic Rochester, MN 55905, USA

Richard J. Shemin, M.D., Professor and Chairman, Department of Cardiothoracic Surgery, Boston University Medical Center Hospital, Boston, MA 02118-2393, USA

Craig R. Smith, M.D. Department of Cardiothoracic Surgery, Columbia-Presbyterian Medical Center, New York, NY 10032, USA

Richard Stennet, M.D., Instructor, Department of Anesthesiology, The New York Hospital-Cornell Medical Center, New York, NY 10021, USA

Patrick R. Treanor, C.C.P., Department of Cardiothoracic Surgery, Boston University Medical Center Hospital, Boston, MA 02118-2393, USA

Ferdinand T. Velasco, M.D., Chief Resident, Department of Cardiothoracic Surgery, The New York Hospital-Cornell Medical Center, New York, NY 10021, USA

Carl F.W. Wolf, M.D., Director, Blood Bank and Transfusion Services, The New York Hospital-Cornell Medical Center, New York, NY 10021, USA

David J. Wolf, M.D., Clinical Associate Professor, Department of Medicine, The New York Hospital-Cornell Medical Center, New York, NY 10021, USA

Part I
Preoperative Considerations in Cardiac Surgery

1
Current Practice of Blood Transfusion in Cardiac Surgery

Carl F.W. Wolf and Jeffrey P. Gold

The History of Transfusion in Cardiovascular Surgery

The use of blood products dates back to the very birth of cardiac surgery. In the earliest days of cross-circulation, systemic hypothermia, inflow occlusion, and subsequently with the development of the heart lung machine, red blood cell transfusion and, later, component therapy have been intimately related to the successful evolution of cardiac surgery. In many large institutions, the activities of the cardiac service determined the majority of the institution's utilization of blood products. Attempts to maintain "normal" circulating blood volume and hematocrit and "normal" coagulation profiles have driven this tremendous demand, and ten to fifteen donor exposures per patient were often required. Donor services needed to be developed to register and screen literally hundreds of donors for a typical cardiac surgery schedule.

Recognition by surgeons and hematologists of the significant trauma to formed elements of the bloodstream, to the red cells and platelets in particular, as well as an overall interest in decreasing patient donor exposure have driven the development of intraoperative hemodilution while on cardiopulmonary bypass. Pump primes that once consisted of whole blood were replaced with smaller volumes of either pure crystalloid solutions or combinations of asanguineous crystalloid and colloid solution, which resulted in no donor exposures. As flow rates, blood pressure, and hematocrit levels on cardiopulmonary bypass were initially set empirically, and as they were blessed with many decades of excellent clinical results, changes came slowly with regard to transfusion therapy in cardiac surgery.

As the surgical risk for even complex open heart procedures declined in the early 1980s, the risk of blood product transfusion suddenly exploded in the nation's medical consciousness. Almost overnight in 1985 the world focused on transfusion-related diseases and in particular, patients were terrified by the threat of the acquired immunodeficiency syndrome (AIDS). This change in mentality further altered the perceived risk-benefit ratios of blood product transfusion and caused the medical community to look at transfusion therapy in a very different way, questioning the need for each donor exposure. The public began to demand changes in the classic paradigms of transfusion therapy and started requesting the availability of autologous and directed donor products. This public awareness prompted patients and families of patients undergoing open heart surgery to question the overall need and wisdom of transfusion at all. Manufacturers of perfusion equipment began to miniaturize blood handling equipment to limit the priming volume and new devices were developed to scavenge and return all shed operative blood. All of these changes and concerns have resulted in the present marketing frenzy that patients, biotechnology manufacturers, and cardiothoracic surgery programs deal with on a daily basis.

The widespread availability of the above-described technology and the mandated utilization of accurate donor testing has shifted the risk-benefit equation toward the direction of overall patient safety, but not to a point that patients or their medical practitioners can relax their vigilance to minimize transfusion therapy. New evidence of long-standing posttransfusion immunoincompetence, and late or "slow" virus infections have recently refueled the fires of patient concern and practitioner cautions. The very need for written informed consent for transfusion therapy in most settings when transfusion of nonautologous blood product is contemplated is further testimony of the level of concern that permeates one of the oldest therapies known to the medical profession.

This book attempts to precisely define the present-day risk of transfusion therapy, and then to meticulously dissect the huge fund of knowledge that has been developed addressing the conservation of blood products in cardiothoracic surgery. Much has changed since the first human was placed on cardiopulmonary bypass in 1953. Blood transfusion and conservation is a rapidly developing and highly dynamic field, marrying the talents of medical scientists ranging from clinicians to molecular biologists. Almost every area of clinical and basic medical science either has been or presently is involved in this Herculean effort.[1-10]

The New York Hospital Protocol for Blood Products in Open-Heart Surgery

At the New York Hospital–Cornell Medical Center, where open-heart surgery has been routinely available since the late 1950s, blood product utilization has evolved dramatically. Pure blood primes gave way to partially asanguineous primes in the mid-1960s and subsequently to asanguineous primes (for adults) in the early 1980s. Attention to transfusion triggers on bypass and after bypass, has further decreased the use of blood products. A comprehensive program of evaluation of blood product utilization for the entire service and for each individual surgeon has allowed

TABLE 1.1. New York Hospital Open-Heart Blood Preparation Protocol.

Adult:	Four units of packed cells; type and cross. Two unit sent to OR with patient. Fresh frozen plasma (FFP), platelets on request only.
Pediatric:	Whole blood, packed cells, FFP, and platelets, individualized per case.

rapid feedback to the program director and to the surgeons, further reducing the volume and diversity of blood products utilized. This comprehensive multidisciplinary approach had been in place and actively utilized since the early 1990s.

The routine availability of antifibrinolytics and mechanical means of blood prime reduction and red cell salvage has had a large impact in the late 1980s and early 1990s. Rapid testing for specific coagulopathic states and specific component therapy has nearly obliterated "shotgun" component therapy. The protocol for blood preparation prior to open heart surgery has evolved over the past three decades as well and currently, as illustrated in Table 1.1, drives all routine blood product preparation in our center for all adult and pediatric patients.

Current Practice of Blood Transfusion in Cardiovascular Surgery

As the morbidity and mortality of cardiac operations have decreased, the risks of the transfusion of allogeneic "bank" blood or directed donor blood have come to represent an increased percentage of the overall risk of cardiac operations.

Currently the practice of blood transfusion in cardiovascular surgery continues to be a topic of considerable interest to many surgeons. This book provides the basis for the interested surgeon to develop a reasonable transfusion plan for each patient, a plan that integrates all currently feasible interventions to minimize allogeneic blood exposure.

The use of blood products in cardiovascular surgery has been studied extensively in recent years in the United States, Europe, and Australia.[11–14] The dominant impression one gets from those studies is that the use of blood products varies widely from institution to institution and from country to country, and that, in turn, suggests that the practice of blood transfusion is primarily determined by the local environment, perhaps by the dominant surgeon(s).

Speiss et al[15] reviewed 1079 mixed cardiac cases done in 1990 and found that 78% received packed red blood cells (PRBC), 53% had platelet transfusions, and 31% received FFP. The overall transfusion rate at his institution was 82%. At the opposite end of the spectrum, Cosgrove et al[16] at the Cleveland Clinic, reviewed in 1985, 441 bypass patients who received an average of 0.3 units per patient with only 10% being transfused. Reviewing Tables 27.1 and 27.2, in Chapter 27, it seems that at most medical centers in the United States at least 50% of patients sent for open heart surgery are exposed to an average of two to four donor units in the form of PRBC, FFP, or platelets. Valvular, mixed, and reoperative cases received more exposures than primary coronary artery bypass (CAB) patients.[17–19]

It has been shown that individual physicians differ in their transfusion decision making.[20,21] Few would argue with the assertion by Bex et al[22]: "The duty of a surgeon is constant self-assessment and determination of what is relevant to his personal practice and applicable to improvement of his personal results. . . . Common sense and the surgeon's subjective personal appreciation of the risks involved in a technique or procedure must play an important role in the final decision reached concerning the patient who has placed his trust in him." Accordingly, appreciation of the risks of giving a transfusion needs to be included in the decision whether to transfuse. The decision to transfuse usually arises from concerns about the risks of not transfusing.[20,21]

In one study, the perception of the risk of not transfusing a patient who potentially needs it was influenced by the ordering physician's personal experience.[20] Physicians who reported having personally treated a patient who suffered an adverse outcome that might have been prevented by transfusion, gave estimates of the risk of myocardial infarction if transfusion were withheld that were twice as high as those given by physicians without such experience.[20] This suggests that the risk of not transfusing, as defined by a panel of experts, is overestimated by physicians with experience of an adverse event, probably resulting in unnecessary transfusions. It would thus appear to be a worthy personal objective for physicians who have experienced such adverse events to reassess the risks that they attach to not transfusing.[3] Perceptions of the risk of transfusing, on the other hand, are not necessarily influenced by personal experience.[20]

From another point of view guidelines for the use of blood products can be helpful in changing physician ordering behavior,[23–26] although some advocate the use of regulations to avoid the delay implicit in the educational approach.[27] It can be argued that "less blood is better" is an unwarranted assumption, and that outcome studies are needed to assure that undertransfusion does not occur.[28] While outcome studies are definitely needed, the current wide variation in use of blood products for similar procedures by different surgical teams suggests that there is a considerable way to go in blood conservation before undertransfusion becomes a significant problem.[12,17] One hopes that by then outcomes data will be available.

The objective of our review of transfusion practices in cardiovascular surgery is to minimize the exposure of patients to allogeneic blood products. Is this single-minded approach cost-effective? In a recent study of preoperative autologous donation in coronary artery bypass grafting (CABG), it was concluded that it was not cost-effective, and the risk of donation before CABG may well outweigh the benefits associated with fewer allogeneic transfusions.[29] But the study did not consider the nonmedical benefits of patient demand for the service, mandates by law in some states that the service be offered to surgical patients, and the fact that litigation has been caused by failure to offer it.[30] In another study, it was calculated that the use of predeposit autologous blood in CABG cost $107 per unit more than a unit of allogeneic "bank" blood.[31] The cost-effectiveness of the practice was estimated at $494,000 per quality-adjusted life year gained. An accompanying editorial, however, still deemed it prudent practice to reduce the transfusion of allogeneic blood whenever possible, including the judicious use of autologous blood.[32] There is no doubt that the primary medical reasons for avoiding allogeneic transfusions have diminished as the risk of transmitting the human immunodeficiency virus (HIV) and other infectious agents has been diminished by current donor testing and screening procedures, but there will always be medical reasons for it, and the risks will never be zero. Indeed, other potentially harmful effects of allogeneic transfusion are only now being explored, such as immunosuppression, and new blood-borne infections can emerge at any time.[33,34]

In our own experience, an extensive use of blood products in cardiac bypass procedures was, over a period of 3 years, markedly modified by providing feedback information on blood use to the responsible surgeons. It may be that a program of information feedback, such as proposed for the European Union hospitals that participated in a recent study of blood utilization, will have a similar salutary effect.[12,28]

Risks of Blood Transfusion

The risks of transfusion can be stated mathematically, but the perception of risks and their significance to the individual patient or physician are much more complex.[35,36] When offered the opportunity to choose between behaviors that have the same ultimate probability of death but that differ in their certainty of death, most people choose the behavior that permits them to live in a state of hopeful uncertainty.[37] That tendency probably explains why people fear HIV infection, with its fatal outcome, more than hepatitis B infection, and it may also explain why fear of other low-probability events, such as being involved in an airplane crash, appears to greatly exceed that of being involved in an automobile crash, even though the probability of injury and death from auto crashes exceeds that from airplane crashes, given that many more auto crashes occur.[37]

In the discussion that follows, the risk of disease transmission is stated as risk per donor exposure, or per blood component unit administered. It is important to realize that a risk so stated of 1 in 420,000 units, for example, becomes 1 in 42,000 if an individual patient is given 10 units (420,000/10), and so on. Since many patients who are transfused are exposed to more than one unit, this is an important factor in assessing risk.

The risks of blood transfusion can be categorized as shown in Table 1.2.[38–42]

TABLE 1.2. The risks of blood transfusion.

- *1. Infectious disease transmission*
  - *Viral Infections*
    - Retroviruses
      - HIV 1/2
      - HTLV-1/II
    - *Hepatitis viruses*
      - Enteric
        - Hepatitis A (HAV)
        - Hepatitis E (HEV)
        - Hepatitis F (HFV)
      - Parenteral
        - Hepatitis B (HBV)
        - Hepatitis C (HCV)
        - Hepatitis D (HDV)
        - Hepatitis G (GBV-C)
    - *Herpesviruses*
      - CMV
      - Human Herpesvirus-6 (HHV-6)
      - Epstein-Barr virus (EBV)
    - *B19 Parvovirus*
    - *Exotic viruses*
      - Rift Valley fever virus, Colorado tick fever virus, Ebola virus, Lassa fever virus, Marburg virus, yellow fever virus, dengue virus
    - *Idiopathic CD-4 lymphocytopenia (ICL)*
    - Creutzfeldt-Jakob disease
  - *Bacteria*
    - *Yersinia enterocolitica; Pseudomonas fluorescens; Serratia liquefaciens; Serratia marcescens* and others
    - Staphylococcus epidermidis, *S. aureus,* Diphtheroids, and others
    - *Treponema pallidum*
    - Lyme disease (*Borrelia burgdorferi*)
    - *Brucella abortus*
    - Rickettsia rickettsiae

(*Continued*)

Screening of Blood Donors

Transmission of blood-borne infections is a most serious complication of allogeneic transfusions. Prospective donors are asked many questions about their health, and especially many questions pertaining to AIDS and AIDS-related symptoms. All donors are given information describing people at risk of exposure to HIV and a method of confidentially excluding themselves if they feel they might fit into one of those high-risk categories. All donors are currently tested for the following (see list in Table 1.3): hepatitis B surface antigen (HBsAg); antibody to hepatitis B core antigen (HBcAb); antibody to hepatitis C virus (HCVAb); antibody to human T-cell lymphocytotropic virus types I and II (anti-HTLV-I/II); antibody to the human immunodeficiency viruses (anti-HIV-1/2); the p24 antigen of

TABLE 1.2. (*Continued*)

Parasites
Malaria (*Plasmodium* species)
Babesiosis (*Babesia microti*) and other piroplasmas
Trypanosoma cruzi
Toxoplasma gondii
Microfilaria
2. *Blood antigen incompatibility*
Acute hemolytic transfusion reaction
Delayed hemolytic transfusion reaction
Alloimmunization
Alloimmunization to red cell, platelet, white cell antigens
Posttransfusion purpura
Neonatal alloimmune thrombocytopenia/neutropenia
Hemolytic disease of the newborn
Refractoriness to platelet transfusions
Graft vs host disease
Febrile reactions (FNHTRs)
Cytokine induced
Leukocyte incompatibility induced
Allergic reactions
Anaphylactoid (urticaria)
Anaphylactic (IgA/anti-IgA)
Noncardiac pulmonary edema (transfusion-related acute lung injury [TRALI])
3. *Nonimmunologic reactions*
Circulatory overload
Iron overload
Depletion of coagulation proteins and platelets
Microaggregate infusion
Metabolic complications
4. *Immunosuppression/immunomodulation*
Immunosuppression
Neoplasia
Infection
5. *Excess morbidity and mortality associated with transfusion*

TABLE 1.3. Tests performed on blood donors.

Hepatitis B surface antigen (HBsAg)
Antibody to hepatitis B core antigen (HBcAb)
Antibody to hepatitis C virus (HCVAb)
Antibody to human T-cell lymphocytotropic viruses types I and II (anti-HTLV-I/II)
Antibody to the human immunodeficiency viruses (anti-HIV-1/2)
HIV-1 p24 antigen
Serum ALT level (SGPT)*
Serologic test for syphilis
ABO and Rh typing
Screen for unexpected red cell antibodies

*The requirement for ALT testing has been eliminated by several regulatory and accrediting bodies but testing continues in many areas to permit salvaged plasma to be used in countries where ALT testing is still required. A value of twice the upper limit of normal or more is commonly used to reject a donation.

HIV[43,44] serologic test for syphilis; ABO and Rh groups; and screen for unexpected anti-red cell antibodies. Because the assays for HCV, HIV, and HTLV were assays for antibody and not for the virus itself, there is a potential "window" period between infection and formation of detectable antibody. As assays for the antibody improve in sensitivity, that window becomes smaller, but cannot reach zero. For that reason, a test for the HIV p24 viral antigen has recently been adopted. The serum ALT [serum glutamic-pyruvic transaminase (SGPT)] level is no longer required, but to satisfy requirements for salvaged plasma users, it is still performed on some donations.

Infectious Complications

Viral Infections

Retroviruses

HIV-1 and HIV-2. HIV infection continues to cause the greatest concern among transfusion recipients even though it is probably one of the least-frequent adverse effects of transfusion. With the advent of donor testing for antibody to HIV in 1985, the risk of transfusion-transmitted HIV decreased dramatically. Subsequently, the assay has been improved in sensitivity, interviewing techniques for the exclusion of high-risk donors have been improved, and new assays for hepatitis C (1990), surrogate assays for non-A, non-B hepatitis (1986), and an assay for HTLV-I/II (1989) have been added to donor screening procedures, all of which also decrease the probability of HIV transmission because of epidemiologic considerations.

With the advent of donor screening for the p24 antigen of HIV, the risk of donation from an HIV-seronegative donor infectious for HIV has been reduced further. Before HIV p24 antigen screening, the risk (presumably due to the donor having a recent infection and not yet having made a detectable antibody, the so-called window period, and not testing positive on any of the other screening tests performed on donor blood) was 1 in 450,000 to 1 in 660,000 units.[44,45] After p24 antigen testing was introduced, it is estimated that the risk has been reduced to 1 in 563,000 to 1 in 825,000 units.[46] If the average recipient receives 5.4 units, the risk becomes 1 in 104,000 to 1 in 153,000 units. Antibody to HIV-1 and a related virus HIV-2 are both tested for with current assays, but HIV-2 is rarely encountered in the U.S., currently being largely confined to Western Africa.

HTLV-I and HTLV-II. HTLV-I, the causative agent of adult T-cell lymphoma-leukemia and the neurologic disease tropical spastic paraparesis (TSP), is endemic in West Africa, parts of Japan, and the Caribbean. A related virus, HTLV-II, is endemic in some native populations in North, Central, and South America. A history of intravenous drug use is commonly found in HTLV-II carriers in the U.S. The viruses are transmitted only by cellular blood products, and infectivity declines with storage time before transfusion. The assay for anti-HTLV-I cross-reacts to some degree but not completely with anti-HTLV-II. In some parts of the country, half of all donors who screen positive for HTLV-I/II are infected with HTLV-II. HTLV-I-infected individuals have a 2% to 4% lifetime risk of developing TSP or leukemia. HTLV-II has not been clearly associated with any diseases, but rare cases of TSP-like illness have been reported. The current residual risk of infection in the U.S. is estimated at 1 in 50,000 to 1 in 70,000.[47,48]

Hepatitis Viruses

Hepatitis A (HAV). Asymptomatic viremia occurs transiently during the incubation period of hepatitis A and thus can theoretically occur in a blood donor, but in practice that rarely occurs. For infection to occur, it is necessary that the recipient be negative for the antibody to HAV. HAV does not cause chronic hepatitis or establish a chronic carrier state and is considered an unlikely infection in routine transfusion practice. Rare examples of HAV transmission by transfused blood have occurred, however,[49] and there have been instances of transmission by coagulation factor concentrate blood derivatives prepared from large pools of donor plasma. Treatment of such pools with the commonly used solvent/detergent technology does not inactivate HAV, since it is not a lipid-enveloped virus.

Hepatitis E (HEV). Like HAV, this virus is not considered to be an important complication of blood transfusion because it does not establish a chronic carrier state. However, it can be a fatal infection in 15% to 20% of pregnant women, and epidemics occur in Africa, Asia, and the former Soviet Union. Since the viremia precedes the development of symptoms as in hepatitis A, parenteral infection from donor blood can theoretically occur.

Hepatitis F (HFV). The agent tentatively designated the hepatitis F virus has been described as a new, enterically transmitted virus, but that finding has not been substantiated. Designation of this isolate as a new hepatitis virus was probably premature.[34,50]

Parenteral Hepatitis Virus

Hepatitis B. The risk of hepatitis B transmission by donor blood is currently estimated at 1 in 200,000,[47] and the incidence rate of acute hepatitis B in blood recipients does not differ from the overall reporting rate for hepatitis B in the nontransfused population.[38]

Hepatitis C. Hepatitis C is responsible for the majority of transfusion-associated hepatitis, about 95%.[51] Only about 1 in 10 to 1 in 20 cases of HCV results from transfusion. A large proportion, about 40%, occur with no identified route of transmission. About 50% of affected patients progress to chronic hepatitis, and cirrhosis develops in 20% of those chronically infected. The residual risk of hepatitis C from blood transfusion is estimated at 1 in 92,000 to 1 in 108,000.[52,53]

Hepatitis D. Hepatitis D is a defective RNA virus that requires hepatitis B virus for replication. It is not transmissible by blood unless hepatitis B viremia is present in the donor; hence, it is screened out by testing for HBsAg.

Hepatitis G and Others. Researchers have recently discovered additional agents that are thought to cause hepatitis and appear to be present in human populations worldwide and in traditionally high-risk populations for parenteral infections such as multiply transfused patients, hemophiliacs, and drug abusers. The G viruses are tentatively identified as hepatitis G,[50] and hepatitis GBV-A, GBV-B, and GBV-C.[54] The latter four appear to be flaviviruses similar to hepatitis C. Their association with significant hepatic disease is not yet established.[50]

Herpesviruses

Cytomegalovirus (CMV). CMV is a member of the herpes virus family, is transmissible by cellular blood products containing infected leukocytes, and is more likely to be transmitted by fresh blood than stored blood.[55] CMV is one of the infectious agents most frequently transmitted by transfusion. Approximately half of all donors are seropositive for CMV, but only 1% to 12% of donors have the potential to transmit the virus.[55] Seronegative donors or blood products depleted of leukocytes are less likely to transmit the infection. In immunocompetent CMV seronegative adults the infection is usually inconsequential, but premature infants weighing less than 1200 to 1500 g can incur significant morbidity, as can immunocompromised adults, such as bone marrow and heart-lung transplant recipients. About 30% of CMV seronegative patients undergoing cardiac surgery with transfusion become infected, usually without clinical manifestations. Less than 10% develop a mononucleosis-like syndrome 3 to 6 weeks after transfusion. Formerly called postperfusion syndrome, it is now referred to as posttransfusion syndrome. It consists of fever, exanthemata, hepatosplenomegaly, enlarged lymph nodes, and atypical lymphocytes in the peripheral blood.[55]

Human Herpesvirus-6 (HHV-6), Herpes Simplex, and Herpes Varicella Zoster. HHV-6 virus is a newly identified human pathogen that causes acute infection in infants and children (roseola infantum, exanthem subiturn, or fourth disease), which can be detected in both the B lymphocytes and serum of acutely infected individuals.[56] HHV-6 is not now a recognized complication of transfusion, but it may be pathogenic in neonatal transfusions.[39]

Herpes simplex and Herpes varicella zoster have never been shown to be transmitted by transfusion.[56]

Epstein-Barr Virus (EBV). Approximately 90% of blood donors have antibody to EBV.[57] They are known to harbor the latent virus in their B lymphocytes. Although most cases of posttransfusion syndrome (see Cytomegalovirus, above) are due to CMV, there have been case reports of the syndrome occurring due to EBV.[56] Posttransfusion infection due to EBV is a rare occurrence. Most donor blood contains antibody along with the virus, which tends to be protective. When infection does occur it is usually asymptomatic. As with CMV, fresh blood less than 4 days old is more likely to transmit the virus. Also as with CMV, leukodepleted blood products are less likely to transmit the infection. In certain patients such as those who are immunosuppressed, for example, graft recipients, it has been suggested that posttransfusion EBV infection may contribute to the development of lymphomas.[56]

B19 Parvovirus

Parvovirus is a nonlipid envelope DNA virus that resists inactivation by the solvent-detergent treatment of plasma products now in common use to inactivate viruses. The acute infection causes temporary suppression of erythropoiesis, which can cause clinically significant anemia in patients with an underlying compensated hemolytic anemia such as in sickle cell disease, hereditary spherocytosis, β-thalassemia, and autoimmuno hemolytic anemia, and if it occurs during pregnancy, it can cause hydrops fetalis. Antibodies to parvovirus are found in 25% to 30% of blood donors. Because antigenemia lasts in an infected donor for only 1 to 2 weeks, the virus is rarely transmitted by transfusion. The virus is the cause of erythema infectiosum, or fifth (exanthematous) disease, in children, which is usually uncomplicated. Parvovirus has not been reported to be a serious problem for transfusion recipients, although knowledge about its effects in susceptible populations is only now emerging.[58]

Exotic Viruses

Exotic viruses include Rift Valley fever virus, Colorado tick fever virus, Ebola virus, Lassa fever virus, Marburg virus, yellow fever virus, and dengue virus. While, based on their occurrence and life cycles, these viruses are theoretically transmissible by blood transfusion, they are not now considered to be important causes of posttransfusion infection.[59]

Idiopathic CD-4 Lymphocytopenia (ICL)

Reports of a few HIV-negative individuals with unexplained low CD-4 lymphocyte counts and diseases or opportunistic infections have raised concerns about the possible existence of an unidentified lymphotrophic virus.[60,61] To date the evidence for such an agent and its distribution in the population has not been interpreted as constituting a threat to the safety of the blood supply. While ICL has occurred in a few individuals whose only commonly accepted AIDS-like risk factor for a transmissible disease is a blood transfusion, it has not been epidemiologically related to transfusion of blood.

Creutzfeldt-Jakob Disease (CJD)

This rare but rapidly progressive dementia is thought to be caused by proteinaceous infectious particles devoid of nucleic acid called prions. Transmission by transplantation of dural or corneal grafts from infected individuals and demonstration of transmission in animals by blood[62] has prompted concern about possible blood-borne transmission.[63] Recently the Food and Drug Administration (FDA) has developed questions for blood donors about familial or transplant-related experience with the disease, which will disqualify donors. A national study has recently been initiated to detect any cases in recipients of blood from newly diagnosed cases of CJD in former blood donors.

Bacteria

Yersinia Enterocolitica, Pseudomonas Fluorescens, Serratia Marcescens, Serratia Liquefaciens, and Others

These organisms proliferate at 2 to 6 °C,[64–66] the temperature at which red cell products are stored. Contamination of donor blood can occur at the time of venipuncture, due to subclinical bacteremia in the donor, or during processing of the donated blood products. Undiscovered contamination and proliferation in the stored blood can cause rigors, fever, hypotension, shock, and death in the recipient.[67] Cases tend to occur sporadically and rarely, and the source of the contamination is usually never found. In one study, fatal bacterial contamination reactions occurred at the rate of 1 per 1.2×10^6 transfusions.[68] Prevention is by visual examination of the blood product for unusual color or darkening. Comparison of the appearance of the tubing segment nearest to the bag (darker when contaminated) with those more distal has been suggested as a marker of an infected unit.[69]

Staphylococcus Epidermidis, Diphtheroids, Staphylococcus Aureus, and Others

These organisms proliferate at room temperature, the temperature at which platelets are stored.[66] Contamination can occur in ways similar to the cold growing organisms described above, and the effects on the recipient are also similar, but usually more mild. Reliable and practical methods for detecting contamination of platelet products before their use have not been developed.

Treponema Pallidum

The serologic test for syphilis was the first test used to prevent transfusion-transmitted infection. The assay, however, is negative during the primary infection with spirochetemia, making detection unlikely. Furthermore, the spirochete is unlikely to survive for more than 3 to 6 days when blood is stored at 2 to 6 °C. Transmission of syphilis by transfusion occurs rarely in the U.S., but the test is useful as a surrogate for promiscuous behavior and contact with the other infectious agents that such behavior implies, such as hepatitis B. In other parts of the world the incidence of syphilis is increasing, making continuation of testing prudent.

Lyme Disease (Borrelia burgdorferi)

Lyme disease is caused by a spirochete, *Borrelia burgdorferi,* which is transmitted by ticks. It has been shown that this organism can survive in stored red blood cells, platelets, and fresh frozen plasma,[70] but no transmission by transfusion has yet been documented.[71]

Brucella Abortus

This organism is known to survive for months in stored blood. Infected donor blood has low concentrations of organism, and is primarily a threat to immunosuppressed patients. There have been no reported cases in the U.S., but cases have been reported elsewhere.[72]

Rickettsia Rickettsiae

This organism, responsible for Rocky Mountain spotted fever, has been reported to cause transfusion-transmitted infection in one case. The rarity of such transmission is probably due to the fact that clinical illness coincides with the period of infectivity.[73]

Parasites

Malaria (Plasmodium Species)

Most transfusion-transmitted malaria in the U.S. has been caused by *P. malariae and P. falciparum.* Between 1972 and 1988 there were 45 cases, or 0.25 cases per million units of whole blood collected, or 2.6 cases per year.[74] Prevention relies primarily on the history of the donor, since anyone with a history of the infection and anyone coming from an endemic area is deferred for 3 years, during which time they must have been free from unexplained symptoms suggestive of malaria.

Babesiosis (Babesia Microti) and Other Piroplasmas

As of 1992 there were only seven reported cases of transfusion-transmitted babesiosis in the literature.[74] *Babesia* infects red cells, primarily in immunosuppressed or splenectomized patients. Red cell products implicated in transmission have been from 3 to 35 days of age. In one study in an endemic area of Massachusetts, 4% to 5% of donors had serologic evidence of infection, but most people with a positive test are not capable of transmitting the infection.[74]

Trypanosoma Cruzi

The protozoan parasite *Trypanosoma cruzi* is the causative agent of Chagas' disease or American trypanosomiasis. In Latin America, Chagas' disease is widespread and at least 16 to 18 million individuals are infected. The prevalence of *T. cruzi* infection in Latin American blood donors is about 3%, ranging from 0.3% in Ecuador to 62% in Santa Cruz, Bolivia. In one blood center in the U.S. 1.1% of donors had a positive serologic test for *T. cruzi*. There have been reports of three cases of transfusion-associated Chagas' disease in North America.[75] Recently an enzyme immunoassay has been developed to screen donors, but it has not yet been licensed and adopted by blood collecting agencies.[76,77]

Toxoplasma Gondii

This zoonosis (members of the cat family are the definitive hosts), due to a ubiquitous parasite, infects as many as 500 million persons worldwide.[78] Its clinical significance lies in seronegative women infected during pregnancy or in immunosuppressed seronegative patients. Toxoplasma occurs rarely in whole blood from asymptomatic donors and has been shown to survive in stored blood up to 50 days.[78] There have been no reported cases of transmission by transfusion of red cells, but there are reports in the older literature of transmission via white cell transfusions from chronic myelogenous leukemia patient/donors to immunosuppressed leukemic patients.[78] Transfusion of white cell-containing blood products to pregnant seronegative patients would appear to be potentially hazardous to the fetus.

The risk of transfusion-transmitted infection per unit of donor blood transfused is summarized in Table 1.4 for the more common and clinically important infectious agents. Also provided is the rate of positive tests found for some of the analytes in the donor population and the general population.

Blood Antigen Incompatibility

Acute Hemolytic Transfusion Reaction

Acute hemolytic reactions occur when red cells are transfused to a recipient with preformed antibody to an antigen on the red cell membrane that is

TABLE 1.4. Risk of transfusion transmitted infection (TTI) per unit transfused.

	TTI risk	Donor prevalence	Population prevalence
HIV	1:563,000	1:10,000	1:250
HBsAg	1:200,000	4:10,000	1:250
HBcAb	-	1:100	5:100
HTLV-I/II	1:50,000	1:10,000	-
HCV	1:92,000	1:200	1:50
Other*	<1:1,000,000	Verylow	-

*Other includes malaria, babesiosis, Chagas' disease, and other rare infections.

capable of fixing complement and hemolyzing the red cell. The usual cause in fatal cases is anti-A or anti-B in the recipient when the red cells are group A, B, or AB and the unit was transfused to the wrong patient due to a clerical error.[79] There are several other blood group systems that involve antibodies and antigens other than A, B, or O that can also cause acute hemolysis, such as Rh, Kell, Kidd, and Duffy. In a large study of 1,784,600 red cell transfusions it was found that 54 ABO-incompatible transfusions occurred (1/33,000) and three were fatal (1/600,000).[80] Forty-three percent of the errors occurred at the bedside where the patient was not properly identified, 11% resulted from phlebotomist error, 25% were due to blood bank error, and the bank with another hospital service together contributed to 17%.[80] In other studies the reported incidence of acute hemolytic transfusion reactions varies from 1 in 1,417 to 1 in 21,000,[81] with a fatality rate of from 17% to 40%. The rate of fatal hemolytic reactions overall was recently estimated at 1 in 100,000 units transfused.[81]

Delayed Hemolytic Transfusion Reaction

Delayed hemolytic transfusion reactions (DHTR) occur when red cells are transfused to a recipient who was previously sensitized to an antigen on the red cell membrane, but at the time of transfusion has no detectable anti-red cell antibody remaining. Following the transfusion an anamnestic response occurs over the ensuing 3 to 14 days, and as the antibody titer rises, the red cell membrane is attacked and the survival of the red cell in the circulation is reduced. The screen for atypical antibodies and the patient's direct antiglobulin test may become positive in such cases. If the survival is not reduced but the phenomenon occurs and is detected, it is termed a delayed serologic transfusion reaction (DSTR) since the only abnormality is in the serologic tests,[82] for example, a positive direct anti-human globulin or Coombs' test. There have been cases with significant intravascular hemolysis with acute renal failure[83] and with fatalities,[84] but in the majority of cases there are no signs or symptoms, or only postoperative fever,[85] perhaps with a decline in hematocrit. The frequency of DHTRs has been estimated at from 1 in 9,100 to 1 in 13,700 units transfused or 1 in 950 to 1 in 2,500 patients transfused. The frequency of DSTRs has been estimated at from 1 in 1,900 to 1 in 3,000 units transfused or 1 in 180 to 1 in 560 patients transfused.[86]

Febrile Reactions [Febrile Nonhemolytic Transfusion Reactions (FNHTRs)]

These reactions are characterized by chills and fever, and some patients also develop back pain, headache, and nausea. Symptoms begin from 5 minutes to 1 to 2 hours after the start of transfusion. They are generally attributed to the presence of antileukocyte antibodies in the recipient,[87] although plasma from the donor may also play a role. In the former instance, the antibodies interact with donor white cells or platelets. Because fever may be a sign of a more serious reaction, such as acute hemolysis, many authorities recommend stopping the transfusion when such reactions occur.[88] Recently the presence of cytokines in the donor plasma has been implicated in some reactions.[89-92] The cytokines apparently come from leukocytes of the donor that disintegrate during storage, releasing the cytokines into the plasma. By removing the leukocytes from the product shortly after collection or removing the plasma from the product shortly before transfusion, it may be possible to prevent many of these reactions.[89]

Allergic Reactions

Following plasma protein transfusion, from 1% to 3% of recipients develop hives or urticaria,[93] an anaphylactoid reaction. Severity varies up to and including anaphylactic shock, characterized by flushing of the skin, hypotension, substernal pain, and dyspnea. The more severe form is rare, about 1 per 20,000 in one series.[93] Preformed antibody to immunoglobulin A (IgA) class-specific antigens in patients lacking IgA is often related to the severe reaction.

Transfusion-Related Acute Lung Injury (TRALI) or Noncardiac Pulmonary Edema

Transfusion-related acute lung injury or TRALI was first recognized as a complication of transfusion during cardiac operations in 1980.[94] It had been reported earlier in other settings, however.[95-96] Current understanding of the phenomenon suggests that donor plasma, and less often recipient plasma, contains a complement-fixing antibody against neutrophil or human leukocyte antigens (HLA) that causes activated complement fragments, possibly from C5, to engender increased permeability of pulmonary capillaries with rapid formation of noncardiac pulmonary edema. The severity of the phenomenon varies from subclinical to fatal. It is characterized by diffuse infiltrates of all lung fields without cardiac enlargement on roentgenogram, dyspnea, nonproductive cough, fever, chills, and hypotension. It has been suggested that multiparous female donors should not be used for plasma-containing blood products for transfusion so as to avoid this infrequent but serious reaction.[96] It is estimated to occur in 0.001% (1/100,000) of blood units transfused, with the frequency of fatality being 0.0004% (1/250,000).[97]

Alloimmunization

Viewed as a complication of transfusion therapy, alloimmunization to red cell, platelet, white cell, and plasma protein antigens looms large. Not only does alloimmunization affect the patient in diverse ways, it can also affect the offspring of the patient who becomes pregnant. Alloimmunization to red cell antigens can delay necessary transfusion, make the finding of compatible blood difficult or impossible, cause acute and delayed hemolytic transfusion reactions, and cause hemolytic disease of the newborn. Alloimmunization to platelet antigens can cause refractoriness to platelet transfusions, posttransfusion purpura, or neonatal alloimmune thrombocytopenia. Alloimmunization to neutrophils and other white cells can cause febrile nonhemolytic transfusion reactions, TRALI, and neonatal alloimmune neutropenia. Alloimmunization to plasma proteins can cause anaphylactic reactions to donor IgA in IgA-deficient patients, refractoriness to factor VIII (antihemophilic factor) in hemophiliacs, urticarial reactions, and coagulopathies in patients exposed to bovine thrombin and factor V when used in fibrin glue. Discussion of each of these phenomena is beyond the scope of this chapter, but suffice it to say that no exposure to alloantigens should be prescribed unless the benefit is clear and necessary.

Graft vs. Host Disease (GVHD)

Graft vs. host disease occurs when immunocompetent donor T and NK lymphocytes engraft in a recipient whose immune system is unable to reject them.[98,99] At from 3 to 30 days after transfusion, fever and rash occur, progressing to erythroderma, pancytopenia, bone marrow aplasia, wasting, diarrhea, and jaundice. Transfusion-associated GVHD is almost universally fatal.[100] Immunosuppressed patients are at greater risk, but immunocompetent patients can acquire the disease. The latter cases usually involve donors who share antigens with the recipient in such a way that the donor cells are not perceived as foreign and eliminated. In homogeneous populations such as Japan, the risk of such an event has been estimated as 1 in 874.[100] In the U.S. the immunologic risk is estimated at 1 in 7174,[101] but the actual rate of the disease has been estimated[102] at 1 in 1×10^6, so clearly other factors, such as the dose of white cells, the age of blood at transfusion, and immunomodulation of the recipients' immune status are important. Cases of GVHD in cardiac surgery patients in Japan,[103] Israel,[104] and the U.S.[105] have involved fresh blood from relatives and anonymous donors that was not irradiated. In addition, it has been suggested that cardiopulmonary bypass patients suffer a functional T-cell immune deficit.[106] Irradiation of blood products with gamma radiation can prevent the phenomenon,[102] but leukoreduction with filters cannot.[107]

Nonimmunologic Reactions

A variety of nonimmunologic reactions or sequelae of transfusion can also occur, such as circulatory overload; iron overload (from chronic transfusion therapy); imbalances due to massive transfusion of blood products lacking certain elements, e.g., packed red cells lacking plasma or platelets (or the concomitant effect of shock causing disseminated intravascular coagulation [DIC]); infusion of microaggregates due to inadequate filtration of blood with resultant pulmonary microembolization; etc.[108]

Immunosuppression/Immunomodulation

For the past 20 years, clinical reports and laboratory studies have suggested that allogeneic blood transfusion causes changes in the recipient's immune system.[109] In various reports, improved renal allograft survival, improvement in patients with Crohn's disease,[110] and decreased "rejection" of the conceptus in women with recurrent abortion[111] have suggested that there is an immunosuppressive effect of transfusion. Similarly, there have been reports of increased cancer occurrence,[112] decreases in survival of cancer patients or tumor-free survival,[113] and increased rates of infection following transfusion.[114–116] In laboratory studies, changes in lymphocyte subsets[117] and activation, decreased NK cell function,[118] decreased antigen-presenting function, and phagocytic cell function have been documented. There is growing evidence that the immunomodulatory effects of allogeneic transfusion are mediated, at least in part, by contaminating leukocytes in the transfused blood product.[119–120]

Excess Morbidity and Mortality Associated witb Transfusion

Studies of long-term survival after blood transfusion in large populations have shown that receipt of a blood transfusion is independently predictive of mortality, adding to the predictive value of age, gender, and previous hospitalization.[121,122] This could lead to the data-derived hypothesis that transfusion per se contributes to the observed increase in morbidity and mortality rates. To assess this hypothesis it would be necessary to investigate the particular causes of death in large transfused populations, e.g., recurrent cancer, infectious complications of surgery, or transfusion-acquired infectious diseases.[109,116] There is as yet no study that provides such evidence, but neither is there any refutation of that hypothesis in the literature.

Conclusion

As is well known to all professionals dealing with patients undergoing cardiothoracic surgical procedures, the use of blood products has been part of the surgical armamentarium since the inception of these procedures and will be used to some extent throughout the foreseeable future. The indications for, as well as the selection of, various types of blood products changes constantly and, as a result, it has become practical to significantly minimize the donor exposures in patients undergoing cardiothoracic surgery. Dramatic changes in blood salvage technology as well as a better understanding of the consequences of hemodilution have allowed for continued clinical and experimental efforts to minimize blood product utilization during these complex operative procedures. Indeed, the ultimate goal of the complete elimination of the use of allogeneic blood products in cardiac surgery and in general thoracic surgery is within reach. It is to that end that the remainder of this text is dedicated, in the hope that clinical caregivers can safely integrate the concepts and technical descriptions in this text into their day-to-day practice.

References

1. Cosgrove D, Thurer D, Lytle B, et al. Blood conservation during myocardial revascularization. *Ann Thorac Suro,* 1979;28:184–189.
2. Zuhdi N, McCollough B, Carey J, et al. Double-helical reservoir heart-lung machine. *Arch Surg* 1961;82:320–325.
3. Spence R. The status of bloodless surgery. *Transfusion Med Rev* 1991; 5;274–286.
4. Viele M, Weiskopf R. What can we learn about the need for transfusion from patients who refuse blood? The experience with Jehovah's Witnesses. *Transfusion* 1994;34:396–401.
5. Cooley D, Crawford E, Howell J, et al. Open heart surgery in Jehovah's Witnesses. *Am J Cardiol* 1964;13:779–781.
6. Ott D, Cooley D. Cardiovascular surgery in Jehovah's Witnesses. *JAMA* 1977;238:1256–1258.
7. Henling C, Carmichael M, Keats A, et al. Cardiac operation for congenital heart disease in children of Jehovah's Witnesses. *J Thorac Cardiovasc Surg* 1985;89:914–920.
8. Cooper J. Perioperative considerations in Jehovah's Witnesses. *Int Anesth Clin* 1990;28:210–215.
9. Spence R, Alexander J, DelRossi A, et al. Transfusion guidelines for cardiovascular surgery: lessons learned from operations in Jehovah's Witnesses. *J Vasc Surg* 1992;16:825–831.
10. Kitchens C. Are transfusions overrated? Surgical outcome of Jehovah's Witnesses. *Am J Med* 1993;94:117–119.
11. Goodnough L. Blood transfusion support in coronary artery bypass graft

surgery. In: Baldwin ML, Kurtz SR, eds. *Transfusion Practice in Cardiac Surgery.* Arlington, VA: American Association of Blood Banks, 1991.
12. The Sanguinis Study Group. Use of blood products for elective surgery in 43 European hospitals. *Transfusion Med* 1994;4:251–268.
13. Wajon P, Walsh R, Symons N. A survey of cardiopulmonary bypass perfusion practices in Australia in 1992. *Anesth Intensive Care* 1993;21:814–821.
14. Goodnough L, Johnston M, Shah T, Chernosky A. A two-institution study of transfusion practice in 78 consecutive adult elective open-heart procedures. *Am J Clin Pathol* 1989;91:468–472.
15. Spiess BS, Gillies SA, Chandler W, Verrier E. Changes in transfusion therapy and reexploration rate after institution of a blood management program in cardiac surgical patients. *J Cardiothorac Vasc Anesth* 1995;9(2):168–173.
16. Cosgrove DM, Loop FD, Lytle BW, et al. Determinants of blood utilization during myocardial revascularization. *Ann Thorac Surg* 1985;40(4):380–384.
17. Goodnough L, Johnston M, Toy P, et al. The variability of transfusion practice in coronary artery bypass surgery. *JAMA* 1991;265:86–90.
18. O'Connor G, Plume S, Olmstead E, et al. A regional prospective study of in-hospital mortality associated with coronary artery bypass grafting. *JAMA* 1991;266:803–809.
19. Myhre, B. To treat the patient or to treat the surgeon. *JAMA* 1991;265:97–98.
20. Salem-Schatz S, Avorn J, Soumerai S. Influence of clinical knowledge, organizational context, and practice style on transfusion decision making. *JAMA* 1990;264:476–483.
21. Salem-Schatz S, Avorn J, Soumerai S. Influence of knowledge and attitudes on the quality of physicians' transfusion practice. *Med Care* 1993;31:868–878.
22. Bex J, Latini L, Durandy Y. The art of cardiac surgery: critical analysis of the limits of statistics in cardiac surgery. *J Cardiovasc Surg* 1994;9:288–291.
23. Goodnough L, Johnston M, Ramsey G, et al. Guidelines for transfusion support in patients undergoing coronary artery bypass grafting. *Ann Thorac Surg* 1990;50:675–683.
24. Despotis G, Grishaber J, Goodnough L. The effect of an intraoperative treatment algorithm on physicians' transfusion practice in cardiac surgery. *Transfusion* 1994;34:290–296.
25. Shanberge J, Quattrociocchi-Longe T. Analysis of fresh frozen plasma administration with suggestions for ways to reduce usage. *Transfusion Med* 1992; 2:189–194.
26. McClelland D. Fresh frozen plasma—opinion and evidence. *Transfusion Med* 1992;2:97–98.
27. Kane R, Garrard J. Changing physician prescribing practices: regulation vs education. *JAMA* 1994;271:393–394.
28. McClelland D. Red cell transfusion for elective surgery: a suitable case for treatment. *Transfusion Med* 1994;4:247–249.
29. Birkmeyer J, AuBuchon J, Littenberg B, et al. Cost-effectiveness of preoperative autologous donation in coronary artery bypass grafting. *Ann Thorac Surg* 1994;57:161–168.
30. Strauss R, Hilsenrath P. Invited commentary. *Ann Thorac Surg* 1994; 57:168–169.
31. Etchason J, Petz L, Keeler E, et al. The cost effectiveness of preoperative autologous blood donations. *N Engl J Med* 1995;332:719–724.
32. Rutherford C, Kaplan H. Autologous blood donation—can we bank on it? *N Engl J Med* 1995;332:740–742.

33. Read E, Leiby D, Dodd, R. Seroprevalence of *Trypanosoma cruzi (T cruzi)* in blood donors with and without risk for infection. *Blood* 1994;84(suppl 1): 467a.
34. Altman L. Researcher reports evidence of a new type of hepatitis virus. *The New York Times* 1995;Jan 11:Al5.
35. Lave L. Health and safety risk analyses: information for better decisions. *Science* 1987;236:291–295.
36. Wilson R, Crouch E. Risk assessment and comparisons: an introduction. *Science* 1987;267:267–270.
37. Schneiderman L, Kaplan R. Fear of dying and HIV infection vs hepatitis B infection. *Am J Public Health* 1992;82:584–586.
38. Dodd R. Infectious complications of blood transfusion. *Hem/Onc Ann* 1994;2:280–287.
39. Vyas G, Gang Y, Murphy E. Transfusion-related transmissible diseases: detection by polymerase chain reaction-amplified genes of the microbial agents. *Trans Med Rev* 1994;8:253–266.
40. Wylie B. Transfusion transmitted infection: viral and exotic diseases. *Anaesth Intensive Care* 1993;21:24–30.
41. Faust R, Warner M. Transfusion risks. *Int Anesth Clin* 1990;28:184–189.
42. DePalma L. Transfusion-transmitted diseases: current status and future directions. *J Int Fed Clin Chem* 1994;6:131–135.
43. American Association of Blood Banks. Policy Statement on HIV Antigen Testing. *Association Bulletin* February 10, 1995; #95-2.
44. Letter, 8/8/95, from Director, Center for Biologics Evaluation and Research (CBER), Food and Drug Administration, DHHS, to All Registered Blood and Plasma Establishments: Recommendations for Donor Screening with a Licensed Test for HIV-1 Antigen.
45. Lackritz E, Satten G, Aberle-Grasse J, et al. Estimated risk of transmission of the human immunodeficiency virus by screened blood in the United States. *N Engl J Med* 1995;333:1721–1725.
46. American Association of Blood Banks. HIV-1 Antigen Test Implementation Guidance. *Association Bulletin* January 4, 1996; #96-2.
47. Dodd R. The risk of transfusion-transmitted infection. *N Engl J Med* 1992;327:419–421.
48. Nelson K, Donahue J, Munoz A, et al. Transmission of retroviruses from seronegative donors by transfusion during cardiac surgery. A multicenter study of HIV-1 and HTLV-I/II infections. *Ann Intern Med* 1992;117:554–559.
49. Noble R, Kane M, Reeves S, et al. Posttransfusion hepatitis A in neonatal intensive care nursery. *JAMA* 1984;252:2711–2715.
50. Alter HJ. The cloning and clinical implications of HGV and HGBV-C. *N Engl J Med* 1996;334:1536–1537.
51. Gill P. Transfusion-associated hepatitis C: reducing the risk. *Transfusion Med Rev* 1993;7:104–111.
52. Busch M. Blood products advisory committee addresses HCV 3.0 terminology; recommends approval of PCR test for HIV RNA. *Council of Community Blood Centers Newsletter*. March 29, 1996;2.
53. Kleinman S, Busch M, Holland P. Post-transfusion hepatitis C virus infection. *N Engl J Med* 1992;327:1601.
54. Simons J, Pilot-Matias T, Leary T, et al. Identification of two flavivirus-like genomes in the GB hepatitis agent. *Proc Natl Acad Sci USA* 1995; 92:3401–3405.

55. Mollison P, Engelfriet C, Contreras M. *Blood Transfusion in Clinical Medicine.* 9th ed. London: Blackwell Scientific, 1993; 765.
56. Mollison P, Engelfriet C, Contreras M. *Blood Transfusion in Clinical Medicine.* 9th ed. London: Blackwell Scientific, 1993; 769.
57. Rubin R, Tolkoff-Rubin N. Post transfusion viral infections. *Transplant Proc* 1988;20:1112–1117.
58. Mosley J. Should measures be taken to reduce the risk of human parvovirus (B19) infection by transfusion of blood components and clotting factor concentrates? *Transfusion* 1994;34:744–746.
59. Smith D, Dodd R, eds. *Transfusion Transmitted Infections.* Chicago: ASCP Press, American Society of Clinical Pathologists, 1991.
60. Laurence J, Debashis M, Steiner M, et al. Apoptotic depletion of CD4+T cells in idiopathic CD4+T lymphocytopenia. *J Clin Invest* 1996;97:672–680.
61. Heredia A, Hewlett I, Soriano V, et al. Idiopathic CD4+T lymphocytopenia: a review and current perspective. *Trans Med Rev* 1994;8:223–231.
62. Manuelidis E, Gorgacz E, Manuelidis L. Viremia in experimental Creutzfeldt-Jakob disease. *Science* 1978;200:1069–1071.
63. Klein R, Dumble L. Transmission of Cruetzfeldt-Jakob disease by blood transfusion. *Lancet* 1993;341:768.
64. Goldman M, Blajchman M. Blood product-associated bacterial sepsis. *Transfusion Med Rev* 1991;5:73–83.
65. Puckett A. Bacterial contamination of blood for transfusion: a study of the growth characteristics of four implicated organisms. *Med Lab Sci* 1986; 43:252–257.
66. Gottlieb T. Hazards of bacterial contamination of blood products. *Anaesth Intensive Care* 1993;21:20–23.
67. Myhre B. Bacterial contamination is still a hazard of blood transfusion. *Arch Pathol Lab Med* 1985;109:982–983.
68. Illert W, Sanger W, Weise W. Bacterial contamination of single-donor blood components. *Transfusion Med* 1995;5:57–61.
69. Kim D, Brecher M, Bland L, et al. Visual identification of bacterially contaminated red cells. *Transfusion* 1992;32:221–225.
70. Badon S, Fister R, Cable R. Survival of *Borrelia burgdorferi* in blood products. *Transfusion* 1989;29:581–583.
71. Aoki S, Holland P. Lyme disease—another transfusion risk? *Transfusion* 1989;29:646–650.
72. Mollison P, Engelfriet C, Contreras M. *Blood Transfusion in Clinical Medicine.* 9th ed. London: Blackwell Scientific, 1993; 772.
73. Mollison P, Engelfriet C, Contreras M. *Blood Transfusion in Clinical Medicine.* 9th ed. London: Blackwell Scientific, 1993; 774.
74. Westphal R. Parasitic disease and blood transfusion. In: Nance S, ed. *Blood Safety: Current Challenges.* Bethesda, MD: American Association of Blood Banks, 1992;97–123.
75. Ramirez L., Lages-Silva E, Pianetti G, et al. Prevention of transfusion-associated Chagas' disease by sterilization of *Trypanosoma cruzi*-infected blood with gentian violet, ascorbic acid, and light. *Transfusion* 1995; 35:226–230.
76. Brashear R, Winkler M, Schur J, et al. Detection of antibodies to *Trypanosoma cruzi* among blood donors in the southwestem and western United States. I. Evaluation of the sensitivity and specificity of an enzyme immunoassay for detecting antibodies to *T. cruzi. Transfusion* 1995;35:213–218.

77. Winkler M, Brashear R, Hall H, et al. Detection of antibodies to *Trypanosoma cruzi* among blood donors in the southwestern and western United States. II. Evaluation of a supplemental enzyme immunoassay and radioimmunoprecipitation assay for confirmation of seroreactivity. *Transfusion* 1995;35:219–225.
78. Wolfe M. Parasites, other than malaria, transmissible by blood transfusion. In: Greenwalt T, Jamieson G. *Transmissible Disease and Blood Transfusion.* New York: Grune & Stratton, 1974.
79. Honig C, Bove J. Transfusion-associated fatalities: review of Bureau of Biologics reports 1976–1978. *Transfusion* 1980;20:653–661.
80. Linden J, Paul B, Dressler K. A report of 104 transfusion errors in New York State. *Transfusion* 1992;32:601–606.
81. Beauregard P, Blajchman M. Hemolytic and pseudo-hemolytic transfusion reactions: an overview of the hemolytic transfusion reactions and the clinical conditions that mimic them. *Trans Med Rev* 1994;8:184–199.
82. Ness P, Shirey R, Thoman S, et al. The differentiation of delayed serologic and delayed hemolytic transfusion reactions: incidence, long-term serologic findings, and clinical significance. *Transfusion* 1990;30:688–693.
83. Holland P, Wallerstein R. Delayed hemolytic transfusion reaction with acute renal failure. *JAMA* 1968;204:149–150.
84. Hillman N. Fatal delayed hemolytic transfusion reaction due to anti-c and E. *Transfusion* 1979;19:548–551.
85. Soper D. Delayed hemolytic transfusion reaction: a cause of late postoperative fever. *Am J Obstet Gynecol* 1985;153:227–228.
86. Case Records of the Massachusetts General Hospital (Case 42–1993). *N Engl J Med* 1993;329:1254–1261.
87. Decary F, Femer P, Giovedoni L, et al. An investigation of nonhemolytic transfusion reactions. *Vox Sang* 1984;46:277–285.
88. Widmann F. Controversies in transfusion medicine: should a febrile transfusion response occasion the return of the blood component to the blood bank? Pro. *Transfusion* 1994;34:356–158.
89. Heddle N, Klama L, Singer J, et al. The role of the plasma from platelet concentrates in transfusion reactions. *N Engl J Med* 1994;331:625–628.
90. Brand A. Passenger leukocytes, cytokines, and transfusion reactions. *N Engl J Med* 1994;331:670–671.
91. Stack G, Baril L, Napychank P, et al. Cytokine generation in stored, white cell-reduced, and bacterially contaminated units of red cells. *Transfusion* 1995;35:199–203.
92. Ferrara J. The febrile platelet transfusion reaction: a cytokine shower. *Transfusion* 1995;331:89–90.
93. Mollison P, Engelfriet C, Contreras M. *Blood Transfusion in Clinical Medicine.* 9th ed. London: Blackwell Scientific, 1993; 690.
94. Culliford A, Thomas S, Spencer F. Fulminating noncardiogenic pulmonary edema: a newly recognized hazard during cardiac operations. *J Thorac Cardiovasc Surg* 1980;80:868–875.
95. Ward H. Pulmonary infiltrates associated with leukoagglutinin transfusion reactions. *Ann Intern Med* 1970;73:689–694.
96. Popovsky M, Chaplin H, Moore S. Transfusion-related acute lung injury: a distress syndrome. *Anaesth Intensive Care* 1993;21:44–49.

97. Malouf M, Glanville AR. Blood transfusion related adult respiratory distress syndrome. *Anaesth Intensive Care* 1993;21:44–49.
98. Linden J, Pisciotto P. Transfusion-associated graft-versus-host disease and blood irradiation. *Trans Med Rev* 1992;6:116–123.
99. Vogelsang G, Hess A. Graft-versus-host disease: new directions for a persistent problem. *Blood* 1994;84:2061–2067.
100. Shivdasani R, Galuska F, Dock N, et al. Brief report: graft-versus-host disease associated with transfusion of blood from unrelated HLA-homozygous donors. *N Engl J Med* 1993;328:766–770.
101. Ohto H, Yasuda H, Noguchi M, et al. Risk of transfusion-associated graft-versus-host disease as a result of directed donations from relatives. *Transfusion* 1992;32:691–693.
102. Anderson K, Weinstein H. Transfusion-associated graft-versus-host disease. *N Engl J Med* 1990;323:315–321.
103. Sakakibara T, Juji T. Post-transfusion graft-versus-host disease after open heart surgery. *Lancet* 1986;2:1099.
104. Thaler M, Shamiss A, Orgad S, et al. The role of blood from HLA-homozygous donors in fatal transfusion-associated graft-versus-host disease after open-heart surgery. *N Engl J Med* 1989;321:25–28.
105. Arsura E, Bertelle A, Minkowitz S, et al. Transfusion-associated-graft-vs-host disease in a presumed immunocompetent patient. *Arch Intern Med* 1988; 148:1941–1944.
106. Marcus J. HLA-homozygous donors and transfusion-associated graft-versus-host disease. *N Engl J Med* 1990;322:1004–1005.
107. Akahoshi M, Takanashi M, Masuda M, et al. A case of transfusion-associated graft-versus-host disease not prevented by white cell-reduction filters. *Transfusion* 1992;32:169–172.
108. Mollison P, Engelfriet C, Contreras M. *Blood Transfusion in Clinical Medicine*. 9th ed. London: Blackwell Scientific, 1993; 62–64, 697–709.
109. Klein H. Immunologic aspects of blood transfusion. *Semin Oncol* 1994; 21:16–20.
110. Williams J, Hughes L. Effect of perioperative blood transfusion on recurrence of Crohn's disease. *Lancet* 1989;2:131–133.
111. Lewis J, Coulam C, Moore B. Immunologic mechanisms in the maternal-fetal relationship. *Mayo Clin Proc* 1986;61:655–665.
112. Cerhan J, Wallace R, Folsom A, et al. Transfusion history and cancer risk in older women. *Ann Intern Med* 1993;119:8–15.
113. Heiss M, Mempel W, Delanoff C, et al. Blood transfusion – modulated tumor recurrence: first results of a randomized study of autologous versus allogeneic blood transfusion in colorectal cancer surgery. *J Clin Oncol* 1994;12:1859–1867.
114. Waymack J. The effect of blood transfusions on resistance to bacterial infections. *Transplant Proc* 1988;20:1105–1107.
115. Mezrow C, Bergstein I, Tartter P. Postoperative infections following autologous and homologous blood transfusion. *Transfusion* 1992;32:27–30.
116. Blumberg N, Heal J. Transfusion and host defenses against cancer recurrence and infection. *Transfusion* 1989;29:236–245.
117. Paglieroni T, Ward J, Holland P. Changes in peripheral blood CD5(B1a) B-cell populations and autoantibodies following blood transfusion. *Transfusion* 1995;35:189–198.

118. Tartter P, Steinberg B, Barron D, et al. Transfusion history, T cell subsets and natural killer cytotoxicity in patients with colorectal cancer. *Vox Sang* 1989; 56:80–84.
119. Bordin J, Heddle N, Blajchman M. Biologic effects of leukocytes present in transfused cellular blood products. *Blood* 1994;84:1703–1721.
120. Bordin J, Bardossy L, Blajchman M. Growth enhancement of established tumors by allogeneic blood transfusion in experimental animals and its amelioration by leukodepletion: the importance of the timing of leukodepletion. *Blood* 1994;84:344–348.
121. Vamvakas E, Taswell H. Long-term survival after blood transfusion. *Transfusion* 1994;34:471–477.
122. Vamvakas E, Taswell H. Mortality after blood transfusion. *Transfusion Med Rev* 1994;8:267–280.

2
Preoperative Evaluation of the Cardiothoracic Surgical Patient for Bleeding Risk

ADAM S. ASCH

Although bleeding and its attendant morbidity is surely a concern of all surgeons, cardiothoracic surgery presents a significant challenge with respect to the diagnosis and management of bleeding. The evaluation of a patient's bleeding risk is an important aspect of the preoperative evaluation. But how much evaluation is appropriate? Where does cost-benefit fit in the equation? There are special concerns related to cardiothoracic surgery patients that are the consequence of coexisting disease and its therapy, and also of the nature of cardiothoracic surgery in this era. This chapter outlines some approaches to these issues, discusses some of the more commonly encountered problems, and offers an algorithm for the cardiothoracic service to use when addressing these questions at the bedside.

The single most important aspect of the clinical evaluation of patients for bleeding risk is the history. There are several points that are critical to this question, particularly the patient's history—recent or past—of epistaxis, easy bruisability, hematomas, heavy or frequent menstrual bleeding, gum bleeding, melena, or hematuria. The date of onset of any of these symptoms helps determine whether any suspected defect might be inherited or acquired. Precipitating factors, frequency, and severity of bleeding must be clarified. Were the bleeding episodes precipitated by trauma, dental extraction, or surgery, or were they spontaneous? If the bleeding is linked to trauma or surgery, did it occur immediately or after several days? Did bleeding necessitate transfusion of blood products? Is there any family history of bleeding? Since bleeding disorders in family members might be undiagnosed, the clinician should not be satisfied by the absence of a history of hemophilia or other bleeding disorders, and specifically inquire about bleeding precipitated by trauma, dental work, or surgery. When the family history is positive, the pattern of inheritance can provide clues to the nature of the bleeding diathesis. Multiple generations of affected individuals of both sexes suggests autosomal dominant inheritance of a bleeding disorder such as von Willebrand's disease or Osler-Weber-Rendu disease. Bleeding limited to males with affected maternal uncles and male cousins is typical of sex-linked disorders such as classic hemophilia. Where affected individuals are limited to a single generation and both sexes are affected, autosomal recessive disorders may be present.

Medications and acquired medical problems and their associated hemostatic defects are the most likely risks for bleeding in cardiothoracic patients, and their presence is therefore a critical point to be established in history taking.[1] Table 2.1 outlines some of these disorders, the nature of the bleeding diathesis, and its pathophysiology. The use of aspirin alone, or included in compound formulations intended for pain relief or treatment of upper respiratory infections, is very common, with a prevalence among

TABLE 2.1. Medications and acquired medical conditions associated with a bleeding risk.

Condition/drug	Bleeding diathesis	Pathophysiology
Coumadin	Multiple factor deficiency	Blocks gamma-carboxylation of vitamin K-dependent factors (II,VII,IX,X)
Aspirin	Platelet defect	Blocks platelet cyclooxygenase
Heparin	Inhibition of II and X	Direct and indirect inhibition of factors II and X
	Thrombocytopenia	Antibody-mediated platelet activiation
Antibiotics	Multiple factor deficiency	Vitamin K malabsorption
Multiple drugs	Thrombocytopenia	Decreased platelet production
Uremia	Platelet defect	Platelet inhibitory metabolites
Liver disease	Multiple factor deficiency	Defective synthesis
	Thrombocytopenia	Hypersplenism
Malabsorption	Multiple factor deficiency	Vitamin K malabsorption
Systemic lupus	Thrombocytopenia	Autoantibodies to platelets
	Thrombocytopathy	Autoantibodies to platelets
	Factor deficiency	Prothrombin deficiency occasionally associated with lupus-type inhibitor
Plasma cell dyscrasias	Decreased fibrin polymerization	Paraprotein inhibition of fibrin monomer polymerization
	Thrombocytopenia	Decreased platelet production
Amyloidosis	Capillary fragility	Vascular amyloid infiltration
	Factor X deficiency	Absorption by amyloid
Myeloproliferative chronic myelogenous leukemia (CML), 1° thrombocytosis, myeloid metaplasia, polycythemia vera	Thrombocytopathy	Abnormal platelet production Decreased platelet production Hyperplenism
Malignancy	Thrombocytopenia	Chemotherapy
	Thrombocytopenia	Marrow infiltration
	Factor deficiency	DIC, some chemotherapy

patients undergoing unplanned surgery perhaps as high as 50%[2] and perhaps higher among patients with previously diagnosed atherosclerotic coronary disease. Does this represent a bleeding risk? Published data suggest not, but among those with a second disorder, such as type I von Willebrand's, bleeding times may be profoundly affected and contribute to a clinically significant bleeding tendency.[3,4] Although bleeding times have been used in the past to evaluate the severity of an aspirin-induced bleeding diathesis, there is little evidence to suggest that bleeding time correlates with subsequent operative blood loss.[5-8]

The aspects of the physical examination that are potentially pertinent to a bleeding diathesis include bruising and, more significantly, hematomas, petechiae, and blood (occult or evident) in the stool. Other findings that may raise concern include splenomegaly, hepatomegaly, lymphadenopathy, joint deformities, and decreased range of motion typical of some inherited bleeding disorders.

There are special problems that are a part of the overall challenge to the hemostatic system that cardiothoracic surgery presents. Specifically, the use of multiple artificial devices such as vascular grafts, catheters, prosthetic valves, intraaortic balloon pumps, ventricular assist devices, and, most important, extracorporeal perfusion,[9] the application of which is a daily reminder of the central role played by the vascular endothelium in maintaining hemostasis, and more specifically the fluid nature of blood. Simply put, blood removed from the antithrombotic effects of endothelium, clots; and, in all of its current forms, extracorporeal perfusion causes large amounts of blood to flow through synthetic vessels that are not lined with endothelial cells.

Contact with the artificial surfaces of these devices leads to activation of the coagulation cascade and the complement pathway that requires heparinization to prevent gross clotting or disseminated intravascular coagulation (DIC). The extracorporeal circuit is generally primed with crystalloid resulting in a dilution of the hematocrit to between 20% and 30%. A heparin dose of 3 mg/kg is generally required to provide adequate anticoagulation. Still, even in the appropriately anticoagulated patient, factors are activated and consumed to some extent.[10] Rarely, a history of heparin-induced thrombocytopenia complicates the management of patients. When suspected, the condition should be investigated with platelet aggregometry tests or surrogates specific for antibody-mediated platelet release, and if present, the use of alternative anticoagulation arranged. Contact results in factor XII activation, and in the presence of factors XI, prekallikrein, and high-molecular-weight kininogen leads to kallikrein formation, which in turn cleaves high-molecular-weight kininogen to form the powerful vasodilator bradykinin. Indeed, this pathway is responsible for the whole body inflammatory response associated with cardiopulmonary bypass.[11] Reversal of heparin anticoagulation with protamine is also associated with the generation of inflammatory mediators: heparin/

protamine complexes lead to the generation of C3a and C5a—both vasoactive.[12-15] The events that occur during bypass lead to the generation of some fibrin emboli, denatured proteins, lipid particles, and platelet and leukocyte aggregates. Repeated platelet activation leads to some platelet loss and to varying degrees of an acquired platelet storage pool defect in which partially degranulated and less hemostatically effective platelets are returned to the circulation.[16,17] Deamino-8-D-arginine vasopressin (DDAVP) may decrease blood loss by improving platelet function in the face of this acquired dysfunction.[18-22]

Modern cell saver systems are used to conserve blood aspirated from the operative field and are responsible for the impressive statistic that less than half of patients undergoing open heart surgery require additional blood transfusions. The recovered blood is heparinized and washed to remove other cellular debris and activated clotting factors and is returned to the patient devoid of plasma factors. The crystalloid and plasma expander dilution of normal blood factors can play a significant role in contributing to a bleeding diathesis, particularly in patients for whom intraoperative blood loss has been higher than expected.[23] Cardiopulmonary bypass can lead to the increased release from vascular endothelium of tissue plasminogen activator and increased fibrinolysis.[24] The protease inhibitor aprotinin (Trasylol) has been shown to decrease postoperative blood loss after open heart surgery.[25-30] Clearly, cardiothoracic surgery represents a major challenge to the hemostatic system.

Rappaport[31] outlines an approach to preoperative assessment (Table 2.2). The assessment is relatively straightforward for level 1 and 2 patients, but the laboratory tests required for an adequate evaluation of patients at higher risk are somewhat more specialized. In addition, there are several disorders associated with abnormal bleeding in which the usual screening tests are likely to be normal. These examples, which include Ehlers-Danlos

TABLE 2.2. Preoperative assessment.

Level*	History/exam	Surgery (hemostatis challenge)	Laboratory assessment
1	Negative	Minor	None
2	Negative	Major	Activated partial thromboplastin time (aPTT), platelet count, bleeding time?
3	Possible	Major	Above and bleeding time, prothrombic time, clot solubility
4	Likely	Any	Above and tests for specific factor abnormalities

*Because of the nature of the surgery, cardiothoracic patients fall into levels 2 through 4. The advice of a hematologic consultant is recommended in helping to assess the risk and in formulating an approach with the surgical team to avoid or minimize potential bleeding complications.

From Rappaport.[31]

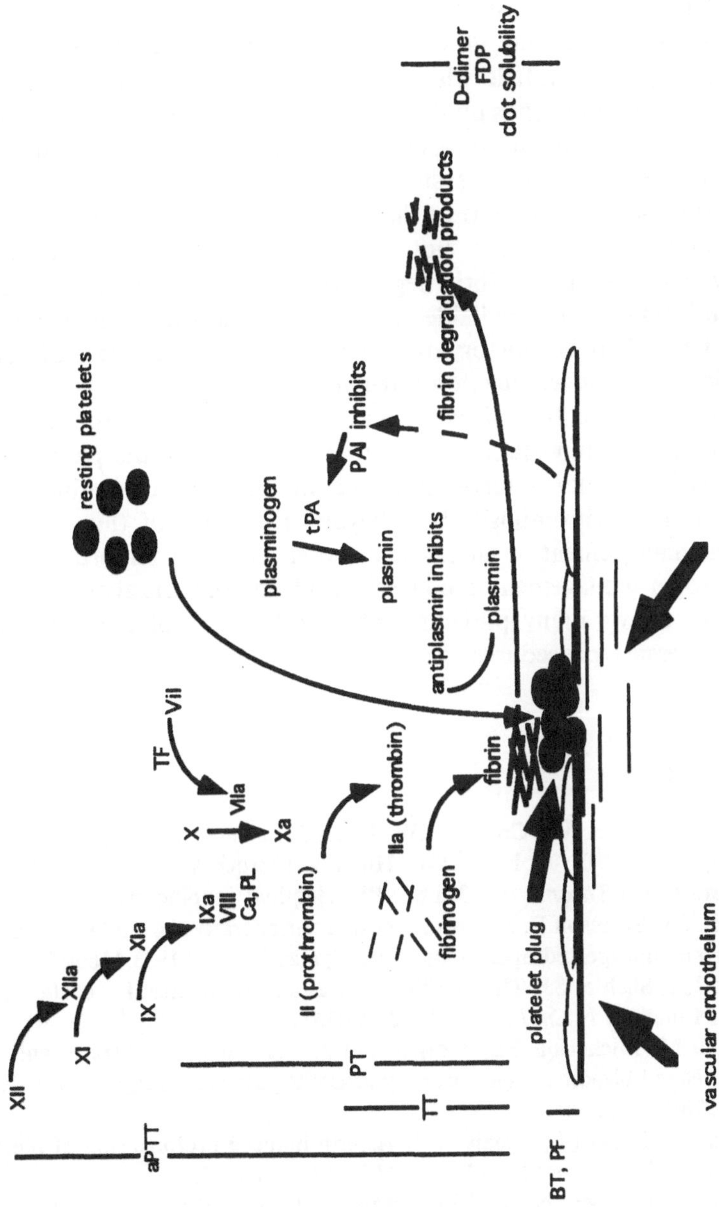

FIGURE 2.1. Vascular hemostatis and its assessment.

syndrome, Henoch-Schönlein purpura, amyloidosis, antiplasmin deficiency, and several other vascular disorders, point to the limitations of our current testing armamentarium. Figure 2.1 illustrates the three arms critical to normal hemostasis and the laboratory tests that help in the evaluation of their function.

Normal hemostasis is a function of platelet function, blood coagulation, and fibrinolysis. The events, although often depicted as occurring in a linear fashion, take place in a field where all reactions are occurring at the same time. The net result depends on the balance between processes. Some of the most blatant holes in our measurement of these processes exist in the assessment of the fibrinolytic system. As Figure 2.1 illustrates, the routine tests measure only a small part of the fibrinolytic pathway. The conversion of plasminogen to plasmin is not accurately assessed by measuring clot solubility or by measuring fibrin degradation products. Commercial assays for α_2-antiplasmin are available in many laboratories, and should be obtained when there is a history of excessive bleeding in the face of normal coagulation and platelet function screening tests.

While the identification of patients at risk for bleeding is the subject of this chapter, it is important to note that for many of the patients who require cardiovascular intervention, the major risk to morbidity and mortality is from thrombosis. It is beyond the scope of this chapter to discuss the management of all of the disorders, but it is important to note that the proper management in concert with hematologists acquainted with these issues allows many patients with true bleeding diatheses to safely undergo necessary procedures.

References

1. White GC, Marder VJ, Colman RW, Hirsh J, Salzman EW. Approach to the bleeding patient. In: Colman RW, Hirsh J, Marder VJ, Salzman EW, eds. *Hemostasis and Thrombosis*. 3rd ed. Philadelphia: Lippincott, 1994.
2. Ferraris VA, Swanson E. Aspirin usage and perioperative blood loss in patients undergoing unexpected operations. *Surg Gynecol Obstet* 1983;156:439.
3. Harker LA, Slichter SJ. The bleeding time as a screening test for evaluation of platelet function. *N Engl J Med* 1972;287:155.
4. Torosian M, Michelson EL, Morganroth J, MacVaugh H. Aspirin and coumadin related bleeding after coronary artery bypass graft surgery. *Ann Intern Mod* 1978;89:325.
5. Amrein PC, Ellman L, Harris WH. Aspirin induced prolongation of bleeding time and perioperative blood loss. *JAMA* 1981;245:1825.
6. Bashein G. Preoperative aspirin therapy and reoperation for bleeding after coronary artery bypass surgery. *Arch Intern Med* 1991;151:89.
7. Lind SE. The bleeding time does not predict surgical bleeding. *Blood* 1991; 77:2547.
8. Rodgers RPC. A critical reappraisal of the bleeding time. *Semin Thromb Hemost* 1990;16:1.

9. Bick RL. Hemostasis defects associated with cardiac surgery, prosthetic devices and other extracorporeal circuits. *Semin Thromb Hemost* 1985;11:249.
10. Davis GC, Sobel M, Salzman EW. Elevated plasmafibrinopeptide A and thromboxane A2 levels during cardiopulmonary bypass. *Circulation* 1980;61:808.
11. Downing SW, Edmunds LH Jr. Release of vasoactive substances during cardiopulmonary bypass. *Ann Thorac Surg* 1992;54:1236.
12. Kirklin JK,, Chenoweth DE, Naftel DC, et al. Effects of protamine administration after cardiopulmonary bypass on complement; blood elements in the hemodynamic state. *Ann Thorac Surg* 1986;41:193
13. Lowenstein E, Johnston WE, Lappas DG, et al. Catastrophic pulmonary vasoconstriction associated with protamine reversal of heparin. *Anesthesiology* 1983;59:470.
14. Morel DR, Sapol WM, Thomas SJ, et al. C5a and thromboxane generation associated with pulmonary vaso and bronchoconstriction during protamine reversal of heparin. *Anesthesiology* 1987;66:597.
15. Weiss ME, Nyhan D, Peng Z, et al. Association of protamine IgE and IgG antibodies with life-threatening reactions to intravenous protamine. *N Engl J Med* 1989;320:886.
16. Harker LA, Maplass TW, Branson HE, et al. Mechanisms of abnormal bleeding in patients undergoing cardiopulmonary bypass: acquired transient platelet dysfunction associated with selected alpha-granule release. *Blood* 1990;75:128.
17. Woodman RC, Harker LA. Bleeding complications associated with cardiopulmonary bypass. *Blood* 1990;76:1680.
18. Hackman T, Gascoayne RD, Naiman SC, et al. A trial of desmopressin to reduce blood loss in uncomplicated cardiac surgery. *N Engl J Med* 1990;322:1085.
19. Sloan EM, Slyono D, Klein HG, et al. DDAVP increases platelet membrane expression of glycoprotein Ib in patients with disorders of platelet function and after cardiopulmonary bypass. *Am J Hematol* 1994;46:199.
20. Temeck BK, Bachenheimer LC, Katz NM, et al. Desmopressin acetate in cardiac surgery: a double blind, randomized study. *South Med J* 1994;87:611.
21. Sheridan DP, Card RT, Pinilla JC, et al. Use of desmopressin acetate to reduce blood transfusion requirements during cardiac surgery in patients with acetylsalicylic acid induced platelet dysfunction. *Can J Surg* 1994;37:33.
22. Beck KH, Mohr P, Bleckmann U, et al. Desmopressin effect on actetylsalicylic acid impaired platelet function. *Semin Thromb Hemost* 1995;21:32.
23. Beck KH, Bleckmann U, Mohr P, Kretschmer V. DDAVP's shortening of the bleeding time seems due to plasma von Willebrand factor. *Semin Thromb Hemost* 1995;21:40.
24. Stibbe J, Kluft C, Brommer EJP, et al. Enhanced fibrinolytic activity during cardiopulmonary bypass in open-heart surgery in man is caused by extrinsic (tissue-type) plasminogen activator. *Eur J Clin Invest* 1984;14:375.
25. Bidistrup BP, Royston D, Sapsford RN, Taylor KM. Reduction in blood loss and blood use after cardiopulmonary bypass with high-dose aprotinin (Trasylol). *J Thorac Cardiovasc Surg* 1989;97:364.
26. Rocha E, Hidalgo F, Llorens R, et al. Randomized study of aprotinin and DDAVP to reduce postoperative bleeding after cardiopulmonary bypass surgery. *Circulation* 1994;90:921.
27. Liu B, Tengvorn L, Larson G, et al. Half-dose aprotinin preserves hemostatic function in patients undergoing bypass operations. *Ann Thorac Surg* 1995; 59:1534.

28. Hendrice C, Schmartz D, Pradier O, et al. Effects of aprotinin on blood loss, heparin monitoring tests, and heparin doses in patients undergoing coronary bypass surgery. *J Cardiothorac Vasc Anesth* 1995;9:245.
29. Mannucci L, Gerometta PS, Mussoni L, et al. One month follow-up of hemostatic variables in patients undergoing aortocoronary bypass surgery. Effect of aprotinin. *Thromb Haemost* 1995;73:356.
30. Rosengart TK, Helm RE, Kemperer J, et al. Combined aprotinin and erythropoietin use for blood conservation: results with Jehovah's Witnesses. *Ann Thorac Surg* 1994;58:1397.
31. Rappaport SI. Preoperative hemostatic evaluation: which tests, if any? *Blood* 1983;61:229.

3
Preoperative Autologous and Directed Blood Donation

ROBERT E. HELM AND KARL H. KRIEGER

Preoperative autologous donation (PAD) is a widely recognized blood conservation strategy that can be defined as the procurement of a specified portion of a patient's blood preoperatively for later use during the intraoperative and postoperative periods. Its appropriate application leads to a direct reduction in homologous transfusion requirement via a unit-for-unit substitution of autologous for homologous blood. Although there was a gradual increase in the use of PAD in cardiac and general surgery from the early 1960s onward, PAD did not achieve a significant role in perioperative transfusion medicine until the advent of AIDS in the early 1980s and the greater transfusion risk awareness that accompanied this disease. But despite educational efforts aimed at increasing physician-patient awareness of the benefits of PAD, it has remained a relatively underutilized resource. Issues that have hampered its more widespread application in cardiac surgery include those of efficacy, safety, and more recently, cost-effectiveness. But perhaps the most important factor limiting the use of PAD in cardiac surgery is the changing character of the cardiac surgical patient pool. The increasingly acute nature of most cardiac operative interventions in the 1990s, in older and sicker patients, severely limits the preoperative time that is available to optimally perform PAD. As will be seen, however, it is the allowance of adequate preoperative time, for both autologous collection and red cell mass regeneration, that provides the key to optimizing PAD. Fortunately, new strategies are becoming available that may decrease the time required to perform PAD, thereby rendering preoperative donation a viable option for a larger number of patients. This chapter defines which patients can benefit from PAD and outlines a safe and effective program for performing PAD on these patients. Consistent with the theme of this book, by identifying those patients who can benefit from PAD, and selectively and optimally applying PAD to these patients, efficient and maximum patient benefit in respect to reduction of homologous blood exposure can be obtained.

An alternative, perceived preoperative blood conservation strategy is the procurement of blood preoperatively from donors known to the patient undergoing surgery, a practice known as directed donation. Despite the psychological comfort provided to the patient, directed donation is nevertheless a form of homologous transfusion, and carries the same risks as well as several unique risks. This chapter reviews the risks and benefits of preoperative directed donation, and makes recommendations for its limited use in cardiac surgery today.

Preoperative Autologous Donation

History and Development of Preoperative Autologous Donation

The use of autologous blood in surgery began with efforts to intraoperatively salvage and reinfuse blood during and following acute blood loss.[1,2] Such use significantly antedated the controlled use of preoperatively donated autologous blood. The first record of the use of preoperatively donated autologous blood appeared in 1921.[3] In this case report, Grant described the removal 24 hours preoperatively of a portion of the blood volume of a patient undergoing resection of a cerebellar tumor. This blood was stored in sodium citrate, refrigerated, and then reinfused immediately following the procedure without incident. The reasons cited for the use of this intentional preoperative autologous technique were the presence of an uncommon blood type, an inability to locate or pay for a suitable donor, and a "large, stout, and plethoric" body type.

Over the ensuing years improvements in the ability to preserve blood and an increase in the understanding of the major erythrocyte antigen systems directed orientation of blood banks and transfusion medicine toward allogeneic blood use. Hemotherapy progressed further in this direction in World War II, with the massive blood requirements of large numbers of acutely injured patients, which could only be satisfied by a large homologous donor pool. It was not until the early 1960s that preoperative autologous donation began to resurface as a means of providing or helping to provide the additional blood required for major surgical procedures. By this time, in the peacetime elective surgical setting, its potential benefits with respect to the decreased risk of incompatibility reaction and transmission of blood-borne disease had become more readily apparent. In 1962 Milles et al reported the use of preoperative autologous donation in 53 patients undergoing a variety of thoracic, gynecologic, and general surgical procedures.[4,5] Removal of up to four units of blood was found to be safe, and resulted in 64% of blood requirements being met by autologous blood. Over the next decade use of PAD slowly but steadily expanded. By 1974 one third of American blood banks offered preoperative autologous donation as an option for patients undergoing surgery.[6] Use of the technique continued to gradually increase, and spread to all forms of major surgery including cardiac surgery, but by the early 1980s less than 5% – and as few as 0.3% – of eligible surgical patients utilized this modality. Preoperative autologous donation clearly remained markedly underutilized, despite its theoretical advantages over allogeneic blood use. Obstacles to more widespread application in all forms of surgery included lack of physician-patient awareness, perceived increases in administrative/organizational complexity and physician-patient inconvenience, and concerns over safety and efficacy. The homologous blood system was well organized, easy to use, and firmly in place.

The advent of HIV and its association with the nation's homologous blood supply greatly altered the unbalanced equilibrium between preoperative autologous and homologous blood use that had come to exist in the early 1980s. The first firm connections between AIDS and the blood supply began to be made in 1983, and that same year the National Blood Bank Association issued a statement recommending that autologous blood transfusions be considered more frequently.[7-9] In 1986 the American Medical Association Council on Scientific Affairs[10] issued a report firmly endorsing the use of preoperative and other autologous donation practices. Editorials and papers supporting the use of autologous blood and outlining ways to further increase its use appeared in many of the major journals.[11] During this time the Association of American Blood Banks (AABB) undertook a concerted nationwide effort to increase physician and public awareness of the availability and benefits of preoperative autologous donation, and formed the National Autologous Blood Resource Center. The lay press helped significantly in these endeavors. In 1982 it was estimated by the AABB that 18,737 units of autologous blood had been collected. By 1987 this number had increased to 282,856 units.[12,13] Despite these individual efforts, however, preoperative autologous donation remained an underutilized resource. One study of 18 tertiary care centers revealed that despite these increases in educational efforts and improvement in public awareness, an average of only 5% of eligible patients utilized PAD, and the AABB revealed that only 4.5% of total donations to member blood banks were autologous in nature.[14] Even with maximum local and regional efforts at physician-patient education recruitment, only 9% to 11% of eligible donors were found to contribute.[7] In 1992, 1.1 million of the 13.7 million blood units collected (8%) were autologous in nature, a 70% increase over the number of autologous units collected in 1989.[15] While such improvement is encouraging, obstacles to more widespread application that existed before the era of HIV have persisted, and the additional problems of cost-effectiveness, appropriate resource utilization, and the general trend toward a reduction in the preoperative time period available, particularly in cardiac surgery, have further hampered progress.[16,17]

Preoperative Autologous Donation in Cardiac Surgery

Efforts to minimize homologous blood use in cardiac surgery began in the 1950s as the large per case homologous blood requirements, coupled with the rapid expansion of the field of cardiac surgery, combined to markedly increase transfusion-related infectious disease transmission and to deplete blood bank stores. General efforts at the use of autologous blood as a means of decreasing homologous use began with the work of Dodrill et al,[18] who espoused the benefits of the technique of intraoperative autologous donation: acute autologous donation prior to cardiopulmonary bypass (CPB) with reinfusion post-CPB. Reports concerning the safe and successful use of preoperative autologous donation for non-cardiac thoracic surgery began to surface as early as 1962, and continued to appear after that time.[5,19–22] It was not until 1967, however, that the use of PAD in cardiac surgery itself was reported.[23] Cuello et al[23] reported the use of PAD in a series of 67 patients undergoing a variety of cardiac and thoracic procedures from 1965 to 1967. Blood was collected between 1 and 21 days prior to planned surgery, and collection was performed at 5- to 6-day intervals, with intramuscular iron supplementation to optimize marrow regeneration capacity. The total blood volume collected varied between 200 and 2000 ml, with an average of two units per patient. Patient ages ranged from 4 to 79 years. The minimum hematocrit for entrance into the study was 35%. The mean admission hematocrit was 41.6%, but, following donation, the mean hematocrit at the time of operation was 37.5%. Twenty-four of these patients underwent procedures requiring cardiopulmonary bypass. Of these patients, 8 were able to be operated on with autologous blood alone, and in the remaining 16 patients autologous blood was able to supply 40% of transfusion requirements.

The extent to which these positive results can be attributed to PAD is difficult to determine, however, as no control group was provided. Of note was that patients experienced an average drop in hematocrit of 4.1%, indicating that only partial red cell regeneration had occurred by the time of surgery. In fact, calculation reveals that the actual net gain in total available red cell mass (red cell mass in the patient plus red cell mass in blood bags) at the time of operation was not two units, but 0.7 unit (Table 3.1). From a mathematical standpoint, therefore, 30% of the first unit drawn and the entire second unit drawn were largely an exercise in waste and inefficiency. In effect, what had taken place was a redistribution of blood from the body to blood collection bags. Unfortunately, the net effect of this form of relatively acute PAD may have actually been detrimental, as the platelets and coagulation factors contained in stored blood experience an obligatory and progressive decrease in function. Additionally, lower hematocrits at the time of operation may compromise the performance of other blood conservation measures, such as the intraoperative removal and reinfusion of fresh whole blood. While this first study of PAD in cardiac surgery

Table 3.1. A summary of studies of PD in cardiac patients.

Study	Population	No. of patients	Control group	Preoperative time interval	Predonation hematocrit	Preoperative hematocrit	No. units "lost" from body	No. units procured	Net autologous unit gain	Rate autologous gain (per wk)	Transfusion results
Cuello (1967)	Mixed cardiothoracic	67	None	1–21 days (14)	41.6%	37.5%	1.3	2.0	0.7	-	-
Newman (1971)	Mixed cardiothoracic	178	None	2–6 days (5)	44.4%	38.4%	2.02	1.92	−0.1	-	-
Lubin (1974)	Mixed cardiac	11	None	21 days	43.9%	36.2%	2.57	3.55	0.98	0.33	36.0% no HB
Cove (1975)	CABG	44	None	1–21 days (14)	43.8%	40.6%	1.25	1.36	0.11		23.0% on HB
Fleming (1977)	Mixed cardiac	147 (10)*	None	60–154 days (92)	41.8%	38.4%	1.13	10	8.87	0.68	52.0% no HB
Mann (1983)	Mixed cardiac	275	None	Not given	41.9%	40.2%	0.6	2.2	1.6		-
Kruskall (1986)	Mixed cardiac	57	Matched	3–105 (28.6)	41.1%	37.1%	1.33	3.1	1.77	0.43	30.0% decreased
Love (1987)	Mixed cardiac	58	Matched	18 days	44.9%	38.3%	2.2	1.97	−0.23	−0.09	36.0% decreased
Owings (1989)	Mixed cardiac	107	Synchronous	33 ± 15.4 days	43.0%	39.5%	1.2	3.0	1.8	0.38	55.0% decreased
Britton (1989)	Mixed cardiac	104	Synchronous	28 days	-	36.6%	-	4.1	-	-	54.4% decreased
Achenbach (1991)	Mixed cardiac	42	Matched	7–21 days (14)	43.5%	39.0%	1.5	2.49	0.9	0.45	72.0% decreased
Dzik (1992)	Aortic valve	79	Synchronous	3–35 (21)	-	-	-	1.6	-	-	37.0% decreased
Goldfinger (1993)	Heart/lung transplant	46	None	-	-	-	-	3.4	-	-	-
Sandrelli (1995)	Mixed cardiac	348	Matched	7–30 (18)	-	42.0%	-	2.2	-	-	-
Total (t)/Mean (m)		1563 (t)		24 (m)	43.0%(m)	38.65%(m)	1.6(m)	3.1(m)	1.5(m)	0.46(m)	

*Ten patients who had 10 units removed had complete data available, which were used to complete this table. CABG, coronary artery bypass graft; HB, homologous blood.

served to illustrate that the technique could be safely and effectively applied in patients with significant cardiac disease, it also provided evidence (suggested) that improved results might be obtained had full red cell regeneration been allowed to occur.

The technique of PAD had actually been in use and under study by Newman et al[22] since 1962, although their report did not appear in the literature until 1971. The authors studied 178 patients undergoing a variety of cardiac and thoracic procedures over a 6 year period, 60 of whom required the use of the open heart apparatus. They confirmed the safety of PAD (one to two units drawn within 2 weeks of surgery), but provided no data regarding its effectiveness in decreasing homologous exposure. Like Cuello et al,[23] they did not allow sufficient time for full red cell regeneration—hematocrit had decreased by three percentage points for each unit drawn—and so a significant net gain in red cell mass was likely not accomplished by the autologous donation process (Table 3.1). Because it is this net gain in autologous mass that allows for a unit-for-unit reduction in homologous red cell use, it is difficult to assess whether any actual benefit was obtained by acutely performing PAD. While it might be argued that the patients did benefit from stimulation of increased bone marrow erythropoiesis preoperatively, their average postdonation hematocrit of 38% probably led to little if any such stimulation.[24] The authors of these early studies are not to be blamed for this shortcoming in technique, however. During this time the maximum storage period for blood was 21 days, and this, therefore, was the maximum period over which blood could be collected. If a red cell regeneration rate of one unit per 2 weeks is assumed, then the maximum volume of net autologous red cell mass that could be gained (using AABB standard minimum donation hematocrit of 33%) is 1.5 units. The preservation mediums that allow for 35- to 42-day storage, were not yet available, nor were methods for longer-term cryopreservation. These early authors were in effect handicapped as to the results that could be achieved with PAD. Greater efficacy would have to await the introduction of techniques for longer-term preservation.

Verska and Larson[25] applied an abbreviated form of PAD to a patient undergoing aortic valve replacement and for whom no compatible homologous blood could be found. Forty-eight hours prior to surgery 500 ml of blood was removed and stored. A second 500-ml volume was removed 24 hours prior to surgery. Hematocrit decreased from 47% prior to the first donation to 34% at the time of operation. The patient's surgery was uneventfully performed without the need for blood. While the authors contend that PAD played a significant role in the successful outcome, clearly, because only 48 hours had elapsed between the first blood draw and the time of operation, no significant red cell production in response to donation could have occurred. The only benefit gained by using PAD was that which could have also been gained had the acute intraoperative autologous donation (IAD) of two units been performed. In fact, performing PAD in the place of IAD was likely detrimental, as previously discussed, because of platelet and coagulation factor loss. Verska and Larson's study highlights this essential point, a concept that has been often passed over in the PAD literature. Nothing is gained by the subacute withdrawal of blood preoperatively that cannot be gained by the far more efficacious IAD. PAD should only be performed when there is sufficient preoperative time for red cell regeneration.

In 1974 Lubin et al[26] applied preoperative autologous donation to 11 patients undergoing open-heart procedures. Up to four units of blood per patient were removed beginning 3 weeks prior to surgery. The authors used a novel approach, known as the "leapfrog" method, to provide relatively fresh autologous blood at the time of surgery. According to this method, the single unit of stored blood removed at the first donation is reinfused immediately following the second donation, this second donation consisting of the removal of two units of blood. At the third donation three units of blood are removed and the two from the second donation are reinfused. This process is continued until the required amount of blood is procured, with the last donation occurring within 24 hours of surgery. The entire quantity of collected blood is therefore relatively fresh, presumably providing for better overall performance. While attractive, the relatively involved and complex nature of this procedure did not lead to widespread acceptance at the time. The authors did show, however, that PAD is safe and effective: 36% of patients did not require any homologous blood, and 66% of transfusion requirements were able to be satisfied with autologous blood. The average drop in hematocrit by the time of operation in this study was 7.8%, indicating that only partial red cell mass regeneration had occurred, and that submaximal benefit was likely obtained. It is interesting to note that along with providing a fresher autologous product, the leapfrog method also for the first time provided the potential to extend the preoperative time available for donation, and therefore to increase the efficacy of PAD.

In 1975 Cove et al[27] focused on the use of PAD in coronary artery bypass surgery. PAD was performed on 44 patients with the only exclusion criteria being those patients with severe left main coronary artery disease and those with preinfarction angina. If two units were to be collected, the first donation was performed 2 weeks prior to surgery. The second unit was collected approximately 3 days prior to surgery, as were single-unit donations. PAD was combined with the use of bloodless prime and the intraoperative donation of one unit of blood. The authors found that 23% of patients were able to be operated on without the use of homologous blood, and that 37% of transfusion requirements could be met with the autologous blood obtained. However, similar to the other early studies of PAD in cardiac surgery (Table 3.1), the relative acute donation schedule utilized by the investigators had decreased hematocrits by two to three percentage points per unit drawn by the time of surgery, and so it is difficult to know whether PAD actually served to decrease homologous blood use.

The study did confirm the safety of PAD in patients with all but the most severe coronary artery disease.

By 1977 the ability to cryopreserve blood had markedly increased the potential for PAD to contribute to the blood conservation effort in cardiac surgery by extending the period of time over which blood could be collected, and therefore over which red cell regeneration could occur. The first to take advantage of PAD with cryopreservation in cardiac surgery was Fleming et al,[28] who evaluated its use in 147 patients undergoing procedures requiring cardiopulmonary bypass. Ten of these patients were able to donate 10 units of blood by cryopreserving blood units that would not be used within 21 days of donation. The average drop in hematocrit by the time of operation in these 10 patients was only 2.5%, indicating that almost full red cell regeneration had occurred by the time of surgery, and that the 10 units of autologous blood represented a true increase in red cell mass. There were no serious adverse events recorded in these 10 donors or in any of the 137 other cardiac surgical patients. The ability to safely procure 10 units of autologous red cells and yet have a normal hematocrit at the time of surgery (and therefore a clear and large net gain in available autologous red cell mass) clearly marked a significant advance in the application of PAD.

In 1983 Mann et al[29] concentrated on evaluating the safety of PAD in a variety of high-risk patients, including 275 patients undergoing procedures requiring cardiopulmonary bypass. There were 197 coronary artery bypass graft (CABG) patients, 63 valvular patients, and 15 patients undergoing surgery for congenital heart disease. The only exclusion criterion used was the presence of preinfarction angina. Patients with left main coronary artery disease were excluded only because the urgent nature of their disease precluded adequate preoperative time. Patients with aortic stenosis were not excluded from donation. An average of 2.2 units of blood was able to be donated (over an unspecified period of time) without serious adverse events in any of the 275 donors. Those minor hypotensive "vasovagal" phlebotomy-related reactions that did occur were judged to be similar in frequency and character to those seen in the general population. Data as to efficacy in reducing homologous transfusion were not provided.

In 1986 Kruskall et al[30] published the first controlled (nonrandomized) study evaluating the use of PAD in cardiac surgery. PAD was applied to 180 patients, 57 of whom underwent cardiac surgery (including CABG, valve, and CABG-valve procedures). Patients donated an average of 3.1 units of blood (range: 1–10 units) over a period of time as long as 105 days prior to surgery. Blood was stored in citrate-phosphate-dextrase (CPD-1) solution (allows for a maximum storage period of 35 days with a minimum of 70% viability), and for delays in surgery or donation beyond this time blood was cryopreserved. That this extended predonation period allowed for at least partial regeneration of red cell mass is evidenced by an average decrease in hematocrit of 4.0% from the time of initial donation to the time of surgery (with an average donation of 3.1 units, the expected hematocrit drop would be 12.3%, therefore the net gain of eight hematocrit points—or the equivalent of $2\frac{2}{3}$ units red cells—can be estimated to be the average benefit provided by PAD). Although two patients died during the period of donation, these deaths were felt to be unrelated to the donation process. The authors found PAD to be safe and effective when results were compared to 100 "comparable" patients not undergoing PAD during the same time period, and they found that the decrease in homologous exposure obtained was directly proportional to the number of units of autologous units procured (Table 3.1).

In 1987 a second more carefully controlled study of PAD was performed by Love et al,[31] who compared 58 cardiac surgical patients undergoing PAD to 58 patients undergoing cardiac surgery without PAD during the same time period. Patients were matched for such factors as age, sex, type of procedure, and length of CPB time. The authors found that collection of one to three units of autologous blood was safe and effective; the percentage of patients exposed to allogeneic blood was decreased by half (from 62% to 36%), and the number of allogeneic units required per patient per group was decreased by 46%. The primary shortcoming of this study was that groups were not matched for predonation hematocrit and red cell mass, two of the primary predictors for the need for homologous transfusion. These parameters may have been significantly higher in the PAD group prior to donation (and may have been one of the reasons why these patients were selected to undergo autologous donation), thereby placing patients in this group at decreased risk for requiring homologous transfusion, regardless of the use of PAD. In addition, it is quite possible that the nonrandomized unblinded nature of this study caused a certain amount of favoritism when withholding transfusions in the PAD group. Because data as to transfusion triggers are not provided, this is difficult to assess.

A similar matched control study was performed by Owings et al[32] in 1989. One hundred and seven patients undergoing elective cardiac procedures (97 CABG, 10 other) had an average of 3.0 ± 1.5 units of autologous blood removed prior to surgery. Excluded from donation were those patients with unstable angina or severe aortic stenosis with a valve area less than 0.8 cm^2. Removal was performed over an average of 33 ± 15.4 days prior to surgery. Such an extended donation period was possible by this time because of the improvements in blood preservation (storage limit increased to 42 days) that had occurred during the prior decade. If donation was extended or surgery was delayed beyond the 42-day preservation limit, the authors mixed the blood with a rejuvenating solution and the blood was then frozen until the time of surgery. Because of the extended donation period, the average drop in hematocrit was between 2.5% and 3%, indicating that significant red cell mass regeneration and a net gain in red cell mass had been achieved through the use of PAD (increase of approximately 2 units; Table 3.1). The authors report that compared to a control population of patients who did not undergo autologous donation, autologous blood donors had a significant decrease in homologous blood exposure. When patients undergoing CABG were analyzed as a separate group, for example, it was seen that 83% of non-PAD patients required homologous blood use versus 27% in the PAD group. Similar to the findings of Kruskall et al,[30] a direct relationship between the number of autologous units drawn and a decrease in homologous exposure was found. For example, if at least three units were drawn, the chance of patients receiving homologous blood decreased to only 10%. While these positive results are undoubtedly due at least in part to the effects of PAD (as though correct application of the technique and increase in total autologous mass had been made available at the time of surgery), they must be interpreted in light of the limited study design. The control group that was "matched" to the PAD group was matched only by the fact that they had similar types of surgery, at the same institution, and during the same time. Similar to Love et al's[31] study, there undoubtedly were reasons why these patients did not undergo treatment with PAD (including age, disease progression, and body size), thereby automatically instilling bias. Control patients were likely at much higher risk for transfusion than patients in the PAD group, regardless of the use of autologous blood. In fact, relative to control patients, patients in the PAD group were older, there were more females, the average hospital stay was longer, and the initial hematocrit was lower relative to patients in the PAD group. Concerns over preferential transfusion treatment hold for this study as well.

A study by Britton et al[33] in 1989 utilized a historic control study format to evaluate PAD. One hundred and four consecutive patients undergoing elective CABG, valve repair or replacement with or without concurrent CABG, and atrial septal defect repair were enrolled in a PAD program. An average of 4.1 units per patient were removed over a period that averaged 28 days. Unfortunately, predonation hematocrit data for the PAD group was not provided, so the degree of red cell regeneration that occurred during the 28-day donation period is difficult to assess. The preoperative hematocrit of 36.6%, compared to 39.4% in historical control patients, suggests that full regeneration had likely not occurred. At least some gain was likely realized, however, as evidenced by a significant decrease in homologous blood exposure as compared to controls. Seventy-six percent of patients in the control group received homologous blood, versus 21% in the PAD group, and the control patients received an average of 2.1 units of red cells, versus 0.6 in the PAD group. This 1.5-unit decrease is consistent with the volume of new red cells expected to be generated by the PAD group given their 4-week preoperative donation time interval (using a 0.46 unit per week mean red cell regeneration rate; Table 3.1). Although somewhat improved as compared to the studies of Love et al[31] and Owings et al[32] (at least the control patients were not drawn from a pool of patients who potentially had been rejected for donation), the limitations of the study design must be considered when evaluating these results.

A study from Europe by Achenbach et al[34] demonstrated that PAD was able to significantly reduce homologous exposure in a group of 42 cardiac surgical patients compared with 42 matched control patients not receiving PAD. As with prior studies, the allowance of insufficient preoperative time resulted in an actual calculated net gain in available autologous mass at the time of surgery of only 0.9 unit, rather than the full 2.5 units drawn as PAD (Table 3.1).

In 1991 the first study evaluating a strategy to improve the ability to collect autologous blood prior to cardiac surgery was performed.[35] Initial studies in baboons in 1988, and in preoperative orthopedic surgery patients in 1989, had demonstrated that recombinant erythropoietin could accelerate the rate and increase the volume of autologous blood collected preoperatively.[36,37] Watanabe et al[35] applied recombinant erythropoietin to PAD in humans undergoing heart surgery in 1991, and found that the volume of blood that was able to be collected preoperatively was increased, presumably through enhanced bone marrow production of new red cells. Other studies soon appeared in the literature, with similar accounts of improved PAD efficacy.[38–41] Common to all these reports was the important finding that not only was the ability to collect red cells improved, but the drop in hematocrit by the time of operation was significantly less in the erythropoietin groups, thereby decreasing the tendency for PAD to actually increase the risk of requiring blood transfusion (i.e., homologous plus autologous).

In 1992 Dzik et al[42] evaluated the safety and efficacy of PAD in patients undergoing aortic valve replacement for aortic valve lesions, including critical aortic stenosis. The physiology of aortic stenosis had led many to believe that it was unsafe to perform PAD in patients with this lesion, although this had never actually been shown to be true in the clinical literature. In fact, Dzik et al noted that in the several studies of PAD performed prior to this time, in which patients with aortic stenosis had not been excluded, no adverse consequences had been encountered.[29,31,33] They therefore enrolled 79 patients undergoing aortic valvular surgery in a PAD program in which a median of two units of blood were drawn over a 3- to 35-day period prior to surgery. Information concerning hematocrit decrease by the time of surgery was not provided, so an estimation of the degree of regeneration that was allowed to occur cannot be made. Clinical features of the 79 patients included a mean aortic valve area of 0.7 cm (range 0.2–2.0) and the mean gradient of 63 ± 24 mm Hg. When the homologous requirements for these 79 PAD patients were compared to a control group consisting of 298 patients undergoing valve replacement during the same time without PAD, a clear benefit was seen. Thirty-seven percent of patients in the PAD group required homologous blood, versus 69% in the control group. Again, as with the previous studies of PAD, care must be taken when interpreting these results, as the chosen control group may have been at higher risk for transfusion (patients with low preoperative hematocrit/red cell mass or those with significant co-morbidities may have been excluded from donation, thereby placing them in the control group). Only one patient in the study experienced a reaction related to transfusion (a syncopal episode 2 hours postdonation and after walking 0.8 km up a gradual incline) but this patient recovered fully and eventually underwent uncomplicated valve replacement. Despite these shortcomings, the authors were able to demonstrate that even in this perhaps "highest" risk population of aortic stenosis patients, autologous donation can be safely and effectively performed, and therefore that these patients should not be denied the option of PAD.

In 1993 Goldfinger et al[43] examined the safety and efficacy of PAD in patients awaiting heart and lung transplantation. Because of unpredictable donation to surgery intervals, collected blood was separated into components and frozen. They found that 64% of patients examined were medically able to donate. While the blood savings realized are difficult to quantify given the study's format, there was a significant decrease in transfusion when the donation and excluded-from-donation groups were compared. This study is important because it serves to establish the rationale behind, and the safety of, PAD in this patient population, and outlines a program for its use. The safety of PAD in this group has subsequently been confirmed by others.[44] The strategy applied is the same strategy that would be applied for any elective surgery planned for a date that is in excess of 42 days postdonation.

In 1995 Sandrelli et al[45] performed a matched control assessment of PAD in a mixed cardiac surgical population. Blood was collected between 30 and 7 days prior to operation and separated into red cell and plasma fractions (subsequently frozen) until reinfusion. The authors recorded parameters regarding the use of other complementary measures including intraoperative autologous blood donation (IAD), residual circuit blood reinfusion, low-dose aprotinin in high-bleeding-risk patients, and shed mediastinal blood reinfusion. They found that 348 consecutive PAD patients experienced a significant decrease in allogeneic transfusion requirement when compared to 344 "matched" control patients undergoing surgery at the same time but not receiving PAD. The authors also found that patients in the PAD group had lower admission hematocrits compared to controls, and confirmed that this led to an inability to remove a comparable volume of IAD blood in the PAD group (127 versus 200 patients, 338 ml versus 403 ml per patient, PAD and control groups, respectively). Unfortunately, as with prior PAD studies, it is difficult to quantitate the contribution of PAD, as important preoperative variables—most notably predonation hematocrit—were not revealed. The PAD group may have had relatively higher hematocrit and red cell mass values, as well as less comorbidity, thereby placing them at lower risk for transfusion. Nevertheless, the difference in allogeneic transfusion requirement suggests that PAD did provide benefit.

The findings of the studies presented in this chronological overview of the literature delineating the clinical application of PAD in cardiac surgery are summarized in Table 3.1 Several issues concerning the appropriate use of PAD become apparent when reviewing this table. First and foremost, these studies do not provide definitive proof that PAD is an effective blood conservation measure. A prospective randomized controlled trial proving the effectiveness of PAD in decreasing allogeneic transfusion has not been performed to date. Data regarding patient versus control selection, as well as criteria describing study groups and their risk factors for transfusion, are generally lacking. The end result is that the benefit of PAD can only be inferred.

These studies do serve, however, to provide important information as to how PAD might be optimized as a blood conservation technique. For example, the earlier studies indicate that performance of PAD shortly before surgery is simply a form of subacute hemodilution, as little or no regeneration of red cell mass is allowed to occur. This is evidenced by the relatively minor net gains in red cell mass seen in Table 3.1. The erythropoietin literature supports the fact that little or no acceleration in red cell production occurs with such short-term donation.[24,46] The result is that a blood product that has suffered a decrement in the percentage of viable red cells, and that is largely or totally devoid of platelet and coagulation function, is provided—at the expense of losing an equivalent volume of blood (which contains full platelet and coagulation function) from the patient. This obviously does not provide for optimal blood conservation. Clearly, for PAD to become a maximally effective blood conservation measure, it is essential that sufficient preoperative time be allowed for full red cell and blood regeneration.

Analysis of these studies also helps provide insight into for whom PAD is best applied from safety, cost, and resource efficiency standpoints. It is clear that PAD can be safely performed in patients undergoing cardiac surgery, even in those with diseases such as aortic stenosis that were previously thought to preclude the use of PAD. It also becomes apparent that PAD is an expensive labor- and resource-intensive endeavor. Clearly it should not be applied to all patients, but only to those predicted to be at risk for transfusion after application of other available measures. The following sections discuss these important issues related to the clinical application of PAD more thoroughly.

Specific Issues Related to the Optimal Use of Preoperative Autologous Donation in Cardiac Surgery

The preceding overview of the major clinical studies performed on the use of PAD in cardiac surgery serves to demonstrate, even despite the notable lack of clear proof in the form of prospective randomized or other optimally controlled studies, that PAD has the potential to serve as a safe and effective blood conservation measure in cardiac surgery. Benefits that can be achieved with PAD are all of those associated with the use of autologous rather than homologous blood. The full potential of PAD to reduce homologous blood requirements can only be fulfilled, however, if it is applied in a logical and optimal manner. Several issues must be addressed when seeking to delineate the optimal way in which to perform PAD. First, the patient group in which PAD can provide the most benefit must be identified. Only by applying PAD selectively to this patient group can an efficient and cost-effective reduction in homologous blood use be achieved. Second, once this target patient group has been determined, PAD must be applied to these patients in a way that maximizes its effectiveness. The literature clearly demonstrates that foremost among the factors important to maximizing the effectiveness of PAD is the allowance of a sufficient preoperative time period for both adequate donation and adequate red cell regeneration. Integrally related to the issues of patient selection *and* technique optimization are those of safety, cost-effectiveness, and appropriate resource allocation. This section addresses these issues, and outlines, based on existing data, the optimal way in which to apply PAD in cardiac surgery today.

Patient Eligibility

Several preoperative patient characteristics identify the cardiac surgical patient who can benefit from PAD (Table 3.2). The first and perhaps the simplest criterion is that the patient must be able to wait the required period of time for both adequate blood volume donation and red cell regeneration. Application of this criterion eliminates a majority of ineligible patients, as the patient group that cannot delay surgery typically includes those patients with disease of sufficient severity to preclude donation. The length of time required for donation depends on both the type of surgical procedure planned and the characteristics of the individual patient. While determination of this time period is the focus of the next section, generally this time period can be assumed to be 2 weeks per unit of blood required (Table 3.1). If a patient cannot tolerate this delay, then PAD should not be performed. It is important to understand that by applying this criterion, PAD is rendered a blood conservation technique applicable to *elective* surgery only, and therefore to an ever-decreasing number of patients in most centers.

TABLE 3.2. Exclusion criteria for PAD.

1. Inability to tolerate a delay in surgery of ≥2 weeks
2. Significant compromise in health or cardiovascular status that precludes donation: (most patients in this category are already excluded by criterion 1)
3. Hematocrit less than 33%
4. Active endocarditis/bacterial infection

Patients undergoing urgent and emergent surgery who cannot have surgery delayed are still candidates for the other blood conservation measures (e.g., intraoperative autologous donation, intraoperative salvage, postoperative shed blood reinfusion, pharmacologic support with the antifibrinolytics, erythropoietin, etc.), and a majority of these patients should still be able to be operated on with the use of little or no homologous blood support.

The second criterion for PAD suitability is that the patient must be healthy enough to undergo donation. As stated, elimination of those patients who cannot tolerate a delay in surgery also eliminates many patients who would be deemed ineligible by this criterion (e.g., patients with symptomatic left main coronary artery disease or unstable or preinfarction angina). Patients who might tolerate a delay but who would be unfit for donation might include those with severe aortic stenosis (AS), idiopathic hyperkinetic heart syndrome (IHHS), or congestive failure.[47] Although Britton's study found that donation in AS patients is safe in general, caution might still be exercised when applying PAD to these severely compromised patients.[33]

A third group of patients who should be disqualified from undergoing PAD are those patients with active endocarditis. The withdrawal, storage, and reinfusion periods allow ample time for bacterial replication should a unit become contaminated. The resulting bacteremia/sepsis incurred at the time of reinfusion can be life threatening.

The fourth and final criteria for donation is adequate preoperative hematocrit and red cell mass. A preoperative hematocrit of less than 33% excludes patients from autologous donation according to current criteria (AABB guidelines), as the risks of adverse donation reaction are thought to outweigh the benefits of decreased homologous transfusion.[50] Patients with hematocrits ≥33% should be considered for donation if other criteria are met. Those patients with mild to moderate anemia (hematocrit between 34% and 38%) of unexplained etiology should have predonation iron studies performed to assess the possibility of iron deficiency anemia, the most common cause of anemia. This would allow appropriate parenteral or intramuscular iron therapy to be initiated prior to donation so that iron status can be more rapidly restored to normal, thereby markedly increasing the red cell regenerative capacity. As with body size, the patient's red cell mass must be taken into consideration when deciding on the use of PAD. The presence of a low red cell mass either through decreased body size and estimated blood volume or decreased hematocrit should lower the threshold for recommending PAD. Conversely, a patient with a large preoperative red cell mass who is at decreased risk for transfusion can probably undergo surgery without homologous blood by using intraoperative and postoperative blood conservation techniques only. The use of PAD in these low transfusion risk patients would not be justified from either a patient-physician effort or cost-effectiveness standpoint. Several strategies are available that seek to increase hematocrit and red cell mass, thereby making PAD a viable option for greater numbers of patients. Recombinant erythropoietin can be used to accelerate red cell production in anemic patients undergoing PAD, although for cost considerations its use currently is limited to those who are unable to tolerate allogeneic transfusion either from a religious or biological (e.g. rare blood type) standpoint.[39] An alternative strategy is to lower the donation hematocrit cutoff. This would allow more patients to donate, and would allow PAD to be applied to a higher transfusion risk patient pool—those patients with anemia. In addition, it would increase the rate of red cell regeneration, as the lower hematocrits experienced by patients during the donation process would lead to increased release of endogenous erythropoietin. The trade-off would be a higher risk of adverse donation-related events.

A perceived but not actual limitation to donation is body size. For homologous donors a minimum weight of 110 lbs has been used as the traditional cutoff for donation. However, the AABB does make specific allowances for autologous donation by people of smaller body size, but recommends that no greater than 15% of the patient's effective blood volume (EBV) be removed at any given donation. A recent study of PAD in children as young as 3 years old clearly demonstrates that body size should affect the volume of blood removed, but not patient eligibility.[48,49] It is important to note here that rather than being avoided, PAD should be more aggressively pursued in these smaller patients, as it is this patient group that is at highest risk for transfusion (adjustments in the amount of anticoagulant should be made for units containing less than 400 ml). On the other end of the spectrum is the patient of large body size, who, assuming a normal hematocrit and bleeding risk, is at relatively low risk for perioperative transfusion. Cost-effective application of PAD might dictate that PAD not be recommended for these patients, even if elective surgery is planned.

Patient age is the final consideration. Previous studies in the blood banking literature have investigated the appropriateness of the elderly as autologous donors and have found no reason for these individuals not to donate blood.[51–54] Simon et al[55] found no increase in adverse events in a group of 244 elderly donors with a mean age of 68 ± 2.3 years. Discussion of this issue is particularly appropriate to the preoperative cardiac surgical patient, as the age of the population continues to increase.[56] Do the risks of the donation process in these patients outweigh the benefits of decreased risk of requiring transfusion? With a limited period of life often remaining (5–15 years), are concerns over the longer term about hepatitis or even HIV disease justified? Our response is that the elderly patient who has passed other criteria for preoperative donation such as elective procedure and adequate cardiovascular status has already been selected out as a relatively healthy individual. This, combined with the basic fact that surgery has been decided on in a patient of advanced age in the first place, usually indicates that the patient is quite viable, despite this advanced age. Nevertheless, the body systems of even these selected, more viable, elderly patients are relatively frail and less able to withstand insult, as indicated by an increased overall mortality as compared to the younger cohort. That these patients are therefore less able to tolerate the sequelae of transfusion such as acute or chronic hepatitis or transfusion reaction, provides an incentive to apply PAD despite the relatively limited remaining lifetime. For these reasons age alone should not be used as a contraindication to donation. The wisest course of action in these patients is to discuss the issue of autologous donation with them, and let them make the decision as to whether to proceed.

Optimal Preoperative Time Interval for PAD

The way in which PAD achieves a reduction in blood use is through the direct substitution of preoperatively donated autologous blood for homologous blood, when, through operative losses, the patient's red cell volume becomes insufficient. Essential to this process is that the preoperatively donated autologous red cell mass must be a volume in excess of what would normally be contained in the body at the time of operation, otherwise the autologous blood must be used to replace *itself* as well as that lost during operation.[57] Mathematically speaking, what this means is that to eliminate the need for homologous red cell transfusion, the red cell mass in the PAD blood units added to the red cell mass in the patient at the start of operation must be equal to or greater than the red cell mass in the patient at the start of operation plus the volume of homologous red cell mass that is required. For example, if an average of three units of homologous red cells are normally required for a 65-kg female undergoing aortic valve replacement, then this would be the number of autologous blood units needed to eliminate the need for these three units of homologous blood. But if three-unit PAD is performed only 2 to 3 days prior to surgery, significant red cell regeneration is now allowed to occur, and so no actual gain in red cell mass is realized by the time of operation. The three units of autologous mass that are needed to replace homologous transfusion requirements in effect do not exist, as they are required to restore the patient's red cell mass back to baseline. The predicted homologous requirements cannot therefore be met. While upon transfusion of these three units of PAD blood, as well as any homologous blood that might be required (e.g., three units), it might misleadingly be stated that three units of the patient's total transfusion requirements were met by autologous blood (i.e., 50% of transfusion needs were met by autologous blood), the reality is that because overall transfusion requirements were increased by three units just by performing PAD, no actual benefit was obtained, despite the efforts exerted withdrawing three units of blood preoperatively. As seen in the previous section, most of the studies of PAD in cardiac surgery at least partially overlooked this simple concept (Table 3.1). In a majority of these studies, the net increase in red cell mass was less than 50% of the stated number of PAD units withdrawn.

Therefore, over 50% of PAD effort was an exercise in cost and resource waste.

As stated previously, the second reason to allow a sufficient preoperative time interval for regeneration of red cell mass is that the higher the hematocrit in the operating room, the greater the volume of blood that can be removed by the blood conservation technique of IAD. This is an essential point. IAD is unit for unit a superior blood product and is theoretically significantly more effective than PAD in supplementing platelet and coagulation function. Blood drawn preoperatively is usually separated into packed red cells and plasma, with the plasma fraction being frozen. The platelets are usually typically discarded as they require special storage not typically performed (PAD blood can also be kept as whole blood, but the platelets and coagulation factors in this whole blood unit are nonfunctional). Additionally red cell viability steadily decreases in PAD blood during storage, so that by 42 days typically only 70% of red cells are viable.[58] In contrast, IAD blood is fresh (reinfused 1–2 hours following donation), it contains near normal levels of functional platelets and coagulation factors, and viability of red cells should approach 100%. IAD is clearly a superior blood conservation modality, and so every effort should be made to allow its preferential application. The allowance of full regeneration of red cell mass is essential when performing PAD, otherwise PAD is simply performed in preference to IAD.

Earlier studies of PAD were understandably handicapped by the limited amount of time for which blood could be stored (21 days), but later surgeons, anesthesiologists, and blood bankers had the capability of almost indefinite storage. Shelf life no longer was the factor limiting the possible predonation time period, and yet investigators repeatedly chose to draw blood within 1 to 3 weeks of operation, resulting in a decrease in hematocrit and body red cell mass at the time of operation, an overall increase in transfusion requirement, and a less effective outcome than might have been obtained by attention to the simple concept of allowing natural restoration of red cell mass. It might be argued that in cardiac surgical patients there often is insufficient time for a longer preoperative delay in surgery. The response to this is simply that any patient who can wait 2 to 3 weeks for surgery can usually wait 4 to 6 weeks for surgery, and those who can't probably should not undergo simple PAD as it is not an effective or cost-effective blood conservation measure for these people. If they in fact can only tolerate a 2-week delay in surgery, then only one unit of blood should be withdrawn.

How long is the optimal preoperative time period required for restoration of red cell mass following donation of blood preoperatively? The data actually exist to help calculate this number. For example, Owings et al[32] drew an average of 3.0 units of blood over an average preoperative period of 33 days, using the AABB minimum hematocrit for donation standard of 34% or greater. Because the average drop in hematocrit from predonation to immediately preoperation was 2.5% to 3%, a net gain of approximately two units was appreciated. It took approximately 33 days to generate two new units of red cell mass equivalents, or one unit every 2 weeks. A similar rate of regeneration is derived when the other studies of PAD in cardiac surgery that provide the necessary data points (predonation hematocrit, postdonation hematocrit, mean length of donation time, mean number of PAD units obtained) are assessed (Table 3.1). In fact, the mean rate of red cell regeneration of the five studies that provided adequate data yields a rate of 0.46 unit per week, or slightly less than one unit every 2 weeks. This rate of regeneration is similar to estimates obtainable from the surgical and hematologic literature, given normal iron stores and oral iron supplementation.[59] Following along with this, the AABB Technical Manual suggests at least a 2-week period be allowed following PAD but prior to surgery to "allow sufficient time to rebuild red cell mass."[60] Other authors have suggested similar rates of red cell regeneration during PAD.[61] Oral iron therapy should be initiated at the time of first donation to ensure adequate iron substrate for subsequent red cell regeneration.

To determine the total length of preoperative time required for optimal PAD for any given patient, the estimated number of blood units required must first be determined (see next section and Table 3.3). This unit number is then multiplied by the length of time required for complete red cell regeneration for each unit drawn (assuming oral iron supplementation, use of a minimum hematocrit of 34%, and no use of recombinant erythropoietin). As discussed, the time period required for regeneration of one unit of red cells is approximately 2 weeks. The resultant number will then be the minimum amount of time that should be set aside for autologous donation.

There are at least three mechanisms for potentially increasing the rate of red cell regeneration. Such an increase is desirable as it should lead to a decrease in the preoperative time required to optimally perform PAD. This will not only decrease operative delays, but will also render PAD a viable option for increased numbers of patients. First, early studies of iron and erythropoiesis suggest that parenteral iron supplementation can stimulate erythropoiesis to two to three to as much as six times normal, even in the presence of normal iron stores.[59,62] The possibility of acute anapbylactic reaction to iron therapy has deterred the widespread use of this enhancement modality, however, and it is difficult to recommend the routine use of a potentially dangerous treatment when it is not of absolute necessity (as it would be for the iron-deficient anemic Jehovah's Witness patient undergoing heart surgery, for example). As stated, however, oral iron supplementation (in conjunction with vitamin C to improve the gastrointestinal absorption of iron) should always be used in the patient undergoing PAD.

The second means of increasing red cell production during PAD is to stimulate increased production of endogenous erythropoietin by decreasing the minimum hematocrit cutoff for donation. Both the rate and magnitude of erythropoiesis are directly related to production of erythropoietin, and

TABLE 3.3. The New York Hospital-Cornell Medical Center schedule of optimal preoperative collection of autologous blood (SOPCAB).

Procedure type	No. units standard patient*	Reoperative procedure (add 1 unit)	No. units needed to adjust hematocrit to 40% (+/− 0.5 per 3% change)	No. units needed to adjust body size to 70 kg (+/− 0.5 per 20 kg change)	Presence of risk factors for bleeding (add 0.5 per risk factor)	Individual patient estimate† (round up to nearest whole number)
1. CABG	1					
2. VALVE-Single	1					
3. VALVE-Double	2					
4. VALVE (single)-CABG	2					
5. VAVLE (double)-CABG	2					
6. ASD Repair	1					
7. Thoracic Aneurism	3					
8. Other complex	2–4					

* = 70kg male or female, hematocrit 40%, no risk factors for bleeding.
† = round upward to nearest whole number.

erythropoietin production is, in turn, directly related to the level of anemia present. Studies have shown, however, that significant stimulation of endogenous erythropoietin production does not begin to occur until hematocrit decreases to below 30%.[46,59] At the AABB minimum hematocrit for donation standard of 33% to 34%, therefore, little or no increase in endogenous erythropoietin production occurs, resulting in little if any increase in red cell production. The patient undergoing PAD according to AABB standards must therefore wait the relatively lengthy 2 weeks per unit blood drawn for adequate regeneration to occur. A strategy to increase the rate of regeneration, therefore, is to decrease the minimum hematocrit for donation.[63] Decreasing this hematocrit would not only allow the removal of more blood (or the more frequent removal of blood), but it would keep hematocrits during the PAD period in a range that would lead to increased production of erythropoietin.[46,59] This would lead to increased red cell production during this period, and to a greater net gain in autologous red cell mass by the time of surgery. The one obvious flaw in this strategy is that lowering the minimum donation hematocrit might also be expected to increase the rate of adverse events, particularly in the cardiac surgical population. The AABB guidelines were set for a reason, and given the basic tenet of do no harm, exposing many cardiac surgical patients to more aggressive donation schedules, and the increased shifts in fluid and oxygen-carrying capacity to which this might lead, cannot be justified. One potential solution, as it is for many aspects of cardiac surgical blood conservation, is to not apply a "blanket" donation trigger, but to individualize donation triggers, as well as donation timing, based on individual health assessment. The healthy 60-kg male with mitral valve disease and a hematocrit of 50% may very well tolerate the acute removal of two units of blood at the time of first donation (with adequate concurrent volume replacement), and subsequent repeated donations to a hematocrit of 28% to 30%. Such front loading of donations would likely be well tolerated by this individual, and would be expected to accelerate erythropoiesis by providing stimulus for increases erythropoietin release. Procurement of blood could therefore be carried out over a shorter preoperative time interval.

The third and final strategy for increasing red cell regeneration during PAD is to exogenously supplement erythropoietin using the recombinant hormone. As mentioned previously this strategy was first utilized in cardiac surgery by Watanabe et al,[35] who found that not only was the volume of blood that could be collected significantly increased in erythropoietin-treated subjects as compared to controls, but that the drop in hemoglobin caused by donation was significantly decreased as well. Not only was more blood available, but because of improved red cell mass recovery, patients had higher hematocrits and were therefore at decreased risk for transfusion at the time of operation. The use of recombinant erythropoietin was found to be safe, and when given subcutaneously was relatively simple to administer. Why then not use erythropoietin for all preoperative autologous donations? The answer very simply is cost. For example, one of the more effective cardiac surgical PAD dosing strategies administered 600 U/kg of r-Hu EPO SQ one time per week. At $90 to $100 per 10,000 units, a 6-week course of therapy in a 70-kg patient would cost $2,520. Obviously it would be difficult to justify these costs except in exceptional circumstances (rare blood type, religious beliefs, etc.). Because of the excessive costs involved, erythropoietin-assisted PAD, although clearly of benefit in respect to blood conservation, will likely not see widespread use in the near future (not until patents held by Amgen expire in the early part of the next century).[59]

Optimum Number of PAD Units

The number of units required for any given procedure varies both with the type of procedure anticipated (i.e., mitral valve versus CABG) as well as the characteristics of the individual patient (e.g., body size, hematocrit, bleeding risk). The number of units required is also affected by the surgeons and anesthesiologists performing each procedure, and therefore institutions vary in their transfusion requirements. The number of units of blood required for each type of operation at any single institution has been termed the schedule of optimal preoperative collection of autologous blood (SOPCAB).[64] Determination of an accurate SOPCAB is an essential part of ensuring maximum allogenic transfusion reduction on the one hand, and minimizing waste and cost/resource inefficiency on the other. If too little blood is ordered, then patients will needlessly be exposed to allogeneic blood. If too much PAD is performed, then this additional blood – and the efforts expended procuring and storing it – will essentially be wasted (unless crossover is practiced, which we do not recommend; see below). The SOPCAB for any institution stands as a critical number. Unfortunately, the SOPCAB is not an easy set of numbers to derive. As indicated, in addition to variation by procedure type and institution, there also exists variation in blood use patterns among surgeons and anesthesiologists. Adding to this complexity are individual patient differences as to transfusion risk. All these factors must be taken into consideration to ensure the most accurate prediction possible. It has been advocated that the SOPCAB for any given procedure should be derived as the number of autologous units required to protect 90% of patients undergoing that particular procedure from allogeneic exposure.[64] While this appears to be an appropriate number, its use alone will result in significant overdrawing of blood, and therefore an unacceptable level of effort, cost, and resource inefficiency. A way in which to render SOPCAB predictions more accurate, while still achieving the 90% allogeneic transfusion reduction mark, is therefore required.

The first step in improving both the accuracy and precision of the SOPCAB is to standardize transfusion triggers, particularly those for red cells. This minimizes individual surgeon and anesthesiologist variability, while at the same time helping to eliminate unnecessary allogeneic exposure.

The second step toward improving SOPCAB accuracy is to individualize numerical predictions based on individual patient transfusion risk characteristics. This is the same concept that underlies the whole of our approach to blood conservation—*individualization based on transfusion risk.* The number of units required for a standard patient with normal red cell mass, hematocrit, and bleeding risk parameters must first be determined for each type of procedure. But rather than stopping there and imposing this number on all patients, this number of units must then be adjusted upward or downward based on alterations in these basic transfusion risk parameters. The 90-kg male patient with a hematocrit of 48% and no bleeding risk factors will clearly require less PAD than a 45-kg female with a hematocrit of 36% who is on aspirin. These are two very different patients, with two very different autologous needs, and the key to maximizing PAD efficiency is to recognize this fact. Table 3.3 lists the number of units of homologous red cells required for each of the major procedural types performed at our institution. Estimates for individual patients can be made by adjusting these numbers upward or downward, as depicted, depending on the relative risk of the patient for requiring transfusion, based on their age, sex, predonation hematocrit red cell mass, and risk of postoperative bleeding. For example, a person undergoing a reoperative CABG can generally be predicted to require 2.5 units of red cells. For a 60-kg female with a starting red cell mass less than 1600 cc and on aspirin at the time of surgery, this number should be increased to four units. This patient would require an 8-week preoperative time period to optimally perform PAD (note that the first one to two donations would have to be cryopreserved). A 70-kg male undergoing combined mitral aortic valve replacement would require predonation of three units and a 6-week preoperative interval. Conversely the 90-kg male with a hematocrit of 48% undergoing two-vessel CABG would not require any PAD in order to undergo successful bloodless surgery if all other blood conservation modalities are appropriately applied.

Safety

The safety of performing PAD in the cardiac surgical population is an issue of primary importance. Traditional criteria for nonautologous blood donation in the general population excluded patients with "heart disease" from giving blood (Table 3.4).[60,65] Presumably because of the self-benefiting nature of PAD, these traditional criteria were modified early on for autologous donors.[57] A subsequent large body of literature has confirmed the safety of allowing PAD in this broader population, particularly in those with cardiac disease.[32,33,42–44,54,66,67] Cardiac disease is no longer itself a contraindication; donation criteria now focus on the type and severity of cardiac disease. Several studies have specifically evaluated the safety of PAD in cardiac surgery, a population subsumed under the general category of high-risk donors (Table 3.5). This investigation has occurred

Table 3.4. Criteria for homologous and autologous blood donation.

	Homologous donation	Autologous donation	
Donor characteristics	AABB standards	AABB standards	BIH policy
Age (years)	17–65	No limit	No limit
Hemoglobin (g/dl)	13.5 (males) 12.5 (females)	11.0 (males and females)	11.0 (males and females) Lower when approved by blood bank medical director
Hematocrit value (%)	41 (males) 38 (females)	33 (males and females)	34 (males and females) Lower when approved by blood bank medical director
Vital signs	BP < 180/100 mm Hg; pulse, 50–100/min	Not specified	Medical director's discretion
Donation frequency	Every 8 weeks	Not specified	As tolerated (usually weekly)
Ongoing bacterial infection; use of antibiotics	Defer	Defer	Defer
Pregnancy	Defer	Not specified	Draw during third trimester
Heart disease	Defer	Not specified	Draw; exclude patients with unstable angina or critical aortic stenosis
Risk group for HIV or HBsAg	Defer	Not specified	Draw
Other criteria for protection of a homologous recipient	Defer	Not specified	Draw

AABB, American Association of Blood Banks; BIH, Beth Israel Hospital; HBsAg, hepatitis B surface antigen; HIV, human immunodeficiency virus.

TABLE 3.5. Safety of PAD in cardiac surgery.

Study	Population	No. of patients	No. units procured per patient	Adverse events		
				Mild	Moderate	Severe
Cuello (1967)	Mixed cardiothoracic	67	2.0	0	0	0
Newman (1971)	Mixed cardiothoracic	178	1.92	0	0	0
Lubin (1974)	Mixed cardiac	11	3.55	2	0	0
Cove (1975)	CABG	44	1.36	0	0	0
Silver (1975)	CABG	15	3	0	0	0
Fleming (1977)	Mixed cardiac	147(10)*	10	0	1	0
Mann (1983)	Mixed cardiac	275	2.2	3	4	0
Kruskall (1986)	Mixed cardiac	57	3.1	0	1	0
Love (1987)	Mixed cardiac	58	1.97	0	0	0
Sassetti (1988)	Mixed cardiovascular	25		3	0	5
Owings (1989)	Mixed cardiac	107	3.0	1	0	0
Britton (1989)	Mixed cardiac	104	4.1	0	0	0
Achenbach (1991)	Mixed cardiac	42	2.49	0	0	0
Dzik (1992)	Aortic valve	79	1.6	0	1	0
Goldfinger (1993)	Heart/lung transplant	46	3.4	0	0	0
Sandrelli (1995)	Mixed cardiac	348	2.2	0	4	0

*Ten patients who had 10 units removed had complete data available, which were used to complete this table.

undoubtedly because it is the cardiac surgical population that stands most to benefit from PAD, given the relatively large allogeneic transfusion requirements, as well as the large numbers of cases performed each year.

A logical and universal exclusion criteria for PAD in patients undergoing cardiac surgical procedures is the presence of unstable or preinfarction angina.[32] Whether to perform PAD in these patients does not typically become an issue clinically, however, as the requirement for rapid surgical intervention precludes the possibility of PAD (Table 3.2). Also traditionally excluded from donation were those patients with critical aortic stenosis.[32] However, several of the early cardiac surgical studies did not exclude these patients, and no adverse events were recorded. More recent studies have specifically addressed the safety of PAD in patients with aortic stenosis (AS). Dzik et al[42] found no increased incidence of adverse events in 79 patients with aortic stenosis undergoing PAD. The average valve area and other hemodynamic data for these patients are given (0.7 cm, 60 mm Hg, respectively), but it is difficult to know exactly how severe the valvular stenoses were in respect to clinical symptomatology. As with unstable angina, however, using the criterion of the patient being able to withstand a delay in surgery of at least 2 weeks should eliminate from consideration those aortic stenosis patients with disease possibly severe enough to render PAD unsafe. In certain patients with severe aortic stenosis who are deemed candidates for PAD, simultaneous volume replacement during blood collection may be prudent in order to maintain ventricular filling and cardiac output. Patients with mitral valve disease and those with dysrhythmias have not been found to suffer an increase in adverse events during PAD. Again, the requirement of a delay in surgery of at least 2 weeks should eliminate the sickest of these patients from consideration.

The safety of PAD in cardiac surgical patients of advanced age has been addressed in the previous section. The general consensus has been that age alone should not prevent one from participating in a PAD program.

An important issue in regard to donation safety in the high-risk cardiac population is where donation should be performed. In most centers autologous donation in non–high-risk patients is performed in blood bank facilities established for volunteer donation purposes. Several studies have suggested that donations in precardiac surgical patients should be performed in a monitored setting with a physician in close proximity, however.[44,67,68] Speiss et al[68] closely monitored high-risk PAD patients, including patients scheduled to undergo cardiac surgery. Previous studies had relied primarily on subjective data to evaluate the safety of PAD, such as the frequency of light-headedness or syncope. By measuring blood pressure, cardiac output, and continuous electrocardiography, Speiss et al found an increase in the incidence of hypotension and electrocardiographic changes during PAD that would have otherwise gone undetected. There was also a significant incidence of systolic and/or diastolic hypotension defined as a drop in blood pressure greater than 20 mm Hg. This was most common in those patients with coronary disease. In most cases the decrease in BP responded to saline administration during or immediately following PAD, but alpha support and/or atropine were administered by anesthesia personnel in five instances. These events may have simply been vasovagal events, but nevertheless they are of concern and indicate that personnel able to effectively deal with such complications should be available for donations by such high-risk patients. For this reason many centers recommend a minimum of at least ECG and intermittent BP monitoring for cardiac PAD patients. This is often performed in the postanesthesia/recovery room setting where critical care nursing and anesthesia personnel are available should they be needed. Because many centers performing cardiac surgery have a procedure room located on the ward that has monitoring capabilities, this would provide an acceptable site. Appointments to use this room for donation could be scheduled for patients and blood bank personnel. Because of its location in or near the cardiac surgical care area, nursing, anesthesia, and surgical personnel would be readily available. Location of the cardiac surgical PAD room near or on the postoperative cardiac care area provides for optimal patient care and maximizes cost and resource effectiveness.

The final issue in respect to safety is the need for saline replacement. A majority of PAD studies did not utilize volume supplementation, with no apparent deleterious sequelae.[33,42] Some investigators replace the withdrawn blood volume with an equal volume of saline.[68] Others utilized a flexible approach, in which saline infusion was applied when clinically indicated, for example, in a patient with suspected intravascular depletion attributable to ambitious diuretic use.[32] We utilize the latter approach at our institution, with only a small percentage of patients receiving volume supplementation.

Donor Recruitment

Recruitment of patients for PAD prior to cardiac surgery is less difficult than recruitment for allogeneic transfusion. In our urban center a preponderant patient concern is blood exposure, and one of the first questions often asked is, "Will I need blood?" Recruitment therefore becomes largely dependent on surgeon awareness of, and involvement in, an institution's PAD program. Once an organized, efficient, and safe PAD program is in place, it becomes the job of the surgeon, at the time that the need for surgery is agreed upon, to assess each patient for (1) the need for PAD, and (2) the suitability for PAD. Suitable patients are consented and enrolled, and the donation process is initiated with planning toward allowing the appropriate preoperative time interval for red cell regeneration. Sample consent forms are found in the AABB technical manual.[69] It is important to add to this form a discussion of the individual institution's policy toward autologous blood testing, discard of infectious units, and crossover of unused autologous blood units into the general blood supply (see the following section).[70] It is emphasized that PAD can only be effectively utilized if the operating surgeon is able to appropriately identify those patients who stand to benefit from PAD, is actively involved in initiating discussion of PAD with these patients, and then ensures optimal donation scheduling relative to the date of surgery. As with other aspects of comprehensive cardiac surgical blood conservation, maximum transfusion reduction can only occur with full surgeon involvement.

Crossover of Unused Autologous Blood

An important logistical issue is the fate of unused autologous units. Much debate has occurred in the literature over this issue, and institutions differ in their approaches to this potential problem.[57,71–74] It has been our contention, however, that if appropriate calculations are made with respect to individual patient needs (Table 3.3), minimum excess blood should be available at the time of patient discharge. By adopting such an approach at our institution, the issue of crossover of autologous units has assumed far less importance.

At the New York Hospital–Cornell Medical Center we have adopted a policy of not allowing crossover of PAD units to the general donor pool. This helps to ensure minimum contamination of the blood supply, while at the same time improving the cost and resource effectiveness of PAD.[73] Donor screening is an essential first step in eliminating potential contaminated donors, and autologous donors who are donating for themselves are less likely to be appropriately screened (a similar problem is seen with screening of directed donors). Safety of autologous units is therefore compromised. Allogeneic blood undergoes a battery of testing, which leads to significant resource consumption and cost. If a PAD unit is transfused to its donor, as it should be, then this testing is rendered unnecessary. Therefore, the essential step in ensuring maximum PAD safety and efficiency from all standpoints is not to transfer unused autologous blood to the general blood supply, but to minimize excess PAD.

Optimal Method of Component Preparation and Storage

The optimal way in which to store PAD blood, like other aspects of PAD, is dependent on the length of preoperative time necessary for (1) collection of the calculated number of units, and (2) appropriate red cell regeneration. As discussed, a 2-week period per unit of blood withdrawn is a useful guideline. Given a maximum 42-day storage period for unfrozen blood (when AS-1 preservative is utilized), a maximum of three units of autologous blood can be procured without a requirement for freezing of the red cell fraction. If AS-1 is not utilized, shelf life for unfrozen red cells is reduced to 35 days. This decreases the number of potential unfrozen PAD units to two from three. If more than three units of blood are predicted to be required for the planned surgical procedure, then these additional units (the first units drawn) should be separated into packed red cells and plasma and both of these components immediately frozen. The last three units should also be separated, but only the plasma fraction frozen. The red cell fraction should only be frozen if more than a 42-day storage period is predicted, as the freezing of red cells consumes additional resources and expense.[75] If surgery is delayed, however, then any red cell unit whose predicted storage time is greater than 42 days should be immediately frozen. These frozen cells can then be held until surgery is performed. Although such freezing adds additional expense (approximately twice the cost of liquid storage) post-thaw red cell viability is at least 80%, even after 21 years of storage.[75] Donated blood should not be kept as whole blood, as all coagulation function will be lost during the 2-week period extending from the last donation to the time of operation. This essentially results in a waste of potential autologous FFP.

Finally, as discussed several times previously, it is of little benefit to perform the last withdrawal within a shorter time interval prior to surgery for the intentional purpose of having whole blood available. Even within a period of 5 days most platelet and coagulation function is absent, and insufficient red cell regeneration is allowed to occur, thereby decreasing the available red cell mass in the patient's body at the time of operation. The ability to perform other superior blood conservation measures (e.g., IAD) is therefore compromised, as is the goal of maximum blood conservation in general.

With appropriate rejuvenation and freezing PAD red cells can be stored indefinitely. Therefore, unused autologous units that have already been frozen can be maintained for future patient use. This would be important for patients with anticipated reoperations or those with staged repairs of complex lesions. The costs of storage would likely have to be assumed by the individual patient unless medical necessity can be proven to his or her insurer. A number of commercial enterprises for long-term storage of blood have arisen.[75] These also present a viable option for patients anticipating surgery in the future and who can afford these services.

Transfusion of Autologous Units

There is, for obvious reasons, a tendency in those caring for intraoperative and postoperative cardiac surgical patients to maintain a lower threshold for reinfusion of PAD blood (versus its allogeneic counterpart). The patient's own blood is available, significant effort and cost have been extended to procure this blood, and it will be discarded (wasted) if not used. It must be remembered, however, that autologous blood is nevertheless a form of transfusion, and many risks accompany its use. These include clerical errors leading to transfusion of the wrong unit of blood, administration of a bacterially contaminated unit, volume overload, and air embolism and other intravenous mishap. It is therefore generally recommended in the blood banking literature that the same guidelines that are used for transfusion of allogeneic blood be used for PAD blood. At our institution we generally adhere to this policy but have implemented an algorithm that prioritizes the reinfusion of the various autologous blood types based on the operative time course and the quality of the blood product (see Figure 11.1; Chapter 11). For example, during CPB, if the hematocrit decreases to below the stated transfusion trigger of 16%, single-unit aliquots of PAD blood are returned after all available Cell Saver blood is returned, but before fresh IAD blood is returned. Thus, the stored red cells of the PAD blood are used to re-elevate whether oxygen-carrying capacity to acceptable levels, while preserving as much fresh whole IAD blood as possible for reinfusion post-CPB, when the benefits of its contained fresh platelet and plasma fraction are needed.

It is important to emphasize that when assessing a patient for the need for transfusion of PAD blood, as with allogeneic transfusion, clinical symptomatology is of primary importance. Numerical transfusion trigger guidelines are useful tools for decreasing unnecessary transfusion, but transfusion does become necessary above these numbers. Assessment of the present and predicted future clinical status of the patients should be the primary indicator for the need for transfusion.

Cost-Effectiveness/Resource Allocation

Two fundamental principles underlie the optimal application of PAD in cardiac surgery: (1) autologous blood should be procured only from those patients who can tolerate a delay in surgery of at least 2 weeks per unit of blood withdrawn, and (2) an accurate prediction of the number of units required, based on type of surgery and individual patient characteristics, must be made and no more than this number of units procured (Table 3.3). By adhering to the first principle ineffective PAD is prevented, and other more effective and cost- and resource-efficient blood conservation measures (e.g., IAD) are not compromised. By adhering to the second principle, needless procurement of blood is avoided, as are the cost, waste, and inefficiency associated with this needless procurement. Although these concepts appear straightforward, the literature is surprising in its disregard for these principles. There is a small but important group of patients who can derive blood conservation benefit from PAD; it is necessary to accurately identify these people, and then to perform PAD in the appropriate manner.

Integration with Other Perioperative Blood Conservation Measures

The technique of PAD is never practiced in isolation. Even in the most rudimentary of blood conservation efforts, it is applied in combination with other measures, such as tolerance of hemodilution and intraoperative salvage. It is a central theme of this book that individual blood conservation modalities must be applied only when they can effect an increment in homologous transfusion reduction. This eliminates waste from both a cost and resource standpoint, and becomes particularly important when the more expensive blood conservation modalities are considered. PAD is one of these. Use of such expensive modalities must be optimized from all standpoints. The key to such optimization is rational integration. The way in which PAD can be optimized as an individual measure has been outlined in the previous section and throughout this chapter. It has been seen that PAD is necessarily linked to IAD, and that IAD should take precedence as it provides a superior and far less expensive blood product. The necessity of performing IAD therefore dictates whether or not PAD should be performed, based on the length of preoperative time that is available. PAD is also linked to other measures by the preference for autologous blood product infusion. This preference should be based on the quality of the blood product, with the lowest quality of blood being reinfused first during CPB (Cell Saver), followed by PAD blood, followed by IAD blood as necessary to raise the hematocrit above 15%. Postoperatively the highest quality autologous product is reinfused first (IAD blood), followed by processed residual circuit blood, followed by PAD blood. As stated, the same transfusion triggers applied for allogeneic red cells and FFP should be used for PAD products, with the ultimate need for transfusion based on assessment of clinical status.

As outlined previously, PAD can also be used with recombinant erythropoietin. Recombinant erythropoietin-assisted PAD received significant attention in the early 1990s, but cost considerations have dampened its widespread application.[35,37–40] Nevertheless it is clear that when erythropoietin is used in effective dosing regimens, it can effect a significant increase in the rate of red cell regeneration. This safely increases the volume of blood that can be obtained during any given time period, rendering PAD a viable option for greater numbers of patients. Erythropoietin will become more affordable for perioperative use when patents expire. Alterations in reimbursement patterns may increase use of erythropoietin in the future as well. For example, it is conceivable that wealthier patients might be given the option of paying to receive erythropoietin in conjunction with their heart surgery, should its use be indicated.

Conclusion

Preoperative autologous donation is a safe and effective blood conservation measure. For it to be so, and to ensure resource- and cost-effectiveness, it must be applied in a logical and optimized manner. This chapter presented the theory underlying optimal application of PAD, and delineated the clinical methodology required for its execution.

Those in the field of general blood banking must encourage the use of PAD in a wide variety of situations and among a variety of surgical specialties with varying perioperative blood needs. Policies and practices are necessarily aimed at the surgical population as a whole, and detail with respect to individual patient populations, such as those undergoing cardiac surgery, may suffer. For PAD to be optimally and comprehensively applied in cardiac surgery, therefore, it is imperative that cardiac surgeons "take the reins" so to speak, and implement measures to ensure that PAD is appropriately applied to each and every eligible patient on which they operate. This is not a difficult task. The surgeon already evaluates each patient preoperatively in the office or clinic. By history, physical examination, and laboratory and diagnostic data he or she already knows which patients can tolerate a delay in surgery, and which, therefore, are candidates for PAD. Finally, by having evaluated his or her personal and institutional needs for transfusion for each of the various procedures, and combining this with an assessment of individual patient characteristics (Table 3.3), the surgeon is already able to accurately assess the number of units of PAD blood required. Having established a safe, monitored, and easily physician-accessible donation area, it remains simply for the surgeon to schedule donations, and then to schedule surgery at the end of the appropriate donation interval.

It is important to understand the limits of PAD as a blood conservation measure. PAD is not a technique that is applicable to all patients, nor do all patients desire to postpone their surgery solely for the purpose of obtaining autologous blood. In addition, new blood conservation techniques and pharmacologic manipulations, as well as improvements in old measures, have and will continue to decrease the necessity of obtaining additional red cell mass preoperatively.[76] We recently reported on the successful coronary artery bypass grafting of 100 consecutive patients using a multimodality blood conservation program that did not incorporate PAD.[77] Nevertheless,

PAD is a valid blood conservation measure. If it is to be applied, however, it must be applied correctly; the health care system will no longer tolerate inefficient and inappropriate use of its resources. The cardiac surgeon stands in a unique position to ensure such optimal application of PAD, and by doing so, be or she can significantly help in efforts to minimize allogeneic transfusion.

Directed Donation

Should a need for transfusion be predicted during the preoperative evaluation of any cardiac surgical patient, then PAD should be performed. Those patients judged to be ineligible for PAD (or do not desire PAD) have two options for meeting their perioperative transfusion requirements: (1) random donor blood from the general blood pool, and (2) directed donor (DD) blood. It is generally perceived by the public that DD blood carries a decreased risk of infectious disease transmission, that it is a source of safer blood. In fact, the reverse may be true. In addition, use of DD blood from first- and second-degree relatives can lead to fatal graft versus host disease, and can harm potential future organ donation between these relatives. Directed donation also adds significant complexity and cost to the general donation process. For these and other reasons, the three major blood bank organizations—the AABB, American Red Cross, the Council on Community Blood Centers—officially discourage the use of directed donations.[78] However, the psychological benefit gained by the patient in knowing the source of his or her blood significantly offsets these potential negative aspects of DD, and demand for this service persists. In a survey performed by the AABB in 1986, 81% of patients expressed preference for DD blood over random donor blood.[78] It is, therefore, imperative for the surgeon recommending transfusion reduction options to fully understand the arguments both for and against the use of DD, so that he or she can help to arrive at an optimal solution for each individual patient. The following section summarizes the negative and positive aspects of DD, and then a recommendation is made for the limited use of DD in cardiac surgery today, based on informed patient demand.

Arguments Against the Use of Directed Donation in Cardiac Surgery

The first and primary argument against the use of DD is the potential for an increased rate of infectious disease transmission. It has been postulated that donor screening is less effective with DD, as patients may be reluctant to disclose questionable past behaviors that may place the donor at increased risk. The cousin who experimented with intravenous drug use or who had a questionable sexual encounter may be reluctant to disclose this information to family members, and yet if they withhold donation (based on personal speculation alone), questions will obviously be asked. In fact it has been demonstrated clinically that the rate of seropositivity for various disease entities [human T-cell lymphotropic virus (HTLV-1), Hepatitis B] is higher in the directed donor population (Table 3.6).[78,79] This is partly because a larger percentage of directed donors are first-time donors, who are known to have a higher rate of seropositivity. Still, the increase in risk is real. In 1996 the estimated risk of hepatitis B in the random donor pool was 1 in 200,000.[78,80] If the risk in the directed donor pool is twice that, then the risk of hepatitis B for directed donors increases to 1 in 100,000. Such an increase in risk, albeit small, must be explained to the patient.

The second argument against the use of DD is the small but real risk of fatal graft versus host disease when blood from first- or second-degree relatives is used (this increased risk does not apply to nonrelated directed donors). Multiple such cases have been reported in the cardiac surgical literature, with the purported mechanism being attack of the recipients stem cells by viable donor white cells, due to human leukocyte antigen (HLA) congruency.[81,82] The risk of graft versus host disease, and its use as an argument against DD, can be eliminated, however, by donor blood irradiation. This is now recommended for all DD blood from any blood relatives. Irradiated blood must be transfused within 28 days of irradiation.[78]

A third related argument against the directed donation of blood from first- or second-degree relatives is that the patient's ability to receive a bone marrow transplant or other organ donation may be compromised in the future.[79] This risk is of course relatively minor, but should be considered, particularly in conjunction with directed donation in children. Similarly, directed donations should not occur from father to mother during pregnancy or during the childbearing years.

The fourth argument against the use of DD in cardiac surgery is the increase in cost and resource allocation required. These costs directly parallel those for PAD, and yet with no reduction in transfusion risk. Because such a cost burden is difficult to justify, except by "soft" parameters, reimbursement for DD by third-party payers may be compromised in the future.

TABLE 3.6. Seroprevalence of infectious disease markers at blood centers, 1991–1992 (rates per 100,000 donations).

	First-time donors		
	Directed (n = 30,778)	Community (n = 384,276)	p
Anti-HIV-1 or -2	13.0	31.0	NS
Anti-HTLV-1	78.0	33.6	<.0001
STS	61.7	54.1	NS
HBsAg	363.9	182.9	<.0001
Anti-HCV	661.1	588.6	NS

HIV, human immunodeficiency virus; STS, serologic test for syphilis; HBsAg, hepatitis B surface antigen; HTLV, human T-cell lymphotropic virus; HCV, hepatitis C virus; NS, not significant. Reprinted with permission.[77]

A fifth consideration is that DD provides a false sense of security in the uninformed patient, and in doing so may lead to a decreased tendency to perform PAD—a blood conservation measure that clearly is of benefit when appropriately performed.[79]

Finally, it should be understood that donor blood type and crossmatching, as well as administrative processing and storage, can take between 24 and 48 hours, depending on the institution. Therefore, while DD blood can be used for those undergoing urgent surgery, it cannot be made available for emergent surgery. The time of surgery should never be affected by the availability of DD blood, as it confers no true advantage over random donor blood.

Arguments for the Use of Directed Donation in Cardiac Surgery

Those in favor of directed donation might suggest that in respect to screening disclosure the opposite may be true, i.e., relatives or close friends are more likely to admit to donation contraindications as they care most about the patient at hand. This is a debate that could never be won, nor does it need to be won on this sociologic level. The fact is that the incidence of infectious disease markers is higher in collective pools of directed donor blood (Table 3.6). It must be remembered, however, that any single individual within this pool harbors one's own independent risk, and a husband married to a wife for 40 years may feel very confident that his wife's blood is safe. He, and any individual like him, should be allowed the option of using this blood (whether society should pay for this option is a matter of debate, however). It remains the responsibility of the surgeon to make this patient aware of the mildly increased infectious and immunologic risks that he may incur by choosing the option of directed donation.

Conclusion

Directed donation is primarily a perceived blood conservation option. While its advantages are limited to increased patient psychological comfort, it has several disadvantages. Although each directed donor is at individual risk for infectious disease transmittal, as a whole the group of directed donors is at greater risk for testing positive for markers of blood-borne illness. It is therefore essential that patients be presented with the facts when determining whether to apply this blood banking modality. The patients should closely consider their potential donors with an understanding of issues such as potential underreporting of risk factors. For those who feel confident of the "safety" of their donor's blood, DD remains a viable blood conservation option. It is an option, however, that should only be considered when preoperative autologous donation is not possible.

References

1. Blundell J. Successful case of transfusion. *Lancet* 1829;431–432.
2. Pineda AA. Review of the history. In: Taswell HF, Pineda AA, eds. *Autologous Transfusion and Hemotherapy.* Boston: Blackwell Scientific, 1991;1–21.
3. Grant FC. Autotransfusion. *Ann Surg* 1921;74(8):253.
4. Langston H, Milles G, Dalessandro W. Further experiences with autologous blood transfusions. *Ann Surg* 1963;158:333–336.
5. Milles G, Langston HT, Dalessandro W. Experiences with autotransfusion. *Surg Gynecol Obstet* 1962; Dec:689–694.
6. Kay LA. The need for autologous blood transfusion. *Br Med J* 1987; 294:137–139.
7. Toy PT, Stehling LC, Strauss RG, et al. Underutilization of autologous blood donation among eligible elective surgical patients. *Am J Surg* 1986;152: 483–486.
8. Amman AJ, Wara DW, Dritz S, et al. Acquired immunodeficiency in an infant. Possible transmission by means of blood products. *Lancet* 1983;1:956–985.
9. Joint statement on acquired immune deficiency syndrome (AIDS) related to transfusion. *Transfusion.* 1983;23:87–88.
10. American Medical Association Council on Scientific Affairs. Autologous blood transfusions. *JAMA* 1986;256(17):2378–2380.
11. Toy PT, McVay PA, Strauss RG, et al. Improvement in appropriate autologous donations with local education: 1987–1989. *Transfusion* 1992;32:562–564.
12. Williamson KR, Taswell HF. Avoiding the hazards of homologous blood transfusion, and other advantages of autologous blood transfusion and hemotherapy. In: Taswell, HF, Pineda AA, eds. *Autologous Transfusion and Hemotherapy.* Boston: Blackwell Scientific, 1991:22–52.
13. Kruskall MS. Autologous blood collection and transfusion in a tertiary-care center. In: Taswell HF, Pineda AA, eds. *Autologous Transfusion and Hemotherapy.* Boston: Blackwell Scientific, 1991;54.
14. Toy PT, Strauss RG, Stehling LC, et al. Predeposited autologous blood for elective surgery: a national multicenter study. *N Engl J Med* 1987;316:517–520.
15. Wallace EL, Churchill WH, Surgenor DM, et al. Collection and transfusion of blood and blood components in the United States, 1992. *Transfusion* 1995; 35:802–812.
16. Goldfinger D, Haimowitz M, Aubuchon JP, et al. Controversies in transfusion medicine. Is autologous blood transfusion worth the cost? Pro, Con. *Transfusion.* 1984;34(1):75–83.
17. Birkmeyer JD, Goodnough LT, Aubuchon JP, et al. The cost-effectiveness of preoperative autologous donation in coronary artery bypass grafting. *Ann Thor Surg.* 1994;57:161–169.
18. Dodrill FD, Marshall N, Nyboer J, et al. The use of the heart-lung apparatus in human cardiac surgery. *J Thorac Surg* 1957;33(l):60–73.
19. Garcia E, Zamora R. Auto transfusion in elective thoracic operations: a preliminary report. *Philippine J Surg Specialties* 1964; 18:33–38.
20. Ascari WQ, Jolly PC, Thomas PA. Autologous blood transfusion in pulmonary surgery. *Transfusion* 1968;8:111–115.
21. Daggett WM, Gada PH, Leape LL, et al. Autologous blood transfusion in pulmonary surgery. *J Thorac Cardiovasc Surg* 1970;59:546–550.
22. Newman MM, Hamstra R, Block M. Use of banked autologous blood in elective surgery. *JAMA* 1971;218(6):861–863.

23. Cuello L, Vasquez E, Rios R, et al. Autologous blood transfusion in thoracic and cardiovascular surgery. *Surgery* 1967;62(4):814–818.
24. Kickler TS, Spivak JL. Effect of repeated whole blood donations on serum immunoreactive erythropoietin levels in autologous donors. *JAMA* 1988; 260(l):65–67.
25. Verska JJ, Larson NL. Autologous transfusion in cardiac surgery: a case report of a patient with a rare antibody. *Transfusion* 1973;13(4):219–220.
26. Lubin J, Greenberg JJ, Yahr WZ, et al. The use of autologous blood in open-heart surgery. *Transfusion* 1974;14(6):602–607.
27. Cove H, Matloff HJ, Sherbcoe R, et al. Autologous blood transfusion in coronary artery bypass surgery. *Transfusion* 1976;16(3):245–248.
28. Fleming AW, Green DC, Radcliffe JH, et al. Development of a practical autologous transfusion program. *Am Surg* 1977;39:194–801.
29. Mann M, Sacks HJ, Goldfinger D. Safety of autologous blood donation prior to elective surgery for a variety of potentially high risk patients. *Transfusion* 1983;23:229–232.
30. Kruskall MS, Glazer EE, Leonard SC, et al. Utilization and effectiveness of a hospital autologous preoperative blood donor program. *Transfusion* 1986; 26:335–340.
31. Love TR, Hendren WG, O'Keefe DD, et al. Transfusion of predonated autologous blood in elective cardiac surgery. *Ann Thorac Surg* 1987;43:508–512.
32. Owings DV, Kruskall MS, Thurer RL, et al. Autologous blood donations prior to elective cardiac surgery: safety and effect on subsequent blood use. *JAMA* 1989;262(14):1963–1968.
33. Britton LW, Eastlund T, Dziuban SW, et al. Predonated autologous blood use in elective cardiac surgery. *Ann Thorac Surg* 1989;47:529–532.
34. Achenbach H, Tanzeem A, Saggau W, et al. Blood use reduction by predonation—how effective is it? In: Friedel N, Hetzer R, Royston D, eds. *Blood Use in Cardiac Surgery.* New York: Springer-Verlag, 1991;171–173.
35. Watanabe Y, Katsuo F, Konoshi T, et al. Autologous blood transfusion with recombinant human erythropoietin in heart operations. *Ann Thorac Surg* 1991;51:767–772.
36. Levine EA, Gould SA, Rosen AL, et al. Perioperative recombinant human erythropoietin. *Surgery* 1989;106(2):432.
37. Goodnough LT, Rudnick S, Price TH. Increased preoperative collection of autologous blood with recombinant erythropoietin therapy. *N Engl J Med* 1989;31:1163–1168.
38. Kulier A, Gombotz H, Fuchs G, et al. Subcutaneous recombinant human erythropoietin and autologous blood donation before coronary artery bypass surgery. *Anest Analg* 1993;76:102–106.
39. Watanabe Y, Katsuo F, Naruse Y, et al. Subcutaneous use of erythropoietin in heart surgery. *Ann Thorac Surg* 1992;54:479–484.
40. Konoshi T, Ohbayashi T, Kaneko T, et al. Preoperative use of erythropoietin for cardiovascular operations in anemia. *Ann Thor Surg*. 1993;56:101–103.
41. D'Ambra MN, Lynch KE, Boccagno J, et al. The effect of perioperative administration of recombinant human erythropoietin (r-HuEPO) in CABG patients: a double blind, placebo-controlled trial. *Anesthesiology* 1992; 77(3a):A159.
42. Dzik WH, Fleisher AG, Ciavarella D, et al. Safety and efficacy of autologous blood donation before elective valve operation. *Ann Thorac Surg* 1992; 54:1177–1181.

43. Goldfinger D, Capon L, Czer L, et al. Safety and efficacy of preoperative donation of blood for autologous use by patients with end-stage heart or lung disease who are awaiting organ transplantation. *Transfusion* 1993;33:336–340.
44. Klapper E, Pepkowitz SH, Czer L, et al. Confirmation of the safety of autologous blood donation by patients awaiting heart or lung transplantation. *J Thorac Cardiovasc Surg* 1995;110:1594–1599.
45. Sandrelli L, Pardini A, Lorusso, et al. Impact of autologous blood predonation on a comprehensive blood conservation program. *Ann Thorac Surg* 1995; 59:730–735.
46. Goodnough LT, Brittenham GM. Limitations of the erythropoietic response to serial phlebotomy: implications for autologous blood donor programs. *J Lab Clin Med* 1991;115(l):28–35.
47. Robblee JA, Crosby E. Transfusion medicine issues in the practice of anesthesiology. *Transfus Med Rev*. 1995;9(l):60–78.
48. Masuda M, Kawachi Y, Inaba S, et al. Preoperative autologous blood donations in pediatric cardiac surgery. *Ann Thorac Surg* 1995;60:1694–1697.
49. Silvergleid AJ. Safety and effectiveness of predeposit autologous transfusions in preteen and adolescent children. *JAMA*. 1987;257(24):3403–3404.
50. Holland PV, Schmidt PH, eds. *Standards for Blood Banks and Transfusion Services*. 13th ed. Arlington VA: American Association of Blood Banks, 1989.
51. Schmidt PJ. Blood donation by the healthy elderly. *Transfusion* 1991; 31(8):681–682.
52. Garry PJ, Vanderjagt DJ, Wayne SJ, et al. A prospective study of blood donations in healthy elderly persons. *Transfusion* 1991;31:686–692.
53. Haugen RK, Hill GE. A large-scale autologous blood program in a community hospital. A contribution to the community blood supply. *JAMA* 1987; 257:1211–1214.
54. Mann M, Sacks HJ, Goldfinger D. Safety of autologous blood donation prior to elective surgery for a variety of potentially "high risk" patients. *Transfusion* 1983;23:229–232.
55. Simon TL, Rhyne SJ, Wayne SJ, et al. Characteristics of elderly blood donors. *Transfusion* 1991;31:693–697.
56. Ko W, Krieger KH, Lazenby WD, et al. Coronary bypass grafting in 100 consecutive octogenarian patients: a multicenter analysis, *J Thorac Cardiovasc Surg* 1991;102(4):532–538.
57. Simon TL, Smith KJ. The issues in autologous transfusion. *Hum Pathol* 1989;20(1):3–5.
58. Beutler E. Liquid preservation of red cells. In: Rossi EC, Simon TL, Moss GS, Gould SA, eds. *Principles of Transfusion Medicine*. Philadelphia: Williams and Wilkins, 1996:58.
59. Helm RE, Gold JP, Rosengart TK, et al. Erythropoietin in cardiac surgery. *J Cardiac Surg* 1993;8:579–606.
60. Walker RH, ed. *American Association of Blood Banks Technical Manual*. 11th ed. Bethesda, MD: American Association of Blood Banks, 1993;494.
61. Goodnough LT, Brittenham GM. Limitations of the erythropoietic response to serial phlebotomy: implications for autologous blood donor programs. *J Lab Clin Med* 1990;115:28–35.
62. Coleman DH, Stevens DR, Doge HT, et al. Rate of blood regeneration after blood loss. *Arch Intern Med* 1953;92:341–349.

63. Levine E, Rosen A, Sehgal L, et al. Accelerated erythropoiesis: the hidden benefit of autologous donation. *Transfusion* 190;30:295–297.
64. Axelrod FB, Pepkowitz SH, Goldfinger D. Establishment of a schedule of optimal preoperative collection of autologous blood. *Transfusion* 1989; 29:677–680.
65. Kruskall MS. Autologous blood collection and transfusion in a tertiary-care facility. In: Taswell HF, Pineda AA, eds. *Autologous Transfusion and Hemotherapy*. Boston: Blackwell Scientific, 1991;60.
66. Popovsky MA, Aubuchon JP. Autologous blood donation in "high-risk" patients. *Transfusion* 1992;32(7):689.
67. Adegboyega PA, Patten ED. A review of presurgical autologous donation by high risk patients. *Trans Mod Rev* 1994;8(3):200–209.
68. Speiss BD, Sassetti R, McCarthy RJ, et al. Autologous blood donation: hemodynamics in a high risk population. *Transfusion* 1992;32:17–22.
69. Walker RH, ed. *American Association of Blood Banks Technical Manual*. 11th ed. Bethesda, MD: American Association of Blood Banks, 1993:401.
70. Kruskall MS. Autologous blood collection and transfusion in a tertiary-care center. In: Taswell HF, Pineda AA, eds. *Autologous Transfusion and Hemotherapy*. Boston: Blackwell Scientific, 1991;58.
71. Silvergleid AJ. Preoperative autologous donation: what have we learned? *Transfusion* 1991;31(2):99–101.
72. Kruskall MS. Autologous blood collection and transfusion in a tertiary-care center. In: Taswell HF, Pineda AA, eds. *Autologous Transfusion and Hemotherapy*. Boston: Blackwell Scientific, 1991;68.
73. Myhre BA. Crossing over of autologous and directed donor blood. *Ann Clin Lab Sci* 1992;22(5):343–352.
74. Yomtovian RA, Schrank JY, Betts YM, Kepner JL. Transfusion of previously donated blood in a community hospital. In: Taswell HF, Pineda AA, eds. *Autologous Transfusion and Hemotherapy*. Boston: Blackwell Scientific, 1991;87.
75. Valeri CR. Frozen red blood cells. In: Rossi EC, Simon TL, Moss GS, Gould SA, eds. *Principles of Transfusion Medicine*. Philadelphia: Williams and Wilkins. 1996:61–66.
76. Silvergleid AJ. Autologous and designated donor programs. In: Petz LD, Swisher SN, Kleinman S, Spence RK, Strauss RG, eds. *Clinical Practice of Transfusion Medicine*. New York: Churchill Livingstone. 1996:287.
77. Page PL. Controversies in transfusion medicine. Directed donations: con. *Transfusion* 1989;29(1):65–70.
78. Schreiber GB, Busch MP, Kleinman SH, et al. The role of transfusion: transmitted viral infections. *N Engl J Med* 1996;334:1685–1690.
79. Jugli T, Takashi K, Shibata T, et al. Post-transfusion graft vs host disease in immunocompetent patients after cardiac surgery in Japan. *N Engl J Med* 1989;321:56.
80. Thaler M, Shamiss A, Orgad S, et al. The role of blood from HLA-homozygous donors in fatal transfusion-associated graft vs host disease after open heart surgery. *N Engl J Med* 1989;321:25.
81. Klein HG. *Standards for Blood Banks and Transfusion Services*. 16th ed. Bethesda, MD: American Association of Blood Banks, 1994.
82. Goldfinger D. Directed blood donations: pro. *Transfusion* 1989;29(1):70–74.

4
Erythropoietin in Cardiac Surgery

Robert E. Helm and Karl H. Krieger

Erythropoietin is an endogenous glycoprotein hormone that serves as the primary stimulus for red blood cell production. Synthesized by the kidney in response to tissue hypoxia, it travels through the bloodstream to the bone marrow, where it increases both the rate and magnitude of red cell production. The recombinant form of erythropoietin became available clinically in 1987 for the treatment of the anemia of chronic renal failure. Its immediate and widespread success in this area prompted application of the drug to other disorders and conditions in which an increase in red cell mass is desirable. One focus of attention has been on the perioperative use of the drug to decrease the need for homologous red cell transfusions. Cardiac surgery, with its consistently high pattern of blood use, has become an important area of investigation and application. This chapter reviews events leading to the discovery and characterization of endogenous erythropoietin, as well as the development and clinical application of the recombinant hormone. It then discusses the basic science and physiology of endogenous erythropoietin, and the erythropoietic response for which it is responsible, in order to provide a firm background for understanding clinical applications of the recombinant hormone. The chapter then reviews the general aspects and pharmacology of the recombinant form of erythropoietin, as well as its general clinical application in the treatment of anemia, and then focuses on experience with recombinant erythropoietin in the perioperative setting, with particular emphasis on the cardiac surgical patient. Finally, potential ways in which the perioperative use of recombinant erythropoietin might be optimized, as well as possible future applications for the drug in the cardiac surgical patient, are discussed. The final section draws all of this information into a concise outline of what the practicing cardiac surgeon needs to know about recombinant erythropoietin, and provides a set of recommendations for use of recombinant erythropoietin in each of the perioperative scenarios that might be encountered.

Historical Background

The acute effect of hypoxia on erythropoiesis was first reported in 1890 by the French histologist Viault,[1] after he noticed an increased number of erythrocytes in his blood following an extended expedition to high altitude regions of Peru. The term *hemopoietin* was applied by Carnot and Deflandre[2] in 1906 to describe the existence of a humoral factor that had the ability to control red blood cell production. This existence was not fully accepted, however, until 1948, when Bonsdorff and Jalavisto[3] reported an increase of red blood cell precursors in the bone marrow of rabbits injected with sera from hypoxic donors, and introduced the term *erythropoietin*. Definitive evidence for the existence of erythropoietin was provided by Reissman and Nomura[4] in 1950 and Erslev[5] in 1953. Reissman and Nomura were able to show that hypoxia of one animal of a parabiotic pair produced marrow hyperplasia and reticulocytosis in the partner, and Erslev demonstrated that serum from hypoxic animals induced a significant reticulocytosis when injected into normal animals. Other experimenters confirmed their results and further characterized the hormone.[6,7] A bioassay was subsequently developed based on measurements of radioiron incorporation.[8] Identification of the source of erythropoietin production rapidly followed. The clinical observation of generalized erythrocytic hyperplasia of the marrow in patients suffering from patent ductus arteriosus suggested a relation between hypoxia of the lower part of the body and stimulus of erythropoiesis.[9,10] In 1957 Jacobson et al[11] were able to localize the site of production to the kidneys when they noticed that nephrectomized animals did not experience an increase in erythropoietin activity in response to hypoxia. Lack of erythropoietin activity was also demonstrated in anemic humans suffering from chronic renal failure.[12] The return of erythropoietin levels to normal following kidney transplantation provided additional evidence for a renal site of production.[13] The renal source of erythropoietin was finally proven by measurement of erythropoietin activity in serum-free isolated perfused rabbit kidneys and in renal extracts of hypoxic rats.[14–16] This was later confirmed by the extraction of erythropoietin messenger RNA (mRNA) from the kidney.[17,18] In addition to the kidneys, by 1972 Fried[19] and others had established the liver as a site of supplemental erythropoietin production. Early on, however, findings in anemic chronic renal failure patients demonstrated that hepatic production alone was insufficient to maintain a normal circulating red blood cell mass.

Development of Recombinant Erythropoietin

With the purification of erythropoietin from urine by Miyake et al[20] in 1977, reliable and specific radioimmunoassays became available for detection of serum erythropoietin levels,[21,22] and in-depth molecular and biochemical studies could be undertaken. These studies led to sequencing of the secreted 165 amino acid protein, cloning of the erythropoietin gene, and, finally, in vitro expression of the gene in mammalian cells.[23,24] The recombinant product (r-HuEPO) has gained rapid clinical acceptance, particularly in the treatment of the anemia of chronic renal failure, for which it received rapid Food and Drug Administration (FDA) approval in 1988. By 1991 it was established that r-HuEPO was being used in 175,000 renal patients in Europe, Japan, and the United States.[25] Recombinant erythropoietin has since received FDA approval also for the treatment of AIDS-related anemia and the anemia associated with cancer chemotherapy.[26] The use of the drug has transcended these approved indications, however, and is currently used to treat a variety of anemias, and to stimulate red cell production in the perioperative setting.[27,28] The history of erythropoietin and development of the recombinant hormone are discussed in depth elsewhere.[29–31]

Endogenous Erythropoietin and the Erythropoietic Response

Biochemistry

Endogenous erythropoietin is a 165 amino acid glycoprotein molecule. Its sequence has been shown to be highly conserved among mammalian species, and it is fully interactive between these species (Figure 4.1).[30] It displays no significant amino acid sequence homology with any other plasma protein,[23,24,32–35] but despite this lack of similarity, erythropoietin appears to have a secondary structure analogous to an entire group of cytokines including growth hormone, prolactin, interleukin-6, and granulocyte-macrophage–colony stimulating factor (GM–CSF) (Figure 4.2).[36–38] Its proposed globular tertiary structure, consisting of four antiparallel alpha helices, is seen in Figure 4.3.[37,38]

Circulating erythropoietin has a total mass of 30 kda, 60% of which is peptide backbone and the remaining 40% carbohydrate.[30,32] In vivo, the carbohydrate moiety is required neither for biologic activity nor target cell specificity, but to prevent the hormone's premature removal from the circulation by the liver.[39,40] Erythropoietin carbohydrate residues also help to make it a relatively hardy molecule that resists denaturation by heat, alkali, and reducing agents.[41] It is very hydrophobic and requires a carrier protein to stay in solution. Current formulations of the recombinant product that are available in the United States utilize human albumin as a carrier, and, therefore, may not be acceptable to certain individuals who object on a religious basis to the use of human blood. For example, the Jehovah's Witness organization has a Medical Hospital Liaison Committee,

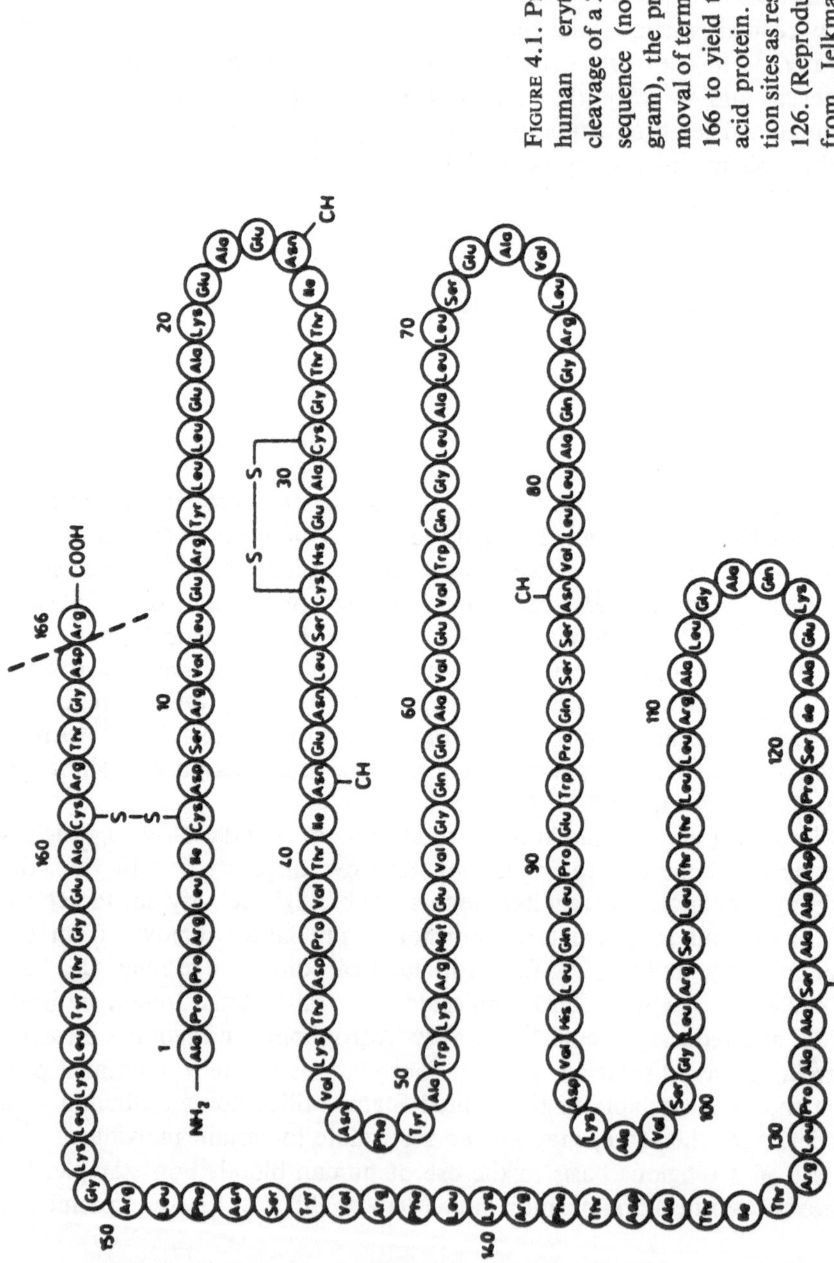

FIGURE 4.1. Primary structure of human erythropoietin. After cleavage of a 27 amino acid leader sequence (not seen in this diagram), the protein undergoes removal of terminal arginine residue 166 to yield the final 165 amino acid protein. Note the glycosylation sites as residues 24, 38, 83, and 126. (Reproduced with permission from Jelkmann,[30] Lappin and Maxwell.[34])

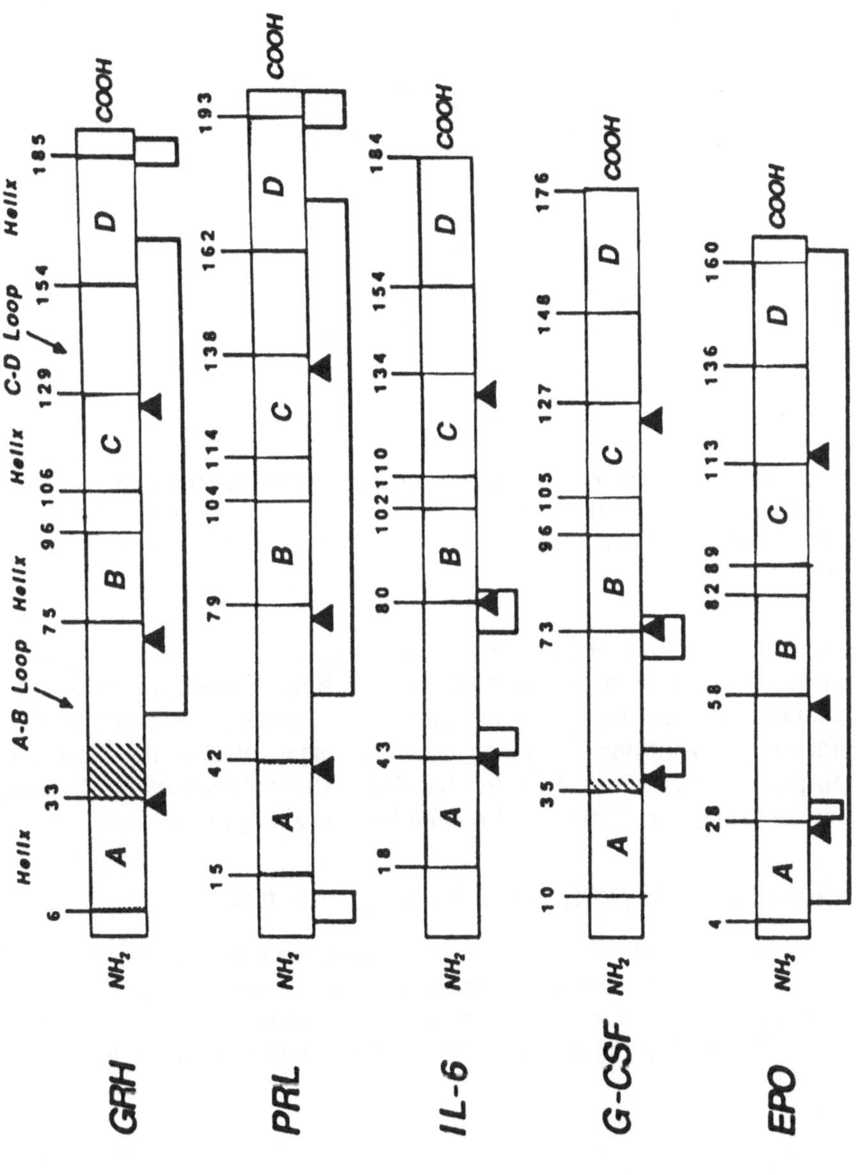

FIGURE 4.2. Secondary structure of five human growth regulating cytokines. Evident is the striking similarity in location of the secondary structural elements, including four alpha helices (A, B, C, and D) and three loops connecting these alpha helices (white areas A-B, B-C, and C-D). (Reproduced with permission from Bazan.[38])

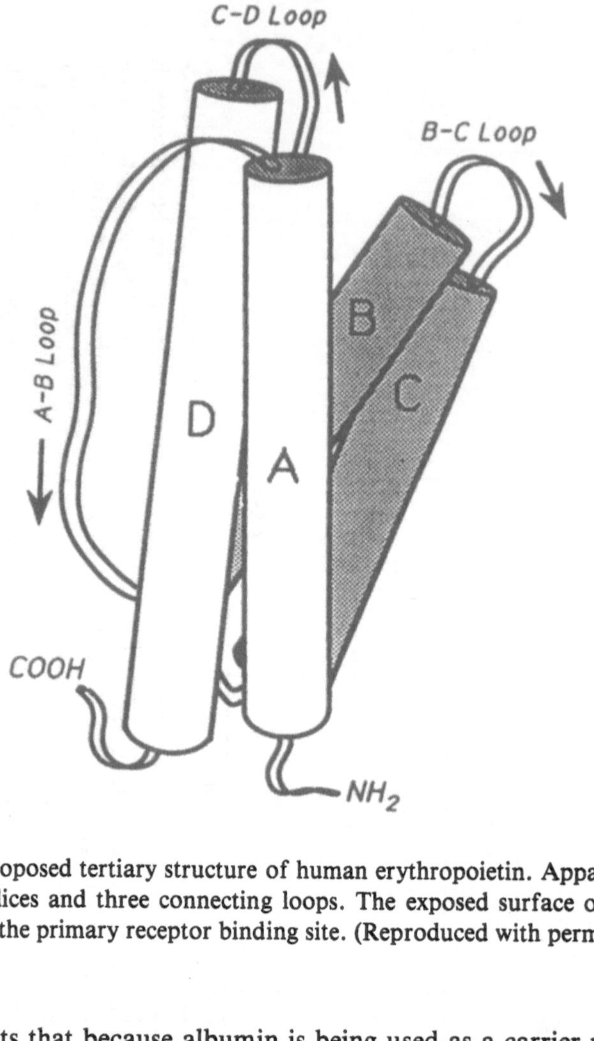

FIGURE 4.3. Proposed tertiary structure of human erythropoietin. Apparent are the four alpha helices and three connecting loops. The exposed surface of helix D is believed to be the primary receptor binding site. (Reproduced with permission from Bazan.[38])

which suggests that because albumin is being used as a carrier protein for purpose of drug administration, and not as blood per se, its use does not contradict its doctrine. The Committee leaves its use, however, up to the individual practitioner.[42] It has been our experience at the New York Hospital-Cornell Medical Center that most Jehovah's Witnesses will accept the use of albumin formulated recombinant erythropoietin.

Site of Production, Metabolism, and Excretion

During fetal life, the liver appears to be the main source of erythropoietin production.[43-45] During late gestation there is a changeover to the kidneys as the primary site of synthesis, and this continues throughout adult life.[18,44,45] While estimates vary, 75% to 90% of erythropoietin is produced by the kidneys, and the majority of the remainder by the liver.[18,19,45-48] Synthesis within the kidney has been localized to the peritubular interstitial cells, and in the liver centrilobular epithelial cells have been shown to produce the hormone.[49-52] The kidney and liver are responsible for the baseline steady-state level of erythropoietin production, as well as increases in erythropoietin production in response to physiologic stimuli. There are no significant tissue stores of erythropoietin, and so all production is by de novo synthesis.[53,54]

It has been proposed by Erslev and Caro[55] that the kidney is ideally suited to be the site of erythropoietin production because of this organ's unique ability to match oxygen demand with oxygen supply. Because the primary energy expenditure of the kidney is in reabsorption of sodium from the renal tubules, changes in the tubular flow directly affect oxygen consumption. In anemic states, cardiac output and renal blood flow typically increase, and so too then does tubular flow and reabsorption. The net result is an increase in oxygen consumption. This increase in oxygen consumption, in the setting of an already decreased oxygen supply, serves to create a relative hypoxic state. This hypoxia is registered by the peritubular oxygen sensor, and an increase in production of erythropoietin ensues. In contrast, in polycythemic states, increased viscosity and decreased glomerular flow typically result in decreased tubular flow and reabsorption, and so oxygen consumption is decreased. This decreased demand, coupled with increased carrying capacity, serves to alleviate the tissue hypoxia that might occur with decreased flow alone (as would be expected to occur in other organs). Erythropoietin production is therefore not stimulated, and can actually be depressed.[56,57]

The normal serum level is 5 to 25 U/ml,[21,27,58] an amount that serves to maintain the body's normal red cell mass (nearly 100 billion new erythrocytes are produced each day).[30] Estimates of endogenous erythropoietin's half-life in the bloodstream in normal individuals have varied between 3 and 8 hours.[30,58-61] A biphasic clearance pattern has been demonstrated.[61-64] Elimination is mainly through hepatic degradation, although renal catabolism and renal excretion also contribute. Marrow uptake and utilization may play a minor role as well.[65]

Physiology of Endogenous Erythropoietin

Stimulation of Erythropoietin Production

The primary physiologic stimulus for increased endogenous erythropoietin production is hypoxia, or decreased availability of oxygen at the tissue level, as determined by (1) *oxygen carrying capacity,* (2) *oxygen tension,* and (3) *oxygen affinity* of the blood (Figure 4.4).[30] Hormonal, paracrine, and pharmacologic agents help modulate this primary response axis. The actual oxygen sensing apparatus, shown to lie in the same cells that produce erythropoietin (renal peritubular interstitial cells), is believed to be a heme

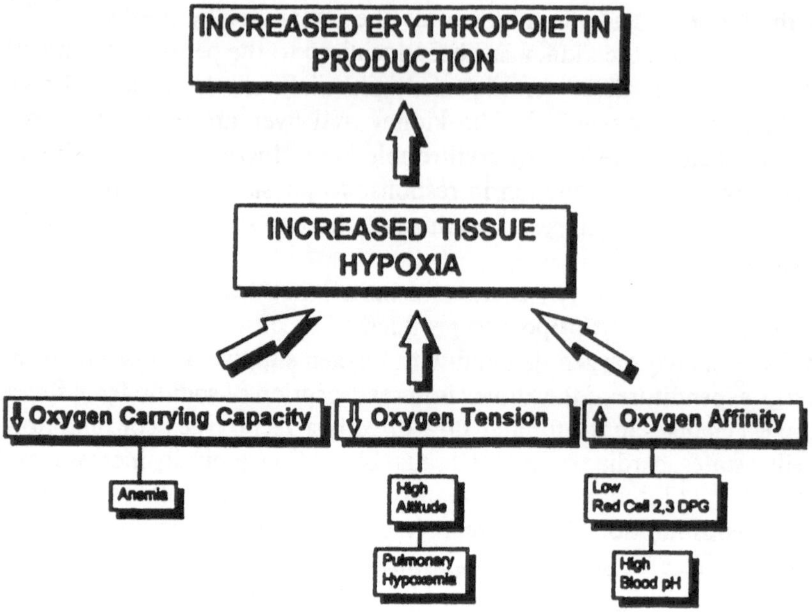

FIGURE 4.4. Tissue hypoxia is the primary stimulus for erythropoietin production. Hypoxia can be attributed to any one or all of three basic abnormalities: (1) decreased oxygen carrying capacity, (2) decreased oxygen tension, and (3) increased oxygen affinity. The most common cause of decreased oxygen carrying capacity is chronic or acute blood loss and anemia. In the perioperative setting depressed oxygen tension is most often attributable to cardiopulmonary dysfunction. Increased oxygen affinity can be found whenever conditions favor binding rather than release of oxygen from hemoglobin.

protein. The leading model utilizes a heme oxygen–sensing molecule, which, when tissue oxygen is low, changes to its deoxy configuration.[66] This then begins the chain of intracellular events that leads to erythropoietin production.

Oxygen carrying capacity is inversely related to erythropoietin production.[55] In many of the chronic anemias (e.g., hemolytic anemias, hemoglobinopathies) erythropoietin levels are increased.[67–72] Similarly, the abrupt decrease in carrying capacity that occurs with acute blood loss leads to an increase in erythropoietin production, with the amount of elevation proportional to the magnitude of the insult.[73–76] Conversely, in hypertransfusion or dehydration-induced polycythemia, erythropoietin levels are found to be decreased.[56,57]

There are two important qualifications that must be made with respect to the relationship between erythropoietin production and changes in oxygen carrying capacity. First, the inverse linear relationship between oxygen carrying capacity and erythropoietin production only applies when the hemoglobin concentration drops below 10.5 g %.[77] For example, patients undergoing autologous blood donation using the American Association of Blood Banks (AABB) minimum hematocrit guideline for donation of 34% experience little if any increase in serum erythropoietin levels.[78–80] As will be seen, this provides the basis for exogenous supplementation with recombinant erythropoietin during preoperative autologous donation. Second, the increase in erythropoietin can only occur if the erythropoietin hormonal axis is intact. It does not hold, for example, in the anemia of chronic renal failure, where low hematocrit is due to inadequate erythropoietin production by the nonfunctioning kidney. It has been demonstrated that the normal relationship between anemia (or hypoxia) and erythropoietin level is lost when serum creatinine rises above 1.5 mg/dl.[41] Other disease states can alter the normal response as well.[81] For example, patients with malignancies, chronic disease, burn injury, and sickle cell disease have been shown to have inappropriately low levels of erythropoietin.[30,82–84] Similarly, the elderly have been found to have depressed levels of erythropoietin relative to that expected for their degree of anemia.[85] This latter relationship may be important in cardiac surgery where the age of the average patient undergoing surgery continues to increase.[86]

Decreases in *oxygen tension* lead to an exponential increase in erythropoietin production.[30,87,88] Travelers to, and the natives of, high-altitude regions demonstrate increased erythropoietin levels, with corresponding increased hematocrits.[89,90] Anemic patients with elevated erythropoietin levels who are exposed to supplemental or hyperbaric oxygen demonstrate a fall in erythropoietin levels.[91] This last demonstration of the importance of oxygen tension is of interest given that the shape of the hemoglobin oxygen binding curve, and hence the oxygen content of fully oxygenated arterial blood, increases by only a small percentage when oxygen tension is increased above normal.[30] The small percentage of arterial oxygen that is in solution and not bound to hemoglobin—and that does increase with increased oxygen tension—may therefore play a significant role in the erythropoietin response. The influence of oxygen tension on erythropoietin production may be clinically important for postoperative anemic cardiac patients who are often ventilated for 6 to 18 hours, and then given supplemental nasal cannula oxygen for an additional period of time. Elevated arterial oxygen pressures during this time may suppress production of the higher levels of erythropoietin necessary for increased bone marrow progenitor cell recruitment and maturation, and thus recovery from postoperative anemia might be significantly compromised.

Finally, the *oxygen affinity* of the blood is directly related to erythropoietin production; increased affinity of hemoglobin for oxygen results in decreased oxygen delivery, increased tissue hypoxia, and increased erythropoietin production. In humans with high oxygen affinity mutant hemoglobin, an erythrocytosis exists, and in rats with high oxygen affinity blood, erythropoietin levels have been shown to rise acutely.[92–94] Red blood cell 2,3-diphosphoglycerate (2,3-DPG) levels inversely affect hemoglobin oxygen affinity. Low 2,3-DPG levels increase oxygen affinity. The decrease in 2,3-DPG levels in banked blood may account for the finding that transfusion of banked blood causes a greater increase in erythropoietin levels than the transfusion of fresh blood.[95] It has been hypothesized that the ability of the red cell to acutely increase its own 2,3-DPG concentration may help to account for the decrease in erythropoietin production found 1 to 3 days following hypoxic insult, despite the fact that hemoglobin levels have not yet begun to rise.[96] Blood pH also affects oxygen affinity, with decreased affinity at low pH. Erythropoietin levels have in fact been shown to decrease with acidosis.[30] A negative effect by acidosis on the oxygen sensing apparatus itself may contribute to this effect.[97] Finally, disorders that decrease blood oxygen affinity, such as sickle cell disease, have been associated with erythropoietin levels that are abnormally low for any given level of anemia.[83]

Serum Erythropoietin Levels

The production of erythropoietin in response to tissue hypoxia—whether it be from decreased oxygen carrying capacity, tension, or affinity—normally occurs in a biphasic fashion. Two to 6 hours after hypoxic insult (e.g., acute blood loss), serum erythropoietin levels rise from baseline, and a peak occurs 12 to 72 hours later, the magnitude and duration of this peak depending on the degree of the hypoxia.[76,98,99] Following this initial peak, erythropoietin levels begin to fall, and over the ensuing weeks levels gradually return to normal as hematocrit returns to normal. Again, the magnitude and duration of this moderate phase of elevation correlate with the degree of hypoxia.[55,76,98] It has been postulated that the moderation of initial peak serum erythropoietin levels 1 to 3 days following hypoxic stimulus results from activation of the body's counterhypoxic mechanisms, such as increase in red cell 2,3-DPG, elevation of cardiac output, and stress release of reticulocytes and sequestered red cells.[96] Figure 4.5 shows the endogenous erythropoietin response (depicted as CONTROL) seen in baboons acutely bled to an average hematocrit of 15%, clearly demonstrating the biphasic nature of this response.[99] In humans with severe acute or chronic anemia, blood levels can reach 6,000 to 10,000 U/L (Figure 4.6).[100] Conversely, in those patients with little anemic stimulus, for example, autologous blood donors adhering to the AABB minimum hematocrit standard of 34%, little if any elevation in erythropoietin production occurs, and consequently red blood cell production is minimally increased (herein lies the rationale for the use of exogenous recombinant erythropoietin in augmenting procurement of autologous blood).[78-80] The biphasic nature of the endogenous erythropoietin response may play a role in the mechanism of action of the hormone at the bone marrow level.

Modulation of Erythropoietin Production

Many substances, including paracrine factors, endocrine hormones, pharmacologic agents, and cytokines, have been shown to help modulate the

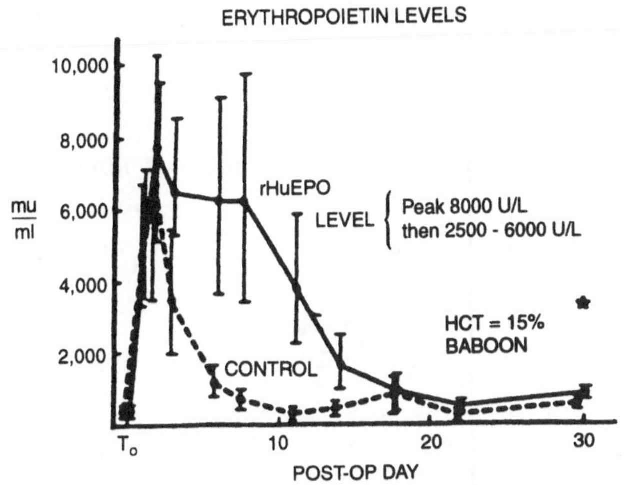

FIGURE 4.5. The typical biphasic endogenous erythropoietin response to acute anemia (hematocrit = 12% to 15%) is evident in the control group of animals. Evident is the initial high peak at 48 to 72 hours post-anemic stimulus onset, which reaches as high as 7500 to 8000 mU/ml. This is then followed by a precipitous decrease in blood levels from day 2 to day 4. Levels then remain persistently elevated until resolution of anemia. The normal endogenous serum erythropoietin level is 4 to 25 μm/ml. (From Levine et al.[99])

amount of erythropoietin produced in response to hypoxia (Table 4.1).[101,102] Among the humoral messengers, thyroid hormone, growth hormone, vasopressin, serotonin, prolactin, and the androgens have been shown to increase erythropoietin levels, and are likely responsible for the circadian pattern of erythropoietin production that has been reported.[30,102–111] Androgens were applied in early attempts to stimulate erythropoietin in anemic individuals.[108,109] Conversely, the estrogens have been shown to inhibit erythropoietin production.[112–115] The opposing effects of androgens and estrogens have been used to theorize that at least part of the difference in normal baseline hematocrit between males and females is due to hormonal influence on erythropoietin.[30]

Several pharmacologic agents have been shown to affect erythropoietin production.[101] The β-adrenergic agonists have been shown to increase production of erythropoietin.[115] β-Adrenergic blocking agents, often used in both pre- and postoperative cardiac surgery patients, have been shown to inhibit production.[103] The mechanism through which β-adrenergic influence occurs may be linked to activation of adenylate cyclase.[102,103] Cobalt has long been known to increase red blood cell production.[116] It has been shown that it exerts its effect by increasing serum erythropoietin levels.[66,116] Cobalt's ability to lock the renal heme oxygen sensor in its deoxy configuration is likely related to this stimulatory effect.[66]

The cytokine group of inflammatory mediators has also been shown to affect production of erythropoietin. Interleukin-1 (IL-1), tumor necrosis

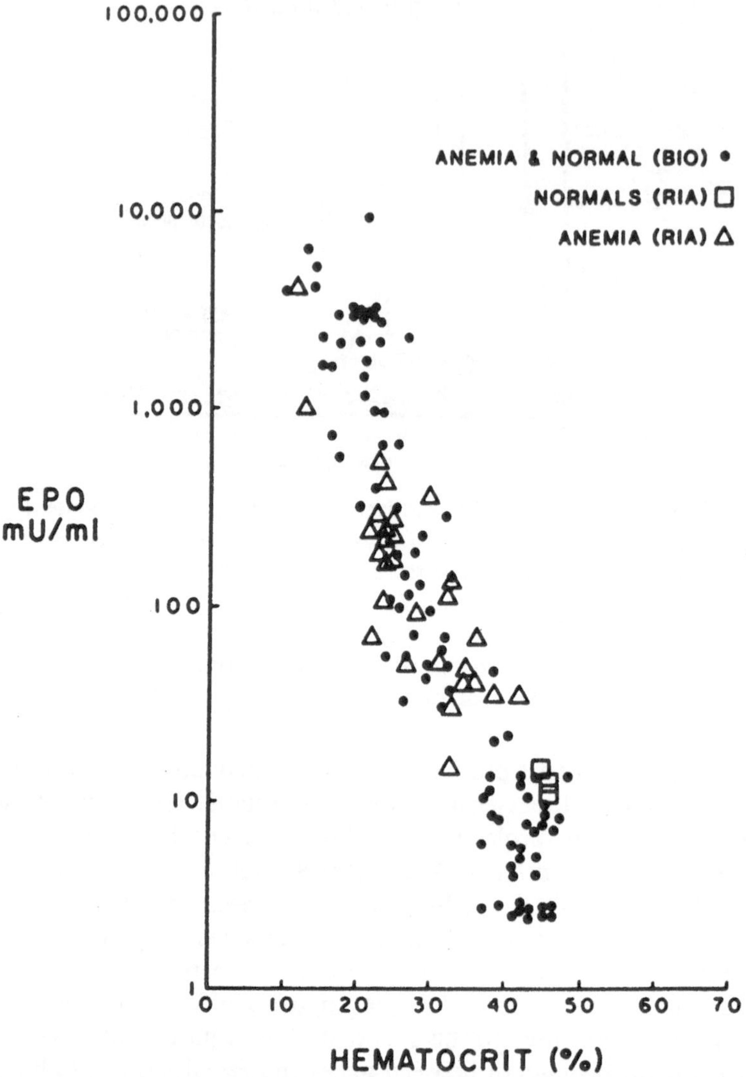

FIGURE 4.6. Serum erythropoietin titers in normal individuals and patients with anemia not attributable to renal disease. Measurements were made using both bioassay (BIO) and radioimmunoassay (RIA). (Reproduced with permission from Erslev et al.[100])

factor, and transforming growth factor-B have all been shown to suppress production of erythropoietin.[117] The relatively low levels of erythropoietin (for the given degree of anemia) seen in the anemias of malignancy, rheumatoid arthritis, and chronic disease, are likely attributable to these cytokine interactions. As will be seen in the following section, these same cytokine interactions can also affect the response of the bone marrow to any erythropoietin that is present, thereby exacerbating the decrease in red cell production.[117]

TABLE 4.1. Factors affecting erythropoietin production.

Increase	Decrease
Endocrine	Endocrine
Thyroid hormone	Estrogen
Growth hormone	
Vasopressin	Cytokine/Paracrine/messenger
Prolactin	IL-1
ACTH	TNF
Testosterone	TGF-β
5α-dihydrotestosterone	
Angiotensin II	Pharmacologic
Vasopressin	β_2-blockers
	Alkylating agents
Cytokine/paracrine/messenger	Mercurial diuretics
Eicosanoids (PGE_1, PGE_2, PGI_2, PGI_2, 6K-PGE_1)	
cAMP	
Pharmacologic	
Cobalt	
Adenosine-A_2 agonists	
Albuterol	
Terbutaline	

ACTH, adrenocorticotropic hormone; cAMP, cyclic adenosine monophosphate; IL, interleukin; PG, prostaglandin; TGF, T-cell growth factor; TNF, tumor necrosis factor.

Stimulation of Erythropoiesis in the Bone Marrow

Among the hemopoietic growth factors, erythropoietin has one of the most restricted ranges of target cell activity.[39] Receptors for erythropoietin have been identified in the placenta,[118] and the megakaryocyte-platelet lineage may be mildly responsive to the hormone.[119–121] Endothelial cell mitosis and migration have been shown to respond to erythropoietin stimulation as well.[122] Otherwise, evidence indicates that erythropoietin interacts almost exclusively with erythroid progenitor cells in the marrow.[30,36] Erythropoietin normally appears to have three major functions in respect to bone marrow red cell progenitors: (1) recruiting and amplifying primitive progenitor cells, (2) permitting survival of these cells in their differentiating forms, and (3) directing a program of terminal differentiation.[36]

The mature red blood cell develops from the pluripotent bone marrow stem cell through a series of changes regulated by several growth factors.[123,124] These changes have been broken down to a series of stages illustrated in Figure 4.7.[43] Development begins with the noncommitted pluripotent stem cell, which at some point becomes committed to the erythroid line, and is then known as a burst forming unit-erythoid (BFU-E) cell. Only a small fraction of these BFU-Es are actively cycling in the marrow, the remainder existing in a dormant state. Once triggered into active cycle, BFU-Es are responsive to multiple growth factors, and their growth factor requirement changes as differentiation proceeds. Very early

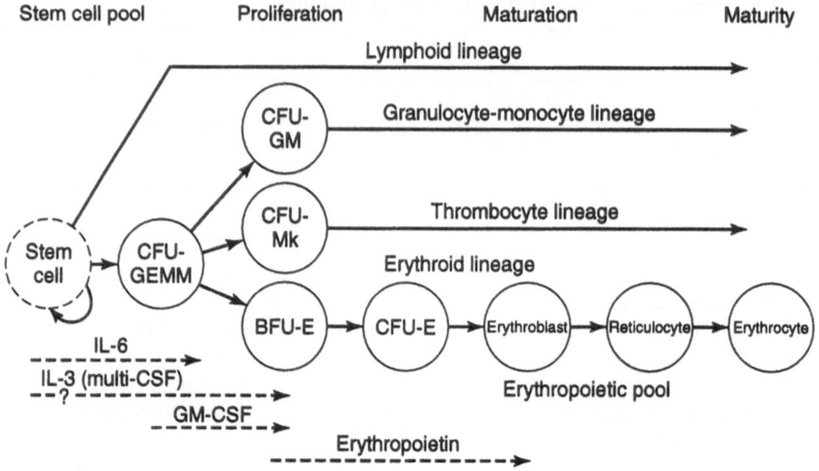

FIGURE 4.7. A model of erythropoietin development from the primitive marrow stem cell. Cytokines such as IL-3, GM-CSF, and IL-6 exert an early influence. Erythropoietin begins to take on importance in the later BFU-E stage, and becomes the predominant growth factor during the CFU-E stage. The hormone's importance then begins to decline, and developing cells no longer require erythropoietin by the time of reticulocyte formation. (Reproduced with permission from Faulds and Sorkin.[43])

BFU-Es are primarily responsive to IL-3, released from T lymphocytes.[123,125] GM-CSF, a multilineage hemopoietin, is able to stimulate BFU-E at more intermediate stages of development.[123,125–127] BFU-Es are initially relatively insensitive to erythropoietin, but sensitivity progressively increases as differentiation proceeds.[123,125,127–129] By the time the developing cell reaches the end of the BFU-E stage, erythropoietin has become its predominant growth factor. It appears that this variation in erythropoietin responsiveness is directly related to the number of receptors expressed on the cell surface. Early BFU-Es—those responsive primarily to IL-3—have been shown to have relatively few erythropoietin receptors. This number steadily increases with development, and parallels the progressive increase in sensitivity.[123,125,127–129] It has been demonstrated that this increase in erythropoietin receptor number may occur through a process of upmodulation, whereby binding by IL-3 and GM-CSF to their own receptors serves to progressively increase the number of erythropoietin receptors expressed.[125] During the BFU-E stage erythropoietin appears to serve primarily in a mitogenic capacity, markedly increasing the number of developing erythroid progenitors.[30,123]

The process by which early noncycling BFU-Es are triggered into active cycle has yet to be elucidated. Because early progenitor cells are relatively insensitive to erythropoietin, it has been hypothesized that high erythropoietin levels might be required to trigger noncycling BFU-Es into activity.[30,130,131] Cell culture experiments showing that high erythropoietin concentrations markedly increase the number of active BFU-Es support this concept.[119,129–132] The natural biphasic erythropoietin response to acute blood loss or hypoxia, with its initial high erythropoietin levels, would lend empiric support to this model.[36] Alternatively, local increases in IL-3 or some other growth factor might be required to trigger increased numbers of cells into replication, but a mechanism relating hypoxic stimulus to such interactions has yet to be uncovered. Because it is estimated that only 5% of primitive erythroid progenitor cells are actually cycling in the marrow, the enormous potential for enhanced erythropoiesis at this stage is readily apparent. Whether it be by a confirmation of the importance of high initial serum levels of erythropoietin, or through the discovery of a novel source of anemia-linked stimulation, the unlocking of this potential will provide an important advance in our ability to control and maximize the erythropoietic response.

It is at the next level of differentiation, the colony forming unit stage (CFU-E), where small clusters of immature cells are found (the progeny of recruited BFU-Es), that erythropoietin is believed to exert its major influence.[126,129,133] By the time progenitor cells reach this stage, their erythropoietin receptor concentration is at its peak, and so too then is their sensitivity to the hormone.[124,126] It is believed that the primary function of erythropoietin at this time is not to stimulate mitosis, but to prevent apoptosis or preprogrammed cell death.[129,134] Studies indicate that erythropoietin may carry out this function by preventing DNA breakdown.[134] Based on this concept a model has been proposed whereby developing CFU-E cells have varying numbers of erythropoietin receptors on their surfaces.[127,129,133,134] Sensitivity to the hormone therefore also varies, and so at normal erythropoietin concentrations only some progenitor cells receive the amount of stimulus that is necessary to prevent DNA breakdown. Under the direction of such normal erythropoietin concentrations enough progenitor cells survive to ultimately form the nearly 100 billion erythrocytes humans produce each day. When the serum erythropoietin concentration is increased due to stimuli such as hypoxia, more progenitor cells are permitted to survive (i.e., those progenitor cells requiring higher concentrations are added to the pool of survivors), and increased red blood cell (RBC) production results. Conversely, in conditions where erythropoietin concentrations are decreased to below normal, as in renal disease, hypertransfusion, hyperoxemia, and starvation, only those progenitor cells able to survive with the least erythropoietin stimulation are able to continue on, and red blood cell production decreases. Interestingly, just as the high initial erythropoietin peak (the first part of the biphasic curve) may correlate with progenitor cell recruitment (the increase in the number of cycling BFU-Es), the second phase of prolonged moderate elevation of erythropoietin levels may correlate with this second period of red cell maturation, in which recruited progenitor cells are allowed to continue on in their development.

As red blood cell passes from the CFU-E stage to the named erythroid precursor stages—proerythroblast, erythroblast, reticulocyte—developing cells again begin to lose their sensitivity to erythropoietin.[124,135–138] By the time the reticulocyte stage is reached erythropoietin receptors are absent, and cells have fully lost their requirement for erythropoietin.[135,136] Changes occurring during this terminal differentiation period include the accumulation of hemoglobin, a decrease in overall size, extrusion of the nucleus, and alterations in the membrane and cytoskeleton that ultimately lead to a biconcave discoid shape.[124] Erythropoietin has been shown to play a role in several of these processes.[124,138,139] Figure 4.8 provides a summary of the relationships in the erythropoietin-erythropoiesis hormonal cycle.[58]

In addition to recruiting, maintaining viability, and directing differentiation of red blood cell precursors, erythropoietin also plays an important role in regulating the rate at which the maturation process as a whole occurs.[100,121,140–145] Although the exact period of time from primitive progenitor cell recruitment to reticulocyte release is difficult to determine, animal studies indicate that this process normally takes 10 to 12 days.[130,146] A 5- to 6-day period has been assigned to the terminal differentiation period (from proerythroblast to marrow reticulocyte release).[143] Reticulocytes normally spend 1 to 2 days maturing in the marrow, and in addition require 1 to 2 days in the circulating blood before their transformation into mature red blood cells is complete.[143] Following hypoxic stimulus, increased erythropoietin levels act to shorten the time between progenitor cell

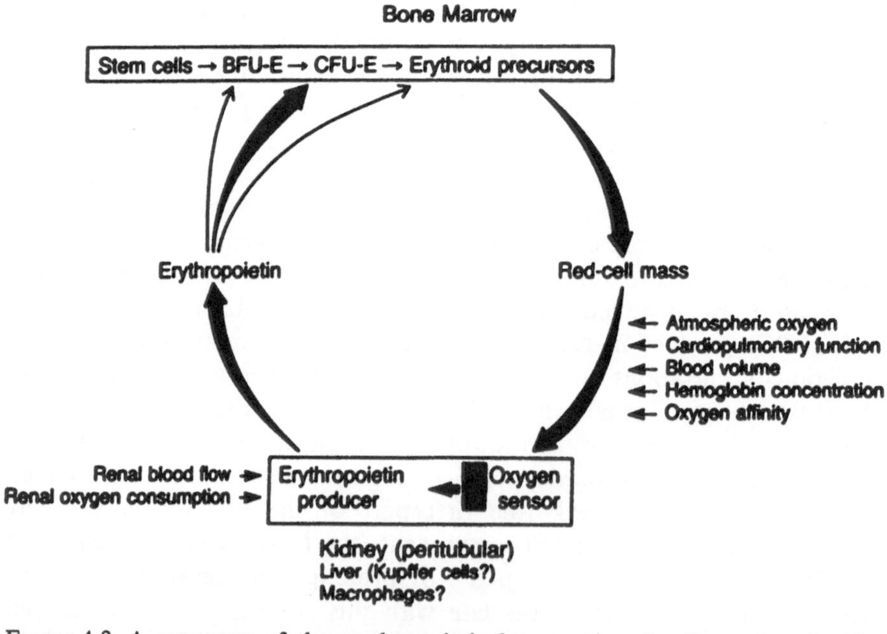

FIGURE 4.8. A summary of the erythropoietin hormonal cycle. (Reproduced with permission from Erslev.[58])

recruitment and bone marrow release by causing cell divisions to be skipped and reticulocytes to enter the blood soon after formation.[130,141–143] A reticulocytosis becomes evident over the first 24 hours after hypoxic stimulus, with the number of reticulocytes typically doubling from 1% to 2%.[142,143] This reticulocytosis becomes more pronounced over the next several days as more reticulocytes are forced into the bloodstream by the expanding marrow, and because the circulating life span of these prematurely released cells is effectively doubled.[71,100,141,147] This obligatory lag period presumably represents the period of time required for the expedited maturation and differentiation of newly recruited marrow progenitor and precursor red cells. The rate of hematocrit rise after this lag period appears to be dependent on the magnitude of the hypoxic stimulus, and the consequent serum erythropoietin level.[141,142] With significant blood loss and adequate iron stores, red blood cell production can increase acutely to two to three times normal, and to as much as eight times normal in chronic anemic states.[148,149]

Abnormalities of the Erythropoietin—Red Cell Relationship and Anemia

The previous sections have focused on the physiology of erythropoietin production—the stimulus for production, the timing and amount of erythropoietin actually produced by this stimulus, and the modulation of this production. With a normal bone marrow capable of the production of normal red blood cells, the presence of anemia (the most common form of hypoxic stimulus) leads to an increase in erythropoietin production, an increase in erythropoiesis, and, over time, a correction of this anemia.

Increased production of erythropoietin does not always lead to an increase in red cell mass and correction of anemia, however. If the bone marrow does not respond normally to erythropoietin stimulation or if the red cells that are produced do not survive normally in the bloodstream, even markedly elevated levels of erythropoietin may not serve to correct anemia. There are three basic abnormalities of the erythropoietin red cell mass relationship that can lead to or propagate anemia: (1) decreased erythropoietin production (anemia of renal disease, anemia of chronic disease), (2) decreased marrow responsiveness (iron deficiency anemia, aplastic anemia, marrow infiltration/obliteration anemia), and (3) decreased red cell survival in the bloodstream (hemolytic anemia, sickle cell anemia, anemia of ongoing blood loss) (Figure 4.9). Anemia can be caused by one of these three primary abnormalities (e.g., anemia chronic renal failure—attributable to decreased renal production), as well as by a combination of these abnormalities (e.g., anemia of chronic disease—attributable to decreased renal production and decreased marrow responsiveness). Understanding which abnormality is the cause of a preoperative patient's anemia can help in delineating appropriate treatment, and in determining responsiveness of this anemia to supplementation with the recombinant hormone.

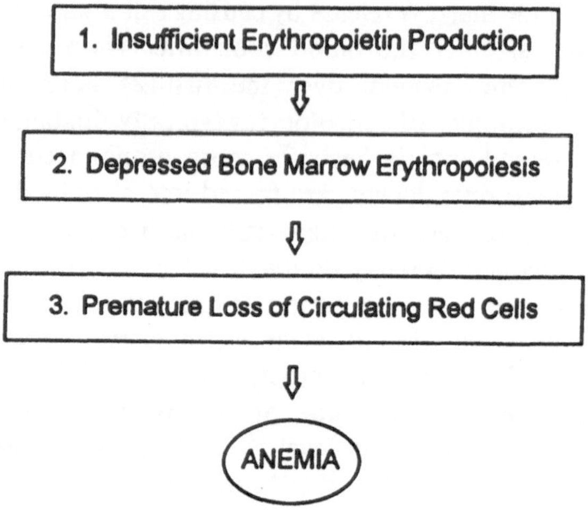

FIGURE 4.9. The three primary abnormalities of the erythropoietin–red cell mass increase relationship. Any specific type of anemia can result from one, two, or all three of these abnormalities.

One anemia involving an abnormality of the erythropoietin axis that deserves particular attention is iron deficiency anemia. Iron deficiency is the most common cause of decreased marrow responsiveness to erythropoietin stimulation, and of anemia in general. In developed countries, 3% of men and 20% of women are iron deficient as judged by circulating iron levels, and an even larger percentage of patients have decreases in iron stores.[150] The percentage of women with iron deficiency decreases after menopause and cessation of menstruation, but this is countered to a large extent in the cardiac surgical population by the increase in iron deficiency that occurs with advanced age and chronic disease. Patients with inadequate iron stores are unable to synthesize adequate amounts of hemoglobin, and a decrease in red cell production results. Serum erythropoietin levels are often appropriately elevated for the degree of anemia, as the failure is not in erythropoietin stimulation, but in hemoglobin and red cell production. Attempts to treat iron deficiency anemia with recombinant erythropoietin supplementation will therefore meet with failure unless iron levels are appropriately restored. A wide variety of conditions can lead to a negative iron balance.[150] The laboratory markers of iron deficiency are listed in Table 4.2.[150,151] These include a serum ferritin less than 10 ng/ml, a total iron binding capacity (transferrin concentration) greater than 350 μg/dl, a plasma iron concentration of less than 50 μg/dl, and a transferrin saturation of 15% or less. These baseline iron studies should be performed on all chronically anemic patients. If iron deficiency is discovered, then attention should be paid to both correction of the underlying cause and adequate iron replacement therapy. Because normal dietary intake is only enough to at most maintain the existing iron levels, supplementation must be instituted.

TABLE 4.2. Laboratory markers of iron deficiency.

Serum iron studies	
	Serum ferritin <12ng/ml
	Serum iron <50 μg/dl
	TIBC (transferrin concentration) >350 μg/dl
Red blood cell indices	
	MCV (Hct/RBC count) <82
	MCHC (Hg/Hct) <32
	MCH (Hg/RBC count) <27
Peripheral smear	
	Microcytosis
	Hypochromia

MCH, mean corpuscular hemoglobin; MCHC, mean corpuscular hemoglobin concentration; MCV, mean corpuscular volume; RBC, red blood cell; HCT, hematocrit; TIBC, total iron binding capacity.

This can take the form of either oral supplementation or parenteral/intramuscular supplementation. Therapy with recombinant erythropoietin results in a functional iron deficiency attributable to an increase in red cell production combined with an inability to rapidly mobilize iron stores, and therefore erythropoietin supplementation should always be accompanied by at least oral iron supplementation.[152,153] Dosing for oral, intramuscular, and intravenous iron supplementation is outlined in Table 4.3.[154,155]

In addition to iron deficiency, deficiencies of folate and vitamin B_{12} can also cause a decreased marrow response to erythropoietin stimulation. Their occurrence in the cardiac surgical population and in the general population is much less common, however. Like iron deficiency, the anemias of folate and B_{12} deficiency readily respond to supplementation therapy.[156] Without such supplementation, anemia and lack of marrow responsiveness will persist, despite appropriate elevations in endogenous

TABLE 4.3. Dosing for oral, intramuscular, and intravenous iron supplementation.

Oral (iron sulfate)	
	Iron sulfate 325 mg PO TID
	Vitamin C 50 mg PO BID (to aid in absorption from the gastrointestinal tract)
	Colace or similar stool softener can decrease the constipating effects of oral iron therapy
Intravenous/intramuscular (iron dextran)	
	Calculate iron deficit (the amount of iron required to restore RBC mass and replenish stores):
	Iron Deficit (mg) = [(normal Hg − patient Hg) × weight (kg) × 2.21] + 1000 mg
	Administer a 0.5 mg test dose iron dextran (Imferon)
	Low but real incidence of severe anaphylaxis, have appropriate Rx available
	Then 100 mg/day (2 ml) Imferon until total target dose (calculated iron deficit) achieved
	Higher daily dosages have been successfully administered; we routinely administer 250 mg/day until total target dose is achieved

Hg, hemoglobin; TID, 3 times per day; BID, 2 times per day; PO, per os or oral; RBC, red blood cell.

erythropoietin levels or implementation of exogenous erythropoietin supplementation.

Recombinant Erythropoietin

In 1985, both Lin et al[23] and Jacobs et al[24] were able to establish in vitro production of biologically active recombinant erythropoietin in mammalian cells transfected with the erythropoietin gene linked to an expression vector. Today, at least two different recombinant erythropoietins (α, β) are clinically available internationally, each produced by a different tumor cell line, and each with slightly different pharmacokinetic properties attributable to minor differences in glycosylation sites (epoietin-β has a longer half-life in the bloodstream).[157,158] Epoietin-α, produced using the Chinese hamster ovary tumor cell line, is the only form that is available clinically in the United States. It is marketed as Epogen (Amgen, Thousand Oaks, CA) for treatment of renal-, HIV-, and cancer chemotherapy—related anemias (the three FDA approved uses as of March 1995), and as Procrit (Ortho Pharmaceutical, Raritan, NJ) for other uses, including perioperative applications (all non-FDA-approved uses). This delineation is a licensing agreement for marketing purposes only, and because the drugs are identical (both Epogen and Procrit are produced by Amgen), they can be used interchangeably for any of the approved or off-label uses.* Epoietin-α is very similar to the endogenous hormone, and with respect to physiology, mechanism of action, and clinical application, the two can be considered identical.[32,159,160]

As discussed in the previous section reviewing the physiology of endogenous erythropoietin and the erythropoietic response, in various disease states endogenous erythropoietin production is insufficient or absent. This leads to marrow hypostimulation, a decrease in red cell production, and anemia. The anemia of chronic renal failure, where the nonfunctioning kidney produces little or no erythropoietin, serves as the classic example of such a deficiency in erythropoietin. Here, the nonfunctioning kidney produces little or no endogenous erythropoietin, resulting in inadequate red cell production, and severe, often transfusion-dependent, anemia. In 1987 patients with dialysis-dependent renal failure served as the ideal patient group on which to evaluate exogenous supplementation with the newly available recombinant product. Its success was immediately apparent, and today transfusion-dependent anemia has been largely eliminated in the chronic dialysis population.

---

*Because many of the applications of recombinant erythropoietin discussed in this and the following sections are "off-label" (non-FDA approved), references providing guidelines for the use of drugs for such off-label indications are provided.[161,162]

This success in the renal failure population prompted application of the drug to other diseases and states in which anemia is an important debilitating feature. In addition to treating those anemias due to decreased endogenous erythropoietin production (anemia of chronic renal failure, prematurity, malignancy, and chronic disease),[163-167] it has been applied to those anemias attributable to decreased responsiveness of the bone marrow to erythropoietin stimulation–anemia of chronic disease, azidothymidine HIV-related anemia, thalassemia, anemia of burn injury, anemia of acute and ongoing blood loss).[168-181] While patients with disorders leading to decreased erythropoietin production generally respond well to recombinant erythropoietin stimulation, patients with decreased marrow responsiveness may or may not respond, depending on the particular disease or deficiency that is present and its ability to be corrected. Correction of iron deficiency, for example, will restore the normal response to erythropoietin. Patients with disease states that lead to production of red cells with decreased intrinsic viability and survival in the bloodstream often respond less well to erythropoietin supplementation, although improvements have been reported. Measurement of endogenous erythropoietin levels can be used to help determine responsiveness. Those patients with markedly elevated levels (e.g., greater than 500 IU/dl) are usually already mounting an appropriate endogenous erythropoietin response,[173,181,182] and are less likely to respond to recombinant supplementation. Patients who suffer from anemia attributable to loss or destruction of normal red cells (e.g., drug-induced hemolysis, valvular hemolysis, gastrointestinal hemorrhage, prolonged ICU stay with frequent laboratory testing) also typically demonstrate appropriate increases in endogenous serum erythropoietin levels and in red cell production. Foremost in the treatment of such patients is the correction of the process leading to red cell loss. If such losses are halted or minimized, and resulting deficiencies corrected (e.g., iron deficiency) then the anemia can be expected to resolve on its own using the endogenous erythropoietin axis. Recovery can be augmented and accelerated, however, with the use of the recombinant product. The ability of the recombinant erythropoietin product to provide *additional* increases in the magnitude and rate of red cell production serves as the basis for much of its use in the correction of anemia in the perioperative setting.

Pharmacology

As might be predicted when using as a model the endogenous erythropoietin response to anemia, the effects of recombinant erythropoietin appear to be dose dependent.[183] The higher the dose, the higher the blood level achieved, and the greater the erythropoietic response. The optimal dose required to stimulate maximum erythropoiesis has yet to be determined, however, because studies in the renal failure population (by far its predominant use) have focused on gradual rather than acute maximum stimulation of erythropoiesis.

Attention to the route of administration is very important when considering optimal use of recombinant erythropoietin. The drug can be administered intravenously (IV), intramuscularly (IM), intraperitoneally (in peritoneal dialysis patients), or subcutaneously (SQ). The intravenous and subcutaneous routes have been primarily used clinically thus far, and it is important to understand their very different pharmacokinetic properties. Intravenous erythropoietin is 100% absorbed and leads almost immediately to peak serum levels. Concentrations then rapidly decrease, with the elimination half-life estimated to be between 3 and 8 hours.[184–189] In contrast, only 25% of subcutaneously administered erythropoietin is absorbed into the bloodstream, but levels remain elevated significantly longer than with intravenous administration. Peak levels are reached 8 to 16 hours after administration, and the half-life has been shown to be between 18 and 30 hours.[185–188] Interestingly, despite its much lower bioavailability, the subcutaneous route of administration appears to be at least as effective as the intravenous route.[186] This may be attributable to the ability of the subcutaneous route to achieve persistent erythropoietin elevation, thereby more closely mimicking the body's natural erythropoietin response (i.e., it serves to prevent progenitor/precursor cell apoptosis by more effectively maintaining erythropoietin levels above the minimum required for cell survival).[25] Clearly, attention must be paid to not only the dose of the drug given, but also the route and timing of administration. Figure 4.10 provides an illustration of the differences in the pharmacokinetics of IV and SQ recombinant erythropoietin dosing.

The finding that SQ administration is at least as effective as IV administration in stimulating gradual erythropoiesis in the renal failure population suggests that attention to the blood levels seen in the endogenous erythropoietin response may also provide the key to development of dosing regimens aimed at acutely and maximally increasing red cell production. Such acute maximum stimulation is essential if recombinant erythropoietin is to have an important role in the perioperative setting. For example, by combining intravenous and subcutaneous administration, at high enough doses and with the correct timing, the biphasic pattern of the blood levels seen in the maximum endogenous erythropoietin response (i.e., to an acute bleed to a hematocrit of 12–15%) can be successfully re-created (Fig. 4.10D). In theory, imposition of this synthetic maximal erythropoietin response on an anemic preoperative patient, or even on a nonanemic preoperative patient in whom large-scale blood loss is anticipated, should lead to initiation of a maximum erythropoietic response in this patient. The resulting rapid increase in red cell production would benefit the patient in the form of decreased homologous blood requirement. Baboon studies indicate that doses as high as 1000 mU/kg/day (with the first dose IV and the remainder SQ) may be required to achieve such "maximum physiologic"

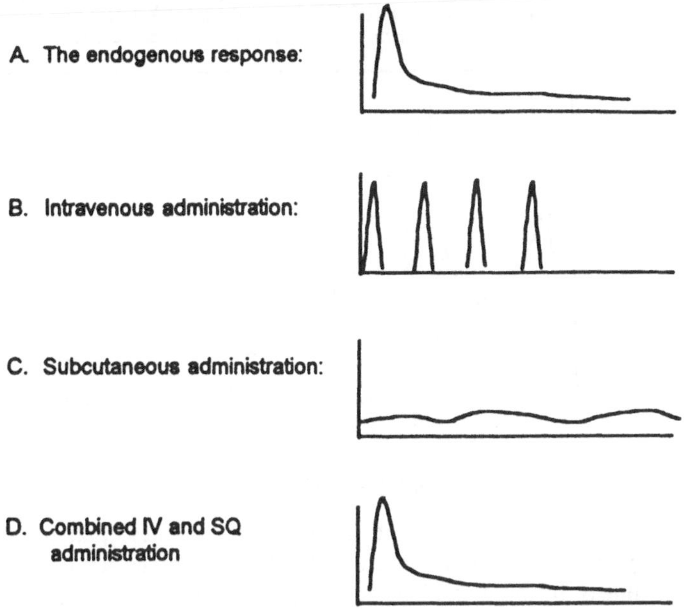

FIGURE 4.10. One potential strategy to improve the efficacy of recombinant erythropoietin for acute perioperative applications. (A) The biphasic endogenous erythropoietin response. These are the serum levels that are seen with an acute anemia of hematocrit = 12% to 15%, and therefore this can be viewed as the natural maximum erythropoietin response that should lead to maximum stimulation of erythropoiesis. (B) Intermittent intravenous administration of the drug provides only brief serum peaks, with levels returning to baseline between peaks. (C) Subcutaneous administration provides for more continuous elevation, but at the cost of lower serum levels, and no high peak in serum levels. (D) The results obtained when intravenous and subcutaneous forms are coadministered. Results of this strategy applied clinically can be seen in Figure 4.11.

biphasic serum levels (Fig. 4.5).[76] In applying this concept clinically to our Jehovah's Witness population undergoing cardiac surgery, we have found that lower doses can achieve the same result if they are appropriately applied. The serum levels attained in 15 patients undergoing urgent and emergent coronary artery bypass graft (CABG) procedures are seen in Figure 4.11. The dosing regimen used to attain these levels included an initial combined IV and SQ dose (300 U/kg and 500 U/kg, respectively) to attain the initial high peak, followed by every other day subcutaneous dosing (500 U/kg) to achieve subsequent prolonged moderate elevation similar to that found during the second phase of the endogenous response. The rapid and large reticulocytosis seen in these patients, coupled with a significant increase in hematocrit when compared to a control population, despite the absence of transfusion, suggests that such levels did indeed provide for a significant and rapid increase in red cell production. Final

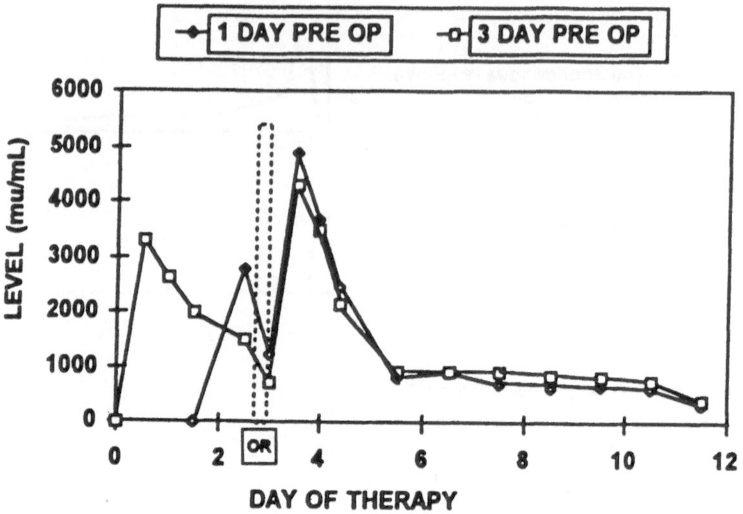

FIGURE 4.11. Erythropoietin levels in 15 Jehovah's Witness patients undergoing CABG. All patients received a 300-U/kg IV dose combined with a 500-U/kg SQ dose at the time of hospital admission (3 days preoperatively in eight patients and 1 day preoperatively in seven patients). Erythropoietin was then continued at 500-U/kg SQ every other day until the time of surgery. A repeat IV/SQ dose (300 U/kg IV, 500 U/kg SQ) was given at the time of arrival in the ICU, and then 500-U/kg SQ doses were repeated on postoperative day 2 and postoperative day 5. OR, operating room. Baseline endogenous EPO levels in all patients were <30 mU/mL.

proof of the efficacy of this approach must await randomized clinical trials, however. These results nevertheless underscore the importance of defining the goals of any given therapeutic intervention (stimulation of gradual erythropoiesis in the renal failure population vs. acute maximum erythropoiesis in the perioperative population), and of attention to the details of the pharmacology involved.

It should be restated here that attention to the iron status of the patient is of utmost importance when applying the recombinant hormone clinically to treat preoperative anemia. It has been clearly demonstrated that iron deficiency is the most common cause of erythropoietin therapy failure. If circulating and stored iron levels are decreased, then little or no response to exogenous supplementation will result. Furthermore, recombinant erythropoietin therapy itself results in iron deficiency, as available iron stores are utilized for increased red cell production. The importance of adequate iron supplementation in ensuring adequate response to erythropoietin, whether it be endogenous or exogenous, cannot be overemphasized.

Safety and Side Effects

Because recombinant erythropoietin is virtually identical to the endogenous hormone, it would be expected to be safe and to have relatively few side effects. Clinically this has indeed been shown to be the case. In the most widely studied patient population, those undergoing erythropoietin therapy for the anemia of chronic renal failure, hypertension, seizures, and thrombosis are among the more serious side effects reported. It remains unclear, however, whether the incidence of these side effects is significantly increased by the use of erythropoietin, as the baseline incidence of these events, such as hypertension and seizures, is relatively high compared to the population in general. In addition, multiple clinical trials indicate that these effects likely appear not as a direct effect of erythropoietin itself, but as a consequence of the changes that occur in the blood as relatively profound anemia is corrected. In the many studies performed on nonuremic individuals, and in patients undergoing perioperative treatment, no serious side effects have been reported.

Several studies of erythropoietin treatment in chronic renal failure have demonstrated a 30% to 35% incidence of new-onset or exacerbated hypertension (defined as diastolic increase greater than 10 mm Hg).[189–191] The increase in blood pressure usually occurs during this initial 2- to 16-week period when hematocrit is increasing, and appears to stabilize and often returns to normal after that point. Hypertension may occur more commonly in patients with preexisting hypertension, particularly unstable hypertension, and is unrelated to erythropoietin dose, rate of RBC increase, or final hematocrit. The underlying mechanism is believed to be increased blood viscosity and decreased hypoxic vasodilatation encountered with higher hematocrits, although other factors may contribute.[191–196] In multiple trials of erythropoietin in normal volunteers, in autologous blood donors, and in other nonuremic patients, an increase in hypertension has never been found, even in the higher-risk cardiac surgery group.

Seizures have also been reported in the renal literature. A phase III clinical trial of erythropoietin revealed a 5.4% incidence of seizures.[189] These were most often encountered in the first 3 to 4 months of therapy and in those with the most rapid rise in blood pressure, suggesting a hypertensive encephalophatic etiology.[192] But because the overall incidence of seizures in this population is 4% to 8%, it is difficult to implicate erythropoietin as an etiologic agent.[197] Several studies support this, and in fact some have found an actual improvement in cerebral blood flow with erythropoietin use and have been able to correlate this with an overall improved sense of well-being in these patients.[198–200] Similarly, seizure activity has not been reported in any studies investigating perioperative uses of erythropoietin.

Early reports in the literature suggested the possibility of an increased incidence of thrombotic events such as venous access failure, deep venous thrombosis, and increased arteriovenous graft and dialyzer clotting.[201–203] This possibility is supported at least theoretically by the characteristics of the erythropoietin-directed correction of anemia in renal patients, including increased viscosity, decreased hypoxic dilatation, mildly increased platelet counts, and a return of platelet function and coagulation toward that found in normal nonuremic patients. Subsequent studies, however, have shown no increased incidence of thrombosis.[101,204–206] For example, Lynn et al[206] found no differences in arterial blood flow velocity, heparin dose required, or fistula function between control and erythropoietin-treated patients. Likewise, a large phase III clinical trial in renal patients revealed a rate of 0.3 thrombotic events per patient year, compared with a rate of 0.5 in non–erythropoietin-treated renal patients.[189] It appears, then, that despite theoretical concerns about thrombosis in renal patients treated with erythropoietin, hematocrit, platelet function and number, and coagulation parameters at most return to normal, and an overall increase in thrombosis is not found. Again, as with hypertension and seizures, thrombosis was not a complication in studies of autologous blood donors and other nonuremic individuals treated with erythropoietin. A single exception is found, however, in Goodnough et al's[147] study of erythropoietin-augmented autologous donation in orthopedic patients, where one subject experienced an acute lower extremity arterial thrombosis. The patient had donated two units of blood over an 8-day period and had a hematocrit of 40% at the time of the event. On angiography, he was subsequently found to have had severe atherosclerotic disease, and so the authors did not attribute the thrombosis to recombinant erythropoietin. Because the hyperviscosity of true polycythemic states has been implicated in blood sludging and thrombosis,[207,208] care must be taken in the cardiac surgery patient to avoid such states. With careful hematocrit monitoring this should not become an issue, particularly in the cardiac surgical setting, where such monitoring is routine.

Other more mild symptoms and side effects of recombinant erythropoietin have been reported as well. Most common are a flu-like syndrome with moderate aches and pains, and headache. Randomized trials have inconsistently shown prevalence of these symptoms over those in controls.[196]

Positive side effects, such as improvement in sexual and neuromuscular function, have been seen in renal failure patients as well.[209,210] Again, however, these are likely related to correction of the relative profound anemia that exists in this patient group. One interesting positive effect, found in the nonuremic population, was recently reported by Hisatomi et al,[197] who demonstrated an improvement in postoperative immune function in cardiac surgical patients treated with erythropoietin for 6 days preoperatively and 7 days postoperatively (200 U/kg/day IV). Cellular immunity was shown to be significantly augmented, as measured by increased numbers of T3 and T4 lymphocytes, and greater production of IL-2. This finding suggests that erythropoietin not only increases red cell production, but also may help to ameliorate or prevent the impairment of cell-mediated immune function that can occur following cardiac surgery.[211,212]

The final question that arises with respect to the safety and side effects of recombinant erythropoietin concerns the maximum safe dosage and overdosage. Theoretically, overdosage could result in a polycythemic state and its attendant complications. Clinically this has not occurred in the non-renal failure population with doses as high as 1200 U/kg three times per week.[173,213] In the dialysis population doses of up to 1500 U/kg TIW have been tolerated for 3 to 4 weeks without adverse effect.[214] Normal male volunteers undergoing autologous blood donation were given doses as high as 1000 U/kg IV 3 times per week without untoward side effects.[215] The maximum dose that can be tolerated, therefore, is unknown. The endogenous response to the most severe anemia that can be consistently tolerated may serve as an appropriate marker for the maximum blood levels that should be obtained using the recombinant product. This upper limit in serum levels can be estimated to be in the range of 10,000 mU/dl (Figs. 4.5 and 4.6).[76,99,100] We have found that a combined 300 U/kg IV and 500 U/kg SQ dose results in sustained peak serum levels averaging 3000 to 5000 mU/kg, suggesting that even higher dosing may be safe and appropriate when attempting to maximally stimulate red cell production.

Costs of Recombinant Erythropoietin

A very important aspect concerning the use of recombinant erythropoietin is relatively high cost. At approximately $90 per 10,000 units (wholesale cost estimate based on a standard hospital account markdown),[216] a single 300-U/kg dose in a 70-kg male (21,000 units) costs about $200. With 9 years still left on the U.S. patent held by Amgen (the 17-year patent expires in the year 2004),[217] and a domestic market closed to competition from the other forms of r-HuEPO produced internationally (erythropoietin-β), costs are not likely to be reduced in the near future. Alternative methods for administration of the drug, such as the use of adenovirus vectors, will likely not be significantly less expensive. In today's health care environment, with its consistent pattern of decreasing reimbursement and support for interventions deemed nonessential by insurers, and private hospital corporations concerned foremost with positive revenues, such costs will likely limit use of the drug to FDA-approved indications. This will occur despite any obvious advantages with respect to reductions in homologous transfusion requirements that would occur with its more widespread application, particularly in the cardiac surgical setting. Off-label non–FDA-approved uses, such as perioperative applications, will be limited to only those patients who need it most, often on an investigational basis, with hospitals often absorbing the costs incurred. A select group of individuals, perhaps those at highest risk for requiring red cell transfusion, or those at highest risk for suffering adverse consequences of transfusions, will therefore have to be more clearly defined, and alternative avenues for reimbursement explored.

Perioperative Use of Recombinant Erythropoietin

Perioperative use of recombinant erythropoietin became attractive because of its theoretical ability to increase perioperative red blood cell mass, thereby decreasing the need for homologous transfusion. Major orthopedic surgery and cardiac surgery have received the most attention in this respect, because of their relative large transfusion requirements, but the recombinant hormone has been applied to other major surgeries as well.[218,219] Erythropoietin has been used to (1) augment autologous blood donation before such procedures, (2) correct preoperative anemia, (3) acutely increase preoperative red cell production, and (4) improve postoperative red cell mass recovery.

Preoperative Autologous Blood Donation

Preoperative autologous donation is an important part of any cardiac surgical blood conservation effort. At a time when urgent or emergent surgical intervention is becoming the norm, however, often the luxury of a 4- to 6-week period for standard autologous donation is not available. Furthermore, the yield after this time is often inadequate. One multicenter study showed an average yield of only 2.2 units.[220] Another found that more than 40% of people could not donate four units of blood, an amount generally believed to shield most cardiac patients from homologous transfusion if other components of blood conservation program are also utilized.[221] As discussed, evidence indicates that a submaximal erythropoietic response is at least partially responsible for the extended length of time required for this often suboptimal autologous collection.[79,80] AABB guidelines state that collection should be withheld if hematocrit is less than 34%.[78] This hematocrit, however, produces little if any tissue hypoxia, and so erythropoietin levels likewise undergo little if any increase. Red cell production is then also minimally increased, and so the autologous blood collection period is prolonged. While utilizing more aggressive donating schedules and lowering minimum hematocrit for donation would improve endogenous erythropoietin stimulation, and thus autologous yield,[79,222] an increase in adverse reactions might also be expected. In this setting, recombinant erythropoietin takes on great attractiveness for its ability to supplement the endogenous response, thereby increasing the rate and volume of autologous donation. By decreasing the time period required for adequate donation, erythropoietin renders preoperative autologous donation a viable alternative for greater numbers of cardiac surgical patients. Several studies to date have examined the use of erogenous erythropoietin for the augmentation of preoperative autologous donation. The following is a brief overview of the important findings in animal and human research, orthopedic and other major noncardiac surgeries, and cardiac surgery.

In an early study of erythropoietin and autologous donation, Levine et al[223] evaluated an "aggressive" autologous donation schedule (three times per week, minimum hematocrit 0.30) in baboons, with and without erythropoietin. They found that this aggressive schedule yielded approximately twice the amount of blood that a standard AABB one time per week, minimum hematocrit 0.34 schedule would have produced, and that erythropoietin (750 U/kg per day IV) increased yield by an additional 35%. Furthermore, the rate of erythropoiesis was markedly increased in the erythropoietin-treated group—in 14 days baboons were able to donate 6.5 units of blood. Abraham et al[215] studied autologous donation in normal human volunteers with and without erythropoietin and found that erythropoietin-treated subjects were able to donate 32% more blood over a period of 26 days. They found no significant difference between doses of 250, 500, and 1000 U/L IV administered three times per week.

Goodnough et al[147] performed a randomized double-blind placebo-controlled multicenter study utilizing erythropoietin to augment autologous donation before elective orthopedic surgery. Forty-seven patients underwent donation two times per week for three weeks preoperatively. Erythropoietin (600 mg/kg IV) was administered two times per week. Donation was deferred for hematocrit according to AABB guidelines. The authors found that the hematocrit of the erythropoietin-treated group was significantly higher by the third visit, and that there were 45 donation deferments in the placebo group versus 12 in the erythropoietin group. Admission and postoperative hematocrits were significantly higher in the erythropoietin treated group, and only one of 23 (4%) erythropoietin patients was unable to donate four or more units of blood, versus seven of 24 (29%) placebo patients. The erythropoietin-treated patients were able to donate 125 total units of blood compared to 99 units by the placebo patients. In a very similar study, Goodnough et al[222] reported that the volume of autologous red cell production was increased by over 50%. Maeda et al[224] administered erythropoietin (6000 units IV) to autologous donors three times per week over a 24-day period prior to their scheduled orthopedic surgery. Autologous blood was then collected on preoperative days 17, 10, and 3. It was found that by the third donation, hemoglobin was significantly higher in the erythropoietin-treated subjects (12.7 vs. 10.7), and that while 40% of the non-erythropoietin-treated individuals required homologous blood, none of the erythropoietin group did. Tasaki et al[225] also evaluated the effects of recombinant erythropoietin on autologous donation and perioperative red cell production in orthopedic surgery. Patients received placebo, 3000 U, 6000 U, or 9000 U IV twice weekly for 3 weeks prior to surgery. During this time three 400-ml phlebotomies were performed. Total RBC volume increased 211, 284, 350, and 383 ml, respectively, over the 21-day period, indicating a dose-dependent relationship. Homologous transfusion requirement was not assessed in this study. Recently, Mercuriali et al[226] evaluated the effect of two different erythropoietin doses on autologous blood donation and transfusion requirement during orthopedic surgery. Fifty randomized patients received either placebo, 300 U/kg, or 600 U/kg IV every 3 to 4 days over an 18-day preoperative period. It was found that the erythropoietin-treated groups donated more blood (4.5 units vs. 2.8 units) and received less homologous product (1.2 units vs. 0.8 units).

The first study of erythropoietin and autologous donation did not appear in the cardiac surgery literature until 1991. Watanabe et al[227] evaluated erythropoietin-assisted autologous donation in 18 preoperative cardiac surgery patients, utilizing 11 retrospective controls. Five hundred milliliters of blood were removed 2 weeks preoperatively, and erythropoietin (100 U/kg/day IV) was administered for 2 weeks prior to surgery and for 1 week afterward. They found that hemoglobin was significantly increased in the erythropoietin-treated group by postoperative day 4, and that while hemoglobin levels in the erythropoietin-treated group were above baseline on the day of operation, these levels remained below baseline in the non–erythropoietin-treated donors. In a second study, Watanabe et al[228] evaluated the subcutaneous administration of erythropoietin in cardiac surgery patients. Group 1 received 100 U/kg/day IV, group 2 received 600 U/kg SQ on preoperative days 14 and 7, and a non–erythropoietin-treated group served as controls. Each patient donated 800 ml of blood over the 2-week period. The authors found that by the time of operation, hemoglobin had returned to at least baseline in both erythropoietin-treated groups, but remained below baseline in control subjects. The authors found no significant difference between the intravenous and much more easily administered subcutaneous routes of administration, confirming the findings of multiple other studies in renal failure patients.[25,229–231] In 1993 Kulier et al[232] studied the efficacy of a simple subcutaneous dosing regimen. Erythropoietin (400 U/kg SQ) was administered one time per week, and autologous blood was collected over a 4-week preoperative period. It was found that patients receiving erythropoietin had a consistently higher hemoglobin level, were able to donate more red blood cells (776 ml vs. 682 ml), and had a significantly decreased homologous blood requirement. Only one patient in the erythropoietin-treated group required homologous transfusion, as compared to 8 of 12 patients in the control group.

Many of these studies of autologous donation in surgery and cardiac surgery confirm the importance of adequate iron supplementation, something that has been emphasized previously in this chapter. For example in the above-cited study by Mercuriali et al,[226] it was found that adequate iron replacement therapy was necessary for a maximal erythropoietic response to occur. Interesting and strong support for the use of iron supplementation during normal and hemachromatosis patients were subjected to erythropoietin-assisted autologous donation, the hemachromatosis patients, with their markedly increased iron stores, were able to produce almost twice as many new red cells (1,764 ml vs. 941 ml). The importance of concomitant iron therapy has been confirmed in multiple other studies.[233-235] Oral iron therapy should be initiated on all patients receiving preoperative erythropoietin for augmentation of autologous donation. The dose for oral iron therapy, as well as those for parenteral and intramuscular supplementation with iron dextran for more severe forms of iron deficiency, are seen in Table 4.3.

Taken as a whole, these studies on the use of recombinant erythropoietin to augment autologous donation serve to illustrate several important points. First, recombinant erythropoietin is effective in increasing both the amount of autologous blood that is able to be collected in a given preoperative time period and the rate of collection of this blood. Second, the increased autologous yield seen with recombinant erythropoietin use, coupled with maintenance of higher hemoglobin levels, results in significant reductions in homologous blood product use. Third, preoperative use of erythropoietin appears to be safe, as no adverse responses attributable to the drug have been seen in any of the autologous donation studies performed thus far. Fourth, use of erythropoietin must be coupled with iron supplementation to achieve a maximum response. Fifth, intermittent subcutaneous administration of erythropoietin appears to be at least as effective as more frequent and logistically difficult intravenous administration. As discussed previously, this may be related to the ability of subcutaneously administered erythropoietin to more closely mimic the persistent elevation in erythropoietin levels that is seen in the body's natural response to anemia. Finally, the relative ease with which subcutaneous erythropoietin can be applied likely will enable increased use of the hormone in both inpatient and outpatient populations.

Several issues regarding recombinant erythropoietin and preoperative autologous donation remain unresolved at this time. First, an optimal dosing regimen has yet to be defined. The widely spaced dosing intervals utilized in many of these studies have likely resulted in submaximal serum erythropoietin levels from a physiologic standpoint. This particularly applies to studies applying IV erythropoietin only one to two times per week. As stated previously, use of these relatively submaximal regimens in the perioperative setting can be understood by realizing that experience with recombinant erythropoietin thus far has been predominantly in the chronic renal failure population. These patients are chronically anemic (with varying degrees of physiologic adaptation), and correction of this anemia can be carried out over an extended period of time. Such gradual correction may result in fewer side effects in this population. The patient undergoing preoperative autologous donation before elective cardiac surgery is in distinct contrast to the renal failure patient, however. While the surgery may be considered elective in a relative sense, most patients with scheduled cardiac surgery have developed clinical symptoms/signs significant enough to warrant surgical intervention. Once the decision to perform surgery has been made, a vast majority of these patients (and their doctors) would prefer to correct the situation as soon as possible in order to minimize the possibility of intervening adverse events, and to restore an often compromised quality of life. Therefore, it is desirable to collect the required amount of autologous blood (should the use of preoperative autologous donation be decided upon) in the shortest possible period of time. The goal is not gradual stimulation of erythropoiesis, but rather maximum erythropoiesis. Transference of dosing regimens used in the chronic renal failure population to the cardiac surgical population is likely not appropriate, as these relatively low-stimulus regimens are in no way meant to acutely and maximally increase red cell production. Regimens aimed at maximal production, such as the one that we have applied more acutely to our Jehovah's Witness population, will need to be developed.[28] By minimizing the time required for successful autologous donation, these regimens will improve safety and patient satisfaction, and, more importantly, make preoperative autologous donation a viable option for a larger percentage of the cardiac surgical population.

The second issue with respect to the use of recombinant erythropoietin for augmentation of autologous donation (and likewise for the other three perioperative indications to be discussed) is the relatively high additional costs incurred by the use of this drug. In today's health care climate, such costs will likely limit use of the drug to only those who need it most (or who are willing to pay for its use). Who these individuals are will have to be more clearly defined, particularly if reimbursement is to be expected. It will likely be a relatively small percentage of patients: those individuals who are candidates for autologous donation and who can wait 2 to 3 weeks for their surgery, but who cannot wait the 5 to 8 weeks required for non-r-HuEPO assisted autologous donation. While an important therapeutic option, erythropoietin-assisted autologous donation is clearly only part of the solution in the quest to avoid homologous transfusion.

Preoperative Correction of Anemia

In addition to assisting autologous blood collection efforts, erythropoietin has also been used to help correct preoperative anemia so that the risk of subsequent intraoperative homologous blood transfusion is lessened. Surprisingly few formal studies have been performed in this area,[236] with most of the literature consisting of case reports relating successful treatment. Several reports have appeared in the cardiac surgery literature about Jehovah's Witnesses with relative preoperative anemia who have successfully undergone heart-lung bypass procedures following a preoperative course of erythropoietin.[28,237,238]

As discussed previously, preoperative anemias can be classified according to which of the three general abnormalities of the erythropoietin–red cell mass hormonal axis are abnormal (insufficient erythropoietin production, bone marrow hyporesponsiveness, and/or shortened red cell survival). A majority of preoperative anemias fall into the latter grouping, and are attributable to blood loss during the preoperative hospital course, e.g., cardiac catheterization, laboratory sampling, central line/intraaortic balloon pump (IABP) placement. If these blood losses are terminated or minimized, and iron and other deficiencies corrected, most preoperative anemias will slowly correct themselves. Typically, however, the luxury of time cannot be afforded in these patients, and rapid correction of anemia is desirable. Supplementation of the endogenous erythropoietin response with the recombinant hormone can accelerate the rate and magnitude of red cell mass regeneration.

Much less commonly an anemia attributable to one of the other abnormalities of the erythropoietin–red cell hormonal axis is encountered in the preoperative setting. Depending on the abnormality present this anemia may or may not respond to recombinant erythropoietin supplementation. For example, in cases of iron deficiency or megaloblastic (folate, B_{12} deficiency) anemia, a good response to recombinant hormone augmentation is seen once these deficiencies are appropriately corrected. Patients with a history of chronic anemia or anemia not attributable to recent blood losses or known iron deficiency should undergo evaluation by a qualified hematologist before erythropoietin therapy is initiated. In this way the type of anemia can be identified, and other appropriate interventions initiated. Assessment of endogenous erythropoietin levels may assist in determining the responsiveness to the type of anemia present to recombinant therapy. All patients in whom preoperative erythropoietin therapy is to be initiated should be started on oral iron supplementation, unless in the rare event the patient has a known or suspected iron overload state, e.g., thalassemia major. More severe iron deficient patients may require parenteral or intramuscular supplementation with iron dextran to obtain a maximal erythropoietic response with recombinant therapy. Table 4.2 provides the laboratory markers for iron deficiency anemia. Table 4.3 provides dosing schedules for oral, intramuscular, and parenteral iron therapy.

Correction of preoperative anemia with recombinant erythropoietin can lead to additional decreases in transfusion requirement by making possible the use of other blood conservation measures as well. If preoperative anemia can be corrected far enough in advance of elective surgery, then patients become eligible to undergo preoperative autologous donation. Restoration of red cell mass to normal or supranormal levels by the time of operation also allows the performance of acute intraoperative autologous donation (IAD) in the operating room, and decreases the degree of obligatory hemodilution that occurs during cardiopulmonary bypass. By allowing the performance of these additional measures, correction of preoperative anemia becomes an essential part of a whole that is greater than the sum of its parts.

The strategy of preoperative correction of anemia followed by intraoperative autologous donation was applied to three Jehovah's Witness patients undergoing surgery at our institution during 1993.[28] Because their admission hematocrit and red cell mass were below our cutoff for excessive risk for requiring red cell transfusion (36% and 1600 ml, respectively),[28] surgery was delayed in these patients for 4, 14, and 17 days while recombinant erythropoietin was administered. This allowed increases in preoperative red cell mass of 12%, 23%, and 12%, respectively. Intraoperatively, higher hematocrits allowed increased volumes of autologous blood to be withdrawn, thereby preserving greater numbers of fresh red cells, platelets, and clotting factors for reinfusion post-bypass. Postoperative bleeding was minimized, and all three patients were discharged home without the need for homologous transfusion. Correction of preoperative anemia with recombinant erythropoietin clearly played an essential role in a successful outcome of these high-transfusion-risk patients.

There are three primary issues regarding the use of recombinant erythropoietin in the correction of preoperative anemia that need to be addressed. First, it must be determined who will and who will not respond to recombinant supplementation. As discussed, most patients with preoperative anemia have a normal erythropoietin–red cell hormonal axis (once continued red cell losses are minimized and iron deficiency is corrected) and will respond to erythropoietin therapy. Eligibility for therapy in this patient group therefore depends on the length of time for which surgery can be delayed for any individual patient. For elective surgery, gradual correction of anemia is possible, and the time, expense, and effort required for recombinant therapy may not be justified. Patients with abnormalities of the erythropoietin–red cell axis not attributable to blood loss or iron deficiency may or may not respond to recombinant therapy. These patients should be assessed by a hematologist to determine their eligibility.

The second issue regarding preoperative erythropoietin therapy is what dosing strategy should be utilized. This, again, depends on the urgency of the surgical procedure required. A majority of cardiac surgical patients with preoperative anemia, however, are likely to be anemic because of a recent involved hospital admission/ICU stay. They are more likely to have been kept hospitalized following an acute cardiac event, e.g., myocardial infarction, unstable angina, acute congestive heart failure (CHF), and surgery is likely either urgent or emergent in character. These patients often cannot wait for preoperative correction of their anemia. Those who can wait and who will respond to erythropoietin therapy require correction of their anemia to be carried out in the shortest possible time period. As discussed previously, such acute maximal stimulation cannot be achieved with the standard erythropoietin regimens employed in the renal failure population, or in patients undergoing relatively long-term preoperative autologous blood donation. Erythropoietin dosing regimens that result in maximum marrow stimulation and red cell production are required and will need to be developed if recombinant therapy is to have a meaningful role in a majority of preoperative anemias.

The third and final issue regarding the use of erythropoietin for the correction of preoperative anemia is whether the costs involved are justified. Delayed surgery for the administration of a very expensive drug to an inpatient is obviously not cost-effective. Reimbursement cannot be expected, particularly when these costs are compared to those incurred by the transfusion of two to four units of banked blood (even when costs of transfusion reactions, acquired hepatitis/HIV disease, etc., are factored in). Use of the drug will likely be limited to those inpatients who are at the highest risk for transfusion-related events (rare blood types, Jehovah's Witnesses), and to those patients who can be treated as outpatients. Efficient outpatient dosing regimens will therefore need to be developed. Again, as with the use of erythropoietin for preoperative autologous donation, use of erythropoietin for correction of preoperative anemia provides a useful means for decreasing transfusion for a select portion of the cardiac surgical population.

Acute Preoperative Stimulation of Erythropoiesis

With the changing nature of cardiac surgery—increased numbers of critically ill patients undergoing urgent and emergent procedures—a majority of nonanemic and anemic patients cannot even wait the 2- to 3-week period required for erythropoietin-assisted autologous donation or for correction of preoperative anemia. This trend is likely to continue in the future. An alternative application for recombinant erythropoietin is to use the hormone to acutely increase red blood cell production to supranormal levels preoperatively, so that intraoperative and postoperative transfusion requirements are decreased, and postoperative recovery from anemia is improved. Because an increase in red cell mass is first seen 5 to 6 days after erythropoietin stimulation, conceivably a 5- to 6-day acute course of erythropoietin therapy could be used to sharply increase the number of developing red blood cells in the marrow, without a significant increase in hematocrit. The subsequent increase in red cell mass could then be taken advantage of intraoperatively in the form of increased potential for intraoperative autologous donation and decreased hemodilution on bypass, and postoperatively in the form of faster recovery from anemia.

Levine et al[76] evaluated the effects of an acute 5-day preoperative course of erythropoietin (1000 U/kg/day IV) in baboons subjected to sham laparotomy and exchange transfusion to 15%. They found that initiation of therapy preoperatively resulted in no change in hematocrit by the time of operation, but significantly improved postoperative recovery. A study by

Hoynck van Papendricht et al[239] utilizing a 6-day preoperative course of erythropoietin (200 U/kg/day SQ) in rats subjected to ileal resection and exchange transfusion to 20% confirmed these findings.

This strategy was first applied clinically by Hisatomi et al,[197] who administered 6 days of preoperative erythropoietin and 7 days of postoperative therapy (200 U/kg/day IV). The authors found that fewer homologous blood transfusions were required in the erythropoietin-treated group (512 ml vs. 721 ml), and that postoperative hemoglobin levels were significantly higher in those treated with erythropoietin. D'Ambra et al[240] administered erythropoietin (150 and 300 U/kg/day SQ) for 5 days preoperatively and 3 days postoperatively. As predicted, postoperative recovery was faster, and fewer homologous blood transfusions were required. Interestingly, despite the lack of elevation of hematocrit at the time of operation, intraoperative red blood cell mass was found to be higher in erythropoietin-treated patients (indicating either a proportional increase in plasma volume so that the percentage of red blood cells remained unchanged, or that the "primed" marrow was able to rapidly unload new red cells as the acute hemodilution of bypass was experienced). This increase in intraoperative mass seen after 5 days of erythropoietin treatment suggests that combining acute preoperative erythropoietin treatment with intraoperative autologous donation might serve as a way to effectively increase red blood cell mass by one to two units. This strategy is attractive for those patients who refuse preoperative blood transfusions on a religious basis, but who will allow intraoperative collection and reinfusion of blood with a continuous closed circuit. It might also prove useful in the increasing numbers of urgent cardiac surgery cases and in those who cannot tolerate autologous blood donation, particularly those at high risk for requiring homologous transfusion.

A trial utilizing this strategy was applied to 15 Jehovah's Witnesses undergoing urgent coronary artery bypass surgery at our institution from 1992 to 1994. Relative to a control group of 100 elective and emergent CABG patients, this group of Jehovah's Witnesses was at particularly high risk for requiring red cell transfusion with respect to established risk factors, including age, sex, preoperative hematocrit, and red cell mass. Because of their religious beliefs, preoperative autologous donation was not possible, and because of the urgent nature of their disease, a delay in surgery to allow full benefit of erythropoietin also was not possible. Therefore, all patients were started on recombinant erythropoietin at the time of admission, and this was continued to the time of surgery. In seven patients a 3- to 4-day preoperative course was able to be given; in the remaining eight patients only a 1-day course was possible. The high-dose "physiologic" regimen (combined IV/SQ) that has been discussed previously was used. Use of erythropoietin was coupled with intraoperative autologous donation (using a continuous closed circuit in accordance with religious specifications) to preserve the maximum number of red cells from destruction and loss during bypass, and with aprotinin to decrease postoperative bleeding. The control group received intraoperative autologous donation only. The results are seen in Figure 4.12. Despite the Jehovah's Witness population's being at much higher risk for requiring red cell transfusion, no patients in this group required red cells as compared with 31% in the control group. And despite this lack of transfusion, postoperative hematocrits in the Jehovah's Witness group were significantly higher than those of the control group at all postoperative time points. The difference in postoperative hematocrits becomes even more apparent when hematocrits in the control group are corrected for transfusions received by subtracting 3% for each red cell unit transfused (Fig. 4.12, dotted line). While part of this difference between groups is undoubtedly attributable to the 30% reduction in postoperative chest tube losses afforded by aprotinin (all patients had shed mediastinal blood reinfusion for up to 18 hours, helping to counter this potential aprotinin effect), the divergent nature of the hematocrit curves and the onset of a reticulocytosis as high as 12.5% 4 to 6 days after initiation of recombinant erythropoietin suggest that

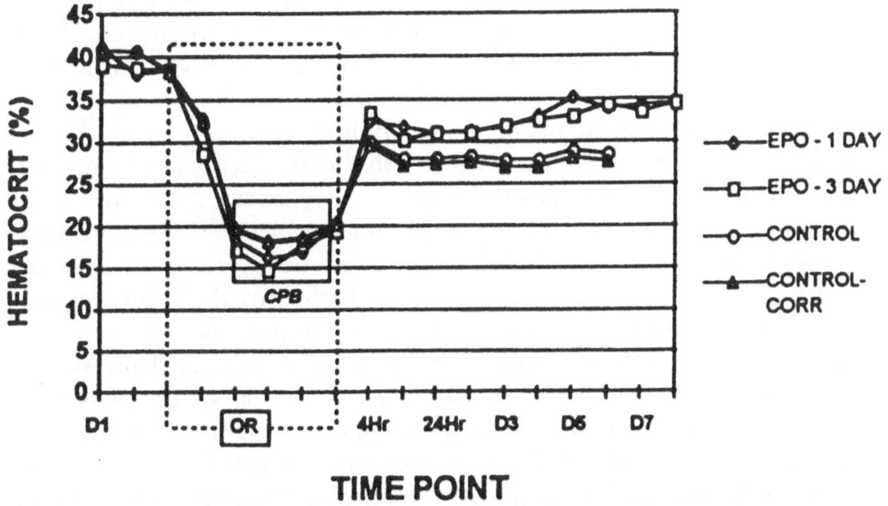

FIGURE 4.12. Preoperative, intraoperative, and postoperative hematocritis of 15 Jehovah's Witness patients undergoing CABG. All patients received a course of acute "maximum physiologic" dose erythropoietin (corresponding serum erythropoietin levels can be seen in Fig. 4.11). The therapeutic regimen was begun 3 days preoperatively in eight patients (solid line, square), and 1 day preoperatively in seven patients (solid line, diamond). No Jehovah's Witness patients required red cell transfusion. Hematocrit data for 100 control CABG patients on whom a similar set of blood conservation techniques was applied but without erythropoietin are also represented (dotted line, circle). These same 100 patients are also seen after correcting their hematocrit for the number of units transfused, by subtracting three percentage points for each unit transfused (dashed line, triangle). CPB, cardiopulmonary bypass; OR, operating room.

erythropoietin use significantly contributed to the successful outcome in these high risk patients.

Postoperative Anemia

Given that the major stimulus for erythropoietin production is decreased tissue oxygen availability, as determined by the three components–oxygen carrying capacity, oxygen tension, and oxygen affinity–with modification by paracrine, endocrine, and pharmacologic factors, there might be envisioned a scenario or combination of circumstances that would provide maximal erythropoietin stimulus, namely, large-volume acute blood loss, marked hypoxia and alkalosis, and decreased 2,3-DPG levels. Together these would act to maximally decrease tissue oxygen availability, and, therefore, to maximally stimulate erythropoietin production. Conversely, there might be envisioned a set of circumstances that would combine to minimize the erythropoietin response to anemia. Unfortunately, several of these are found in the routine postoperative cardiac surgical patient. Postoperative hematocrits after standard cardiac procedures at our institution average 28% to 30%. While below 34%, this level may still not be sufficiently low to stimulate significant erythropoietin production. These patients are on ventilators 4 to 12 hours postoperatively, with arterial oxygen pressures often elevated during this time. As discussed, this increased oxygen tension might damp erythropoietin production.[86] The continued supplemental use of oxygen 1 to 3 days after extubation might further blunt the erythropoietin response. Hypoventilation, or, more commonly, mild acidosis would compound the problem.[33,92] Beta-blockers, commonly used postoperatively, would also be expected to suppress production.[102,105] Hypoperfusion and hypothermia of the kidneys during bypass might directly compromise the renal erythropoietin response. Finally, all of these effects would be additive to the overall depression in erythropoietin production seen in the elderly.[85] The possibility of such an iatrogenic deficiency is supported by a study comparing erythropoietin levels in cardiac surgical and cholecystectomy patients.[241] Postoperative erythropoietin levels were significantly lower on postoperative day 1 in the cardiac patients, and never surpassed those in the cholecystectomy group despite much greater levels of anemia (30% vs. 36%). This suggests that erythropoietin may benefit virtually all anemic postoperative cardiac surgical patients by correcting the relative deficiency of the hormone that is present in these patients. Several studies have looked at the use of recombinant erythropoietin in the treatment of postoperative anemia.

Levine et al[99] administered 1000 U/kg per day for 14 postoperative days to baboons whose operation consisted of sham laparotomy and exchange transfusion to 15%. They found that the rate of erythropoiesis in the erythropoietin group was 2.1% as compared with 1.3% in a placebo group, and that the time required for return to a hematocrit of 30% was 9.9 days and 17.4 days, respectively. In a second study, Levine et al[76] looked at the effect of both pre- and postoperative erythropoietin (1000 U/kg IV) on erythropoiesis.[76] Animals were given placebo, 5 days of preoperative erythropoietin, or 5 days of preoperative erythropoietin and 14 days of postoperative erythropoietin. They found the time required for return to a hematocrit of 30% was 17.7, 12.4, and 8.0 days, respectively. In other words, it took over 50% less time for hematocrit to return to normal with both pre- and postoperative erythropoietin versus placebo, and both pre- and postoperative erythropoietin were superior to preoperative erythropoietin alone. The authors found that a postoperative peak in erythropoietin levels was absent in those animals treated with preoperative erythropoietin only, while this peak reached almost 4000 U/L in nonerythropoietin-treated animals. This suggested a suppression of the normal erythropoietin response by preoperative exogenous erythropoietin use, and provides support for the use of postoperative erythropoietin if preoperative erythropoietin has been used to augment autologous donation or to correct preoperative anemia. Tasaki et al,[225] in their study of autologous donation in orthopedic surgery, clinically confirmed Levine et al's finding that endogenous erythropoietin production is relatively suppressed immediately postoperatively in patients treated with preoperative erythropoietin. In line with this, postoperative red cell mass recovery rate was found to be higher in control subjects than in individuals treated with preoperative erythropoietin only. This suggests that if exogenous erythropoietin is used to supplement autologous donation, then it should be continued at least through the immediate postoperative period.

Watanabe et al's[227] study on erythropoietin-augmented preoperative autologous donation in cardiac surgery also evaluated the effects of continuing erythropoietin postoperatively. They found that postoperative erythropoietin therapy resulted in a significant increase in hemoglobin by the seventh postoperative day. With the discontinuation of erythropoietin at that time, hemoglobin gradually returned to control levels, suggesting that continuation of erythropoietin beyond 7 postoperative days would have been beneficial (particularly in those with continued anemia or transfusion requirement).

As with the use of erythropoietin for preoperative autologous donation, there are still several issues in respect to postoperative erythropoietin that will need to be resolved. First, an acceptable level of postoperative anemia will need to be more clearly defined. Erythropoietin will not be needed in patients above this level unless a future transfusion requirement can be predicted (e.g., ongoing blood loss, prolonged ICU stay, severe renal insult). Second, the proper length of postoperative therapy needs to be evaluated. Again, this will likely be closely related to the degree of postoperative normovolemic hemodilution that is acceptable. Finally, the question exists as to whether erythropoietin should be started on patients postoperatively only after they are found to be critically anemic, or should it be started preoperatively on those patients who are at known risk for requiring transfusion (e.g., low red blood cell mass, double valve procedures, reoperations, bleeding disorders), or who cannot easily receive transfusions (e.g., Jehovah's Witnesses, rare blood types). Clearly the need for transfusion is greatest in the first 5 to 6 postoperative days, and only by starting therapy preoperatively can red cell mass be increased during this crucial time. One possible strategy might be to begin erythropoietin therapy preoperatively (at the time of admission, for example) in all high-transfusion-risk patients, and then continue its use postoperatively only if the hemoglobin level is below a certain value, or if ongoing transfusion requirements can be predicted. Such an approach applies erythropoietin therapy only to those who need it most, and by doing so, maximizes cost-effectiveness.

Summary: Optimizing Use and Future Applications

This chapter began with a review of the endogenous erythropoietin and the erythropoietic response, to provide the reader with an understanding of the physiology and mechanism of action of the natural hormone. It then moved on to discuss the recombinant hormone, and reviewed its general clinical use in the treatment of anemia. Application of the recombinant hormone in surgery and cardiac surgery was then reviewed, with an emphasis on its clinical efficacy in preserving hematocrit and reducing homologous blood use. The present section provides a concise summary of these findings, and discusses the potential ways in which perioperative use of the drug might be optimized with respect to blood conservation in the cardiac surgical patient.

Endogenous Erythropoietin and the Erythropoietic Response

Erythropoietin is a glycoprotein hormone that is produced in the kidneys in response to tissue hypoxia, the most common form of which is decreased oxygen carrying capacity, or anemia. Serum levels begin to rise within minutes of a hypoxic stimulus, and peak 12 to 28 hours afterward, the magnitude and breadth of this peak being directly related to the magnitude of the hypoxic stimulus. Levels then decline as counterhypoxic mechanisms begin to take effect, and then slowly return to normal as hematocrit returns to normal. This biphasic endogenous serum erythropoietin response leads to changes in its target organ – the bone marrow – that ultimately leads to an increase in the rate and magnitude of red cell production. This is first evidenced by a reticulocytosis that can appear within 24 hours after the onset of hypoxic stimulus. This early reticulocytosis results from the early release of reticulocytes from the marrow stimulated by the elevation in serum erythropoietin. Recruitment and proliferation of red cell progenitors, and acceleration of the rate of red cell maturation, through shortening of the cell cycle time and skipping of generations, yields a maximum reticulocytosis and the first increase in hematocrit in as few as 4 to 6 days after the onset of hypoxic stimulus. Over the ensuing days and weeks, as increased red cell production leads to a correction in hematocrit, erythropoietin levels slowly return to normal. Again, the magnitude and rate of these occurrences is dependent on the magnitude of the hypoxic stimulus. Above hematocrits of 34%, little hypoxic stimulus for increased erythropoietin production occurs, and erythropoietin levels are only mildly elevated. Correction of such a mild anemia therefore requires a prolonged period of time. Severe anemia, however, leads to a prompt and precipitous rise in serum erythropoietin levels, resulting in maximum marrow stimulation and a maximum rate of red cell mass and hematocrit increase.

Several factors or conditions can modulate the amount of erythropoietin that is produced in response to hypoxia, including local and paracrine messengers (seratonin), pharmacologic agents (beta-blockers, adenosine), and humoral messengers (thyroid hormone, growth hormone, prolactin, sex hormones) (Table 4.1). Other factors or disease states can affect how well the marrow responds to erythropoietin stimulation, or how long these newly produced red cells survive in the bloodstream. Depressed erythropoietin production (e.g., renal failure, chronic disease), decreased marrow responsiveness (e.g., iron deficiency, aluminum toxicity, aplastic anemia, myelofibrosis, chronic disease), and decreased red cell survival in the bloodstream (e.g., sickle cell disease, thalassemia, ongoing blood loss) are the three basic abnormalities of the erythropoietin–red cell mass axis that can lead to anemia. The most common cause of anemia in the perioperative setting is that attributable to acute or ongoing blood loss.

Recombinant Erythropoietin

Recombinant erythropoietin became available for clinical use in 1988. Produced by recombinant technology using a human tumor cell line, the recombinant product is nearly identical to the endogenous form, and therefore it has few side effects and an excellent safety profile, particularly in the nondialysis population. Biochemically, it is a very hydrophobic molecule, and therefore it is formulated with human albumin as a carrier protein (in the U.S.). Most patients who reject the use of allogeneic blood product transfusion on a religious basis (one of the principal non–FDA-approved indications for its perioperative use at present) will accept the use of human albumin for this purpose, however. Pharmacologically, erythropoietin's bioavailability, peak serum levels, and serum half-life are dependent on its route of administration. The intravenous route results in 100% bioavailability and instantaneous peak levels, but its half-life is only 3 to 6 hours. Conversely, the other most common route of erythropoietin administration, the subcutaneous route, has only a 25% bioavailability, but peak levels are not achieved until 18 to 24 hours after administration, and the half-life is extended to 24 to 30 hours. Studies in renal failure patients have demonstrated that despite the lower serum levels achieved with subcutaneous dosing, it is at least as effective as the intravenous form. These results have been confirmed in the perioperative setting, where intermittent and logistically much simpler subcutaneous injection has yielded similar results to intravenous use of the drug. This finding may be attributable to the fact that subcutaneous administration of the hormone more closely mimics the persistent elevation in serum erythropoietin levels seen in the endogenous response, and suggests that greater attention to this natural response may lead to more efficacious use of the drug in the future.

The success of recombinant erythropoietin in the clinical arena is clear. Today it is used in over 200,000 renal failure patients worldwide. In addition to treatment of the anemias of renal failure, HIV disease, and cancer chemotherapy, for which the drug is FDA approved, recombinant erythropoietin has been used on an investigational basis to treat the other types of anemia in which production or maintenance of red cell mass is insufficient due to abnormalities of the erythropoietin–red cell hormonal axis. The response of any of these anemias to exogenous erythropoietin supplementation depends on the anemia's underlying etiology. Endogenous erythropoietin levels can generally be used as a guide to judge the response that will be obtained. High serum levels (e.g., greater than 500 mU/dl) generally predict poor response. Such high levels indicate that an adequate endogenous erythropoietin response to the anemia is present, and therefore that the defect lies in either decreased marrow responsiveness or decreased red cell survival. If surgery is anticipated in any anemic patient whose anemia cannot be attributed to recent blood loss or iron deficiency, the consultation of a hematologist should be obtained before erythropoietin therapy is instituted. Intervention may or may not include the use of recombinant erythropoietin, depending on the type of anemia encountered.

By far the most common form of anemia encountered in the perioperative setting is that attributable to acute or chronic blood loss. Once blood loss decreases or ceases, such anemia will correct itself over time, using the body's endogenous erythropoietin response. These patients demonstrate appropriate rises in endogenous erythropoietin levels, an appropriate bone marrow response (given adequate iron stores), and, without additional blood losses, an appropriate increase in red cell mass. This normal erythropoietic response to anemia can be modified, however. By using the recombinant hormone to additionally increase serum levels, marrow stimulation and red cell production can be further increased. The ability of the endogenous erythropoietin response to be augmented in these patients provides the basis for use of the recombinant product in the perioperative setting.

The most common cause of failure of recombinant erythropoietin therapy is iron deficiency. Therefore, baseline iron studies should be performed on all patients with preoperative anemia in whom the use of erythropoietin is anticipated (Table 4.2). Appropriate oral or parenteral supplementation can then be initiated to correct any deficiency that is present (Table 4.3). Because many patients treated with recombinant erythropoietin develop a functional iron deficiency, owing to the marked increase in red cell production and an inability to mobilize iron stores rapidly enough, all patients started on erythropoietin should be started on oral iron therapy. Folate and vitamin B_{12} supplementation may be given at the start of erythropoietin treatment as well.

Finally, recombinant erythropoietin therapy has been shown to be safe, particularly in the non–renal-failure population. This is likely due to its very strong similarity with the endogenous form of the hormone.

Perioperative Application of Recombinant Erythropoietin in the Cardiac Surgical Patient

The perioperative use of recombinant erythropoietin is not FDA approved, and its use for this purpose is considered investigational. According to FDA regulations, however, the physician can prescribe erythropoietin or any FDA-approved drug for non–FDA-approved indications at his or her own discretion. There are four basic ways in which recombinant erythropoietin can be applied perioperatively to the surgical and cardiac surgical patient: (1) augmentation of autologous donation, (2) correction of preoperative anemia, (3) acute preoperative marrow stimulation, and (4) correction of postoperative anemia.

Studies investigating the use of recombinant erythropoietin to augment preoperative autologous donation have clearly revealed that use of the recombinant hormone can increase both the rate and volume of autologous blood collection. This is attributable to the minimal endogenous erythropoietin response that occurs when using the AABB sanctioned minimum hematocrit of 34%. While the use of a lower minimum hematocrit would be expected to increase the endogenous response and therefore the autologous yield, it might also be expected to result in a higher incidence of complications. The use of the recombinant hormone to supplement the endogenous response serves as an alternative way to increase autologous yield, but without this risk of additional donation-related complications. At least 10 studies evaluating autologous donation in cardiac surgery have appeared in the literature. Erythropoietin augmented autologous donation has been shown to be both safe and effective by these studies. The cost-effectiveness of autologous donation itself remains in question,[242,243] and until such cost issues are resolved, erythropoietin augmentation will likely enjoy only limited use.

Recombinant erythropoietin has been used to correct preoperative anemia in the cardiac surgical patient. The anemia most commonly encountered in the perioperative setting is that of acute or ongoing blood loss, typically attributable to procedural losses (e.g., cardiac catheterization) and laboratory sampling. Less commonly encountered anemias include those of decreased erythropoietin production, decreased bone marrow responsiveness, and production of abnormal red cells with decreased viability. Anemias due to one of these three abnormalities may or may not respond to recombinant erythropoietin supplementation. Measurement of endogenous erythropoietin levels may help to differentiate responders from nonresponders. Unless the anemia is clearly due to recent blood loss, the consultation of a hematologist should be obtained so the etiology of the anemia can be identified and appropriate interventions initiated as early in the preoperative course as possible. This intervention may or may not include the use of recombinant erythropoietin to augment endogenous erythropoietin blood levels. The dosing and length of time required for recombinant therapy, if applied, depends on the type of anemia that is to be treated, and the degree of anemia present. A set hematocrit/red cell mass should be established as the end point for therapy. At our institution a hematocrit of greater than 36% and red cell mass greater than 1600 cc generally decrease the risk for requiring red cell transfusion and this is used as the therapeutic end point for preoperative erythropoietin therapy. Correction of those factors that lead to marrow hyporesponsiveness can markedly improve outcome when recombinant therapy is used. The most important of these correctable factors is iron deficiency, due to its prevalence in the general population. Iron stores must be assessed and appropriately corrected prior to initiation of recombinant erythropoietin therapy. Laboratory diagnosis of iron deficiency and guidelines for supplementation are found in Tables 4.2 and 4.3, respectively.

In addition to the treatment of anemia, recombinant erythropoietin has demonstrated usefulness in providing an acute "supranormal" increase in red cell production in nonanemic precardiac surgical patients. Such an increase in production leads to an increase in red cell mass at the time of surgery that can then be taken advantage of intraoperatively in the form of increased volume of intraoperative autologous donation and decreased hemodilution during cardiopulmonary bypass (CPB), and postoperatively in the form of faster recovery from anemia. Studies indicate that such therapy should be initiated 5 to 8 days prior to surgery. In this way a substantial marrow-priming effect can occur without an appreciable increase in hematocrit (and the increased risk of polycythemia). Because such postoperative therapy can suppress endogenous erythropoietin production postoperative, use of the recombinant hormone should be continued postoperatively in those patients who remain at risk for requiring red cell transfusion.

The fourth general perioperative application of recombinant erythropoietin is the correction of postoperative anemia. In the cardiac surgical patient such anemia typically results in intraoperative blood loss. Suppression of endogenous production (attributable to appropriate suppression of perioperative tissue hypoxia by postoperative caregivers) may contribute to and prolong this anemia. Recombinant erythropoietin has been successfully applied to help correct this problem. Because a delay in hematocrit rise of 4 to 6 days occurs with recombinant therapy, the major issue that arises is how can the drug be administered so that its benefits (increased red cell mass) are seen at the time they are needed most—during the first 24 hours postoperatively (typically when the most severe anemia is experienced and the most transfusions given). One strategy is to begin the drug preoperatively on those patients at highest risk for transfusion, continuing it postoperatively only for the continued presence of transfusion risk (e.g., low hematocrit, continued bleeding). If the drug is given preoperatively, a suppression of endogenous production will occur postoperatively, and therefore the drug should be continued at least through the immediate postoperative period. A second question that arises in respect to postoperative erythropoietin therapy is the length of time that it should be continued. A useful rule of thumb would be to continue therapy until existing and predictable future patient risk factors for red cell transfusion have been eliminated. A typical postoperative course consists of 5 to 7 days of therapy.

Development of Optimal Dosing Regimens

Clinical application of recombinant erythropoietin in the renal failure population has involved the use of dosing regimens aimed at a gradual increase in red cell mass. This is so because these patients are chronically anemic, often with appropriate physiologic adaptation to the chronic anemic state, and so the need for a rapid correction of anemia is considered unnecessary. In contrast, the pre- and postoperative cardiac surgical patient requires a rapid and maximum increase in red cell production if homologous blood use is to be avoided. Dosing regimens that can achieve such increases are therefore required if the drug is to have any significant role in the perioperative setting. A potentially useful approach to the development of such regimens is to use the serum levels seen in the endogenous erythropoietin response to acute severe anemia (e.g., to a hematocrit of 10–15%) as a model for the levels that need to be achieved. This maximum endogenous response is characterized by an initial 24- to 36-hour peak in erythropoietin levels, followed by more moderate persistent elevation that continues, slowly decreasing, until hematocrit returns to normal. Dosing regimens utilizing either IV or SQ administration alone cannot pharmacologically re-create these levels. For example, if an initial high peak in serum erythropoietin concentration is required for early (committed red cell) progenitor recruitment and replication, then subcutaneous dosing schedules, which can only provide low to moderate elevation in serum levels, will fall short of providing for maximal marrow stimulation. Similarly, if persistent elevation of serum erythropoietin levels above a certain minimum is necessary to prevent preprogrammed cell death, then relatively little benefit is obtained from the brief serum peaks obtained with intermittent IV administration. Because the attainment of persistent elevation is more clearly essential to erythropoietin's stimulatory function, and because subcutaneous administration is simpler than intravenous administration, at present the subcutaneous route is preferred, particularly when outpatient use is anticipated.

If using the endogenous response as a model for the development of regimens for the recombinant hormone is valid (and it appears to be by successfully predicting the superiority of SQ vs. IV administration), then more closely copying this model may provide for further improvement in efficacy. One possible way to re-create both the initial high peak in serum levels and the period of persistent elevation is to use both the SQ and IV routes of administration (Fig. 4.10). At New York Hospital we have developed a regimen that initially administers both IV and SQ erythropoietin at the initiation of therapy to re-create the initial extended high peak, and then continues therapy as SQ only, to mimic the period of persistent elevation. This regimen has been successfully applied to our Jehovah's Witness population (Fig. 4.11).

Cost

The cost of erythropoietin provides probably the most formidable obstacle to its widespread use. At the present time its application to the treatment of non-renal failure, non-HIV uses will likely continue to be restricted by lack of insurance coverage for these applications. Investigational use (e.g., its use for all Jehovah's Witness patients undergoing cardiac surgery at our institution) will provide the drug to some patients. More widespread application must await FDA and insurance company approval. Private reimbursement by patients who have a strong personal preference to avoid the use of homologous blood is another payment possibility.

The Future of Recombinant Erythropoietin in Cardiac Surgery

Recombinant erythropoietin has shown tremendous clinical efficacy in correcting or helping to alleviate the anemias of chronic renal failure, AZT-induced AIDS-related anemia, and cancer chemotherapy. It has also shown utility in many non–FDA-approved applications, including perioperative applications aimed at reducing or eliminating homologous transfusion requirement. A review of the literature reveals this success, but also demonstrates that optimal dosing regimens and strategies that allow the drug to provide maximum perioperative benefit have yet to be fully realized. Successful future approaches will likely customize use of the drug to the individual patient. Use of erythropoietin will be based on assessment of each patient's preoperative characteristics, and on their postoperative hospital course. By applying erythropoietin in a logical and individualized fashion, the full potential of the drug in cardiac surgery will be realized.

Predicting the future uses of erythropoietin is difficult and its application may be directed by forces not readily apparent. In Europe, for example, unfortunate experiences with HIV-contaminated blood in the late 1980s prompted approval of recombinant erythropoietin for augmentation of autologous blood donation. The appearance of forms of HIV resistant to standard blood bank screening is a recent cause for concern with our own blood supply, and new blood-borne diseases might surface at any time. Were the blood supply to be contaminated in the future, public demand for perioperative blood conservation would dramatically increase. Perioperative use of recombinant erythropoietin would then become an important part of most major surgeries, and research performed on optimal application of the drug in this setting will have proven itself worthwhile.

Recombinant Erythropoietin: General Information and Guidelines for Use

General Information

Nomenclature

Epoietin-α (the only form available in the U.S.) is produced by Amgen (Thousand Oaks, CA). It is produced through recombinant DNA technology using a mammalian tumor cell line. Epoietin-α is marketed by Amgen as Epogen for the three FDA-approved uses: (1) the anemia of renal failure, (2) the anemia of HIV disease, (3) the anemia of cancer chemotherapy.

Through a licensing agreement with Amgen, Ortho Biotech (Raritan, NJ) also markets the drug as Procrit for all non–FDA-approved indications. Epogen and Procrit are identical and both are manufactured by Amgen. Other names for epoietin-α commonly encountered in the literature include r-HuEPO and Epo.

Epoietin-β is the other major form of recombinant erythropoietin that is produced. Only available outside the U.S., it differs from erythropoietin-α primarily in minor glycosylation sites and pharmacokinetics.

Pharmacology

The half-life and bioavailability of epoietin-α are dependent on the route of administration. The most commonly used routes are intravenous and subcutaneous. Intravenous administration results in rapid high peak serum levels (100% bioavailability), but serum levels rapidly dissipate (half-life of 3 to 8 hours). Conversely, subcutaneous administration results in much lower serum levels (25% bioavailability), but levels remain elevated longer (peak levels reached 8 to 16 hours postdose, half-life of 18 to 30 hours). Subcutaneous administration is at least as effective as intravenous administration, and is more easily applied on an outpatient basis. Elimination occurs primarily by hepatic degradation.

Side Effects

Epoietin-α is virtually an exact copy of the endogenous hormone (minor differences in glycosylation sites) and thus few side effects are encountered, particularly in the perioperative non-renal-disease setting. Mild flu-like symptoms might occasionally be seen. An increased incidence of venous access thrombosis has been debated in the renal literature. This complication has not been seen in the perioperative setting. An increased incidence of hypertension seen in the dialysis population is likely related to viscosity changes that occur as hematocrit rises. This side effect has not been documented in the perioperative setting.

Costs

Wholesale costs for erythropoietin at our institution in 1993 was approximately $90 per ten thousand units. A 300 unit per kg dose in a 70 kg patient therefore costs $190.

Indications for Perioperative Use of Recombinant Erythropoietin

Recombinant erythropoietin is FDA approved only for the treatment of the anemia of chronic renal failure, AZT-induced AIDS-related anemia, and anemia following cancer chemotherapy. A physician is free, however, to apply any FDA-approved drug to other nonapproved uses at his/her and the patient's own risk (reimbursal should not be expected, however).

In the Department of Cardiothoracic Surgery at the New York Hospital-Cornell Medical Center we feel justified in using erythropoietin in the Jehovah's Witness population undergoing cardiac surgery, where its use can be lifesaving. These regimens might also be applied in the following cases:

1. Patients in whom augmentation of preoperative autologous donation is predicted to be of necessity because of an inadequate preoperative time period for sufficient donation.
2. Patients with the anemia of chronic renal failure who have been either not treated or inadequately treated with erythropoietin prior to surgery.

3. Patients with preoperative anemias known to be responsive to erythropoietin.
4. Patients at high risk for adverse reactions to allogeneic transfusion.
5. Patients with rare blood types.
6. Patients who strongly object to allogeneic blood use, and are willing to accept the costs of recombinant erythropoietin.

Recommendations for Erythropoietin Dosing

Should it be decided that a patient is a candidate for perioperative use of erythropoietin, the following is a set of recommendations for its application in each of the four perioperative scenarios that might be encountered by the cardiac surgeon or cardiac anesthesiologist: (1) augmentation of preoperative autologous donation, (2) preoperative correction of anemia, (3) acute preoperative marrow stimulation, and (4) correction of postoperative anemia. For each scenario, two possible dosing strategies are outlined. The first is the dosing regimen that has been generally applied in the literature to date. If several were available, those strategies that were shown most effective have been chosen. The second dosing strategy for each perioperative scenario is the one used at the New York Hospital-Cornell Medical Center (NYH-CMC) for patients undergoing cardiac surgery. This regimen is based on mimicking the physiology of the natural maximum erythropoietin-erythropoietic response. We have found it to be safe and effective in the high-risk Jehovah's Witness population.

Augmentation of Preoperative Autologous Blood Donation

Preoperative autologous donation should be initiated as far in advance of surgery as possible to allow for regeneration of red cell mass by the time of operation. Full regeneration of red cell mass by the time of operation allows the performance of other important blood conservation measures such as intraoperative autologous donation and decreases the degree of obligatory hemodilution that occurs during CPB (for a more in-depth discussion of optimal preoperative autologous donation refer to Chapter 3). The use of recombinant erythropoietin can accelerate red cell mass regeneration and therefore allow optimal application of preoperative autologous donation in the patient with limited preoperative time.

Standard Regimen 1

1. Administer erythropoietin 600 U/kg SQ 1 week prior to the first donation or at the time of the first donation.
2. Repeat 600 U/kg SQ dose one time per week during the time of autologous blood collection.
3. Oral iron therapy initiated at the time of first evaluation.

Standard Regimen 2

1. Administer erythropoietin 150 to 600 U/kg SQ 1 week prior to the first donation or at the time of the first donation. Higher doses will lead to a greater increase in red cell mass, but will also be more expensive. The longer the period of preoperative time available, therefore, the lower the dose that should be utilized.
2. Repeat SQ dose following each blood donation.
3. Oral iron therapy initiated at the time of first evaluation.

The NYH–CMC Regimen

1. Administer a combined IV/SQ erythropoietin dose (300 U/kg IV and 500 U/kg SQ) at the time of the first donation.
2. Repeat 500 U/kg SQ dose at the time of each autologous blood collection.
3. A repeat combined IV/SQ dose can be substituted for the regular 500 U/kg dose every 2 weeks.
4. Oral iron therapy initiated at the time of first evaluation.

Preoperative Correction of Anemia

Unless a patient's anemia is clearly due to acute preoperative blood loss (e.g., recent cardiac catheterization, voluminous laboratory blood sampling, IABP use), then the consultation of a hematologist should be obtained before initiation of recombinant erythropoietin therapy. This is particularly true if there is any indication by history or family history of the existence of a chronic anemic state. Patients should be evaluated for an ongoing source of occult blood loss (stool guaiac), and a baseline set of iron studies should be obtained. If iron deficiency is demonstrated (Table 4.2), appropriate replacement therapy should be initiated as soon as possible. The use of parenteral iron will accelerate restoration of iron stores and facilitate subsequent recombinant erythropoietin therapy, but its use carries the small but real risk of anaphylaxis. Guidelines for the use of acute parenteral iron replacement are found in Table 4.3.

Standard Regimen

Initial dose of erythropoietin (300 to 500 U/kg SQ) as soon as the appropriateness of erythropoietin therapy is decided on.

Maintenance doses of 300 to 500 U/kg SQ three times per week until the time of surgery.

Continue therapy for postoperative hematocrit less than 25%.

Initial parenteral iron supplementation if significant iron deficiency exists.

Maintenance oral iron therapy during the entire pre- and postoperative period.

The NYH–CMC Regimen

1. Administer a combined IV/SQ erythropoietin dose (300 U/kg IV and 500 U/kg SQ) as soon as recombinant erythropoietin therapy is decided upon.
2. Repeat 500 U/kg SQ dose every other day until the time of surgery. If possible, delay surgery until hematocrit rises to greater than 36%, as this will allow the use of intraoperative autologous donation, decrease the extent of obligatory hemodilution during CPB, and reduce the overall risk for requiring homologous transfusion.
3. Continued therapy for postoperative hematocrit less than 25%.
4. Maintenance oral iron therapy during the entire pre- and postoperative period.

Acute Preoperative Marrow Stimulation

Standard Regimen

This regimen is the same as for the acute correction of preoperative anemia.

1. Initial dose of erythropoietin (300 to 500 U/kg SQ) as soon as the appropriateness of erythropoietin therapy is decided upon.
2. Maintenance doses of 300 to 500 U/kg SQ three times per week until the time of surgery.
3. Monitor hematocrit to guard against development of preoperative polycythemia.
4. Continue therapy for postoperative hematocrit less than 25%.
5. Maintenance oral iron therapy during the entire pre- and postoperative period.

The NYH–CMC Regimen

This regimen is the same as for acute correction of preoperative anemia.

1. Administer a combined IV/SQ erythropoietin dose (300 U/kg IV and 500 U/kg kg SQ) as soon as recombinant erythropoietin therapy is decided upon.
2. Repeat 500 U/kg SQ dose every other day until the time of surgery. If possible, delay surgery until hematocrit rises to greater than 36%, as this will allow the use of intraoperative autologous donation and reduce the risk for requiring homologous transfusion.
3. Continue therapy for postoperative hematocrit less than 25%.
4. Maintenance oral iron therapy during the entire pre- and postoperative period.

Correction of Postoperative Anemia

Standard Regimen

1. Initial postoperative dose (300 to 500 U/kg SQ) for hematocrit less than 25%.
2. Maintenance dose of 300 to 500 U/kg three times per week until desired hematocrit is obtained.
3. Maintenance oral iron therapy during the entire postoperative period.

The NYH-CMC Regimen

1. Administer a combined IV/SQ erythropoietin dose (300 U/kg IV and 500 U/kg SQ) as soon as recombinant erythropoietin therapy is decided upon.
2. Maintenance dose of 500 U/kg SQ dose every other day until the desired hematocrit increase is obtained.
3. Maintenance oral iron therapy during the entire pre- and postoperative period.

References

1. Viault F. Sur l'augmentation considérable du nombre des globules dans le sang chez les habitantes des hautes plateux de l'Amérique du Sud. *CR Acad Sci Paris* 1890;111:918–919.
2. Carnot P, Deflandre C. Sur l'activité hemopöiétique des différents organes au cours de la régeneration du sang. *CR Hebd Acad Sci* 1906;143:432–435.
3. Bonsdorff E, Jalavisto E. A humoral mechanism in anoxic erythrocytes. *Acta Physiol Scand* 1948;16:150–170.
4. Reissman KR, Nomura T. Studies on the mechanism of erythropoietic stimulation in parabiotic rats during hypoxia. *Blood* 1950;5:372–380.
5. Erslev A. Humoral regulation of red cell production. *Blood* 1953;8:349–357.
6. Gordon AS, Piliero SJ, Kleinburg W, et al. A plasma extract with erythropoietic activity. *Proc Soc Exp Biol Med* 1954;86:255–258.
7. Hodgson G, Toha J. The erythropoietic effect of urine and plasma of repeatedly bled rabbits. *Blood* 1954;9:299–309.
8. Plzak LF, Fried W, Jacobson LD, Betharol WF. Demonstration of stimulation of erythropoiesis by plasma from anemic rats using Fe^{59}. *J Lab Clin Med* 1955;46:671–678.
9. Schmid R, Gilbertsen AS. Fundamental observations on the production of compensatory polycythemia in a case of patent ductus arteriosus with reversed blood flow. *Blood* 1955;10:247–251.
10. Stohlman F, Rath CE, Rose JC. Evidence for a humoral regulation of erythropoiesis. *Blood* 1954;9:721–733.
11. Jacobson LO, Goldwasser E, Fried W, Plzak L. The role of the kidney in erythropoiesis. *Nature (Lond)* 1957;179:633–634.
12. Gallagher NI, McCarthy JM, Hart KT, et al. Evaluation of plasma erythropoietic-stimulating factors in uremic patients. *Blood* 1959;14:662–667.

13. Denny WF, Flanigan WJ, Zuckoski CF. Serial erythropoietin studies in patients undergoing renal homotransplantation. *J Lab Clin Med* 1966;67:386.
14. Erslev AJ. In vitro production of erythropoietin by kidneys perfused with serum-free solution. *Blood* 1974;44:77–85.
15. Fried W, Barone-Varelas J, Berman M. Detection of high erythropoietin titers in renal extracts of hypoxic rats. *J Lab Clin Med* 1981;97:82–86.
16. Jelkmann W, Bauer C, Fisher JW. Demonstration of high levels of erythropoietin in rat kidneys following hypoxic hypoxia. *Pfleugers Arch* 1981; 392:34–39.
17. Schuster SJ, Wilson JH, Erslev AJ, et al. Physiologic regulation and tissue localization of renal erythropoietin messenger RNA. *Blood* 1987;70:316–318.
18. Bondurant MC, Lind RN, Loury MJ, et al. Anemia induces accumulation of erythropoietin mRNA in the kidney and liver. *Mol Cell Biol* 1986;6:2731–2733.
19. Fried W. The liver as a source of extrarenal erythropoietin production. *Blood* 1972;40:671–677.
20. Miyake T, Kung CKH, Goldwasser E. Purification of human erythropoietin. *J Biol Chem* 1977;252:5558–5564.
21. Sherwood JB, Goldwasser E. A radioimmunoassay for erythropoietin. *Blood* 1979;54:885–893.
22. Egrie JC, Cotes PM, Lane J. Development of radioimmunoassays for human erythropoietin using recombinant erythropoietin as tracer and immunogen. *J Immunol Methods* 1987;90:235–241.
23. Lin FK, Suggs S, Lin CH, et al. Cloning and expression of the human erythropoietin gene. *Proc Natl Acad Sci USA* 1985;82:7580–7584.
24. Jacobs KC, Shoemaker C, Rudersdorf R. Isolation and characterization of genomic and cDNA clones of human erythropoietin. *Nature (Lond)* 1985;313:806–810.
25. Eschbach JW. Erythropoietin 1991—an overview. *Am J Kidney Dis* 1991;18(4):3–6.
26. Drug information from packaging insert for Epogen. Thousand Oaks, CA: Amgen, 1996.
27. Spivak JL. Erythropoietin: basic and clinical aspects. *Hematol Oncol Clin North Am* 1994;8(5):863–1043.
28. Rosengart TK, Helm RE, Klemperer JD, et al. Combined aprotinin and erythropoietin use for blood conservation: results with Jehovah's Witnesses. *Ann Thorac Surg* 1994;58:1397–1403.
29. Erslev A. Blood and mountains. In: Wintrobe MM, ed. *Blood Pure and Innocent.* New York: McGraw-Hill, 1980;257.
30. Jelkmann W. Erythropoietin: structure, control of production, and function. *Physiol Rev* 1992;72(2):449.
31. Zon LI. History of erythropoietin. In: Garnik MB, ed. *Erythropoietin in Clinical Application.* New York: Marcel Dekker, 1990;1.
32. Lai Pit, Everett R, Wang FF, et al. Structural characterization of human erythropoietin. *J Biol Chem* 1986;261:3116.
33. Recny MA, Scoble HA, Kim Y. Structural characterization of natural human urinary and recombinant DNA-derived erythropoietin. *J Biol Chem* 1987; 262:17156–17163.
34. Lappin TRJ, Maxwell AP. Chemistry and assays of erythropoietin. In: Jelkmann W, and Gross AJ, *Erythropoietin.* Berlin: Springer, 1989;7–18.
35. Davis JM, Arakawa T, Strickland TW, et al. Characterization of recombinant

human erythropoietin produced in Chinese hamster ovary cells. *Biochemistry* 1987;26:2633–2638.
36. Spivak JL. Erythropoietin: a brief review. *Nephron* 1989;52:289–294.
37. Bazan JF. A novel family of growth receptors: a common binding domain in the growth hormone, prolactin, erythropoietin and IL-6 receptors, and the P75 IL-2 receptor β chain. *Biochem Biophys Res Commun* 1989;164:788.
38. Bazan JF. Haemopoietic receptors and helical cytokines. *Immunol Today* 1990;11:350–354.
39. Dordai MS, Wang FF, Goldwasser E. The role of carbohydrate in erythropoietin action. *Endocrinology* 1985;116:2293–2299.
40. Goldwasser E, Kung CKH, Eliason J. On the mechanism of erythropoietin induced differentiation. XIII. The role of sciatic acid in erythropoietin action. *J Biol Chem* 1974;249:4202.
41. Spivak JL. The mechanism of action of erythropoietin. *Int J Cell Cloning* 1986;4:139–166.
42. Personal Communication: Brother John Mountain of the Medical Liaison Committee for The Watchtower Bible and Tract Society, New York, NY.
43. Faulds D, Sorkin EM. Epoetin (recombinant human erythropoietin) a review of its pharmacodynamic and pharmacokinetic properties and therapeutic potential in anaemia and the stimulation of erythropoiesis. *Drugs* 1989; 38(6):863–899.
44. Clemons GK, Fitzsimmons SL, Demanincor D. Immunoreactive erythropoietin concentrations in fetal and neonatal rats and effects on hypoxia. *Blood* 1986;68:892–899.
45. Zanjani ED, Ascensao JL, McGlave PB, et a]. Studies on the liver to kidney switch of erythropoietin production. *J Clin Invest* 1981;67:1183–1188.
46. Tan CC, Eckardt KU, Ratcliffe PJ. Organ distribution of erythropoietin mRNA in normal and uremic rats. *Kidney Int* 1991;40:69–76.
47. Fandry J, Bunn HF. In vivo and in vitro regulation of erythropoietin mRNA: measurement by competitive polymerase chain reaction. *Blood* 1993; 81(3):617–623.
48. Jacobson LO, Marks EK, Gaston EO, et al. Studies on erythropoiesis. XI. Reticulocyte response of transfusion induced polycythemic mice to anemic plasma from nephrectomized mice and to plasma from nephrectomized rats exposed to low oxygen. *Blood* 1959;14:635.
49. Kourey ST, Bondurant MC, Koury MJ. Localization of erythropoietin synthesizing cells in murine kidneys by in situ hybridization. *Blood* 1988; 71:524–527.
50. Lacombe C, DaSilva JL, Bruneval P. Peritubular cells are the site of erythropoietin synthesis in the murine hypoxic kidney. *J Clin Invest* 1988; 81:620–623.
51. Suzuki T, Sasaki R. Immunocytochemical demonstration of erythropoietin immunoreactivity in peritubular endothelial cells of the anemic mouse kidney. *Arch Histol Cytol* 1990;53:121–124.
52. Lacombe C, DaSilva JL, Bruneval P, et al. Erythropoietin: sites of synthesis and regulation of secretion. *Am J Kidney Dis* 1991;18(4):14–19.
53. Schooley JC, Mahlmann LJ. Evidence for the de novo synthesis of erythropoietin in hypoxic rats. *Blood* 1972;40:662–670.
54. Jelkmann W. Temporal pattern of erythropoietin titers in kidney tissue during hypoxic hypoxia. *Pflugers Arch* 1982;393:88–91.

55. Erslev AJ, Caro J. Physiologic and molecular biology of erythropoietin. *Med Oncol Tumor Pharmacother* 1986;3:159–164.
56. Misago M, Chiba S, Kikuchi M, et al. Effect of absolute and relative changes in hematocrit on erythropoiesis in mice. *Int J Cell Cloning* 1986;4:320–330.
57. Adamson JW. The erythropoietin/hematocrit relationship in normal and polycythemic man: implications of marrow regulation. *Blood* 1968;32:597–609.
58. Erslev AJ. Erythropoietin. *N Engl J Med* 1991;324(19):1339.
59. Eckardt KU, Boutellier U, Kurtz A. Rate of erythropoietin formation in humans in response to acute hypobaric hypoxia. *J Appl Physiol* 1989; 66:1785–1788.
60. Fu JS, Lertora JL, Brookins J, et al. Pharmacokinetics in intact and anephric dogs. *J Lab Clin Med* 1988;111:669–676.
61. Mladenovic J, Eschback JR, Koup JR. Erythropoietin kinetics in normal and uremic sheep. *J Lab Clin Med* 1985;105:659–663.
62. Emmanuel DS, Goldwasser E, Katz AI. Metabolism of pure human erythropoietin in the rat. *Am J Physiol* 1984;247:Fl68–FI76.
63. Urabe A, Takaku F, Mizoguchi H, et al. Effect of recombinant human erythropoietin on the anemia of chronic renal failure. *Int J Cell Cloning* 1988;6:179–180.
64. Kindler J, Eckardt KU, Ehmer B, et al. Single-dose pharmacokinetics of recombinant human erythropoietin in patients with varying degrees of renal failure. *Nephrol Dial Transplant* 1989;4:345–349.
65. Lim VS, DeGowin RL, Zavala D, et al. Recombinant human erythropoietin treatment in pre-dialysis patients: a double-blind placebo controlled study. *Ann Intern Med* 1989;110:108–114.
66. Goldberg MA, Dunning SP, Bunn HF. Regulation of the erythropoietin gene: evidence that the oxygen sensor is a heme protein. *Science* 1988;242:1412–1415.
67. Baer AN, Dessypus EN, Goldwasser E, et al. Blunted erythropoietin response to anemia in rheumatoid arthritis. *Br J Haemotol* 1987;66:559–564.
68. DeKlerk G, Rosengarten CJ, Vet RJWM, et al. Serum erythropoietin (ESF) titers in anemia. *Blood* 1981;58:1164–1170.
69. Erslev AJ, Wilson J, Caro J. Erythropoietin titers in anemic, non uremic patients. *J Lab Clin Med* 1987;109:429–433.
70. McGonigle RJ, Ohene-Frempong K, Lewy JE, et al. Erythropoietin response to anemia in children with sickle-cell disease and Fanconi's hypoproliferative anemia. *Acta Haematol* 1985;74:6–9.
71. Spivak JL, Barnes DC, Fuclis E, et al. Serum immunoreactive erythropoietin in HIV-infected patients. *JAMA* 1989;261:3104–3107.
72. Takeuchi M, Ememura T, Nishimura J, et al. Regulation of erythropoietin and burst-promoting activity production in patients with aplastic anemia and iron deficiency anemia. *Acta Haematol* 1988;80:145–152.
73. Rosen AL, Gould SA, Seghal LA, et al. Erythropoietin response to normovolemic anemia. *Fed Proc* 1985;44:1266.
74. Miller ME, Cronkite EP, Garcia JF. Plasma levels of immunoreactive erythropoietin after acute blood loss in man. *Br J Haematol* 1982;52:545–549.
75. Miller ME, Rorth M, Stohlman F, et al. The effects of acute bleeding on acid-base balance, erythropoietin (EP) production and in vivo P50 in the rat. *Br J Haematol* 1976;33:379–385.
76. Levine EA, Gould SA, Rosen AL, et al. Perioperative recombinant human erythropoietin. *Surgery* 1989;106(2):432.

77. Spivak JL, Hogans BB. Clinical evaluation of a radioimmunoassay for serum erythropoietin using reagents derived from recombinant erythropoietin. *Blood* 1987;70(suppl 1):143a (abstract).
78. Holland PV, Schmidt PH, eds. *Standards for Blood Banks and Transfusion Services.* 13th ed. Arlington, VA: American Association of Blood Banks, 1989.
79. Goodnough LT, Brittenham GM. Limitations of the erythropoietic response to serial phlebotomy: implications for autologous blood donor programs. *J Lab Clin Med* 1991;115(1):28–35.
80. Kickler TS, Spivak JL. Effect of repeated whole blood donations on serum immunoreactive erythropoietin levels in autologous donors. *JAMA* 1988; 260(1):65–67.
81. Barosi G. Inadequate erythropoietin response to anemia: definition and clinical relevance. *Ann Haematol* 1994;68(5):215–222.
82. Sherwood JB, Goldwasser E, Chikote R, et al. Sickle cell anemia patients have low erythropoietin levels for their degree of anemia. *Blood* 1986;67:46–49.
83. Miller CB, Jones RJ, Plantoidosi S, et al. Decreased erythropoietin response in patients with the anemia of cancer. *N Engl J Med* 1990;322:1689–1692.
84. Robinson H, Monafo WW, Saver SM, et al. The role of erythropoietin in the anemia of thermal injury. *Ann Surg* 1972;178(5):565–572.
85. Carpenter MA, Kendall RG, O'Brien AE, et al. Reduced erythropoietin response to anemia in elderly patients with normocytic anemia. *Eur J Haematol* 1992;49:119–121.
86. Ko W, Krieger KH, Lazenby WD, et al. Coronary bypass grafting in 100 consecutive octogenarian patients: a multicenter analysis. *J Thorac Cardiovasc Surg* 1991;102(4):532–538.
87. Abrecht PH, Littell JK. Plasma erythropoietin in men and mice during acclimatization to different altitudes. *J Appl Physiol* 1972;32:54–58.
88. Pagel H, Jelkmann W, Weiss C. Isolated serum-free, perfused rat kidneys release immunoreactive erythropoietin in response to hypoxia. *Endocrinology* 1991;128:2633–2638.
89. L'Enfant G, Sullivan K. Adaptation to high attitude. *N Eng J Med* 1971; 284:1298–1309.
90. Milledge JS, Cotes PM. Serum erythropoietin in humans at high attitude and its relation to plasma renin. *J Appl Physiol* 1985;59:360–364.
91. Embury SH, Garcia JF, Mohanas N, et al. Effects of oxygen inhalation on endogenous erythropoietin kinetics, erythropoiesis, and properties of blood cells in sickle-cell anemia. *N Engl J Med* 1953;311:291–295.
92. Adamson JW, Finch CA. Hemoglobin function, oxygen affinity, and erythropoietin. *Annu Rev Physiol* 1975;37:351–369.
93. Hebbel RP, Eaton JW, Kronenberg RS, et al. Human plasmas. Adaptation to altitude in subjects with high hemoglobin oxygen affinity. *J Clin Invest* 1978;62:593–600.
94. Lechermann B, Jelkmann W. Erythropoietin production in normoxic and hypoxic rats with increased blood O_2 affinity. *Respir Physiol* 1985; 60:1–8.
95. Napier JAF. Effect of age and 2,3-DPG content of transfused blood on serum erythropoietin. *Vox Sang* 1980;39:318–321.
96. Finch CA. Erythropoiesis, erythropoietin, and iron. *Blood* 1982;60(6)1241–1246.
97. Eckardt KU, Kurtz A, Baver C. Triggering of erythropoietin production by hypoxia is inhibited by respiratory and metabolic acidosis. *Am J Physiol* 1990;258:R-678–R-683.

98. Rosen AL, Gould SA, Seghal LR, et al. Erythropoietin response to acute anemia. *Crit Care Med* 1990;18(3):298–302.
99. Levine EA, Rosen AL, Seghal LR, et al. Treatment of acute postoperative anemia with recombinant human erythropoietin. *J Trauma* 1989;29(8):1134–1139.
100. Erslev AJ, Wilson J, Caro J. Erythropoietin titers in anemic, nonuremic patients. *J Lab Clin Med* 1987;109(4):429–433.
101. Fisher JW. Pharmacologic modulation of erythropoietin production. *Annu Rev Pharmacol Toxicol* 1988;28:101–102.
102. Fisher JW, Nakashima J. The role of hypoxia in renal production of erythropoietin. *Cancer Suppl* 1992;70(4):928–929.
103. Gross DM, Fisher JW. Effects of terbutaline, a synthetic beta adrenoceptor agonist, on in vivo erythropoietin production. *Arch Int Pharmacodyn Ther* 1978;236:192–201.
104. Fink GD, Fisher JW. Erythropoietin production after renal denervation or beta-adrenergic blockade. *Am J Physiol* 1976;230:508–513.
105. Fisher JW, Roh BL, Halvorsen S. Inhibition of erythropoietic effect of hormones by erythropoietin antisera in mildly plethoric mice. *Proc Soc Exp Biol Med* 1967;126:97–100.
106. Peschle C, Sasso GF, Mastroberardino G, et al. The mechanism of endocrine influence on erythropoiesis. *J Lab Clin Med* 1971;70:20–29.
107. Jepson JH, Friesen HG. The mechanism of human placental lactogen on erythropoiesis. *Acta Haematol* 1968;15:465–471.
108. Peschle C, Zanjani ED, Gidari AS, et al. Mechanism of thyroxine action on erythropoiesis. *Endocrinology* 1971;89:609–612.
109. Alexanian R. Erythropoietin and erythropoiesis in anemic man following androgens. *Blood* 1969;33:564–571.
110. Coates PM, Brozovic B. Diurnal variation of serum immunoreactive erythropoietin in a normal subject. *Clin Endocrinol* 1982;17:419–422.
111. Wide L, Bengtsson C, Birgegård G. Circardian rhythm of erythropoietin in human serum. *Br J Haematol* 1989;72:85–90.
112. Paulo LG, Fink GD, Roh BL. Effects of several androgens and steroid metabolites on erythropoietin production in the isolated perfused dog kidney. *Blood* 1974;43:39–47.
113. Dukes PP, Goldwasser E. Inhibition of erythropoiesis by estrogens. *Endocrinology* 1961;69:21–29.
114. Mirand EA, Gordon AS. Mechanism of estrogen action in erythropoiesis. *Endocrinology* 1966;78:325–332.
115. Jelkmann W, Beckman B, Fisher JW. Enhanced effects of hypoxia on erythropoiesis in rabbits following beta-2 adrenergic actuation with albuterol. *J Pharmacol Exp Ther* 1979;211:99–103.
116. Goldwasser E, Jacobson LO, Fried W, et al. Studies on erythropoiesis. V. The effect of cobalt on the production of erythropoietin. *Blood* 1958;13:55.
117. Means RT. Clinical application of recombinant erythropoietin in the anemia of chronic renal disease. In: Spivak JL, ed. *Hematology Oncology Clinics of North America: Erythropoietin: Basic and Clinical Aspects.* Philadelphia: W.B. Saunders, 1994;8(5):934–935.
118. Koury MJ, Bondurant MC, Grabes SE, et al. Erythropoietin messenger RNA levels in developing mice and transfer of ^{125}I-erythropoietin by the placenta. *J Clin Invest* 1988;82:154–159.
119. Dessypres EN, Graber SE, Krantz SB, et al. Effects of recombinant erythro-

poietin on the concentration and cycling status of human marrow hematopoietic progenitor cells. *Blood* 1988;72:2060–2062.

120. Harina JH, Schmid CR, Rob JM. Bone marrow changes following treatment of renal anemia with erythropoietin. *Kidney Int* 1991;40:917–922.
121. Dessypres EN, Gleaton JH, Armstrong OL. Effect of human recombinant erythropoietin on human marrow megakaryocyte colony formation in vitro. *Br J Haematol* 1987;65:265–269.
122. Anagnostov A, Lee ES, Kessimian N, et al. Erythropoietin has mitogenic and positive chemotactic effect on endothelial cells. *Proc Natl Acad Sci USA* 1990;87:5978–5982.
123. Erickson N, Queensberry PJ. Regulation of erythropoiesis. The role of growth factors. *Med Clin North Am* 1992;76(3):745–755.
124. Kourey MJ, Bondurant MC, Atkinson JB. Erythropoietin control of terminal differentiation: maintenance of cell viability, production of hemoglobin, and development of the erythrocyte membrane. *Blood Cells* 1987;13:217–226.
125. Testa U, Pelosi E, Gabbiarelli M. Cascade transactivation of growth factor receptors in early human hematopoiesis. *Blood* 1993;81(6):1442–1456.
126. Sawada K, Krantz SB, Kai CH, et al. Purification of human blood burst-forming units—erythroid and demonstration of the evolution of erythropoietin receptors. *J Cell Physiol* 1990;142:219.
127. Sonada Y, Yang YC, Wong, GG, et al. Analysis in serum-free culture of the targets of recombinant human hemopoietic growth factor: interleukin 3 and granulocyte/macrophage-colony-stimulating factor are specific for early developmental stages. *Proc Natl Acad Sci USA* 1988;85:4360.
128. Migliaccio G, Migliaccio AR, Adamson JW. In vivo differentiation of human granulocyte/macrophage and erythroid progenitors: comparative analysis of the influence of recombinant human erythropoietin, G-CSF, CM-CSF, and IL-3 in serum-supplemented and serum-deprived cultures. *Blood* 1988; 72:248–256.
129. Krantz SB. Erythropoietin. *Blood* 1991;77(3):419–434.
130. Papayannopoulou T, Abkowitz J. Biology of erythropoiesis, erythroid differentiation, and maturation. In: Hoffman R, Benz JE Jr, Shattil SJ, et al., eds. *Hematology, Basic Principles and Practice.* New York: Churchill Livingstone, 1991;252–263.
131. Dessypres EN, Graber SE, Krantz SB, et al. Effects of recombinant erythropoietin on the concentration and cycling status of human marrow hemopoietic progenitor cells in vivo. *Blood* 1968;72:2060.
132. Dessypres EN, Krantz SB. Effect of pure erythropoietin on DNA synthesis by human marrow day 15 erythroid burst forming units in short-term liquid culture. *Br J Haematol* 1984;56:295.
133. Koury MJ, Bondurant MC. The mechanism of erythropoietin action. *Am J Kidney Dis* 1991;18(4):20–23.
134. Koury MJ, Bondurant MC. Erythropoietin retards DNA breakdown and prevents programmed death in erythroid progenitor cells. *Science* 1990; 248:378–381.
135. Kourey MJ, Bondurant MC. Maintenance by erythropoietin of viability and maturation of murine erythroid precursor cells. *J Cell Physiol* 1988;137:65.
136. Wickrena A, Krantz SA, Winkelmann, et al. Differentiation and erythropoietin receptor gene expression in human erythroid progenitor cells. *Blood* 1992;80(8):1940–1949.

137. Sawyer ST. The physiology and biochemistry of erythropoietin receptors. In: Erslev AJ, Adamson JW, Eschbach JW, Winearls CG, eds. *Erythropoietin Molecular, Cellular and Clinical Biology*. Baltimore: Johns Hopkins University Press, 1991;120.
138. Hillman, RS, Finch CA. Erythropoiesis: normal and abnormal. *Semin Hematol* 1967;4:327–336.
139. Papayannopulu T, Finch CA. On the in vivo action of erythropoietin: a quantitative analysis. *J Clin Invest* 1972;51:1179–1185.
140. Udupa KB, Crabtree HM, Lipshitz DA. In vitro culture of proerythroblasts: characterization of proliferative response to erythropoietin and steroids. *Br J Haematol* 1986;62:705–714.
141. Hanna IRA, Talbutt RG, Lamerton LF. Shortening of the cell-cycle time of erythroid precursors in response to anemia. *Br J Haemotol* 1969;16:381.
142. Rosen AL, Gould SA, Seghal LA, et al. Erythropoietic response to normovolemic anemia. *Fed Proc* 1985;44:1266.
143. Rapaport SI. Erythropoiesis. In: Rappaport SI, ed. *Introduction to Hematology*. New York: J.B. Lippincott, 1987;1–9.
144. Major A, Bauer C, Breymann C, et al. rh-Erythropoietin stimulates immature reticulocyte release in man. *Br J Hematol* 1994;87:605–608.
145. Hillmann RS. Characteristics of marrow production and reticulocyte maturation in normal man in response to anemia. *J Clin Invest* 1969;48:443–453.
146. Abkowitz JL, Holly RD, Hammend WP. Cyclic hematopoiesis in dogs: studies of erythroid burst forming cells confirm an early stem cell defect. *Exp Hematol* 1988;16:941.
147. Goodnough LT, Rudnick S, Price TH. Increased preoperative collection of autologous blood with recombinant erythropoietin therapy. *N Engl J Med* 1989;31:1163–1168.
148. Coleman DH, Stevens AR, Dode HT, Finch CA. Rate of blood regeneration after blood loss. *Arch Intern Med* 1953;92:341 – 349.
149. Kushner JP. Normochronic normocytic anemias. In: Wyngaarten JB, Smith LH, Bennett JC, eds. *Cecil Textbook of Medicine*. 19th ed. Philadelphia: W.B. Saunders, 1992;838.
150. Kushner JP. Hypochromic anemias. In: Wyngaarten JB, Smith LH, Bennett JC, eds. *Cecil Textbook of Medicine*. 19th ed. Philadelphia: W.B. Saunders, 1992;843.
151. Baker WF, Bick RL. Iron deficiency anemia. In: Bick RL, Bennet JM, Byrnes RK, et al., eds. *Hematology: Clinical and Laboratory Practice*. Boston: Mosby, 1993;257–279.
152. Rutherford CJ, Scheider TJ, Dempsey H, et al. Efficiency of different dosing regimens for recombinant human erythropoietin in a simulated perisurgical setting:the importance of iron availability in optimizing response. *Am J Med* 1994;96:139–145.
153. Brugnara C, Chambers LA, Malynn E, et al. Red blood cell regeneration induced by subcutaneous recombinant erythropoietin: iron deficient erythropoiesis in iron replete subjects. *Blood* 1993;81(4):956–964.
154. Fairbanks VF, Hines JD, Mazza JJ, et al. The anemias. In: Mazza JJ, ed. *Manual of Clinical Hematology*. New York: Little, Brown, 1995;32–36.
155. Gailani D. Anemia and transfusion therapy. In: Woodley M, Whelan A, eds. *The Washington Manual of Medical Therapeutics*. New York: Little, Brown, 1992;343–344.

156. Allen RH. Megaloblastic anemias. In: Wyngaarten JB, Smith LH, Bennett JC, eds. *Cecil Textbook of Medicine.* 19th ed. Philadelphia: W.B. Saunders, 1992;846–854.
157. Storring PL, Gaines Das RE. The international standard for recombinant DNA-derived erythropoietin: collaborative study of four DNA-derived erythropoietins and two highly purified human urinary erythropoietins. *J Endocr* 1992; 134:459–484.
158. Abraham PA, St Peter WI, Redic-Kill KA, et al. Controversies in determination of epoietin (recombinant) human erythropoietin dosages. *Clin Pharmacokinet* 1992;22(6):409–415.
159. Egrie JC, Strickland TW, Lane J, et al. Characterization and biological effects of recombinant human erythropoietin. *Immunobiology* 1986;172:213–214.
160. Egrie JC, Strickland TW, Lane J, et al. Characterization of pure-recombinant erythropoietin. *Exp Hematol* 1985;13(5):458.
161. Nightingale SL. FDA perspective: use of drugs for unlabeled indications. *Fam Physician* 1986:269.
162. Use of approved drugs for unlabeled indications. *FDA Drug Bull* 1982;12:4–5.
163. Spivak JL. Recombinant human erythropoietin and the anemia of cancer. *Blood* 1994;84(4):997–1004.
164. Abels RI. Use of recombinant human erythropoietin in the treatment of anemia in patients who have cancer. *Semin Oncol* 1992; 19(suppl 8):29–35.
165. Ohls RK, Wirkus PE, Christensen RD. Recombinant erythropoietin as treatment for the late hyporegenerative anemia of RH hemolytic disease. *Pediatrics* 1992;90:678–680.
166. Ohls RK, Christensen RD. Recombinant erythropoietin compared with erythrocyte transfusion in the treatment of the anemia of prematurity. *J Pediatr* 1991;119:781–788.
167. Henry DH. Recombinant human erythropoietin in the treatment of the anemia associated with solid tumors. In: Baver C, Koch KM, Selgalla P, Wieczorek L, eds. *Erythropoietin—Molecular Physiology and Clinical Applications.* New York: Marcel Dekker, 1993;293–298.
168. Tefferi A, Silverstein MN. Recombinant human erythropoietin therapy in patients with myelofibrosis with myeloid metaplasia. *Br J Hematol* 1994; 86:893–896.
169. Ayash LJ, Elias A, Hunt M, et al. Recombinant human erythropoietin for the treatment of the anemia associated with autologous bone marrow transplantation. *Br J Hematol* 1994;87:153–161.
170. Turba RM, Lewis VL, Green D. Pressure sore anemia: response to erythropoietin. *Arch Phys Med Rehabil* 1992;73:498.
171. Henry DH, Beall GN, Benson CA, et al. Recombinant human erythropoietin in the treatment of anemia associated with human immunodeficiency virus (HIV) infection and zidovudine therapy. Overview of four clinical trials. *Ann Intern Med* 1992;117(9):739–748.
172. Bowen D, Culligan D, Jacobs A. The treatment of anemia in the myelodysplastic syndromes with recombinant human erythropoietin. *Br J Hematol* 1991;77:419–423.
173. Mittleman M, Lessin LS. Clinical application of recombinant erythropoietin in myelodysplasia. In: Spivak JL, ed. *Hematology/Oncology Clinics of North America:Erythropoietin: Basics and Clinical Aspects.* Philadelphia: W.B. Saunders, 1994;8(5):993–1009.

174. Zeigler ZR, Rosenfeld CS, Shadduck RK. Resolution of transfusion dependence by recombinant erythropoietin (r-Hu EPO) in acquired pure red cell aplasia (PRCA) associated with myeloid metaplasia. *Br J Haematol* 1993; 83:28–29.
175. Carnielli V, Montini G, DaRiol R, et al. Effect of high dose human recombinant erythropoietin on the need for blood transfusion in pre-term infants. *J Pediatr* 1992;121:98–102.
176. Lopez J, Steegman JL, Perez G, et al. Erythropoietin in the treatment of delayed hemolysis of a major ABO-incompatible bone marrow transplant. *Am J Hematol* 1994;45:237–239.
177. Rodgers GP, Dover GJ, Uyesaka N, et al. Augmentation by erythropoietin of the fetal hemoglobin response to hydroxyuria in sickle cell disease. *N Engl J Med* 1993;328:73.
178. Olivieri NF, Freedman MH, Perrine SP, et al. Trial of recombinant human erythropoietin: three patients with thalassemia intermedia. *Blood* 1992; 80(12):3258.
179. Law EJ, Still JM, Gattis CS. The use of erythropoietin in two burned patients who are Jehovah's Witnesses. *Burns* 1991;17(1):75–77.
180. Kornowski R, Schwartz D, Jaffe A, et al. Erythropoietin therapy obviates the need for recurrent transfusions in a patient with severe hemolysis due to prosthetic valves. *Chest 1992;102(1):315–316.*
181. Glaspy JA, Chap L. The clinical application of recombinant erythropoietin in the HIV infected patient. In: Spivak JL, ed. *Hematology/Oncology Clinics of North America: Erythropoietin: Basics and Clinical Aspects.* Philadelphia: W.B. Saunders, 1994;8(5):993–1009.
182. Jacobs A, Janoswska-Wieczbrek A, Caro J. Circulating erythropoietin in patients with myclodysplastic syndromes. *Br J Haematol* 1989;73:36.
183. Eschbach JW, Egrie JC, Downing MR, et al. Correction of the anemia of end-stage renal disease with recombinant human erythropoietin. Results of a combined phase I and II clinical trial. *N Engl J Med* 1987;316(2):73–78.
184. Brune TH, Schindel-Kunzel F, Behringwerke AG. Pharmacokinetics and bioavailability of r-Hu-erythropoietin (EPO) expressed in C-127 mouse cells after subcutaneous application. *Am J Kidney Dis* 1991;18(4):105(abstract).
185. Brune TH, Schindel-Kunzel F. IV kinetics of r-Hu-erythropoietin (EPO) expressed in C-127 mouse cells: dose dependent and linear. *Am J Kidney Dis* 1991;18(4):105(abstract).
186. Ladeforged SD, Friedberg M, Eidmok I, et al. Subcutaneous versus intravenous administration of recombinant erythropoietin. *Am J Kidney Dis* 1990; 18(4):109(abstract).
187. McMahon FG, Vargas R, Ryan M, et al. Pharmacokinetics and effects of recombinant human erythropoietin after intravenous and subcutaneous injection in healthy volunteers. *Blood* 1990;76(9):1717–1722.
188. Flaherty KK, Caro J, Whalen J, et al. Pharmacokinetic and pharmacodynamic evaluation of human recombinant erythropoietin in healthy men. *Pharmacotherapy* 1989;abstract 9191.
189. Eschbach JW, Abdulhadi MH, Brown JK, et al. Recombinant human erythropoietin in anemic individuals with end-stage renal disease: results of a phase III multicenter clinical trial. *Ann Thorac Surg* 1989;11:992–1000.
190. Klingermann HG, Shepard JD, Eaves CJ, et al. The role of erythropoietin and other growth factors in transfusion medicine. *Transfusion Med Rev* 1991; 5(1):33–47.

191. Raine AEG, Phil D, Roger SD. Effects of erythropoietin on blood pressure. *Am J Kidney Dis* 1991;18(4)suppl:76–81.
192. London GM, Zins B, Ponnier B, et al. Vascular changes in hemodialysis patients in response to recombinant human erythropoietin. *Kidney Int* 1989;36:878–882.
193. Deschodt G, Granolleras C, Alsabadini B, et al. Changes in cardiac output, blood pressure, and peripheral resistance following treatment of renal anaemia by recombinant human erythropoietin. *Nephrol Dial Transplant* 1988;3:494–495.
194. Schaefer RM, Leschke M, Strauer BE, et al. Blood rheology and hypertension in hemodialysis patients treated with erythropoietin. *Am J Nephrol* 1988; 8:449–453.
195. Varl J, Ponikvor R, Drinovec J, et al. Complications and advantages during long term SC application of recombinant erythropoietin. *Am J Kidney Dis* 1991;18(4):115(abstract).
196. Bennett WM. Side effects of erythropoietin therapy. *Am J Kidney Dis* 1991;18(4):84–86.
197. Hisatomi K, Isomura T, Galli SJ, et al. Augmentation of interleukin-2 production after cardiac operations in patients treated with erythropoietin. *J Thorac Cardiovasc Surg* 1992;104:278–283.
198. Stifter S, Ludvik B, Watzinger U, et al. Erythropoietin improves regional cerebral blood perfusion in patients on chronic hemodialysis. *Am J Kidney Dis* 1991;18(4):108(abstract).
199. Horina JH, Fazekas F, Niederkorn K, et al. Cerebral hemodynamic changes following treatment with erythropoietin. *Nephron* 1991;58:407–412.
200. Johnson WJ, McCarthy JT, Yanagihara T, et al. Effects of recombinant human erythropoietin on cerebral and cutaneous blood flow on blood coagulability. *Kidney* 1990;38:919–924.
201. Casati S, Passenni P, Campise MR, et al. Benefits and risks of protracted treatment with human recombinant erythropoietin in patients having hemodialysis. *Br Med J* 1987;295:1017–1020.
202. Schaefer RM, Kuerner B, Zech M, et al. Treatment of the anemia of hemodialysis patients with recombinant human erythropoietin. *Int J Artif Organs* 1988;11:249–254.
203. Eschbach JW, Adamson JW. Recombinant human erythropoietin: implications for nephrology. *Am J Kidney Dis* 1988;11:203–209.
204. Anderson R. Recombinant human erythropoietin (EPO) effect on heparinization and dialyzer clotting in the chronic hemodialysis patient. *Am J Kidney Dis* 1991;18(4):103(abstract).
205. Martin-Lester M. Does the use of erythropoietin lead to increased risk of access failure? *Am J Kidney Dis* 1991;18(4):110(abstract).
206. Lynn KL, Shand BI, Buttimore AL, et al. Placebo-controlled study of blood viscosity and arteriovenous access in hemodialysis patients following erythropoietin administration. *Am J Kidney Dis* 1991;18(4):109(abstract).
207. Romijn JA. Erythropoietin. Letter to the editor. *N Engl J Med* 1991; 325(16):1176–1177.
208. Adamson JW, Vapnek D. Recombinant human erythropoietin to improve athletic performance. *N Engl J Med* 1991;324:698–699.
209. Sobh MA, Abdel-Hamid IA, Atta MG, et al. Sexual potency in uraemic patients before and after correction of anaemia with erythropoietin. *Am J Kidney Dis* 1991;18(4):113(abstract).

210. Sobh M, El-Tantawy A, Said E, et al. Effect of correction of anaemia by erythropoietin(EPO) in chronic haemodialysis patients on neuromuscular functions. Erythropoietin abstracts. *Am J Kidney Dis* 1991;18(4):113.
211. Ide H, Kakiuchi J, Furuta N, et al. The effect of cardiopulmonary bypass on T cells and their subpopulations. *Ann Thorac Surg* 1987;44:277–282.
212. Hisatomi K, Isomura T, Kawara T, et al. Changes in lymphocyte subsets, mitogen responsiveness, and interleukin-2 production after cardiac operations. *J Thorac Cardiovasc Surg* 1989;98:580–591.
213. Bessho M, Jinnai I, Matsuda, et al. Improvement of anemia by recombinant erythropoietin in patients with myelodysplastic syndromes and aplastic anemia. *Int J Cell Cloning* 1990;8:445–451.
214. Eschbach JW, Egrie JC, Downing MR, et al. The use of recombinant human erythropoietin (r-Hu EPO): effect in end stage renal disease (ESRD). In: Friedman HL, Beyer BS, DeSanto D, Giordano M, eds. *Prevention of Chronic Uremia.* Philadelphia: Field and Wood, 1988;148–155.
215. Abraham PA, Halstenson CI, Macres MM, et al. Epoietin enhances erythropoiesis in normal men undergoing repeated phlebotomies. *Clin Pharmacol Ther* 1992;52:205–213.
216. Red Book 1993. Montclair, NJ: *Medical Economics Data,* 1993;466.
217. Personal communication. Ortho Biotech Drug Information Line (1-800-325-7504).
218. Connor JP, Olsson CA. The use of recombinant erythropoietin in a Jehovah's Witness requiring major reconstructive surgery. *J Urol* 1992;147(l):131–132.
219. Atubek U, Spence RK, Pello M, et al. Pancreaticoduodenectomy without homologosy blood transfusion in an anemic Jehovah's Witness. *Arch Surg* 1992;127(1):349–351.
220. Toy PT, Strauss RG, Stehling CC, et al. Predeposited autologous blood for elective surgery: a national multicenter study. *N Engl J Med* 1987;316:517–520.
221. Goodnough LT. Autologous blood donation. *JAMA* 1988;259:2405.
222. Goodnough LT, Price TH, Rudnick S, et al. Preoperative red cell production in patients undergoing aggressive autologous blood with and without erythropoietin therapy. *Transfusion* 1992;32:441–445.
223. Levine EA, Rosen AL, Gould SA, et al. Recombinant human erythropoietin and autologous blood donation. *Surgery* 1988;104:365–369.
224. Maeda H, Hitomi Y, Hirata R, et al. Erythropoietin and autologous blood donation. *Lancet* 1989;2(8657):284.
225. Tasaki T, Ohto H, Hashimoto C, et al. Recombinant human erythropoietin for autologous blood donation: Effects on perioperative red-blood-cell and serum erythropoietin production. *Lancet* 1992;339:773–775.
226. Mercuriali F, Zaneila A, Barosi G, et al. Use of erythropoietin to increase the volume of autologous blood donated by orthopedic patients. *Transfusion* 1993;33:55–60.
227. Watanabe Y, Katsuo F, Konoshi T, et al. Autologous blood transfusion with recombinant human erythropoietin in heart operations. *Ann Thorac Surg,* 1991;51:767–772.
228. Watanabe Y, Katsuo F, Naruse Y, et al. Subcutaneous use of erythropoietin in heart surgery. *Ann Thorac Surg* 1992;54:479–484.
229. Bommer J, Samherber W, Koch WM, et al. Variations of recombinant human erythropoietin applications in hemodialysis patients. *Contrib Nephrol* 1989; 76:149–158.

230. Besarb A, Vlasses P, Caro J, et al. Subcutaneous (SC) administration of recombinant human erythropoietin (H-rEPO) for treatment of ESRD anemia. *Kidney Int* 1990;37:236(abstract).
231. Graf H, Barnas U, Loibel U, et al. Subcutaneous versus intravenous administration of recombinant erythropoietin. A prospective study of effectiveness and side-effects. *Nephrol Dial Transplant* 1989;4:473(abstract).
232. Kulier Alt, Gombotz H, Fuchs G, et al. Subcutaneous recombinant human erythropoietin and autologous blood donation before coronary artery bypass surgery. *Anesth Analg* 1993;76:102–106.
233. Brugnara C, Chambers LA, Malynn E, et al. Red blood cell regeneration induced by subcutaneous recombinant erythropoietin. *Blood* 1993;81(4): 956–964.
234. Finch CA. Erythropoiesis, erythropoietin, and iron. *Blood* 1982;60(6): 1241–1246.
235. Van Wyck DB, Stivelman JC, Ruiz J. Iron status in patients receiving erythropoietin for dialysis-associated anemia. *Kidney Int* 1989;35:712–716.
236. Konoshi T, Ohbayashi T, Kaneko T, et al. Preoperative use of erythropoietin for cardiovascular operations in anemia. *Ann Thorac Surg* 1993;56:101–103.
237. Fullerton DA, Campbell DN, Whitman GJR. Use of human recombinant erythropoietin to correct severe preoperative anemia. *Ann Thorac Surg* 1991;51:825–826.
238. Guadini VA, Mason HDW. Preoperative erythropoietin in Jehovah's Witnesses who require cardiac operations. *Ann Thorac Surg* 1991;51:823–824.
239. Hoynck van Papendricht MA, Jeekel H, Busch OR, et al. Efficacy of recombinant erythropoietin for stimulating erythropoiesis after blood loss and surgery. *Eur J Surg* 1992; 158:83–87.
240. D'Ambra MN, Lynch KE, Boccagno J, et al. The effect of perioperative administration of recombinant human erythropoietin (r-HuEPO) in CABG patients: a double blind, placebo-controlled trial. *Anesthesiology* 1992; 77(3a):A159(abstract).
241. Levine EA, Rosen AL, Sehgal LR, et al. Erythropoietin deficiency after coronary artery bypass procedures. *Ann Thorac Surg* 1991;51:764–766.
242. Etchason J, Petz L, Keeler E, et al. The cost effectiveness of preoperative autologous blood donation. *N Engl J Med* 1995;332:719–724.
243. Rutherford CJ, Kaplan HS. Autologous blood donation—can we bank on it? *N Engl J Med* 1995;332:740–742.

5
AIDS Risk in Cardiac Surgery

NASSER K. ALTORKI, THOMAS W. NASH, AND CARL F.W. WOLF

Since its initial recognition in 1981, the acquired immune deficiency syndrome (AIDS) has become a nationwide as well as a worldwide pandemic reported from practically every continent. In the United States, 80,961 AIDS cases were reported in 1994 alone and the cumulative AIDS cases since 1981 are over 440,000.[1] More importantly, it is estimated that 1 in 250 Americans is infected with the human immunodeficiency virus (HIV).[2] Although initial epidemiologic reports identified homosexual men as a high-risk group for acquiring HIV infection, it is now apparent that practically every segment of society is vulnerable regardless of its race, gender, or lifestyle. Indeed, the number of AIDS cases attributed to heterosexual contact increased by 21% from 1990 to 1991. While the majority of AIDS cases are still reported in major urban areas, more than 5% have been reported from nonmetropolitan areas. The rate of reported AIDS cases in nonmetropolitan areas is increasing faster than that in urban areas.

The almost universally fatal outcome of patients in the early years of the epidemic instilled an irrational fear among all segments of society in dealing with HIV-infected individuals to the extent that victims of the disease became social pariahs stigmatized by society and shunned by family and friends. Physicians in general and surgeons in particular were faced, for perhaps the first time since the black deaths of the Middle Ages, with the ethical issues of caring for patients who have a potentially communicable and a frequently highly lethal disease. Concerns over the possibility of disease transmission from patients to health care workers (HCWs) and vice versa have fueled a frenzied and often hysterical political and social debate improperly aimed at mandatory physician testing and even penalization of seropositive health care workers. Like all irrational arguments, this had no foundation in factual knowledge or scientific methodology. Perhaps the major benefit of that social and political hysteria was the initiative undertaken by the medical community as a whole to rationally evaluate the potential threat to patient and physician alike and thus establish rational guidelines of care. This medical debate has been guided by the basic tenets of Hippocratic medicine as expressed by the recommendations of the Governor's Committee on AIDS for the American College of Surgeons (ACS). The series of recommendations developed at the ACS Clinical Congress in Chicago in October 1991 begin by stating that "Surgeons have the same ethical obligation to render care to HIV-infected patients as they have for other patients."

This chapter examines several relevant questions:

1. What is the risk of occupational HIV transmission to the health care worker from an infected patient?
2. What is the risk of HIV transmission to a patient from an infected health care worker?
3. What is the risk of HIV transmission to a patient from transfusion of blood and blood products?
4. What is the role of intraoperative protective measures?
5. What are the guidelines for patient and physician testing?
6. What is the management of an individual following documented HIV exposure?

Occupational Risk of Viral Transmission to Health Care Workers

Hepatitis B Virus Exposure

Despite the anxiety generated by the possibility of occupational transmission of HIV, the hepatitis virus remains the leading occupationally acquired blood-borne pathogen.[2] Viral hepatitis is caused by several viral strains among which the hepatitis B virus (HBV) poses the greatest threat to HCWs. HBV is transmitted via transfusions, percutaneous blood exposure, or sexual intercourse. In actively infected individuals as many 10^9 viral particles may be present in a milliliter of serum. Although the disease resolves in the great majority of patients without significant sequelae, 5% develop chronic active hepatitis and become chronic carriers of the disease.[3] Approximately 0.5% to 5% of all hospitalized patients are HBV carriers.[4] It is this pool of patients who are HBV-Ag positive that should be the main concern of HCWs. The Centers for Disease Control (CDC) estimates that 5100 HCWs were infected by the HBV in 1991 through occupational exposure and that 125 of them will eventually die from their disease.[4] A recent study reported that the prevalence of HBV antigen positivity among surgeons was 17%, more than threefold higher than the 5% prevalence noted for the population at large.[4] None of the surgeons who tested positive for HBV antigen reported nonoccupational risk factors. The high viral titers in the blood of HBV carriers accounts for a 30% probability of acquiring the infection following occupational exposure.[5]

Conversely, over 300 patients developed HBV antigenemia following treatment by an HBV-infected HCW[6]—dentists, general practitioners, general surgeons, as well as cardiothoracic surgeons.[7-12] In the majority of cases infection could have been prevented if customary infection control guidelines such as glove use were adhered to. Nonetheless transmission still occurred despite glove use in cases linked to obstetricians, general surgeons, and cardiovascular surgeons.[10,12] Presumably in such instances undetected sharp instrument injury to the surgeon resulted in contamination of the operative field.

The introduction of a hepatitis B vaccine derived through recombinant technology should, together with strict application of infection control guidelines, result in a significant improvement in reported transmission rates.[13] The vaccine should be given to all surgeons who are HBV antigen negative. A 10-μg dose is given intramuscularly in the deltoid region and repeated at 1 and 6 months. A booster dose may be required at 5- to 7-year intervals. HBV antigen positive surgeons should be guided by the CDC recommendations governing practice guidelines (Table 5.1).

HIV Exposure

Risk to Health Care Workers

To date 57 HCWs had documented seroconversion following exposure to HIV infected blood.[14] That group includes one surgeon, as well as other physicians, phlebotomists, nurses, and laboratory staff. Interestingly, the majority of injuries that resulted in seroconversions in an HCW have occurred on the ward rather than in the operating room. A serostudy of surgeons working in 21 hospitals in or adjacent to two major metropolitan areas with a high prevalence of HIV showed that out of 770 voluntary participants only one was HIV infected.[4] The seropositive surgeon, a general surgeon, reported three percutaneous injuries involving patients with AIDS and did not report nonoccupational risk factors for HIV. Clearly the probability of nosocomial transmission of HIV from patient to HCW in general is low and from patient to surgeon in particular is even lower. The risk is estimated at 0.2% to 0.5% per year compared to 30% for HBV transmission.[14,15] The risk of HIV transmission to surgical personnel was calculated at a major metropolitan hospital with a high prevalence of HIV-infected patients.[16] The estimated risk was 0.125 infections per year or 1 infection every 8 years.[16] The authors stated that the risk would be even lower (1 in every 80 years) in areas of the country where the prevalence of HIV infection is less than 3%. None of the previous studies, however, has included cardiothoracic surgeons.

The risk of viral transmission from patients to HCWs depends on the nature of the injury (parenteral vs mucous membrane exposure) and on the infectivity of the virus, which varies from one patient to the other and

TABLE 5.1. Recommendations for preventing transmission of human immunodeficiency virus and hepatitis B virus to patients during exposure-prone invasive procedures.

1. All HCWs should adhere to universal precautions, including the appropriate hand washing, use of protective barriers, and care in the use and disposal of needles and other sharp instruments. HCWs who have exudative lesions or weeping dermatitis should refrain from all direct patient care and from handling patient-care equipment and devices used in performing invasive procedures until the condition resolves. HCWs should also comply with current guidelines for disinfection and sterilization of reusable devices used in invasive procedures.
2. Currently available data provide no basis for recommendations to restrict the practice of HCWs infected with HIV or HBV who perform invasive procedures not identified as exposure-prone, provided the infected HCWs practice recommended surgical or dental technique and comply with universal precautions and current recommendations for sterilization/disinfection.
3. Exposure-prone procedures should be identified by medical/surgical/dental organizations and institutions at which the procedures are performed.
4. HCWs who perform exposure-prone procedures should know their HIV antibody status. HCWs who perform exposure-prone procedures and who do not have serologic evidence of immunity to HBV from vaccination of from previous infection should know their HBsAg status and, if that is positive, should also know their HBeAg status.
5. HCWs who are infected with HIV or HBV (and are HBeAg positive) should not perform exposure-prone procedures unless they have sought counsel from an expert review panel and been advised under what circumstances, if any, they may continue to perform these procedures. Such circumstances would include notifying prospective patients of the HCW's seropositivity before they undergo exposure-prone invasive procedures.
6. Mandatory testing of HCWs for HIV antibody, HBsAg, or HBeAg is not recommended. The current assessment of the risk that infected HCWs will transmit HIV or HBV to patients during exposure-prone procedures does not support the diversion of resources that would be required to implement mandatory testing programs. Compliance by HCWs with recommendations can be increased through education, training, and appropriate confidentiality safeguards.

by the stage of the disease in the same patient. Notwithstanding the low rate of transmission, the outcome is likely to be fatal, and every attempt should be made to further reduce the probability of occupationally acquired HIV.

Risk to Patients

The first confirmed HIV transmission from an HCW to a patient was reported by the CDC in 1990.[17] The case involved a female patient of an HIV-infected dentist. Five additional patients of the same dentist with no other apparent risk factors for HIV had since seroconverted as well.[18] Nucleotide sequencing of the virus from all five patients indicated genomic relatedness to the dentist's virus. To date these remain the only confirmed cases of seroconversion of patients treated by an infected HCW. HIV testing of approximately 18,000 patients treated by 57 other HIV-positive HCWs, including surgeons, revealed that 92 patients were seropositive.[14]

Eighty-five patients had significant risk factors for HIV while seven were infected prior to being treated by the HCW. HIV nucleotide sequencing was done in 27 patients treated by three HCWs, none of whom had genetically related virus to those of the HCW.

Several look-back studies investigated the risk of HIV transmission from HIV-infected surgeons to their patients. Most had a small sample size and HIV testing was not commonly performed, particularly in the earlier studies. Over 7,500 patients were reported in seven studies and approximately 33% were HIV tested.[19–25] Only two patients were seropositive, one with known risk factors and another whose infection was traced to an unscreened blood transfusion. In the only report involving an HIV-positive cardiothoracic surgeon, 612 patients were examined, none of whom developed AIDS or an AIDS-related complex.[25] Specifically, among 189 patients tested for HIV, no positive results were obtained. The probability of HIV viral transmission from surgeon to patient has been mathematically estimated based on (1) the rate of intraoperative injury to the surgeon or their assistants (0.008), (2) the probability of the surgeons being HIV positive (0.004), and (3) the risk of transmission of HIV infection after a single puncture wound.[26] In such a mathematical construct the risk was estimated at $0.008 \times 0.004 \times 0.0015 = 4.8 \times 10^{-8}$, or 1 chance in 21 million per hour of surgery. Despite a nonzero risk, it is estimated that the risk of contracting HIV from a surgeon with unknown HIV status is ten times less likely than being struck by lightning and twice as likely as being hit by a falling aircraft.[27] The risk of acquiring HIV from an HIV-positive surgeon is one-tenth the chance of dying from anesthesia.[28] This is a stark contrast to the risk posed by HBV-infected surgeons. Over 330 patients have acquired HBV infection following treatment by 33 HBV-infected HCWs including 20 surgeons.[29] Thus HBV remains the single most common and most serious nosocomially transmissible viral agent for patient and surgeon alike.

Risk of Blood Transfusion

As described in Chapter 1, the current risk to a recipient of a blood transfusion of either hepatitis B or HIV is very small. The risk of hepatitis C is much higher, being estimated at 1 in 2,000 to 1 in 6,000.[30] The hepatitis B risk is currently estimated at 1 in 200,000,[31] and the incidence rate of acute hepatitis B in blood recipients does not differ from the overall reported rate for hepatitis B in the nontransfused population.[32]

HIV infection continues to cause the greatest concern among transfusion recipients even though it is probably one of the least frequent adverse effects of transfusion. With the advent of donor testing for antibody to HIV in 1985, the risk of transfusion-transmitted HIV decreased dramatically. Subsequently, the assay has been improved in sensitivity, interviewing techniques for the exclusion of high risk donors have been improved, and new assays for hepatitis C (1990), an assay for human T-cell lymphotropic virus (HTLV)-I/II (1989), and surrogate assays for non-A and non-B hepatitis (1986) have been added to donor screening procedures, all of which also decrease the probability of HIV transmission.

The risk of HIV infection from transfusion is currently cited as 1 in 225,000.[31,33] In a prospective study of cardiac surgery patients transfused between 1985 and 1991 in Texas and Maryland, there were two seroconversions in a group of patients who received 120,301 units of blood, for a rate of infection of one in 60,000 units.[34] Because the assays for HIV are currently assays for antibody and not for the virus itself, there is a potential "window" period between infection and formation of detectable antibody. As assays for the antibody improve in sensitivity, that window becomes smaller, but cannot reach zero. For that reason, a test for the HIV antigen is currently under consideration.[35] Recent data suggest that the risk of a donation from an HIV-seronegative donor being infectious for HIV (presumably due to the donor having a recent infection and not yet having made a detectable antibody—the so-called window period—and not testing positive on any of the other screening tests performed on donor blood) has now declined to less than 1 in 440,000 units.[36] If the average recipient receives four units, the risk becomes one in 110,000 units.

Intraoperative Preventive Measures

As stated previously, viral transmission occurs primarily through parenteral exposure either through direct inoculation into the vascular space or by exposure through broken skin (such as dermatitis) to HIV-infected blood. Interestingly only a few studies have evaluated the frequency of exposure to blood and other body fluids in the operating room. An observational study involving over 1300 consecutive surgical procedures was undertaken at San Francisco General Hospital (SFGH), an institution where the prevalence of HIV among surgical patients approaches 25%. Accidental overall blood exposure occurred in 8.3% of cases, with parenteral exposure in 1.7%.[16] The risk of exposure was highest for procedures lasting more than 3 hours and those associated with blood loss exceeding 300 ml. Interestingly, a preexisting knowledge of the patient's HIV status did not alter the exposure rate. The high prevalence of HIV infection among surgical patients within the institution may have prompted strict adherence to high standards of infection control. This may not necessarily be the case at institutions with a lower HIV prevalence where awareness of preexisting seropositivity may have an impact on decreasing exposure rates. In fact, at least two other studies have shown that overall blood exposure rate was significantly higher than that reported at SFGH. Blood-skin contact was reported by 87% and percutaneous injury by 40% of orthopedic surgeons surveyed by the American Academy of Orthopedic Surgeons.[37] In another study, Quebbeman et al[38] reported a 50% intraoperative cutaneous exposure rate and 15% injury rate among surgical personnel at the Medical College of Wisconsin. Blood contamination was particularly frequent in cardiothoracic procedures, with finger injuries and splash facial exposures being the most common pattern. Furthermore, it appears that exposure risk is higher for the surgeon and first assistant than for the other members of the operating team.

The majority of percutaneous injuries occur as a result of suture needles when personnel manually handle the needle for loading onto a needle holder or by suturing within the depth of a body cavity and using the index finger of the nondominant hand to locate the needle. Most intraoperative exposure and injuries can be reduced to a minimum by enforcing strict adherence to infection control practices, improved barrier protection, and modification of surgical techniques. Beyond the usual use of surgical caps and masks, the use of face shields essentially eliminates any chance of facial or conjunctival splashes when compared with the protection conferred by glasses or goggles. The use of double gloves and wearing waterproof gowns drastically decreases, but does not totally eliminate, finger injuries from suture needles and forearm and chest blood exposure.[39] Sleeve covers should be routinely used to minimize forearm cutaneous blood exposure while the use of waterproof high boots decreases the odds of the often unrecognized foot or ankle exposure.

Technique modification is the single most effective means of intraoperative protection.[14] Sharp instruments should be placed in a neutral zone between the surgeon and the scrub nurse so that they do not handle instruments at the same time. Needles should preferably be loaded onto needle holders using a forceps and should never be located in the depth of a wound by finger palpation. The surgeon must, whenever possible, handle the tissue with instruments, thus minimizing direct manual manipulations. Overall high levels of vigilance in intraoperative maneuvers should be practiced in every case regardless of the serostatus of the patient.

Management of Occupational Exposure

Rational management of HCWs exposed to HIV depends on the risk that a particular occupational exposure can transmit HIV from the patient to the HCW. In the 1980s, studies of occupational exposure suggested that in 1 in 250 to 1 in 300 exposures resulted in HIV transmission to the HCW. The analysis did not take into account factors that can greatly increase or decrease that transmission rate. Studies in Europe and North America of HCWs occupationally exposed to HIV have identified risk factors that, if present, significantly increase the likelihood that a particular exposure can transmit HIV.[40–45] The decision to institute postexposure prophylaxis depends in large measure on the presence or absence of these factors.

Type of Exposure

Deep needlestick exposures present the greatest risk to the HCW. Mucocutaneous exposures are much less hazardous. In the CDC study of 42 infected HCWs, 36 acquired infection via needlestick exposure and four were infected following mucocutaneous exposure to HIV (one had both types of exposure and one had an undetermined type of exposure). Of 1143 mucous membrane exposures compiled from multiple studies, only one resulted in HIV infection (0.09%). A National Institutes of Health study reported that none of the 2712 HCWs who had skin-only contact with HIV-infected blood became infected. HIV infection has been rarely reported from skin contact only; in these cases the skin involved was not intact (abrasion, skin disorders). Therefore, these cases should more accurately be classified as unapparent percutaneous exposures. The risk for skin-only contact is therefore negligible unless the contact is prolonged and/or the skin integrity is compromised.

Volume of Inoculum

The quantity of infected blood transmitted to the HCW is a major issue. A hollow-bore needle can transmit twice as much blood as a similarly sized suture needle. Gloves can reduce the blood inoculum by a significant factor. The CDC has analyzed multiple needlestick exposures and found that two critical risk factors increased the inoculum volume and therefore greatly increased the chance of HIV infection:

1. Visible blood on the needle;
2. Procedure involving the needle being placed directly into an artery or vein (i.e., venipuncture, and not a needle used for administering medication through IV tubing).

The inoculum introduced via percutaneous injury from sharps and scalpels is much smaller and HIV risk is correspondingly far less. Of the 37 percutaneous exposures that resulted in HIV infection that were reported in the CDC study, 34 involved hollow-bore needles, one a scalpel, one a broken vial, and one an unspecified sharp object.

HIV Viral Load of the Infected Blood or Body Fluid

The possibility that a particular percutaneous exposure will transmit HIV also depends on the amount of circulating HIV in that patient's blood. The number of virions per milliliter of blood (the viral load) can range from near zero in patients successfully treated with newer combination antiretroviral therapies, to more than one million in patients in the terminal stages of HIV who have not responded to or who have not received effective therapy. The highest viral loads are typically seen in patients in the late, terminal stages of HIV *and* in patients who are newly infected with HIV (in the first 6 to 12 weeks after infection). In one survey, no needlestick from an asymptomatic HIV-infected patient resulted in HIV infection in HCWs, but 0.4% of needlestick exposures (4 cases following 889 needlesticks) from symptomatic late-stage HIV patients caused HIV infection in HCWs.

Nonbloody fluids have not been shown to transmit HIV in the health care setting except after accidental research laboratory exposure to high titers of HIV in culture fluid. HIV infection has been reported in HCWs via nonblood exposure after a needlestick injury with a needle that had been used for the thoracentesis of bloody pleural fluid. HIV is primarily cell associated in body fluids (these fluids also contain varying amounts of cell free virus). So, body fluids with a cellular component (especially lymphocytes and macrophages), are more likely to be infectious. Semen, vaginal secretions, cerebrospinal fluid, saliva following dental work or oral trauma, and pleural and peritoneal fluid should be considered capable of transmitting HIV, albeit at a low rate. Urine, nonbloody saliva, tears, and feces pose an extremely low (probably zero) risk of HIV transmission.

Management Following Occupational Exposure

Standard local wound care should be provided to the area of exposure, although there is no reason to believe that local disinfectants will impair the ability of inoculated HIV to initiate an infection.

The HCW should be tested for HIV at the time of exposure. Informed medical personnel should provide supportive counseling about the medical and psychological issues surrounding HIV exposure. This counseling should include:

1. A review of the likelihood of occupational transmission of HIV to reduce the anxiety that is likely to ensue before serologic tests can document whether HIV infection has or has not occurred. The HCW should be told that experience and research have shown that 99.7% or so of HCWs who are occupationally exposed to HIV do not develop HIV infection, even if the HCW does *not* take postexposure prophylaxis.
2. A review of the pros and cons of immediate antiviral therapy (see below).
3. A review of the exposure event to make sure that the HCW understands if any breach of universal precautions occurred and how this may be prevented in the future.
4. A discussion about the minuscule potential for transmission of HIV by the HCW to household contacts (other than sexual partners) and coworkers.
5. A review of safe sex practices with strong recommendation that these practices be followed until the "window" period has passed and there has been documentation of noninfection with HIV.

There is no scientific reason to curtail the clinical duties of potentially infected HCW during this window period. Numerous large studies[14–16] have failed to demonstrate that an HIV-infected HCW poses a risk of HIV infection to patients, with the possible exception of the cluster of HIV-infected patients associated with a Florida dentist in 1990.[17] Notwithstanding that event, the case for HCW-to-patient transmission has not been firmly established. Some restrictive hospital regulations regarding HIV-infected HCWs have been influenced by the fear and emotion surrounding the potential for HIV infections rather than a careful assessment of the relative risk of transmitting this infection to patients.

The question about whether HCWs exposed to HIV should receive postexposure prophylactic antiretroviral therapy was a controversial and unanswered one until late 1995. There were until then a number of well-documented cases in which zidovudine, administered to HCWs immediately after HIV exposure failed to prevent HIV infection. These cases mirrored similar data in macaque (chosen for their immunologic similarity to humans) models in which postexposure administration of zidovudine did not reliably prevent similar immunodeficiency viral infection.

Four important developments in antiretroviral research dramatically changed the outlook and recommendations for postexposure prophylaxis:

1. A 1995 case control study[40] done in the United States, France, and Great Britain of HCWs occupationally exposed to HIV blood demonstrated that those who took zidovudine immediately after exposure had a 79% lower risk of infection with HIV.
2. The use of zidovudine monotherapy as a therapeutic standard for years had resulted in the emergence of zidovudine-resistant HIV strains. These strains were found both in patients who had been on zidovudine for months or years and in newly infected patients who had never received zidovudine. These latter patients had been primarily infected with zidovudine-resistant strains. This prevalence of zidovudine-resistant HIV strains undermined the potential effectiveness of zidovudine as a single drug in postexposure prophylaxis.
3. In late 1995 and through 1996, a number of studies demonstrated that combination therapy with two or three antiviral agents (sometimes including zidovudine) was far more effective than the previous standard therapy of zidovudine alone and was effective even in patients with zidovudine-resistant HIV.
4. Studies performed in early 1996 demonstrated that protease inhibitors (a class of drugs that can inhibit the activity of HIV protease enzymes) were impressively potent anti-HIV agents.[46,47] These drugs had the capacity, especially in combination with one or two of the older agents to produce up to 2-log reduction in viral load. Multiple studies demonstrated that in approximately 85% of patients treated with these protease containing

drug combinations, circulating viral loads were reduced to nonmeasurable levels.

These findings have formed the foundation for the following recommendations for postexposure antiviral therapy (adapted from the CDC, the U.S. Public Health Service, and the International AIDS Society)[42,44,48]:

1. Postexposure prophylaxis should be strongly recommended to HCWs who have had HIV exposures that can be described as high risk (e.g., hollow-bore needle puncture, deep tissue injury, etc.). HCWs who had low-risk occupational HIV exposure (e.g., mucocutaneous exposure) should be offered antiviral therapy. Postexposure antiviral therapy is not appropriate for those HCWs who have had occupational exposure with a negligible risk of transmitting HIV (e.g., needlestick exposure that cannot transmit blood, such as a needle used for administering fluids or medication through an intravenous line or Heplock).
2. Prophylaxis should be started as soon as possible after exposure, preferably within 1 to 3 hours after exposure. Postexposure prophylaxis administered more than a few hours after exposure should not be considered futile. In the animal models in which postexposure prophylaxis effectively thwarted HIV infection, antiviral therapy was successful only if administered immediately after infection. These animal model results have limited applicability to the human situation because the mode of animal infection (usually direct intravenous inoculation of virus) and the mechanics of infection (these experiments used mice and cats and HIV, or macaques and the simian immunodeficiency virus) are quite different from the circumstances of HCW exposure. There are no human studies that show when it is too late to administer effective postexposure prophylaxis. Even if HIV infection has been possibly established by the time postexposure prophylaxis is considered, antiviral therapy should be vigorously recommended. New studies have shown that the prognosis in HIV infection depends in part on the viral load that develops shortly after initial infection. Aggressive antiviral therapy early after the initial HIV infection may therefore improve prognosis by reducing this viral load.
3. HCWs who receive postexposure prophylaxis should receive a two- or three-drug regimen of antiviral agents. Zidovudine should be included in this regimen because the formal studies on postexposure prophylaxis have examined only the impact of zidovudine. It is likely that any other anti-HIV drug or regimen that has been shown to be clinically effective would also be effective in the postexposure setting, but there are no data yet to support this assumption. Zidovudine should be combined with lamivudine, and a protease inhibitor, preferably inandivir, should be added to the regimen if there is a reasonable possibility that the patient has zidovudine- or lamivudine-resistant HIV or if the exposure is a

high-risk one. Dideoxyinosine (DDI) may be substituted for zidovudine if the source patient has received zidovudine (especially in monotherapy) for more than 12 months or if the patient had exhibited clinical deterioration or biologic signs of drug resistance (e.g., rising serum viral titers over the preceding few months) while on a zidovudine containing antiviral regimen. If there is a reason to suspect drug resistance to lamivudine or inandivir (for example, if the source patient had been on these drugs for months), a different regimen should be selected with the advice of an infectious disease consultant. The doses for these drugs are as follows: zidovudine 200 mg every 8 hours, lamivudine 150 mg every 12 hours, and inandivir 800 mg every 8 hours. Inandivir must be taken on an empty stomach; the q8h dosing must be followed closely and the HCW should drink at least 48 ounces of fluid per day.

The optimal duration of this postexposure regimen has not been established, but a 4-week course is reasonable as 4 weeks of zidovudine has been shown to be effective. The antiviral drugs listed above are usually well tolerated, especially for a short, 4-week course. The major side effects of these antiviral drugs are the following:

1. Zidovudine—nausea, headache, fatigue, anemia.
2. Lamivudine—nausea.
3. Inandivir—nausea, hyperbilirubinemia, renal stones, flank pain. Up to 4% of patients on inandivir therapy may develop kidney stones and/or flank pain. Ample fluid intake can reduce this risk. The risk during 4 weeks of therapy is less than 1%.
4. DDI—nausea, diarrhea, neuropathy, pancreatitis. Neuropathy usually occurs after months of therapy.

Zidovudine has not been reported to produce any problems when administered during pregnancy. The safety of the other agents during pregnancy is unknown.

Patient/Physician Testing

The presence or absence of HIV infection in either patients or physicians can be determined accurately by serologic tests; the enzyme-linked immunoabsorbant assay (ELISA), and the Western blot tests are most commonly used. These assays detect serum antibodies directed against the core and envelope proteins of HIV. The most widely used ELISA kit uses a recombinant HIV viral lysate as an antibody target. Antibodies directed against HIV can be produced as early as 2 weeks after infection, but are not present in reliably detectable amounts until at least 3 and certainly by 6 months after infection.

The most recent versions of the ELISA and Western blot tests have a sensitivity and specificity on the order of 99%. The predictive accuracy of both of these tests depends on the pretest probability that the person to be tested has a high or low likelihood of actually having the HIV virus. The likelihood that a negative ELISA test is falsely negative (that is, the patient being tested actually has the HIV virus, but the ELISA test remains negative) has been estimated at 1 in 40,000 to 1 in 1,000,000. Given the newest modifications of the ELISA test, the latter is likely to be the more accurate figure. Western blot tests can be falsely negative very early in the course of HIV infection and rarely during the terminal stages of HIV infection when overall antibody production wanes. The estimated false-negative rate for Western blot is approximately 1 in 250,000.

If the ELISA assay is positive, a confirmatory test, usually the Western blot test, is routinely done. False-positive Western blot tests are extremely rare (approximately 1 in 20,000). These false-positive cases are usually attributable to cross-reacting antibodies seen in patients with excess antibody production (e.g., gammopathies). When run together, the ELISA and Western blot tests are virtually always in concordance. Both the ELISA and Western blot tests must be positive before one can make a reliable *serologic* diagnosis of HIV.[49-53]

If the ELISA or Western blot tests are nondiagnostic or controversial (some ELISA test results can be marginally positive, and confirmatory Western blot tests are indeterminate), there are a number of strategies that can be employed to determine if a valid HIV infection exists:

1. The Western blot test can be repeated in 3 and 6 months. If there is a true HIV infection, more antibodies to HIV antigens will develop over this time and the Western blot will become overtly positive.
2. Direct measurement and approximate quantitation of circulating HIV-RNA can now be done using recombinant techniques, either the polymerase chain reaction (PCR) or branched DNA (bDNA) chain signal amplification. These tests represent a major advance in the early and accurate detection of HIV-RNA in serum. Both are superior to p24 antigen testing and direct viral culture. The PCR and bDNA assays are equivalently sensitive and can detect as low as 200 to 1,000 copies of HIV-RNA per milliliter of serum. Both are highly reproducible and reliable assays. HIV-RNA has been detected by these assays *before* seroconversion has been documented. If these recombinant methods are fully validated by ongoing studies, they will be a useful supplement to the ELISA test in the early detection of HIV infection.[51,54] The FDA approved the PCR test in June 1996.
3. The serum in question can be tested directly for HIV by viral culture. This is a time-consuming and potentially dangerous process that is

susceptible to laboratory contamination and therefore false-positive tests. Given the low levels of viremia seen during much of the course of the HIV infection, the chance of detecting early HIV infection by viral culture ranges from only 65% to 100%.[49]

4. HIVp24 (core) antigen can be assayed directly from serum samples. P24 antigenemia occurs early in the course of HIV infection, before antibodies to HIV are formed. Serum samples drawn during the acute retroviral syndrome (see below) are most likely to contain detectable p24 antigen, but not all samples will. P24 antigen is detected unreliably and inconsistently during most of the course of the HIV infection. When anti-HIV antibodies appear (including anti-p24 antibodies), p24 antigenemia decreases to often undetectable amounts, only to rise again during the terminal stages of the HIV infection. The p24 antigen test has been replaced by the more accurate HIV-RNA assays.

The interval between infection with HIV and the detection of diagnostic levels of anti-HIV antibody is commonly termed the window period. The ELISA test is more likely to become positive earlier in the course of HIV infections than the Western blot. Patients tested during this typically 4- to 6-month period usually do not have detectable antibody to HIV or their ELISA and/or Western blot tests are indeterminate. The ELISA test is more likely to become positive earlier in the course of bona fide HIV infections than the Western blot. Six months after exposure (occupational or otherwise) to HIV, antibodies can be detected to HIV in virtually all cases in which HIV infection has occurred. There are extremely rare and unusual circumstances in which anti-HIV antibodies cannot be detected until 9 to 12 months after infection. For practical purposes, if their ELISA and Western blot tests remain negative 6 months after exposure, the HCW should assume that he or she has not been infected with HIV.

Although many patients or HCWs newly infected (not simply exposed) with HIV are asymptomatic, at least one half (and, in some series, up to 90%) of patients will experience a flu-like syndrome 6 weeks or so after infection, known as the acute retroviral syndrome. The severity of this illness can vary considerably; many patients with this disorder do not feel ill enough to seek medical attention. The syndrome can be quite severe with a broad range of signs and symptoms that may include fever, aphthous ulceration, headache, adenopathy, rash, arthralgias, pharyngitis, and occasionally hepatosplenomegaly, diarrhea, or neuropathy. Laboratory evaluation may reveal leukopenia, thrombocytopenia, lymphopenia, and elevated liver function tests. This illness is virtually indistinguishable from a number of viral syndromes (e.g., mononucleosis, measles, or rubella) as well as secondary syphilis. During this acute retroviral syndrome, circulating titers of HIV are at very high levels, higher than at any other stage of the HIV infection except for the late, terminal stages. Given the intense viremia of the acute retroviral syndrome, circulating HIV-RNA can usually be detected at this time by the PCR or branched DNA assays even if there is still no detectable antibody to HIV.

Recommendations for Patient Testing

Health care workers who have had occupational exposure to serum or body fluids from a patient who may have the HIV virus should request, through an appropriate intermediary, that the patient be tested for HIV antibody. Regulations regarding HIV testing typically require that the patient give informed consent for an HIV antibody test. Given the anxiety and emotional overlay that can accompany an HCW's occupational exposure, someone other than the exposed HCW should approach the patient for consent for this test. If the patient's serologic test for HIV antibodies is negative, the patient, in all likelihood, is not infected with HIV. False-negative HIV serologic tests only occur if the patient has recently (within the past 6 months) been infected with HIV. If a seronegative patient falls into the high-risk category for HIV infection, a test for circulating HIV-RNA by PCR or branched DNA should be done. A positive result identifies a true HIV infection. The predictive value of a negative HIV-RNA in serum combined with a negative serologic assay means that there is an overwhelming likelihood that the patient's blood cannot transmit HIV.

Recommendations for HCW Testing

HCWs who believe that they have been exposed to blood or body fluids from a patient infected or potentially infected with HIV should have an ELISA done shortly after that exposure to establish a baseline value (Table 5.2). If this test is positive, a confirmatory test should be run (e.g., Western blot). If the HCW develops a syndrome consistent with the acute HIV syndrome in the ensuing 6 to 12 weeks, an assay for HIV-RNA should be done at that time. If the patient remains symptomatic during the 6 months following potential occupational exposure, then ELISA tests should be run on the HCW at 6 weeks, 12 weeks, and 3 and 6 months after exposure. If these tests are negative, the HCW can conclude that he or she has not acquired HIV.

In one recently reported case, an HCW who suffered a superficial needlestick injury was tested for HIV antibody at the time of HIV exposure as well as 3, 6, and 8 months later.[55] Antibodies to HIV were detected only at the 8-month test. Despite multiple attempts, HIV could not be cultured

TABLE 5.2. The provisional Public Health Service recommendations for chemoprophylaxis after occupational exposure to HIV–1996.

Type of exposure	Source material*	Antiretroviral prophylaxis
Percutaneous	Blood, plus . . .	
	Highest risk	Recommend
	Increased risk	Recommend
	No increased risk	Offer
	Fluid containing visible blood, other potentially infectious fluid†, or tissue	Offer
	Other body fluid (e.g., urine)	Not offer
Mucous membrane	Blood	Offer
	Fluid containing visible blood, other potentially infectious fluid†, or tissue	Offer
	Other body fluid (e.g., urine)	Not offer
Skin, increased risk‡	Blood	Offer
	Fluid containing visible blood, other potentially infectious fluid, or tissue	Offer
	Other body fluid (e.g., urine)	Not offer

Source: Adapted from ref 48.

*Any exposure to concentrated HIV (e.g., in research laboratory or production facility) is treated as percutaneous exposure to blood with highest risk. Recommend–postexposure prophylaxis (PEP) should be recommended to the exposed worker. Offer–PEP should be offered to the exposurd worker with counseling. Not offer–PEP should not be offered because there are not occupational exposures to HIV.

Highest risk–*both* larger volume of blood (e.g., deep injury with large-diameter hollow needle previously in source patient's vein or artery, especially involving an injection of source-patient's blood) *and* blood containing a higher titer of HIV (e.g., source with acute retroviral illness or end-stage AIDS; viral load measurement may be considered, but its use in relation to PEP has not been evaluated).

Increased risk–*either* exposure to larger volume or blood *or* to blood with a higher titer of HIV.

No increased risk–neither exposure to larger volume of blood nor to blood with higher titer of HIV (e.g., solid suture needle injury from source patient with asymptomatic HIV infection).

†Includes semen, vaginal secretions, cerebrospinal, synovial, pleural, peritoneal, pericardial, and amniotic fluids.

‡For skin, risk is increased for exposures involving a high titer of HIV, prolonged contact, an extensive area, or an area in which skin integrity is visibly compromised. For skin exposures without increased risk, the drug toxicity outweighs the benefit for PEP.

from this HCW's serum even 1 year later, raising the possibilities that the delayed seroconversion was due to an aborted HIV infection, infection with an attenuated HIV strain, or infection with a non-HIV virus that produces cross-reacting antibodies. This case stands alone in possibly demonstrating delayed (beyond the usual 6 months) seroconversion. For practical purposes, if the ELISA, Western blot, and HIV-RNA tests are negative 6 months after exposure, the HCW should assume that he or she has not been infected with HIV. In cases of shallow, superficial inoculation of HIV, another set of antibody tests may be run at 9 months to allay any remaining concerns about undiagnosed infection.

If an HCW's serum tests positive for HIV-RNA and/or if the ELISA and confirmatory Western blot tests are repeatedly reactive, the HCW has been infected with HIV. If only the serologic tests are positive, additional confirmatory tests (direct viral cultural and/or HIV-RNA assays) must be done. If the diagnosis of HIV infection is confirmed, the HCW should receive medical and psychological counseling to consider the merits and disadvantages of antiviral therapy and to take appropriate precautions to avoid further transmission of this virus (safe sex practices, no blood donations, etc.).

References

1. Centers for Disease Control. *CDC Semiannual HIV/AID Surveillance Report.* Altanta: CDC, December 1994.
2. Centers for Disease Control. Guidelines for prevention of transmission of human immunodeficiency virus and hepatitis B virus to health care and public safety workers. *MMWR* 1989;38:121–163.
3. Seef LB, Kaff RS. Evolving concepts of the clinical and serologic consequences of hepatitis B virus infection. *Semin Liver Dis* 1986;6:11–22.
4. Panlilio A, et al. Serosurvey of human immune deficiency virus, hepatitis B virus and hepatitis C virus infection among hospital based surgeons. Serosurvey Study Group. *J Am Coll Surg* 1995;180:16–24.
5. CDC. *Hepatitis Surveillance Report No. 48.* Atlanta: U.S. Department of Health and Human Services, Public Health Service, 1982;2–3.
6. CDC. Recommendations for preventing transmission of human immunodeficiency virus and hepatitis B virus to patients during exposure-prone invasive procedures. *MMWR* 1991;40:1–9.
7. Lettau LA, Smith JD, Williams D, et al. Transmission of hepatitis B with resultant restriction of surgical practice. *JAMA* 1986;255:934–937.
8. Rimland D, Parkin WE, Miller GB, Schrack WD. Hepatitis B outbreak traced to an oral surgeon. *J Engl J Med* 1977;296:953–958.
9. Grob PJ, Pischof B, Naeff F. Cluster of hepatitis B transmitted by a physician. *Lancet* 1981;2:1218–1220.
10. Coutinho RA, Albrecht-van Lent P, Stoutjesdijk L, et al. Hepatitis B from doctors (letter). *Lancet* 1982;1:345–346.
11. Haeram JW, Siebke JC, Ulstrup J, Geiram D, Helle I. HBsAg transmission from a cardiac surgeon incubating hepatitis B resulting in chronic antigenemia in four patients. *Acta Med Scand* 1981;210:389–392.
12. Flower AJE, Prentice M, Morgan G, et al. Hepatitis B infection following cardiothoracic surgery (Abstract). 1990 International Symposium on Viral Hepatitis and Liver Diseases, Houston, 1990;94.
13. Centers for Disease Control. Guidelines for prevention of transmission of human immunodeficiency virus and hepatitis B virus to health care and public safety workers. *MMWR* 1989;38:121–163.

14. Raahave D, Bremmelgard A. New operative techniques to reduce surgeon's risk of HIV infection. *J Hosp Infect* 1991;Suppl A:177–182.
15. Henderson DK, Fahey BJ, Willy M, et al. Risk for occupational transmission of human immunodeficiency virus type 1 (HIV-1) associated with clinical exposures: a prospective evaluation. *Ann Intern Med* 1990;113:740–746.
16. Gerberding MD, Littell C, Tarkington A, Brown A, Schecter WP. Risk of exposure of surgical personnel to patients blood during surgery at San Francisco General Hospital. *N Engl J Med* 1990;322:1788–1793.
17. Centers for Disease Control. Possible transmission of human immunodeficiency virus to a patient during an invasive dental procedure. *MMWR* 1990; 39:489–493.
18. Ceisielski, C, Marianos D, Chin-Yih O, et al. Transmission of human immunodeficiency virus in a dental practice. *Ann Intern Med* 1992;116:798–805.
19. Mishu B, Schaffner W, Horan JM, et al. A surgeon with AIDS. *JAMA* 1990; 264:467–470.
20. Danila RN, MacDonald KL, Rhame FS, et al. A look-back investigation of patients of an HIV-infected physician. *N Engl J Med* 1991;325:1406–1411.
21. von Reyn CF, Gilbert TT, Shaw FE, et al. Absence of HIV transmission from an infected orthopedic surgeon: a 13 year look-back study. *JAMA* 1993; 269:3807–1811.
22. Dickinson GM, Morhart RE, Klimas NG, et al. Absence of HIV transmission from an infected dentist to his patients. *JAMA* 1993;269:1802–1806.
23. Rogers AS, Froggatt JW, Townsend T, et al. Investigation of potential HIV transmission to the patients of an HIV-infected surgeon. *JAMA* 1993; 269:1795–1801.
24. Longfield JN, Brundage J, Badger G, et al. Look-back investigation after human immunodeficiency virus seroconversion in pediatric dentist. *J Infect Dis* 1994;169:1–8.
25. Babinchak TJ, Renner C. Patients treated by a thoracic surgeon with HIV: a review. *Chest* 1994;106:681–683.
26. Lowenfels AB, Wormser G. Risk of transmission of HIV from surgeon to patient. *N Engl J Med* 1991;325:888–889.
27. Wilson R. Analyzing the daily risks of life. *Techno Rev* 1979;81:41–44.
28. Daniels N. HIV infected professionals; patients rights and the "switching dilemma." *JAMA* 1992;267:1368–1371.
29. Bell D, Shapiro C, Martone W, et al. HIV-positive health-care professionals: Should they still provide patient care? *Int Conf AIDS* 1992;8:C266 (abstract no. PoC 4130).
30. Kleinman S, Alter H, Busch M, et al. Increased detection of hepatitis C virus (HCV)-infected blood donors by a multiple-antigen HCV enzyme immunoassay. *Transfusion* 1992;32:805–813.
31. Dodd R. The risk of transfusion-transmitted infection. *N Engl J Med* 1992;327:419–421.
32. Dodd R. Infectious complications of blood transfusion. *Hem/Oc Ann* 1994; 2:280–287.
33. Busch M. Retroviruses and blood transfusions: The lessons learned and the challenge yet ahead. In: Nance S, ed. *Blood Safety: Current Challenges.* Bethesda, MD: American Association of Blood Banks, 1992;1–44.
34. Nelson K, Donahue J, Munoz A, et al. Transmission of retroviruses from

seronegative donors by transfusion during cardiac surgery. *Ann Intern Med* 1992;117:554–559.

35. American Association of Blood Banks. Policy statement on HIV antigen testing. *Association Bulletin* 1995;95(2).
36. Kenrad Nelson quoted in *CCBC Newsletter,* January 27, 1995, p. 4, and Eve Lackritz in *CCBC Newsletter,* January 13, 1995, p. 5.
37. Tokars JI, Chamberland ME, Schable CA, et al. A survey of occupational blood contact and HIV infection among orthopedic surgeons. The American Academy of Orthopaedic Surgeons Serosurvey Study Committee. *JAMA* 1992; 268:489–494.
38. Quebbeman EJ, Telford GL, Hubbard S, et al. Risk of blood contamination and injury to operating room personnel. *Ann Surg* 1991;214:614–620.
39. Matta H, Thompson AM, Rainey JB. Does wearing two pairs of gloves protect operating theatre staff from skin contamination? *Br J Med* 1988;297:597–598.
40. CDC. Case control study of HIV seroconversion in healthcare workers after percutaneous exposure to HIV infected blood—France, United Kingdom and United States, January 1988–August 1994. *MMWR* 1995;44:929–933.
41. Gerberding J. Management of occupational exposures to blood borne viruses. *J Engl J Med* 1995;322:444–451.
42. Bell DM. Occupational risk of HIV infection in healthcare workers. In: *Improving the Management of HIV Disease.* New York. International AIDS Society-USA, 1996;4:7–10.
43. Tokars JL, Marcus R, Culover DH, et al. Surveillance of HIV infection and zidovudine use among healthcare workers after occupational exposure to HIV infected blood. *Ann Intern Med* 1993;118:913–919.
44. Gerberding JL. Prophylaxis for occupational exposure to HIV. *Ann Intern Med* 1996;125:497–501.
45. Ippolito G, Puro V, DeCarli G. The risk of occupational human immunodeficiency virus infection in healthcare workers—Italian multicenter study. *Arch Intern Med* 1993;153:1451–1458.
46. Mathez D, De Truchis P, Gorin C, et al. Ritonivir, AZT, DDC as a triple combination in AIDS patients. Nat Conf Retroviruses & Opportunistic Infections, 1996 (abstract 285).
47. Gulick R, Mellors JW, Havlir D, et al. Potent and sustained antiretroviral activity of indinavir (IDV), zidovudine (AZT) and lamuvidine (3TC). Int Conf AIDS, 1996 (abstract ThB931).
48. Update. Provisional Public Health Service recommendations for chemoprophylaxis after occupational exposure to HIV. *MMWR* 1996;45:468–472.
49. Schleupner C. Detection of HIV-1 infection. In: Mandell G, Bennett J, Dolin R, eds. *Principles and Practice of Infectious Diseases.* New York, Churchill Livingstone, 1995;1253–1267.
50. Phair J, Wolinsky S. Diagnosis of infection with the human immunodeficiency virus. *Clin Infect Dis* 1992;15:13–16.
51. Rogers MF, Ou CY, Rayfield M, et al. Use of the polymerase chain reaction for early detection of the proviral sequences of human immunodeficiency virus in infants born to seropositive mothers. *N Engl J Med* 1989;320:1649–1654.
52. Niu MT, Stein DS, Schnittman SM. Primary human immunodeficiency virus type 1 infection review of pathogenesis and early treatment intervention in humans and animal retrovirus infections. *J Infect Dis* 1993;168:1490–1501.

53. CDC. Update: serological testing for antibody to the human immunodeficiency virus. *MMWR* 1988;36:833–845.
54. Mulder J, et al. rapid and simple PCR assay for the quantitation of human immunodeficiency virus type 1 RNA in plasma: application to acute retroviral infection. *J Clin Microbiol* 1994;32:292–300.
55. Lafrere J, et al. Time to seroconversion after needlestick injury. *Lancet* 1995;345:1634–1635.

6
Cardiac Surgery in Jehovah's Witnesses

TODD K. ROSENGART

The Jehovah's Witnesses are members of a religious organization that was founded in the 1870s as a nondenominational Christian study group by a Pennsylvanian named Charles Taze Russell.[1] The WatchTower Bible and Tract Society was formed in 1881. The WatchTower Society was headquartered in Brooklyn, New York in 1909, and has subsequently grown into an international organization with more than 5 million followers worldwide. The name "Jehovah's Witnesses," adopted by the Society in 1931, was derived from the Biblical passage, "You are my witnesses, saith Jehovah" (Isaiah 43:10).

From a medical standpoint, a critical component of the Jehovah's Witnesses practice is their belief that blood transfusions are absolutely prohibited by God. This belief was first mentioned in the December 1927 edition of the Jehovah's Witnesses publication, *The Watchtower,* in which the sanctity of blood was addressed. A more stringent requirement to avoid blood transfusion was initiated after this practice became common during World War II. Although Jehovah's Witnesses abstain from accepting the transfusion of whole blood or its principal components—packed red cells, platelets, and fresh frozen plasma—many will accept the transfusion of such minor blood products as albumin, immune globulin, or even fibrinogen (cryoprecipitate).[2] Furthermore, although the transfusion of stored, predonated autologous blood is not accepted, extracorporeal circulation and other similar procedures (hemodialysis) are generally considered permissible by the Jehovah's Witnesses since these procedures are viewed as extensions (via artificial conduits) of the natural blood circulation.[3]

The Jehovah's Witnesses' avoidance of blood transfusions stems from their interpretation of several Biblical passages. In a passage from Genesis, there is the divine commandment following Noah's survival of the Great Flood that "every moving animal that is alive may serve as food for you. . . . Only flesh with its soul—its blood—you must not eat" (Genesis 9:3,4). This passage is interpreted by the Jehovah's Witnesses to mean that blood is equated with the soul, and since animal blood is deemed in the Bible to be sacred, human blood is of even greater significance. The "eating," or intake, of human blood is thereby strictly forbidden. Since, obviously, the Bible does not specifically prohibit blood transfusions, the interpretation that blood transfusions are unacceptable is a generalization from these specific Biblical passages. The Jehovah's Witnesses infer that if oral acceptance of blood is prohibited, then any means of administering blood is similarly proscribed.[4] The severe penalty for blood transfusions is consistent with a subsequent divine command, "I shall certainly set my face against the soul that is eating the blood and I shall indeed cut him off from this people" (Leviticus 17:10).

The Jehovah's Witnesses' refusal of blood transfusions has been viewed as an extremist abstention from modern medical care, but the Jehovah's Witnesses are, in fact, otherwise strong advocates for the advances in medical therapy and in particular are quite aware of and embrace alternative blood therapies. Provocatively, they would note that the human act of dying for one's beliefs is not outside the range of normal human behavior, and in fact in the case of the military, it is an expected and honored societal conduct.[1,5]

The right of a competent adult to refuse blood transfusions as a matter of firmly held religious beliefs has been substantially validated through legal judgments.[1,5,6] One such judgment by the Illinois Supreme Court stated that "even though we may consider a patient's beliefs unwise, foolish or ridiculous, in the absence of an overriding danger to society we may not permit interference therewith in the form of conservatorship established in the waning hours of . . . life, the sole purpose of [which would be] compelling [the patient] to accept medical treatment forbidden by . . . religious principles and previously refused by [the patient] with full knowledge of the probable consequences."[1] On the other hand, another court ruling, more recently questioned, determined that a male Jehovah's Witness patient could be compelled to receive a transfusion if his death and subsequent loss of income could lead to the patient's offspring becoming wards of the state.[1] Similarly, essentially every state has legal requirements that minors may be given transfusions in life-threatening situations or as consistent with standard medical practice.

Approximately 20% of the more than 5 million Jehovah's Witnesses reside in the United States. Therefore, this population represents a significant potential number of patients at risk for blood transfusion, especially in cardiac surgery. Furthermore, successful techniques developed in taking care of Jehovah's Witnesses may also prove to be extremely useful in the development of blood conservation strategies for the general population. Partly as a response to this need to be able to safely perform open heart surgery in Jehovah's Witnesses, and as part of our emphasis on blood conservation at New York Hospital, we have developed a multimodality blood conservation program that has been utilized for cardiopulmonary bypass in Jehovah's Witness patients since 1992. We reported our original results in 1994 for our first 18 patients.[7] To the end of 1995, a total of 50

TABLE 6.1. Blood conservation measures in the Jehovah's Witnesses population.

1. Aprotinin (full Hammersmith regimen)
2. Erythropoietin (800 U/kg IV/SQ load, 500 U/kg SQ QOD)
3. *Minimum* CPB circuit volume (1200 cc)
4. *Maximum* volume IAD (calculated on-bypass hematocrit 18%)
5. Retrograde autologous priming of the bypass circuit (up to 900 ml crystalloid withdrawal)
6. Cell saver "skin to skin"
7. Hemostatic operative technique
8. Shed mediastinal blood reinfusion
9. Reduced laboratory sampling

patients have been operated upon utilizing this protocol, the results for whom were recently presented.[8] This blood conservation protocol consists of a series of basic components (Table 6.1) that are directed toward reversing the two principal sources of blood transfusion requirements in open heart surgery, namely, an inadequate preoperative red blood cell mass, and excessive postoperative bleeding.[7,9]

Blood Conservation Protocol

A critical initial component of the conservation protocol is to ensure that the patient will have an adequate hematocrit while on bypass. To determine the preoperative hematocrit needed to achieve an adequate hematocrit on bypass, we utilize a nomogram based on the patients' gender, height, and weight, to determine the total blood volume, multiplied by their baseline hematocrit to determine preoperative red cell mass. This value is the input of an equation that includes the anticipated pump prime volume and thereby allows calculation of the hemodilution effects of the crystalloid pump prime.[10] This equation has proven to be quite accurate in estimating the hematocrit on bypass. If the estimated on-bypass hematocrit is inadequate (less than 18%), then surgery is delayed until adequate erythropoietin therapy can be administered. If the hematocrit is adequate, then surgery is not delayed.

Based upon our review of the literature, we have elected to use a high-dosage erythropoietin (epo) regimen of 300 U/kg intravenous load, followed by maintenance therapy of 500 U/kg subcutaneously every other day.[11] This regimen is supplemented by oral or intravenous iron, folate, and vitamin C. We have noted a dynamic, early rise in hematocrit and sustained increases in erythropoiesis above that obtained with a standard dosage regimen with this protocol. In our experience, we can anticipate hematocrit increases of 2% to 3% per day within approximately 5 to 7 days after initiating this epo regimen. Erythropoietin therapy is continued postoperatively until a hematocrit of 30% is obtained. In our recent experience, however, we have found that the initial postoperative hematocrit so often approximates the preoperative hematocrit, which is normally greater than 30%, that postoperative epo therapy is usually not required.

The crystalloid pump prime volume is the variable other than red cell mass that determines on-bypass hematocrit, as validated by the hemodilution equation noted above. Decreases in hematocrit with the institution of bypass are directly proportional to the dilution of the red cell mass caused by the asanguineous pump prime volume. For patients with a body mass of less than 65 kg, the crystalloid prime volume can be decreased to 1200 to 1400 ml from 2000 ml by utilizing a small volume oxygenator and small diameter tubing. Furthermore, we have recently adopted the practice (not in the original Jehovah's Witnesses protocol) of withdrawing approximately 900 cc of the crystalloid prime from the pump circuit as bypass is initiated, a process called retrograde autologous priming (RAP). The RAP process has dramatically decreased the hemodilution associated with bypass, and accordingly, minimized the demands for preoperative epo therapy to boost the preoperative red cell mass.[12]

The success of the RAP protocol in fact often creates an on-bypass red cell mass that can be considered excessive—that which contributes to hematocrits greater than 18%. Furthermore, RAP can produce hematocrits on bypass that may be potentially deleterious in the setting of hypothermia, generally considered to be levels greater than 30%, because of the adverse rheologic properties of blood with hypothermia at these hematocrit levels. Opportunistically, we are therefore able, and essentially required, to withdraw blood prior to heparinization, often in quantities up to one third of the total blood volume, in order to bring on-bypass hematocrits to a more appropriate target range of 18% to 25%. This process, called large-volume intraoperative autologous donation (IAD), has been demonstrated by our group in separate studies to significantly reduce red cell transfusion requirements, possible by optimizing intraoperative red cell conservation.[10] The majority of this IAD blood is reinfused following the administration of protamine, but is, however, kept in continual connection to the patient via indwelling intravenous lines and slowly reinfused throughout the case. This technique allows for the maintenance of a continuous circuit without extracorporeal blood storage, in compliance with the religious considerations of the Jehovah's Witnesses.

The second major component of our multimodality blood conservation strategy is the use of several modalities to minimize or avoid blood loss. The use of the antifibrinolytic agent aprotinin is considered by us to be a critical component of this strategy. We utilize a full Hammersmith regimen of aprotinin to reduce coagulopathic postoperative blood loss.[13] Aprotinin administration is critical not only in minimizing postoperative bleeding, but also to "dry up" the surgical field prior to closure, which facilitates the verification of complete surgical hemostasis. Half-dosage aprotinin therapy and the administration of α-amino caproic acid (Amikar) are also effective treatment regimens for post-bypass coagulopathies.[14] In reviewing the literature and in view of our own experience, it is nevertheless our consideration that the full-dose aprotinin regimen yields optimal antifibrinolytic and hemostatic effects, which is essential for these high-risk patients.[13–15]

The major technical components of the blood-conserving arm of our protocol includes meticulous hemostatic technique, avoidance of the use of lap pads, which can absorb a significant amount of unrecoverable blood, and exclusive use of the cell saver intraoperatively. The cell saver blood is reinfused via a continuous circuit in a manner analogous to that for autologously donated blood. Unlike the IAD blood, the cell saver blood is usually exposed to heparin and to the bypass circuit prior to collection. The cell saver blood, lacking the potential benefit of being unexposed to these coagulopathic sources, as is the case with IAD blood, is therefore reinfused as needed to maintain an acceptable minimum hematocrit.

The reinfusion of shed mediastinal blood, collected via specialized pleural and mediastinal drains, is a potentially lifesaving technical innovation that we include in our protocol for postoperative conservation. This shed mediastinal blood can be administered back to the patient in a continuous circuit, as described above. In reality, the intraoperative use of aprotinin and the attention to hemostasis has minimized postoperative blood loss to the point that shed blood autotransfusion has rarely been required, and serves mainly as a safeguard against unanticipated postoperative bleeding.

Perhaps the most important postoperative conservation strategy we employ is the simple technical intervention of minimizing blood draws for laboratory determinations, which can account for up to 250 ml of blood loss, a full unit of packed red blood cells, over the course of a hospitalization. By utilizing pediatric blood tubes and by eliminating unnecessary testing, we found that we could significantly reduce this source of blood loss.

Experience in the Jehovah's Witnesses Population

We have to date performed nearly 60 open-heart procedures in our Jehovah's Witnesses population, and we have recently reviewed our experience with the first 50 of these patients.[16] Although open-heart surgery in Jehovah's Witnesses has been described in a number of previous reports, at least one of which represents a much larger series of patients than ours, none of these previous cohorts has involved the application of a comprehensive blood conservation protocol as described here.[17–19] Most previous reports in fact describe efforts at bloodless surgery in which the primary blood conservation technique is surgical hemostasis, and in which the safeguards against the potentially lethal effects of coagulopathy or hemodilution in this population have been extremely limited. The significant risks imposed by these constraints are demonstrated by low hematocrits postoperatively and at the time of discharge, and the number of deaths related to anemia in these reports.

Despite the recent advent of the many blood conservation techniques included in our blood conservation protocol, our initial patient selection was nevertheless conservative, and primarily included relatively low-risk procedures such as coronary bypass. We have since expanded our selection criteria to essentially all cardiothoracic procedures, because of the encouraging results in our initial experience. Our reviewed experience now includes 30 coronary bypass patients, and 20 patients who have undergone other, more complex or prolonged procedures that represented increased transfusion risks (Table 6.2). Several of these cases, including reoperations, multiple valve replacements, and aneurysm repair, generally would have been considered to represent prohibitive transfusion risks.

Our most recent experience has included an extension to the pediatric population, as well, where the hemodilution imposed by the pump prime volume compared with the child's diminutive red cell mass imposes a formidable obstacle to the performance of open-heart surgery without transfusion. This experience has included the successful performance of several complex procedures in the pediatric population, including an aortic root reconstruction in one child, but a lower limit of red cell mass still remains as a barrier to bloodless open-heart surgery in the neonate and young child. Because of the large relative volume of pump prime in these pediatric patients, the utilization of hemoconcentration in the operating room has significantly enhanced the post-bypass hematocrits that can be achieved in these patients. Through the use of RAP and hemoconcentration, the pediatric patient with an adequate initial red cell mass can, in fact, often be discharged without transfusion with hematocrits generally equal to that on admission.

There have been two deaths in this group of 50 Jehovah's Witnesses patients, both at an extended time interval postoperation and neither related to the prohibition of blood transfusion. There has been no evidence of increased thromboembolic complications such as renal failure, stroke, or myocardial infarction in these patients, despite their receiving full dose aprotinin in combination with erythropoietin as part of the treatment regimen.

TABLE 6.2. Jehovah's Witnesses population: 50 patients, 1992–1995.

Procedures	Number of reoperations
27 Coronary artery bypass graft (CABG)	4
13 Valve/multiple valve	4
3 Valve-CABG	1
7 Other (aneurysm, atrial septal defect, pediatric, etc.)	2
50	11 (22%)

To further quantify our experience in the Jehovah's Witnesses population, we compared our results with the 30 Jehovah's Witnesses coronary bypass patients with 100 non-Witnesses, primary coronary bypass patients who were not part of the comprehensive blood conservation program. The two groups were well matched for preoperative transfusion risks, including age, gender, and red cell mass. Control patients received Amikar if they were at risk of coagulopathic bleeding because of aspirin use, underwent intermediate volume IAD (one to two units), and received cell saver blood, although not on the strict, exclusionary basis employed for the Witnesses patients. The control patients did not undergo RAP, or receive aprotinin or erythropoietin.

Chest tube outputs were significantly less in the Witness group than in the control group (Fig. 6.1). Fifty-six percent of the control group received homologous blood transfusions, a mean of 1.8 units per patient, compared with no transfusions for the Witnesses patients. In spite of this transfusion requirement in the control patients, discharge hematocrits were equivalent between the two groups (Fig. 6.2). Furthermore, the diagnostic-related group (DRG)-matched lengths of stay and ancillary costs were similar, and in many cases decreased, in the Witnesses patients compared with the control population.

Summary

Open-heart surgery can be performed in essentially any patient without blood transfusions, utilizing the multimodality blood conservation regimen discussed above. In patients in whom blood transfusion is not as great a risk as in Jehovah's Witnesses, a variation of this conservation program can be

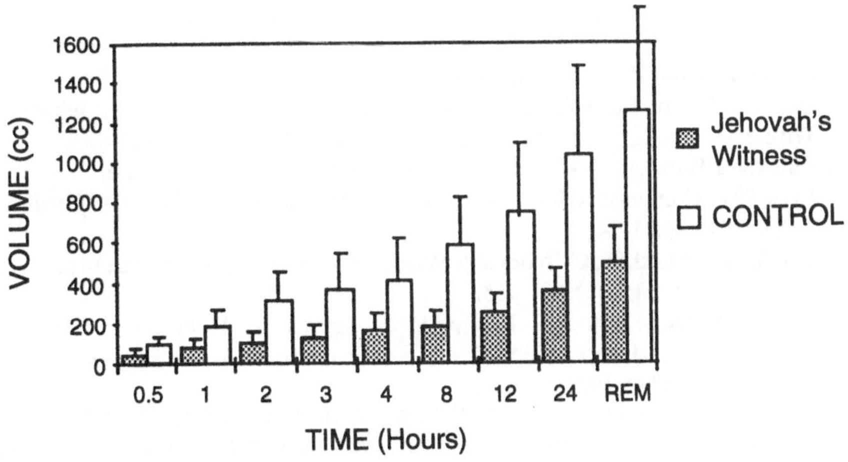

FIGURE 6.1. Chest tube outputs in 30 Jehovah's Witness patients versus 100 non-Jehovah's Witnesses control patients.

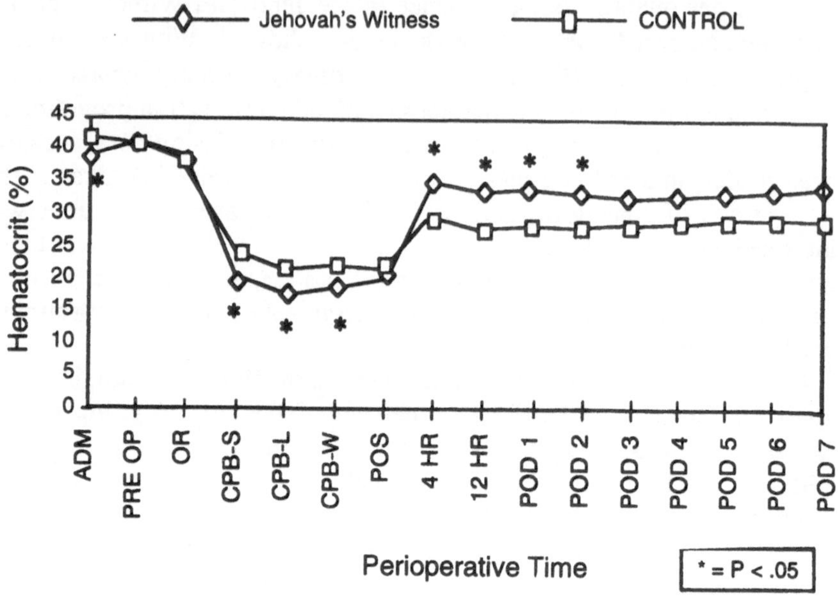

FIGURE 6.2. Hematocrits at various time intervals during hospitalization in 30 Jehovah's Witness patients versus 100 non-Jehovah's Witness control patients.

employed, as is discussed elsewhere in this text. We anticipate and hope that this blood conservation program will in fact be of significant benefit in decreasing transfusions in all open-heart surgery patients.

References

1. Vercillo AP, Duprey SV. Jehovah's Witnesses and the transfusion of blood products. *NY State J Med* 1988;88(9):493–494.
2. Questions from Readers. *The WatchTower* June 1, 1990;30–31.
3. Questions from Readers. *The WatchTower* March 1, 1989;30–31. Jehovah's Witnesses—the surgical ethical challenge. *JAMA* 1981;246:2471.
4. Jehovah's Witnesses—The surgical ethical challenge. *Awake* 1986;5.
5. Byrn RW. Compulsory lifesaving treatment for the competent adult. *Fordham L Ren* 1975;44:23–24.
6. Findley LJ, Fletcher JC. Jehovah's Witnesses and the right to refuse blood. *NY State J Med* 1988;88(9):464–465.
7. Rosengart TK, Helm RE, Klemperer J, Krieger K, Isom OW. Combined aprotinin and eyrthropoietin use: results with Jehovah's Witnesses. *Ann Thorac Surg* 1994;58:1397–1403.
8. Rosengart TK, Helm B, Velasco F, et al. Open heart surgery without transfusion: a multimodality strategy in over forty consecutive Jehovah's Witness patients. *J Am Coll Cardiol* 1996;27(2)(suppl A):231A.
9. Rosengart TK. Risk analysis of primary versus reoperative coronary bypass surgery. *Ann Thorac Surg* 1993;56:S74–77.

10. Helm RE, Klemperer JD, Rosengart TK, et al. Intraoperative autologous donation: volume-dependent red cell preservation. *Am Coll Surg Surg Forum* 1994;45:249–252.
11. Helm RE, Gold JP, Isom OW, Rosengart TK, Zelano JA, Krieger KH. Erythropoietin in cardiac surgery. *J Cardiovasc Surg* 1993;8:579–606.
12. Rosengart TK, DeBois B, Helm R, et al. Retrograde autologous priming (RAP) for cardiopulmonary bypass: a safe and effective means of decreasing hemodilution and transfusion requirements. *Circulation* 1995;92(8 Suppl):I763.
13. Levy JH, Pifarre R, Schaff H, et al. A multicenter, double-blind, placebo-controlled trial of aprotinin for reducing blood loss and the requirement for donor blood transfusion in patients undergoing repeat coronary artery bypass grafting. *Circulation* 1995;92:2236–2244.
14. Fremes SE, Wong BI, Lee E, et al. Metaanalysis of prophylactic drug treatment in the prevention of postoperative bleeding. *Ann Thorac Surg* 1994; 58:1580–1588.
15. Blahut B, Harringer W, Bettelheim P, Doran JE, Spath P, Lundsgaard-Hansen P. Comparison of the effects of aprotinin and tranexamic acid on blood loss and related variables after cardiopulmonary bypass. *J Thorac Cardiovasc Surg* 1994;108(6):1083–1091.
16. Rosengart TK, Helm B, Velasco F, et al. Open heart surgery without transfusion: a multimodality strategy in fifty consecutive Jehovah's Witness patients. *J Am Coll Surg* (in press).
17. Ott DA, Cooley DA. Cardiovascular surgery in Jehovah's Witnesses: report of 542 operations without blood transfusion. *JAMA* 1977;238:1256–1258.
18. Gaudiani VA, Mason HDW. Preoperative erythropoietin in Jehovah's Witnesses who require cardiac procedures. *Ann Thorac Surg* 1991;51:823–824.
19. Mann MC, Votto J, Kambo J, McNamee M. Management of the severely anemic patient who refuses transfusion: lessons learned during the case of a Jehovah's Witness. *Ann Intern Med* 1992;117:1042–1048.

7

Blood Conservation in Cardiopulmonary Transplantation

Nabeel G. El-Amir, Justin S. Kang, and Craig R. Smith

In 1964 performance of a valve replacement without transfusion was a reportable event.[1] The rapid growth of cardiac surgery in the late 1970s placed increasing demands on the blood supply, leading to a proportional increase over the next decade in literature describing techniques for blood conservation in routine cardiac surgery.[2–5] It was logical that these techniques would be applied to cardiac transplant as that procedure entered a period of exponential growth in the 1980s, and it was not long before case reports marked the performance of cardiac transplants without blood or blood products in Jehovah's Witnesses.[6,7]

With more than 22,000 cardiothoracic transplants performed worldwide as of 1993,[8] issues of blood conservation specific to heart, heart-lung, and lung transplant have assumed increasing importance. This chapter begins by examining the transfusion-related adverse effects specific to transplant recipients that make blood conservation a priority. Next, features of cardiothoracic transplant that make conventional techniques for blood conservation difficult to apply are discussed. Finally, the available strategies for blood conservation in this population are reviewed.

Transfusions and Transplant Patients

Problems Associated with Transfusions

Infection remains the largest single cause of early mortality in cardiothoracic transplant recipients.[9,10] With two rare exceptions, the risks associated with transfusion in transplant recipients (Table 7.1) are primarily those of infection.

Graft-Versus-Host Disease

Graft-versus-host disease (GVHD) is uncommon but is almost universally fatal in immunosuppressed patients.[11–13] Simply stated, GVHD is defined

Table 7.1. Risks associated with transfusions in thoracic transplant recipients.

Infection	Other
Cytomegalovirus	Graft-versus-host disease
Toxoplasmosis	Donor-mediated hemolysis
Human immunodeficiency virus (HIV)	
Bacterial	

as the clinical manifestations of a rejection reaction mounted against the host by transfused allogeneic lymphocytes. The mechanism of GVHD involves the activation of donor T-lymphocytes directed against host antigens, and induction of cytotoxic damage via a wide variety of cytokines.[11] In transfusion-associated GVHD, the clinical picture varies from maculopapular rash, anorexia, and abnormal liver-function tests to pancytopenia and marrow aplasia. In addition to immunosuppressed patients, persons at risk for GVHD include immunocompetent adults who share a human leukocyte antigen (HLA) haplotype with an HLA-homozygous blood donor, premature infants, and neonates with hemolytic disease. Curiously, although immunosuppression seems to be a clear risk factor, transfusion-associated GVHD has not been described in AIDS patients, suggesting that the exact nature of immunosuppression may play a key role.[13] There is no effective treatment of GVHD once the disease is established. Gamma irradiation of blood products is the most effective method of prevention. Problems associated with this option, however, include the release of K^+ in the irradiated blood, possible pathogenicity of the radiation damaged lymphocytes, and significant expense. Considering the rarity of GVHD and the frequency of blood transfusion, this method of prevention is not recommended at the present.

Donor-Mediated Hemolysis

An interesting variant on GVHD has been seen in heart-lung transplant recipients who receive ABO compatible rather than ABO identical organs. In a series reported from the University of Minnesota, 70% of such patients expressed donor-derived anti-ABO antibodies and developed severe hemolysis.[14] The problem is thought to be related to the large lymphocyte load carried in the carinal and peritracheal lymph nodes on the heart-lung organ block. The problem appears to be less common in lung-only recipients and has not been described in heart-only recipients. The transfusion policy recommended by the Minnesota group is to use donor ABO blood products in all lung or heart-lung recipients receiving ABO compatible, nonidentical donor organs.

Infection

Transfusion-related viral, bacterial, and protozoal infections are well-recognized adverse effects. The most common examples are hepatitis B, hepatitis C, cytomegalovirus (CMV), toxoplasmosis, and human immunodeficiency virus (HIV).

Cytomegalovirus

From 30% to 80% of the general population has CMV infection, with a small minority symptomatic. In contrast, CMV infection is a significant source of morbidity and mortality in solid organ transplant recipients.[15] There are three potential sources of CMV infection: endogenous reactivation, the donor organ, and cellular blood products. Endogenous reactivation occurs in CMV seropositive transplant recipients when the latent form of the virus multiplies in the immunosuppressed host. In CMV seronegative recipients, transplantation of thoracic organs from a CMV seropositive donor carries a 73% to 100% risk of primary CMV infection.[16,17] Blood from a seropositive donor transfused into a seronegative transplant recipient conveys similar CMV infection risks.[16] In a review of experience at 12 heart transplant centers, the frequency of CMV infection in heart transplant recipients ranged from 29% to 100% (mean 58%).[18]

A relationship between the age of transfused blood and the risk of CMV transmission has been suggested.[19] Blood elements transmitted with the donor organ are fresher than any received from the blood bank. As a result, the viability of "passenger leukocytes," which are the presumed carriers of CMV, is greater in the donor organ than in banked blood. Given the likely mechanism of CMV transmission, it is possible that transmission of donor leukocytes could be minimized by aggressive donor organ flush with preservation solution during organ procurement or by resection of lymphatic tissue on the organ block.

Among CMV seronegative patients that receive seropositive organs or blood products, only a small minority (0–27%) remain seronegative.[16,17] The majority became infected and seroconvert without developing clinical disease, while approximately 27% develop clinically symptomatic CMV disease.[9] In one report, symptomatic CMV disease occurred in 40% of heart and heart-lung transplant recipients.[17] The frequency of infection, disease, and mortality is at least as high, and in some series higher, when seronegative single- or double-lung transplant recipients receive seropositive organs.[20,21]

Pneumonitis is the most frequent and serious form of CMV disease. Other manifestations include retinitis, gastrointestinal ulceration, marrow suppression, and central nervous system disease. CMV disease depresses cell-mediated immunity and increases the likelihood of opportunistic infections (such as *Pneumocystis carinii*) and bacterial abscesses.[22] CMV may potentiate graft atherosclerosis in heart transplants and obliterative bronchiolitis in lung transplants.[23,24]

CMV disease is treated with Ganciclovir and immune globulin. Ganciclovir is effective treatment for CMV pneumonitis in heart, kidney, and liver transplant recipients, but has been less effective in heart-lung recipients.[19] Use of CMV hyperimmune globulin may confer additional benefit. Novick et al[25] showed that CMV hyperimmune globulin prevented the development of CMV disease in their study group, even though it failed to decrease viral titers.

Prevention of CMV disease is based on reducing the frequency of CMV transmission. Strict avoidance of CMV mismatching (donor positive, recipient negative) would reduce the risk of infection from the donor organ and its passenger lymphocytes. This approach, however, is not an accepted practice because the prevalence of CMV in the general population would impose a significant waiting list disadvantage on CMV-negative recipients. Since registry data for heart, heart-lung, and lung transplant have never shown a 1-year survival disadvantage for mismatched patients,[26] the waiting list disadvantage would clearly outweigh any potential benefit. Standard practice is to use Ganciclovir and immune globulin prophylaxis in mismatched patients.

Because the supply of blood products greatly exceeds that of donor organs, it is usually possible to observe a policy of using CMV-negative blood products for CMV-negative transplant recipients. When it is necessary to use CMV-positive products, or when CMV screening of blood products cannot be done, it is appropriate to use Ganciclovir and immunoglobulin prophylaxis to reduce morbidity associated with CMV disease.

Microfilters and photoactive compounds can also be used to reduce CMV transmission in blood products. Transfusion through a microaggregate blood filter with appropriate pore size (Leuko-gard 6, Pall Biomedical, Glen Cove, NY) depletes leukocytes, which are the primary CMV vector.[27,28] De Graan-Hentzen et al[29] showed that CMV infection occurred in 10 of 86 control patients but in none of 59 patients receiving leukocyte-depleted blood.[29] Microfilters do not allow rapid infusion rates and can be associated with complement activation, but are generally safe and constitute accepted practice in most transplant centers. Photoactive dyes (hematoporphyrin derivatives, benzoporphyrin derivatives, and various cyanines) bind to viral envelopes and destroy them after illumination with a xenon light source or a tunable dye laser. Although most blood components are spared from irreversible damage, the technique does cause transient dysfunction of platelets.[30] Photoactive treatment is complex and not widely available, and is generally reserved for specific critically ill patients.

Toxoplasmosis

Taking into account regional variations, the incidence of positive antibody serology to *Toxoplasma gondii* in the United States and the United Kingdom ranges from 15% to 50%, with an annual infection rate of 1.0% to 1.5% in the general population.[31,32] However, in the immunosuppressed transplant patient, *T. gondii* infection can result in significant morbidity and mortality.[33,34] As with CMV, the transplant recipient can acquire toxoplasmosis from infected blood products, from infected donor organs, or from reactivation of latent infection in the recipient. Although most infections are asymptomatic, clinical manifestations of disease involve three main organ systems: cardiovascular, pulmonary, and (most importantly) the central nervous system (CNS). In the CNS, toxoplamosis presents as encephalitis, meningoencephalitis, and mass lesions. Diagnosis is based on a combination of data provided by cerebrospinal fluid (CSF) profile, serology, magnetic resonance imaging (MRI) scanning, biopsy, and polymerase chain reaction (PCR) technology. Disease is treated with pyrimethamine, sulfadiazine, and folinic acid. In those seronegative patients receiving seropositive products, pyrimethamine prophylaxis has been extremely useful in reducing the incidence of clinical disease.[33]

Studies of toxoplasmosis in heart[34] and heart-lung[35] recipients have been reported in both the United Kingdom and the United States. Wreghitt et al[35] noted that four of seven (57%) patients who were mismatched for *T. gondii* who did not receive prophylaxis with pyrimethamine developed primary donor-acquired *T. gondii* infection, whereas 2 of 14 (14%) patients who received prophylactic treatment developed primary infection. Likewise, Luft et al[36] also demonstrated a high incidence of infection among three of four (75%) mismatched patients.

Human Immunodeficiency Virus

Despite the general level of concern about the risk of HIV infection, the problem has been extremely uncommon in cardiothoracic organ transplant recipients. This is probably due in part to the fact that the vast majority of such transplants have been performed after serotesting for HIV in donors and recipients became widely available. To date, there is only one case report describing HIV infection after heart transplantation.[37] The transplant took place in 1984, and the HIV status of the donor and recipient were unknown. The authors presumed that both were negative because of the absence of clear risk factors, and concluded that the virus was transmitted via infusion of clotting factors. HIV serotesting of blood and of organ donors has proven to be an effective method of prevention in the transplant population.

Bacterial Infections

Several studies have demonstrated that animals transfused with uncontaminated blood products are more susceptible to bacterial infections and have a higher mortality than controls.[38–40] This is thought to be explained by alterations in T-lymphocyte and macrophage function observed in the transfused animals.[38] Although the incidence of bacteremia in heart transplant recipients is similar to that in nonimmunosuppressed patients,[18] transplant patients have decreased resistance to bacterial infections specifically related to blood transfusions,[41] perhaps because T-lymphocyte and macrophage alterations are further amplified by immunosuppression. Fortunately, bacterial contamination of blood components is rare. However, organisms such as *pseudomonas* species, *Escherichia coli,* and *Yersinia* species are capable of growing at cold storage temperatures and are potential sources of infection.[42] Meticulous adherence to standard methods for blood component processing and transfusion are prudent strategies to reduce the risk of bacterial contamination and sepsis in cardiothoracic organ transplant recipients when transfusion cannot be avoided.

Limits to Blood Conservation in Thoracic Transplantation

Table 7.2 outlines several features of thoracic transplantation that increase the difficulty of blood conservation.

Emergency Status

Virtually all cardiopulmonary transplantation procedures are performed as emergencies. This eliminates the opportunity to correct coagulopathies (discussed below), and to apply most preoperative techniques for blood conservation, such as autologous donation, because the waiting period is

TABLE 7.2. Translant recipient characteristics associated with increased bleeding risks.

Emergency status
Mechanical support
Ventricular assist devices
Intraortic balloon pumping
Extracorporeal membrane oxygenation
Iatrogenic anticoagulation
Coumadin
Aspirin
Warfarin
Heparin
Noniatrogenic anticoagulation
Hepatic congestion
Technical factors
Reoperative status
Highy vascular surgical planes
Heart-lung transplantation
Double-lung transplantation
For cystic fibrosis
Size mismatch or organs
Pericardial and pleural spaces

variable, unpredictable, and rarely short enough to fall within the 21- to 35-day storage time for banked blood.[43]

Need for Mechanical Support

An increasing number of patients require some form of mechanical circulatory support as a bridge to transplant. Support devices encountered include intraaortic balloon pumping, ventricular assist devices, and extracorporeal membrane oxygenation. These critically ill patients frequently have hepatic dysfunction producing an underlying coagulopathy, amplified by a need for continuous anticoagulation with heparin and other agents. Not surprisingly, the most common complication during the bridging period is bleeding.[44,45] In addition, platelet dysfunction and thrombocytopenia are universal consequences of extracorporeal perfusion.[46,47]

Iatrogenic and Noniatrogenic Coagulopathy

The emergent nature of organ transplantation precludes elective elimination of aspirin, warfarin, and related anticoagulants. Because aspirin acts by irreversibly acetylating platelet cyclooxygenase,[5] and because the half-life of platelets is about 5 days, aspirin should ideally be discontinued a week before surgery. Warfarin must be discontinued for 2 to 5 days to restore effective function of vitamin K–dependent procoagulant factors (II, V, VII, IX, and X), and vitamin K injection does not act rapidly enough to correct coagulation in less than 24 hours. Infusion of platelets (aspirin) or fresh frozen plasma (warfarin) will correct coagulation more rapidly but works against the goal of blood product conservation, and may not be well tolerated just prior to transplant in patients with congestive heart failure. Heart transplant candidates with mechanical valve prostheses must remain on warfarin during their waiting period, and warfarin is often considered important for patients with atrial arrhythmias and dilated cardiac chambers. Aspirin is frequently used by candidates with end-stage ischemic heart disease and those with cerebrovascular disease. Warfarin is considered important for lung transplant recipients with primary pulmonary hypertension. Noniatrogenic anticoagulation is usually the result of hepatic congestion accompanying the end-stage heart failure frequently encountered in heart, heart-lung, or lung transplant candidates. Correction requires infusion of blood products.

Pretransplant approaches to coagulopathy are limited. Indications for iatrogenic anticoagulation in the medical treatment of waiting patients should be carefully considered and conservative. One alternative to consider is the acceptance of a lower prothrombin time (PT) for patients without mechanical valves who still require continuous warfarin anticoagulation. Several alternatives have been applied at Columbia-Presbyterian Medical Center; patients with primary pulmonary hypertension on warfarin are strictly maintained at a PT of 14 to 15 seconds. Warfarin-dependent heart transplant candidates are converted to intravenous heparin anticoagulation when they become status I on the waiting list. Some patients have been effectively managed as outpatients with subcutaneous heparin injections.

Technical Factors: Reoperative Status, Vascular Adhesions, Empty Space

In a large series from the United Kingdom, 26% of heart transplants and 34% of heart-lung transplants had prior thoracic surgery, and required significantly more blood products than patients without previous surgery. In the same series, heart-lung or double-lung transplants with inflammatory diseases required 15 to 30 units of blood and blood products perioperatively.[48] Heart-lung transplantation requires extensive dissection through highly vascular planes in the middle mediastinum, which become virtually inaccessible once the organs are implanted, and makes surgical hemostasis difficult to achieve after reversal of heparin. With all types of thoracic transplant, size mismatch often results initially in empty space between the organs and surrounding structures. This takes away the benefit of gentle tamponade by adjacent structures, which can be an important natural mechanism for controlling diffuse small vessel bleeding.

Strategies for Blood Conservation in Thoracic Organ Transplantation

Preoperative Considerations

The nonelective nature of transplantation negates most preoperative options available in routine cardiac surgery. While predonation and freezing of autologous plasma to obtain clotting factors and platelet concentrates has produced inconsistent benefits in cardiac surgery,[49] preoperative methods to increase red cell mass can reduce the need for perioperative blood transfusion. In a randomized, controlled trial, erythropoietin given to patients about to undergo elective surgery increased their red cell mass by 41% over controls.[50] In transplant patients, however, the unpredictable time on the waiting list introduces timing problems that may make preoperative erythropoietin impractical. Erythropoietin has been used effectively to treat anemia in children following cardiac transplantation,[51] but has not been studied in transplant recipients preoperatively.

Intraoperative Considerations

Intraoperative Predonation

The technique for pre-bypass intraoperative autologous donation has been well described in routine cardiac surgery.[52] Blood is withdrawn before cardiopulmonary bypass and normovolemia is restored by infusion of colloid or crystalloid. The amount of blood to be phlebotomized is calculated by the following formula:

$$\text{Autologous Blood (ml)} = \{(V1 \times C1) - (V2 \times C2)\}/C1$$

where V1 = the calculated blood volume of the patient,
V2 = the total prime solution in the extracorporeal circuit,
C1 = the patient's hematocrit preoperatively, and
C2 = the desired level of the hematocrit during bypass (15%–20%).

Moderate normovolemic anemia (hematocrit between 18% and 20%) is well tolerated in the absence of acute cardiac ischemia.[52,53] Schonberger et al[52] found that reinfusion of autologous blood withdrawn before bypass reduced postoperative blood loss, and requirements for banked homologous blood, in 33 of 50 patients (66%) undergoing coronary bypass. Others have found higher platelet counts and higher coagulation factor concentrations in patients receiving predonated blood.[54,55] This has not been studied specifically in transplant recipients. The technique depends on adequate red cell mass, which is frequently lacking in very seriously ill patients receiving intensive life support. Cyanotic lung and heart-lung transplant patients, such as those with Eisenmenger's syndrome, are more favorable because of polycythemia.

Surgical Hemostasis

In theory, use of foreign materials for hemostasis, such as Surgicel, Gelfoam, or Teflon felt, should be minimized in immunosuppressed patients, although in practice a clear disadvantage is difficult to demonstrate. The operative fields in thoracic transplantation, particularly in heart-lung and double-lung transplantation, are very large, and frequently contain broad areas of profuse small vessel bleeding. A patient, systematic, and thorough approach to surgical hemostasis is important from start to finish.

In heart-lung transplantation Novick et al[56] advocate suture closure of pleural and pericardial tissues overlying the bloody posterior dissection, and incorporation of posterior mediastinal tissue in the back wall of the tracheal anastomosis to improve hemostasis (Fig. 7.1). They report that this technique has eliminated reoperations for bleeding, decreased transfusion requirements, and decreased chest tube losses from 4.3 L to 1.4 L during the first postoperative day.

Vouhé and Dartevelle[57] have also described modifications of the technique for heart-lung transplant that they claim have reduced bleeding. The soft tissues accompanying the donor organ block are carefully inspected for backbleeding that might not be expected. Dissection in the mediastinum is very limited, and mechanical stapling is used extensively to achieve hemostasis of recipient tissues.

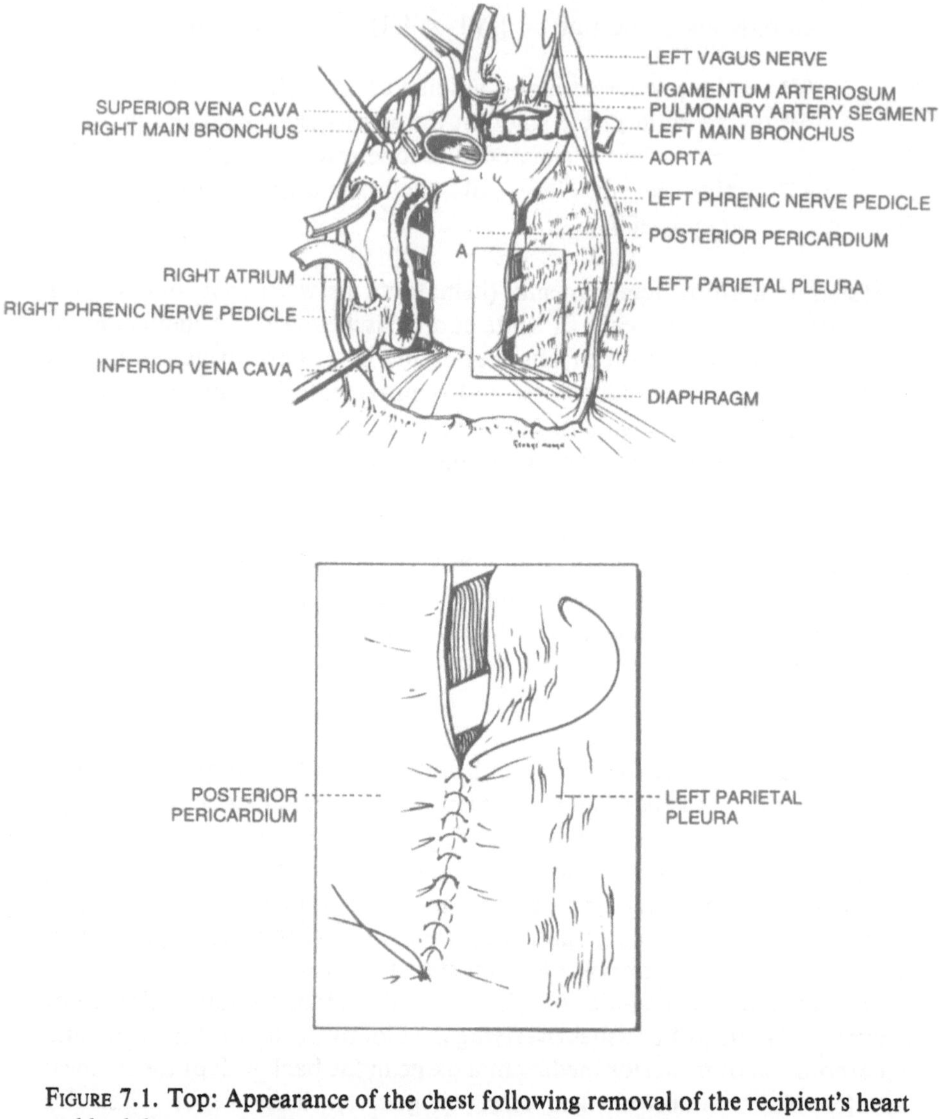

FIGURE 7.1. Top: Appearance of the chest following removal of the recipient's heart and both lungs. As much posterior pericardium as possible is left in situ. Both main bronchi will be subsequently excised and the trachea trimmed to one ring above the carina. Bottom: Using a running 4-0 polypropylene suture, the posterior mediastinal pleura is sutured to the posterior pericardium from the diaphragmatic surface to the cephalad aspect of the pericardial reflection on each side. Subsequently, large bites of the posterior mediastinal tissues will be incorporated in the posterior aspect of the tracheal anastomosis to obtain better hemostasis in that region. (From Novick et al.[56])

Other Intraoperative Techniques

Use of an asanguineous prime, return of bypass circuit contents to the patient, cell separators (Haemonetics Cell Saver, Haemonetics, Braintree, MA), and ultrafiltration are well-established techniques in cardiac surgery[5,8] that are equally useful in thoracic transplantation. Ultrafiltration can be especially advantageous in patients who start with substantial fluid overload, which is characteristic of many heart and heart-lung transplant recipients. Blood products infused during the procedure are usually given through a leukocyte-depleting microfilter (Leuko-gard 6, Pall Biomedical, Glen Cove, NY) to minimize CMV transmission. This may provide immunologic benefits as well by removing activated leukocytes and their cytokines. For this reason the placement of a microfilter in the arterial line of the bypass circuit has been suggested. For such a filter to accommodate average adult flow rates, however, the pore size must be increased, and the effectiveness of leukocyte filtration diminishes proportionally. Clinical trials addressing these issues are incomplete.

Pharmacologic Agents

Most thoracic transplant procedures require cardiopulmonary bypass, although it can be avoided in most single-lung transplants and in some double-lung transplants. Even with assiduous application of blood-conserving techniques, well-described effects of cardiopulmonary bypass on the coagulation systems contribute to a bleeding tendency. There has been a continually increasing interest in pharmacological approaches[49–51,58–60] (Table 7.3) to counteract these effects.

Heparin Reduction

Standard practice in cardiac surgery and in thoracic transplantation includes continuous heparin anticoagulation during cardiopulmonary bypass, adjusting the heparin dosage to maintain an activated clotting time (ACT) of at least 400 seconds. Excessive anticoagulation produces excessive postoperative mediastinal bleeding.[61] Insufficient heparinization results in coagulation factor and platelet consumption and thrombus formation. Use of a reduced heparin loading dose combined with maintenance of an ACT between 250 to 300 seconds has been reported to be safe for cardiac surgery,[62] but the consequences of inadequate

TABLE 7.3. Pharmacological approaches to blood conservation in transplant recipients.

Heparin dose reduction	Antifibrinolytic agents
Aprotinin	Epsilon amino caproic acid (Amicar)
Desmopressin acetate (DDAVP)	Tranexamic acid
Prostacyclin	

anticoagulation can be far more serious than bleeding, and such approaches should be adopted with caution. Recently there has been interest in the use of heparin-bonded bypass circuits and oxygenators in the hope these would allow reduction or elimination of systemic heparin requirements. One series has been reported in which patients perfused through heparin-bonded circuits required fewer perioperative blood transfusions than controls. Merits of this approach, however, have not been examined in a large patient population.

Aprotinin

Aprotinin is a serine protease inhibitor that was initially used to treat pancreatitis. Since the late 1980s, aprotinin has been shown to significantly decrease blood loss during open-heart surgery.[63–65] The mechanisms of action are not fully understood, but it is known that aprotinin preserves platelet function and inhibits complement, plasmin, and kallikrein activation, and attenuates the proinflammatory response to extracorporeal circulation.[8,66] There have been relatively few serious problems associated with the use of the drug. Anaphylaxis is rare (<1%) in patients receiving the drug for the first time, although more common in patients who receive the drug more than once. Prothrombotic effects producing a trend toward coronary bypass graft thrombosis have been suggested in some studies but remain highly controversial.[67,68] A trend toward mild and reversible renal dysfunction has also been reported.[69,70]

The group at Harefield Hospital has reported the largest experience with aprotinin in thoracic organ transplantation.[71] In 17 of 57 heart transplant recipients designated as a high-risk group for perioperative bleeding, blood loss was reduced by one third, transfusion requirements were decreased, and platelet requirements were eliminated. Similar results were evident in heart-lung, single-, and double-lung recipients.[49]

In thoracic transplantation, it should be kept in mind that cyclosporine and aprotinin could have synergistic effects on renal function. Dosage of both drugs should be considered carefully, and renal perfusion should be maximized with good hydration and low-dose dopamine.

At many centers using left ventricular assist devices (LVAD) as a bridge to transplant, aprotinin is used routinely during LVAD insertion and during LVAD removal when the transplant is performed.[72,73] As aprotinin becomes more widely used, there may be other patients presenting for transplant who have received the drug at previous operations. In any patient who has received the drug before, it is prudent to withhold the aprotinin infusion until the patient is cannulated for cardiopulmonary bypass. Skin testing for immediate hypersensitivity can be done, and assays exist for detection of aprotin-specific antibody, although guidelines for interpretation of the findings remain to be developed.[74]

Desmopressin-Acetate (DDAVP)

DDAVP is a synthetic analogue of arginine vasopressin that has been shown to decrease bleeding in certain forms of von Willebrand's disease, hemophilia, uremia, and chronic liver disease. Initial reports suggested that DDAVP reduced bleeding and use of blood products in high-risk cardiac surgery patients.[75,76] The postulated mechanism was an increase in levels of von Willebrand factor combined with augmentation of platelet function. There appeared to be few adverse reactions, although there was concern about possible antidiuretic properties. However, a more recent double-blind, randomized, placebo-controlled trial clearly failed to support these initial findings.[77] The investigators also reviewed 20 previous trials and found that 14 did not show any benefit from DDAVP. DDAVP has not been studied in a thoracic transplant population, but would seem unlikely to be of value.

Prostacyclin

In vitro, prostacyclin has protective effects on platelets.[59] In a randomized, prospective trial, prostacyclin appeared to reduce blood transfusion requirements in cardiac surgery patients, but was associated with significant hypotension. Some patients with primary pulmonary hypertension presenting for single-lung, double-lung, or heart-lung transplant have been maintained on chronic prostacyclin infusion pretransplant. Too little evidence exists to speculate about the role prostacyclin might play in blood conservation in such patients.

Antifibrinolytic Agents

Epsilon amino caproic acid (Amicar) and tranexamic acid are agents that interfere with plasmin-mediated fibrinolysis. A recent summary of published experience concluded that both agents are effective in reducing blood loss and transfusion requirements in cardiac surgery.[78] There has been no experience reported with either agent in a thoracic transplant population. Effects on renal function have not been identified with either drug. This might prove to be an advantage over aprotinin in a transplant population receiving other nephrotoxic drugs, but it is important to remember that neither drug has been as thoroughly studied as aprotinin.

Postoperative Considerations

Mediastinal blood loss in the first 24 to 48 hours can be very high in thoracic transplantation, averaging 3100 ml in one series of heart-lung transplants.[49] Such volumes are an important potential source of blood replacement through reinfusion. Autotransfusion of shed mediastinal blood has been shown to reduce requirements for transfusion of exogenous blood by 50%.[79] This technique has not been studied specifically in a thoracic transplant population, but it is widely practiced.

Summary

Bleeding and blood conservation are significant issues in thoracic transplantation. The infectious risks of blood transfusion are especially threatening to immunosuppressed patients, with CMV pneumonia in single-lung, double-lung, or heart-lung recipients as the best example. At the same time, iatrogenic and noniatrogenic coagulopathies are very common in thoracic transplant patients, which makes avoidance of transfusion even more of a challenge. The nonelective nature of transplant procedures further increases the difficulties by eliminating preoperative strategies for blood conservation that can be very effective in an elective surgical population. These circumstances increase the importance of pharmacologic agents, such as aprotinin, in a thoracic transplant population. All standard intraoperative and postoperative blood-conserving techniques in cardiac surgery, such as reinfusion of shed mediastinal blood, are equally appropriate in thoracic transplant patients.

References

1. Cooley DA, Bloodwell RD, Beall AC. Cardiac valve replacement without blood transfusion. *Am J Surg* 1964;112:743–751.
2. Toy PTCY, Strauss RG, Stehling LC, et al. Predeposited autologous blood for elective surgery. *N Engl J Med* 1987;316:517–520.
3. Love TR, Hendren WG, O'Keefe DD, et al. Transfusion of predonated autologous blood in elective cardiac surgery. *Ann Thorac Surg* 1987; 43:508–512.
4. Moran JM, Babka R, Silberman S, et al. Immediate centrifugation of oxygenator contents after cardiopulmonary bypass. *J Thorac Cardiovasc Surg* 1978;76:510–517.
5. Cosgrove DM, Loop FD, Lytle BW. Blood conservation in cardiac surgery. *Cardiovasc Clin* 1982;12:165–175.
6. Corno AF, Laks H, Warner Stevenson L, et al. Heart transplantation in a Jehovah's Witness. *J Heart Transplant* 1986;5:175–177.
7. Lammermeier DE, Duncan JM, Kuykendall RC, et al. Cardiac transplantation in a Jehovah's Witness. *Tex Heart Institute J* 1988;15:189–192.
8. Kemkes BM. Hemostatic failures and heart-lung transplantation: assessing the current situation. *J Heart Lung Transplant* 1993;12:3–6.
9. Miller LW, Naftel DC, Bourge RC, et al. Infection after heart transplantation: a multiinstitutional study. *J Heart Lung Transplant* 1994;13:381–393.
10. Kaye MP. The registry of the International Society for Heart and Lung Transplantation: tenth official report—1993. *J Heart Lung Transplant* 1993; 12:541–548.
11. Deeg HJ. Graft-versus-host disease: host and donor views. *Semin Hematol* 1993;30:110–118.
12. Herman JG, Beschorner WE, Baughman KL, et al. Pseudo-graft-versus-host disease in heart and heart-lung recipients. *Transplantation* 1988;46:93–98.
13. Anderson KC, Weinstein HJ. Transfusion-associated graft-versus-host disease. *N Engl J Med* 1990;323:315–321.

14. Burdine J, Perry EH, Kshettry VR, et al. Donor derived antibodies and hemolysis after ABO compatible but non-identical heart-lung and lung transplantation. Presented at the International Society for Heart and Lung Transplantation, April 5–8, 1995, San Francisco, CA.
15. Preiksaitis JK. Indications for the use of cytomegalovirus-seronegative blood products. *Transf Med Rev* 1991;5:1–17.
16. Preiksaitis JK, Rosno S, Grumet C, et al. Infections due to herpesviruses in cardiac transplant recipients: role of the donor heart and immunosuppressive therapy. *J Infect Dis* 1983;147:974–981.
17. Pollard RB. Cytomegalovirus infections in renal, heart, heart-lung and liver transplantation. *Pediatr Infect Dis J* 1988;7:97–102.
18. Linder J. Infection as a complication of heart transplantation. *J Heart Transplant* 1988;7:390–394.
19. Prince AM, Szmuness W, Millian SJ, David DS. A serologic study of cytomegalovirus infections associated with blood transfusions. *N Engl J Med* 1971; 284:1125–1131.
20. Duncan AJ, Dummer JS, Paradis IL, et al. Cytomegalovirus infection and survival in lung transplant recipients. *J Heart Lung Transplant* 1991; 10:638–646.
21. Maurer JR, Tullis E, Scavuzzo M, et al. Cytomegalovirus infection in isolated lung transplantations. *J Heart Lung Transplant* 1991;10:647–649.
22. Onorato IM, Morens DM, Martone WJ, et al. Epidemiology of cytomegaloviral infections: recommendations for prevention and control. *Rev Infect Dis* 1985;7:479–497.
23. Koskinen PK, Krogerus LA, Nieminen MS, et al. Cytomegalovirus infection-associated generalized immune activation in heart allograft recipients: a study of cellular events in peripheral blood and endomyocardial biopsy specimens. *Transpl Int* 1994;7:163–171.
24. Normann SJ, Salomon DR, Leelachaikul P, et al. Acute vascular rejection of the coronary arteries in human heart transplantation: pathology and correlations with immunosuppression and cytomegalovirus infection. *J Heart Lung Transplant* 1991;10:674–687.
25. Novick RJ, Menkis AH, McKenzie FN, et al. Should heart-lung transplant donors and recipients be matched according to cytomegalovirus serologic status? *J Heart Transplant* 1990;9:699–706.
26. Hosenpud JD, Novick RJ, Breen TJ, et al. The Registry of the International Society for Heart and Lung Transplantation: eleventh official report—1994. *J Heart Lung Transplant* 1994;13:562–570.
27. Sayers M. Prevention of cytomegalovirus infection by using leukocyte-depleted components. *Curr Stud Hematol Blood Transf* 1994;60:41–52.
28. Lane TA. Leukocyte reduction of cellular blood components: effectiveness, benefits, quality control, and costs. *Arch Pathol Lab Med* 1994;118: 392–404.
29. De Graan-Hentzen YCE, Gratama JW, Mudde GC, et al. Prevention of primary cytomegalovirus infection in patients with hematologic malignancies by intensive white cell depletion of blood products. *Transfusion* 1989;29:757–760.
30. Matthews JL, Sogandares-Bernal F, Judy M, et al. Inactivation of viruses with photoactive compounds. *Blood Cells* 1992;18:75–89.
31. McCarty M. Of cats and women. *Br Med J* 1983;287:445–446.
32. Fleck DG. Toxoplasmosis. *Public Health* 1969;83:131–135.

33. Holliman RE, Johnson JD, Adams S, et al. Toxoplasmosis and heart transplantation. *J Heart Transplant* 1991;10:608–610.
34. Ryning FW, McLeod R, Maddox JC, et al. Probable transmission of *Toxoplasma gondii* by organ transplantation. *Ann Intern Med* 1979;90:47–49.
35. Wreghitt TG, Hakim M, Gray JJ, et al. Toxoplasmosis in heart and heart and lung transplant recipients. *J Clin Pathol* 1989;42:194–199.
36. Luft BJ, Naot Y, Araujo FG, et al. Primary and reactivated *Toxoplasma* infection in patients with cardiac transplants: clinical spectrum and problems in diagnosis in a defined population. *Ann Intern Med* 1983;99:27–31.
37. Anthuber M, Kemkes BM, Heiss MM, et al. HIV infection after heart transplantation: a case report. *J Heart Transplant* 1991;10:611–613.
38. Scorza LB, Waymack JP, Pruitt BA. The effect of transfusions on the incidence of bacterial infection. *Milit Med* 1990;155:337–339.
39. Waymack JP, Robb E, Alexander JW. Effect of transfusion on immune function in a traumatized animal model. II. Effect on mortality rate following septic challenge. *Arch Surg* 1987;122:935–939.
40. Waymack JP, Warden GD, Alexander JW, et al. Effect of blood transfusion and anesthesia on resistance to bacterial peritonitis. *J Surg Res* 1987; 42:528–535.
41. Tartter PI, Quintero S, Barron DM. Perioperative blood transfusion associated with infectious complications after colorectal cancer operations. *Am J Surg* 1986;152:479–482.
42. Larison PJ, Cook LO. Adverse effects of blood-transfusion. In: Harmening DM, ed. *Modern Blood Banking and Transfusion Medicine.* 3rd ed. Philadelphia: F.A. Davis, 1994;351–374.
43. Stoelting RK, Miller RD. Fluid and blood therapy. In: Stoelting RK, Miller RD, eds. *Basics of Anethesia.* 3rd ed. New York: Churchill Livingstone, 1994;233.
44. Pennington DG, McBride LR, Swartz MT, et al. Use of Pierce-Donachy ventricular assist device in patients with cardiogenic shock after cardiac operations. *Ann Thorac Surg* 1989;47:130–135.
45. Schiessler A, Friedel N, Weng Y, et al. Mechanical circulatory support and heart transplantation: pre-operative status and outcome. *ASAIO J* 1994;40:476–481.
46. Aster RH, George JN. Thrombocytopenia due to sequestration of platelets. In: Williams WJ, Beutler E, Erslev AJ, Lictman MA, eds. *Hematology.* 4th ed. New York: McGraw-Hill, 1990;1398–1400.
47. Aster RH, George JN. Thrombocytopenia due to platelet loss. In: Williams WJ, Beutler E, Erslev AJ, Lictman MA, eds. *Hematology.* 4th ed. New York: McGraw-Hill, 1990;1401–1402.
48. Hunt BJ, Sack D, Amin S, et al. The perioperative use of blood components during heart and heart-lung transplantation. *Transfusion* 1992;32:57–62.
49. Royston D. Aprotinin therapy in heart and heart-lung transplantation. *J Heart Lung Transplant* 1993;12:19–25.
50. Goodnough LT, Rudnick S, Price TH, et al. Increased preoperative collection of autologous blood with recombinant human erythropoietin therapy. *N Engl J Med* 1989;321:1163–1168.
51. Blackburn MEC, Kendall RG, Gibbs JL, et al. Anaemia in children following cardiac transplantation: treatment with low dose human recombinant erythropoietin. *Int J Cardiol* 1992;36:263–266.
52. Schonberger JPAM, Bredée JJ, Tjian D, et al. Intraoperative predonation contributes to blood saving. *Ann Thorac Surg* 1993;56:893–898.

53. Okita Y, Miki S, Ueda Y, et al. Reduction of homologous blood transfusion in reoperative valve surgery. *J Heart Valve Dis* 1994;3:411–416.
54. Wagstaffe JG, Clarke AD, Jackson PW. Reduction of blood loss by restoration of platelet levels using fresh autologous blood after cardiopulmonary bypass. *Thorax* 1972;27:410–414.
55. Kaplan JA, Cannarella C, Jones EL, et al. Autologous blood transfusion during cardiac surgery: a re-evaluation of three methods. *J Thorac Cardiovasc Surg* 1977;74:4–10.
56. Novick RJ, Menkis AH, McKenzie FN, et al. Reduction in bleeding after heart-lung transplantation: the importance of posterior mediastinal hemostasis. *Chest* 1990;98:1383–1387.
57. Vouhé PR, Dartevelle PG. Heart-lung transplantation: technical modifications that may improve the early outcome. *J Thorac Cardiovasc Surg* 1989; 97:906–910.
58. Hackmann T, Gascoyne RD, Naiman SC, et al. A trial of desmopressin (1-desamino-8-D-arginine vasopressin) to reduce blood loss in uncomplicated cardiac surgery. *N Engl J Med* 1989;321:1437–1443.
59. Addonizio VP, Fisher CA, Jenkin BK, et al. Iloprost (ZK36374), a stable analog of prostacyclin, preserves platelets during simulated extracorporeal circulation. *J Thorac Cardiovasc Surg* 1985;89:926–933.
60. Dietrich W, Barankay A, Dilthey G, et al. Reduction of homologous blood requirement in cardiac surgery by intraoperative aprotinin application: clinical experience in 152 cardiac surgical patients. *Thorac Cardiovasc Surg* 1989; 37:92–98.
61. von Segesser LK, Weiss BM, Garcia E, et al. Reduction and elimination of systemic heparinization during cardiopulmonary bypass. *J Thorac Cardiovasc Surg* 1992;103:790–799.
62. Cardoso PFG, Yamazaki F, Keshavjee S, et al. A reevaluation of heparin requirements for cardiopulmonary bypass. *J Thorac Cardiovasc Surg* 1991; 101:153–160.
63. Royston D, Bidstrup BP, Taylor KM, et al. Effect of aprotinin on need for blood transfusion after repeat open heart surgery. *Lancet* 1987;2:1289–1291.
64. Fraedrich G, Weber C, Bernard C, et al. Reduction of blood transfusion requirement in open heart surgery by administration of high dose of aprotinin: preliminary results. *Thorac Cardiovasc Surg* 1989;37:89–91.
65. Dietrich W, Barankay A, Dilthey G, et al. Reduction of homologous blood requirement in cardiac surgery by intraoperative aprotinin application. Clinical experience in 152 cardiac surgical patients. *Thorac Cardiovasc Surg* 1989; 37:92–98.
66. Wachtfogel YT, Kucich U, Hack CE, et al. Aprotinin inhibits the contact, neutrophil, and platelet activation systems during simulated extracorporeal perfusion. *J Thorac Cardiovasc Surg* 1993;106:1–10.
67. Cosgrove DM, Heric B, Lytle BW, et al. Aprotinin therapy for reoperative myocardial revascularization: a placebo-controlled study. *Ann Thorac Surg* 1992;54:1031–1038.
68. Bidstrup BP, Underwood SR, Sapsford RN, et al. Effect of aprotinin (trasylol) on aorta-coronary bypass graft patency. *J Thorac Cardiovasc Surg* 1993; 105:147–153.
69. Blauhut B, Gross C, Necek S, et al. Effects of high-dose aprotinin on blood loss,

platelet function, fibrinolysis, complement, and renal function after cardiopulmonary bypass. *J Thorac Cardiovasc Surg* 1991;101:958–967.

70. Sundt TM, Kouchoukos NT, Saffitz JE, et al. Renal dysfunction and intravascular coagulation with aprotinin and hypothermic circulatory arrest. *Ann Thorac Surg* 1993;55:1418–1424.
71. Royston D. High-dose aprotinin therapy: a review of the first five years experience. *J Cardiothorac Vasc Anesth* 1992;6:76–100.
72. Pae WE, Aufiero TX, Weldner PW, et al. Aprotinin therapy for insertion of ventricular assist devices for staged heart transplantation. *J Heart Lung Transplant* 1994;13:811–816.
73. Goldstein DJ, Seldomridge JA, Chen JM, et al. Use of aprotinin in LVAD recipients reduces blood loss, blood use, and perioperative mortality. *Ann Thorac Surg* 1995;59:1063–1068.
74. Levy JH. Antibody formation after drug administration during cardiac surgery: parameters for aprotinin use. *J Heart Lung Transplant* 1993;12:26–32.
75. Salzman EW, Weinstein MJ, Weintraub RM, et al. Treatment with desmopressin acetate to reduce blood loss after cardiac surgery: a double-blind randomized trial. *N Engl J Med* 1986;314:1402–1406.
76. Czer LS, Bateman TM, Gray RJ, et al. Treatment of severe platelet dysfunction and hemorrhage after cardiopulmonary bypass: reduction in blood product usage with desmopressin. *J Am Coll Cardiol* 1987;9:1139–1147.
77. Temeck BK, Bachenheimer LC, Katz NM, et al. Desmopressin acetate in cardiac surgery: a double-blind, randomized study. *South Med J* 1994;87:611–615.
78. Fremes SE, Wong BI, Lee E, et al. Metaanalysis of prophylactic drug treatment in the prevention of postoperative bleeding. *Ann Thorac Surg* 1994; 58:1580–1588.
79. Schaff HV, Hauer JM, Bell WR, et al. Autotransfusion of shed mediastinal blood after cardiac surgery. *J Thorac Cardiovasc Surg* 1978;75:632–641.

8
Blood Conservation for Infants and Children Undergoing Surgery for Acquired and Congenital Heart Diseases

Jeffrey P. Gold

The Challenge of Blood Conservation in Congenital Cardiac Surgery

Surgery for congenital heart disease dates to the very birth of the practice of clinical cardiac surgery in the early 1930s. In spite of this fact, the ability to conserve the use of blood products and to preserve the patient's own circulating red blood cell mass has been one of the major challenges facing cardiac surgeons today. Although many lessons have been learned and applied from the practice of adult cardiac surgical blood conservation including mechanical, pharmacologic, and adjunctive measures, professionals treating children with congenital heart disease realized very quickly that they are not small adults, and therefore special challenges and special technical and pharmacologic considerations are required.

The major challenge is related to patient size and associated circulating red cell mass. As only approximately 7% of an average neonate's body mass is circulating blood volume, the effects of dilution, exposure to foreign surfaces, and destruction of formed elements related to the conduct of cardiopulmonary bypass become paramount considerations.[1-3]

The pathophysiology of many congenital cardiac disease states that produces cyanosis and associated polycythemia can assist in successful blood conservation measures as patients who carry these categories of disease have higher circulating red cell masses and a highly stimulated erythropoietic system.

Significant attempts have been made to conserve blood products in many forms of pediatric surgery, including orthopedic surgery, burn surgery, liver surgery, and various forms of transplantation.[4-9] All of these revolve around preoperative and intraoperative technical considerations.[10-12] By combining the fund of knowledge gleaned from these other areas of pediatric surgery with the specific issues related to congenital heart surgery, can one strive to minimize and ultimately eliminate the use of transfusion in the practice of congenital heart surgery.[13-15]

Preoperative Patient Preparation for Cardiac Surgery

The size and weight of patients is a major predictor of transfusion requirement in all cardiopulmonary bypass, and is particularly relevant in pediatric patients undergoing this form of surgery. The patient's circulating blood mass represents between 5% and 7% of their body weight. A 70-kg adult having elective coronary surgery is a very different consideration from a 2.5-kg neonate having an emergent arterial switch for transposition of the great vessels. Appreciation of the small circulating red blood cell mass, and calculating the dilutional effects of cardiopulmonary bypass are paramount in controlling the minimum safe hematocrits as well as predicting safe postoperative levels of circulating red cell mass. Preoperative hematocrit and hemoglobin concentrations are therefore also important in calculating these parameters.[16] The following standard equation predicts the effect of dilution on cardiopulmonary bypass hematocrit in infants, children, and young adults:

$$\underline{\mathrm{Hct}_{cpb} = (\mathrm{RBC\ Vol}_{P_t} + \mathrm{RBC\ Vol}_{\mathrm{CBP\ Machine}})/(\mathrm{Blood\ Vol}_{Pt} + \mathrm{Blood\ Vol}_{\mathrm{CBP\ Machine}})}$$
$$\mathrm{Hct}_{cpb} = (\mathrm{body\ wt}_{kg} \times f \times 1000 \times \mathrm{Hct}_{pt})/(\mathrm{body\ wt}_{kg} \times f \times 1000) + \mathrm{Vol}_{\mathrm{CBP\ Machine}}$$

where Hct_{cpb} is the approximate hematocrit on cardiopulmonary bypass, RBC Vol is the volume of red blood cells in the patient and/or bypass circuit, and f is an age-related factor that is 0.08 for neonates and infants, falling to 0.065 for teenagers and young adults. Unfortunately, this mathematical relationship tends to somewhat overestimate the minimal hematocrit and hemoglobin on cardiopulmonary bypass, but it does provide a rough frame of reference.

Preoperative platelet count and the status of the coagulation system is of great importance as well. Patients who are thrombocytopenic or are coagulopathic should be normalized as much as possible in an attempt to minimize intraoperative and postoperative blood loss. Either preoperative platelet transfusion or factor repletion (as applied to intraoperative) as defined by a full coagulogram are useful in controlling these parameters.

The use of preoperative and postoperative recombinant erythropoietin has been suggested and employed in limited studies.[17,18] The impact of limited preoperative supplemental erythropoietin on long-term growth and development of the hematopoietic system is unknown, and therefore is not routinely used in children. In patients with preexisting physiologic polycythemia due to underlying cyanotic congenital heart disease, the use of preoperative erythropoietin is generally considered unnecessary and is at times contraindicated.[19,20] Protocols employing routinely administered preoperative etythropoietin with specific targeted preoperative red cell masses have been successfully selectively employed in high-risk patients in many centers including ours.[21–23]

Blood product preparation is essential for all infants and children undergoing cardiac surgery. Although one continually strives for a bloodless surgical procedure, the availability and use of appropriate products can limit the number of donor exposures should transfusions become necessary. Many centers have successfully employed fresh warm blood products carrying the highest possible degree of platelet function and durability of red cell function as their primary resource for transfusion following pediatric cardiac surgery.[24] Indeed, our center has long had a preference for fresh whole warm blood rather than the use of component therapy. This is based on patient body weight, prior surgery, and on cardiac diagnosis.

Figure 8.1 shows the blood preparation for a routine pump case. A type I unit is less than 5-day-old packed cells, a type II unit is less than 24-hour-old whole blood, and a type III unit is fresh warm whole blood (less than 2 hours old and frequently from a directed donor). Component

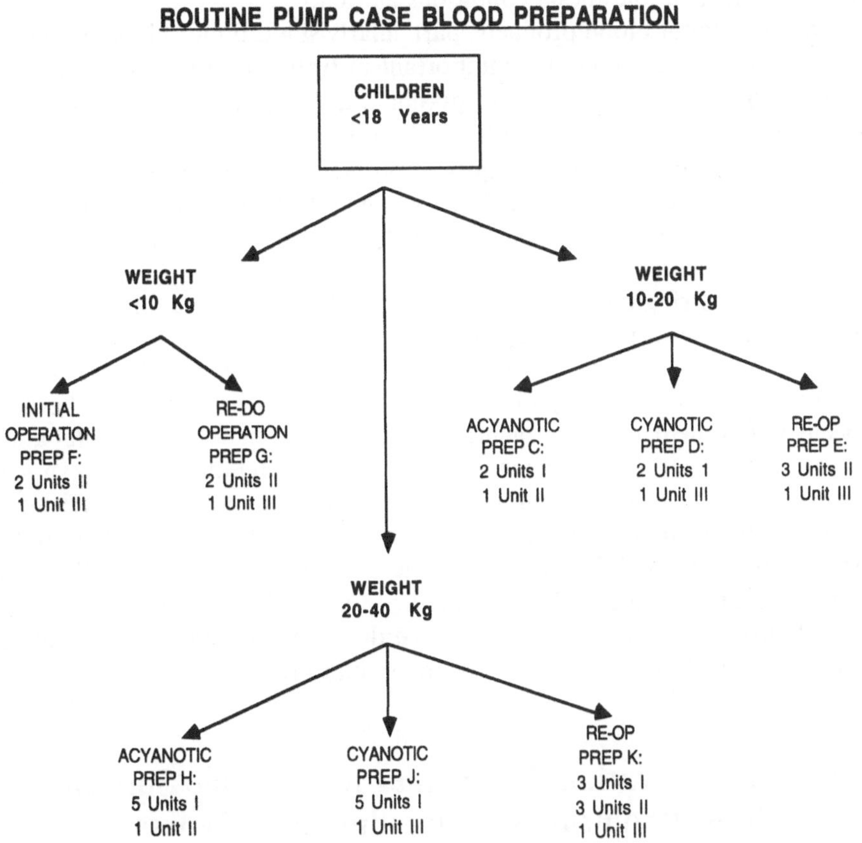

FIGURE 8.1. Blood preparation protocols for neonates, infants, and children undergoing cardiopulmonary bypass for repair of congenital heart disease. These vary as a function of patient weight, presence, or absence of cyanosis, and history of prior transternal cardiac surgery.

therapy is relegated only to specific measured hematologic deficiencies rather than simply red cell and volume expansion in the immediate postoperative period.

Directed and autologous donor products have become an increasingly prevalent source of transfusion products and continue to supply a very large percentage of the blood products required for elective congenital cardiac surgery.[25] Easing of restrictions on donor age and body mass have facilitated this process.[26,27] The use of autologous blood products particularly in polycythemic patients has been very successful in the pediatric population. One can harvest many small units of red cell or other components without any significant physiologic impact on the patient's underlying cardiopulmonary stability. This predonation by the patient in many cases can provide for all of the perioperative blood product requirements as well as those occurring in the postoperative period. The technology exists to do this type of multicomponent pheresis in the operating room under controlled anesthesia conditions as well.

Directed donor blood products, particularly single donor blood products, have also become increasingly important in transfusion therapy. With the ability to do platelet pheresis, plasma pheresis, and to selectively do erythropheresis on parents or other relatives, it is possible over a period of time when planning elective surgery to produce a spectrum of single donor blood products up to and including a single unit of fresh warm whole blood for use on the day of intended surgery.[28] With improved preservation techniques, including long-term cryopreservation technology, it is possible to store these single donor products (as well as others) for indeterminate periods of time while planning surgery.

The timing of surgery for congenital heart disease is particularly important as it relates to ongoing physiologic, hematologic, and hormonal events occurring in the patient. As mentioned above, reversal of all coagulopathic defects and treatment of any vitamin deficiencies and anemic states should be completed prior to scheduling elective surgery. If cardiac catheterization is necessary prior to surgical intervention, the catheterization procedure should be separated in time from the surgical procedure to allow for repletion of any blood loss occurring during the catheterization, and metabolism of any anticoagulants given during the diagnostic procedures. This is particularly important in neonates and infants.

Blood Conservation Techniques for Cardiac Surgical Procedures Requiring Cardiopulmonary Bypass

The widespread use of percutaneous monitoring lines has minimized the blood loss during the preincision patient-preparation phase of surgery. Cut-downs are now rarely necessary and attendant blood loss associated with these procedures is therefore minimized. Great vigilance needs to be maintained by the surgical, anesthesia, and perfusion teams to minimize hemodilution during all phases of surgery. This is particularly important in the pre-bypass, as large amounts of hemodilution may occur during this portion of the operative preparation and therefore can mandate the use of red cell transfusions at a later time.[28]

Technical aspects of the operation unquestionably form the cornerstone of all blood conservation techniques. An appropriately placed suture can minimize large amounts of postoperative blood loss and hemodynamic instability, and indeed frequently save a child's life. One needs to be meticulous about the selection of suture size, needle size, as well as suture placement particularly with complex, lengthy suture lines in high-pressure vessels and chambers of the cardiovascular system. Surgery for transposition of the great arteries underscores this concept. The neocoronary anastomosis and great vessel reconstructions are lengthy, and complex suture lines and have been a source of blood loss and hemodynamic instability in the past. Considerable time and attention has been dedicated to the development of techniques to minimize this technical problem. The use of tissue-like conduits, which include autografts, homografts, as well as native and gluteraldehyde-preserved pericardial patches and conduits, further serves to mimimize blood loss as compared with other types of prosthetic material used for conduit and patch material.

Topical hemostatic agents have been widely used over time, including topical thrombin, thrombin-soaked collagen material such as microfibullary collagen, or sponge-like collagen pledgets, which are transiently effective when applied over complex high-pressure suture lines. The use of a tissue glue-like material created by equal quantity mixtures of topical thrombin and autologous or homologous cryoprecipitate can form good-quality typical hemostatic plugs for isolated tiny bleeding points that are not assessable or technically amenable to suture placement.[29]

The use of topical aprotinin, when sprayed across the surgical field has also been reported to limit topical fibrinolysis and improve platelet function.[30–32] This has been successfully used in numerous studies of decreased postoperative blood loss. Mechanical forms of topical hemostatis such as packing materials, even if absorbable, can be quite deleterious if not removed. In the closed chest situation, they can place pressure on small delicate blood vessels and indeed be the underlying cause of either cardiac tamponade-like syndromes or localized cardiac compression syndromes. Therefore, their permanent use should be avoided whenever possible, and they should be removed if at all possible prior to chest closure.

Adequate drainage of the mediastinum and pleural spaces is important in all patients undergoing cardiothoraic surgery, but is particularly important in infants and neonates. Broad-caliber, mediastinal and pleural drains with wide mediastinal access to the pleural space should be utilized in order to minimize the collection of even small amounts of blood in the confined regions. Small amounts of regional fibrinolysis can produce more significant blood loss by its topical effect and lead to regional or global tamponade. Good-quality drainage without cardiac compression minimizes this problem.

Congenital heart surgery particularly in the neonate, has traditionally required the use of significant time periods of hypothermia, which may include deep hypothermic circulatory arrest. This technique, although applicable to large categories of adult patients, is much more widely used in children due to the technical circumstances of cannula placement, and the exposure of small and delicate intracardiac anatomic details. If preferred hyperthermia is utilized, a meticulous control of acid-base balance and thorough rewarming are necessary prior to separation from cardiopulmonary bypass in order to minimize bleeding associated with the profound degrees of systemic hypothermia.

Intraoperative Techniques for Congenital Heart Surgery Not Requiring Cardiopulmonary Bypass

Many of the techniques utilized for open congenital heart surgery are suitable for closed congenital heart surgery and procedures performed without cardiopulmonary bypass. Several specific considerations are worthy of mention. The closed procedures, which include coarctation repair, banding of the pulmonary artery, Blalock-Taussig shunts, ductal ligations and a number of other limited procedures, are all frequently performed without the requirement of cardiopulmonary bypass. The use of systemic anticoagulation including heparin has been widely used successfully for Blalock-Taussig shunts and other types of systemic to pulmonary artery shunts. With good mechanical hemostasis and the judicious use of topical agents, it is frequently not necessary to reverse the heparin at the end of the procedure.

Patients with long-standing cyanotic heart disease tend to have large-caliber and significant numbers of mediastinal- and pleural-based bronchopulmonary collateral vessels. These are extremely friable, thin-walled vessels that can be collectively the source of a significant amount of intraoperative and postoperative blood loss if not carefully controlled. Judicious use of electrocautery, metal clips, and other topical hemostatic agents is important in obtaining excellent control of these vessels prior to closure. As they have a tendency to be pleural based, simple maneuvers including placement of chest tubes and limited degrees of mediastinal dissection can frequently be associated with large amounts of blood loss if special care is not taken. Even occult rib fractures associated with retractor placement can bleed profusely if not recognized and appropriately dealt with in the operating room.[33] Topical hemostatic agents as described above can be extremely useful in controlling this form of surgical blood loss in patients who by nature of their age or cardiac changes are somewhat coagulopathic.[34]

Cardiopulmonary Perfusion Techniques for Infants and Children with Congenital Heart Disease

A requirement for cardiopulmonary bypass and the associated dilution with a purely asanguineous prime has focused attention on the cardiopulmonary bypass apparatus as the primary consideration for blood conservation in this challenging group of patients.[35,36] Efforts need to be made to minimize the size of the blood path in the entire circuit.[37-39] Small oxygenator volumes as well as fine-bore cardioplegia tubing, oxygenators, and other elements all serve together to limit the dilution associated with the bypass interval.[40] Keeping tubing length as short as possible and utilizing the minimal caliber tubing for table connection, as well as thin-walled high drainage cannulas, produce excellent results without requiring further hemodilution.

The hematocrit on cardiopulmonary bypass as described in the mathematical relationship above will vary as a function of patient body weight, patient age, starting hematocrit, and total amount of asanguineous prime. Much has been debated about the minimum safe hematocrit on cardiopulmonary bypass. Many have advocated the use of intentional hemodilution such that the hematocrit on bypass roughly parallels the temperature in varying degrees of hypothermia.[41] A minimum safe hematocrit of approximately 15–20% has been widely targeted for most forms of congenital heart surgery particularly at moderately decreased temperatures. Further investigation of these parameters and the relationship of the minimum safe hematocrit on bypass to the patient's baseline hematocrit needs to be further evaluated, as it may depend much more on oxygen delivery index, blood pH, flow rate, perfusion pressure, and other considerations than on the actual temperature.[42-44]

Adjunctive measures to conserve red cell mass, including cell saver-type technology and modified ultrafiltration, have been widely used with mixed results.[45,46] Many centers have successfully used cell salvage technology in children and small adults, whereas they have relied almost exclusively on modified ultrafiltration in infants and very small children.[47-49] Modified ultrafiltration is most successful in patients under 15 kg in body weight because of the small patient blood volume relative to the fraction of ultrafiltered fluid and the contents of the volume residual within the blood oxygenator system.[48-50] Although this technique adds approximately 10 to 15 minutes to the operative procedure, and is performed prior to heparin reversal, many centers have deemed this to be a safe, effective, and appropriate use of time. We have incorporated this routinely into the intraoperative regime (Fig. 8.2). Not only is hematocrit dramatically increased, and total body water reduced, but the inflammatory mediator in the circulatory blood seems to be dramatically reduced as well.[50-52]

Heparin-coated circuits, either ionically or covalently bound, have been used in many centers on adult patients and have been utilized in a limited number of children as well. A clear-cut therapeutic benefit has not been identified in infants and children but may be more important in surgical procedures requiring longer perfusion times and in reoperations.

The control of anticoagulation as monitored through the use of activated clotting times, thrombo-elastograms, and heparin concentration titrations has become more popular in children in recent years.[53-58] With larger amounts of anticoagulation required for high-efficiency membrane oxygenators, if one uses adjuncts such as aprotinin or other factor concentrates, the anticoagulation and its reversal become more challenging and somewhat less precise.[59,60] Many centers have switched to protamine titrations as well as the use of routine activated clotting times.[61,62] Simple stoichiometric reversal of heparin with protamine sulfate, which works quite frequently in adults, is often inaccurate in infants and children and underestimates the total required protamine doses even though heparin dosage is routinely and adequately employed at 200 U/kg. The protamine dosage therefore needs to be titrated to postoperative activated clotting time (ACT) and to residual circulating heparin levels.[59-65]

Parenteral Adjunctive Hemostatic Therapy for Infants and Children Undergoing Cardiopulmonary Bypass

Many adjunctive hemostatic agents have been employed in corrective and palliative surgical procedures for infants and children with congenital heart disease. Although initial enthusiasm has been present for almost all of these agents, there has been considerable waxing and waning in ensuing years. Suffice it to say that none of these agents has become standard therapy for all pediatric patients undergoing congenital heart surgery.

Desmopressin acetate [1-deamino-8-D-arginine desmopressin acetate (DDAVP)] has been utilized in adults as well as infants and children undergoing cardiac surgery.[66-69] Although initial enthusiasm was quite widespread for the dramatic impact of this agent on minimizing postoperative blood loss and minimizing transfusion requirement, it has become much less widely used recently with the development of better agents, with the realistic recognition of the therapeutic benefits, and with the reporting of some adverse reactions to the drug.[70-73] It clearly is effective for patients with underlying von Willebrand's syndrome, some other platelet disorders, and a handful of metabolic associated diseases. It has also been shown to be

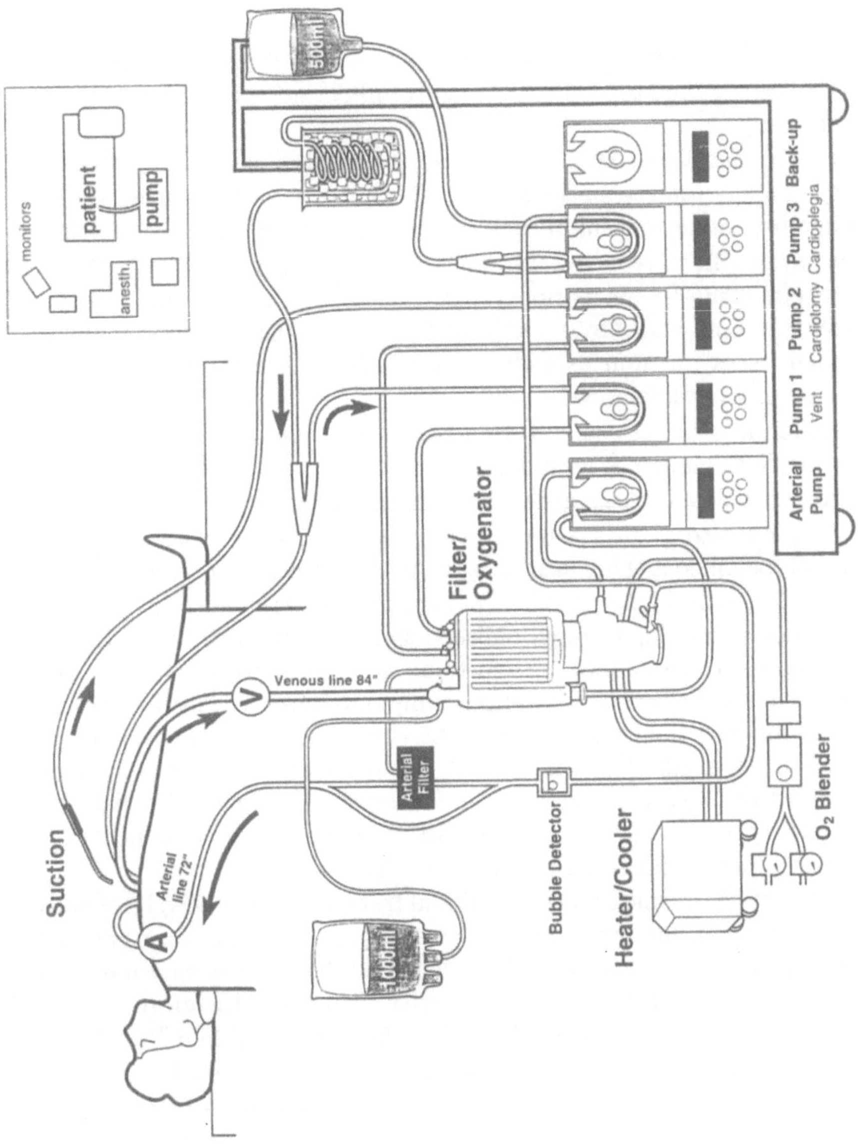

FIGURE 8.2. Modified ultrafiltration system employed at New York Hospital–Cornell Medical Center for infants and children under 20 kg.

effective in infants and children with severe renal insufficiency.[74] Many patients on long-term aspirin therapy also seem to benefit from intraoperative DDAVP.[74] Although once widely used routinely, its use has become more restrictive recently. Its advantages are that it is not particularly expensive, although it does add somewhat to the cost of these procedures and has a few rare side effects. The drug should be administered slowly to a total dosage of 0.3 μg/kg and can be repeated at a later time if necessary.[75,76] The benefit of DDAVP has also been suggested to improve upon the systemic and topical effect of aprotinin or other agents when given synergistically.[77,78]

Aprotinin has been reported recently in children undergoing cardiac surgery in many centers, particularly in Europe.[74,79-82] Widespread use of aprotinin in routine congenital heart procedures has been associated with a significant benefit in reducing intraoperative blood loss as well as transfusion requirements in the perioperative period.[83-86] The dosage remains controversial, and varies by a factor of four across the literature. Clearly, the initial bolus infusion as well as any maintenance infusion must be calculated in a per kilogram fashion.

Aprotinin may be associated with a significant number of side effects as well as the development of antibodies in a fixed percentage of patients. This is a serious problem if repeat exposures occur at a later time,[87] given the need for subsequent cardiac surgical procedures. Given the staged nature of surgery for many types of congenital heart disease, particularly for the univentricular heart, starting with either systemic to pulmonary artery shunts, or pulmonary artery banding, moving through bidirectional cavopulmonary anastomosis up through total cavopulmonary anastomosis.[88] The need for multiple surgical procedures and therefore multiple pump runs raises the risk of exposure to this agent, and therefore increases the risk of allergic/anaphylactic reaction. A secondary drawback is presently the cost of the drug; however, given many of its benefits, it seems to be a worthwhile investment for patients requiring reoperation surgery, patients with underlying coagulopathic states, and other patients with complex congenital heart disease.

Epsilon amino caproic acid (Amicar) and tranexamic acid (TA) have both been widely used in adult settings and have been applied to pediatric patients with varying degrees of success.[89-91] Large controlled studies have not been performed with any of these latter adjunctive agents, and therefore demonstrable value has not been established in infants and children.[92-94] These agents are relatively inexpensive and are generally considered to be safe.[95-97]

The use of preoperative and postoperative vitamin K to replenish the vitamin K-dependent clotting factors that were deficient either due to the patient's nutritional status and depressed hepatic function, or due to the administration of sodium warfarin preoperatively should be selectively employed. Oral medication is regarded as safer than intravenous or intramuscular use of vitamin K compounds.

Perioperative transfusion of platelets, fresh frozen plasma, cryoprecipitate, and other hemostatic adjuncts should be only selectively utilized in patients known to be qualitatively or quantitatively deficient of the specific factor.[98] The "shotgun" approach to postoperative bleeding with platelets, cryoprecipitate, and other materials is not only dangerous, but is frequently unsuccessful and certainly very expensive. Selective use of these agents to correct specific patient deficiencies is a far more effective means. Furthermore, empiric transfusion of platelets and factors, mild to moderate postoperative thrombocytopenia, transient postoperative elevation in prothrombin time, or partial thromboplastin time should also be aggressively avoided. In the nonbleeding hemodynamically stable patient, postoperative thrombocytopenia and mild defects in fluid-phase coagulation are not at all uncommon and will frequently resolve rapidly as the patient completely rewarms and metabolic function stabilizes. Only patients with evidence of coagulopathic bleeding or profound hematologic laboratory abnormalities should be transfused and with selected products as indicated.

Postoperative Blood Conservation Techniques for Patients Undergoing Congenital Heart Surgery

The establishment of safe transfusion triggers based on postoperative hemoglobin and hematocrit concentrations, platelet counts, and markers of fluid-phase coagulation are important to minimize the use of blood products in this group of patients.[99] Formerly one targeted hematocrits in the high 30s to low 40s, but we now understand well that hemodynamically stable patients without evidence of ongoing bleeding can be very safely allowed to have hematocrits in the mid- to high 20s without any consideration for transfusion whatsoever. Lower values may be equally safe. One needs to assess the oxygen delivery index prior to considering red cell transfusion. If the patient is warm and well perfused, and otherwise stable, even hematocrits in the low 20s can be accepted without any adverse impact on the postoperative recovery.[100–101]

The reinfusion of shed mediastinal blood, although quite popular in the adult setting, has only been minimally applied in infants and small children because of the technical considerations surrounding the use of this technology. As smaller and better collection systems and reinfusion systems are developed, the routine reinfusion of postoperative shed blood at least during the first 4 to 6 hours postoperatively will become more prevalent. If topical hemostatic agents have been employed, including any thrombin-like material, cryoglue or aprotinin, the mediastinal effluent should be discarded and not reinfused.

The increasing use of delayed sternal closure in critically ill infants and children has posed special problems related to blood conservation. In this instance the sternum is left unapproximated and sometimes the skin itself is left open, and closed only with a plastic barrier drape to prevent bacterial contamination. This allows the swollen mediastinal tissue to not be compressed by the rigid bony confines of the chest closure and therefore also allows for better postoperative cardiac and pulmonary function. With the lack of ability to completely and securely close the chest, bleeding tends to be a greater problem as the mediastinal structures are cooler and are exposed to foreign surfaces. Subsequent surgery is necessary to later close the chest.[102,103]

Unfortunately, patients requiring delayed sternal closure tend to be those with the greatest degrees of hemodynamic instability, longer and more complex procedures, longer intervals requiring cardiopulmonary bypass, greater degrees of intraoperative hypothermia, as well as many of the other risk factors for considerable postoperative bleeding. Excellent mediastinal and pleural drainage, as well as careful plastic barrier drape closure of the mediastinal incision, should be important considerations prior to transporting these critically ill children from the operating room. At the time of delayed closure all abnormal coagulation parameters, platelet counts, and circulating red cell mass should be corrected prior to returning the child for further surgery to close the chest.

Complications of Transfusion Therapy in Infants and Children Undergoing Congenital Heart Surgery

Just as the challenges of preventing blood loss and minimization of transfusion in infants and children are different and much more demanding than they are in adults undergoing cardiac surgery, the complications associated with transfusion therapy are more pronounced, rapid in onset, and indeed quite distinct in many ways from those associated with adult transfusion therapy.

A particular problem relates to the development of transfusion-induced significant hypocalcemia, and its associated metabolic and hemodynamic sequelae. This is due to red cell infusion of stored blood products. Calcium chelating agents have been widely utilized such as Adsol and ASD-1 as the anticoagulant and preservation medium of choice for most red cell products.[104] As the amount of calcium chelating activity is not calculated to match exactly the amount of collected blood, an additional amount of calcium-binding activity is present within the nonneutralized chelating agent. This will therefore rapidly reduce ionized serum calcium concentration and in particular do so very rapidly in patients with small body surface areas and small circulating blood volumes. Calcium metabolism is frequently abnormal or immature in critically ill neonates and infants. In addition, parathormone levels may be low or absent because of DiGeorge syndrome, which may be associated with the underlying congenital heart disease.

Either empiric or preferably measured repletion of ionized calcium needs to be associated with all red cell transfusion therapy. Frequently, unexplained hypotension or evidence of low cardiac output is associated with red cell transfusion therapy and almost invariably this relates to this change in serum ionized calcium.

Temperature changes in infants and children associated either with room temperature or less than room temperature blood products is also an important consideration. Although a unit of room temperature or cooler red cells in a 70-kg adult would produce a very minimal systemic temperature change, this might produce a profound temperature change in a neonate or infant. With the advent of technologically improved fluid and blood warming systems, it is possible to bring all transfusion therapy to body temperature prior to infusion into the patient.[105–106] This has become standard in situations where rapid transfusion of blood products is required.

Specific factor inhibition due to the use of topical agents has been reported in infants and children undergoing cardiac surgery. In particular, factor V inhibitors, which are due to antibody production, have been reported.[107] Theoretically, this can occur with many other types of factors and platelets.

Transfusion-mediated infection is also a concern associated with transfusion and particularly so in young children with immature immune systems. Although the number of donor exposures tends to be smaller, the incidence of infection, particularly with viral agents, including hepatitis and HIV, does not appear to be lessened compared with adults having a similar number of donor exposures.[108–109] There does not appear to be any degree of immune tolerance associated with transfusing infants and children, and may be quite the opposite.[110,111] The use of blood products that are free of agents such as cytomegalovirus (CMV) and other benign agents is important. The role of leuko-reduced blood products and leuko-reduction filters in the operating room and postoperatively are presently being explored, and may likely be important in these patients with immature and depressed immune systems.[112–115]

Exposure of operating room and intensive care unit personnel to blood products is a frequently unrecognized complication of transfusion therapy.[116] Although the incidence of exposure is far less than that of the patient, efforts directed at decreasing patient exposure will also decrease personnel exposure as well.

New York Hospital–Cornell Medical Center Protocols for Blood Conservation in Infants and Children Undergoing Cardiac Surgery

New York Hospital–Cornell Medical Center over the past 12 years has evolved a simple and straightforward algorithm for the management of patients undergoing cardiothoracic surgery for congenital heart disease. Rigorous algorithmic steps are taken for every patient in order to attempt to successfully complete "bloodless" surgical procedures in almost all patients.

All patients undergo extensive and complete preoperative hematologic evaluation, which not only includes an assessment of the hemoglobin, hematocrit, platelet count, and coagulation status, but may involve platelet function testing as well as a formal coagulogram as indicated. Programs of directed and/or autologous donation, and if necessary, single donor preferred blood products, are scheduled prior to necessary diagnostic and surgical procedures. If a patient is not cyanotic with significant polycythemia, recombinant erythropoieten is selectively employed on a protocol basis. Many patients are phlebotomized in the operating room employing high-volume hemodilution protocols as their blood volume, circulating red cell mass, and hemodynamic stability permits. Such phlebotomy precedes the administration of antifibrinolitic agents such as Amicar and aprotinin. All products are stored at room temperature and administered through a standard filter and blood warmer at later stages of the procedure following protamine administration and normalization of the ACT.

Ultraminiaturization of all components of a cardiopulmonary bypass circuit are utilized (Fig. 8.3). Each feature of the bypass circuit from cannula to cannula has been critically evaluated and the prime volume reduced. Retrograde arterial priming of the arterial pump line, the filter, and other components of the miniature circuit is performed as hemodynamically tolerated immediately before initiating cardiopulmonary bypass (Fig. 8.4). Patients are anticoagulated with 200 units of heparin per kilogram with a target ACT of 500 seconds. The only exception to this rule is when aprotinin is used, and then the initial dosage is increased to 300 units per kilogram with a target ACT of 750 seconds.

Hypothermia used during the operative procedures is minimized and as much of the procedure as possible is done at normothermic or near normal conditions. Rewarming to a core temperature of 36.5° to 37.0°C is completed in every patient prior to separation from bypass whenever possible. Deep hypothermic circulatory arrest and deep hypothermia "low flow" and "trickle flow" is avoided whenever possible. Topical hemostatic agents, which include thrombin-soaked Gelfoam, cryoglue, and aerosolized aprotinin, are selectively utilized as indicated. None of them is routinely employed. Every attempt is made to remove these materials prior to chest closure.

Controlled hemodilution on cardiopulmonary bypass and subsequent cell salvage and/or modified ultrafiltration are utilized in every patient. A minimum hematocrit of 15% at normothermic bypass, and lower hematocrits are frequently tolerated based on closely monitored venous oxygen saturations, particularly at hypothermic temperature levels.

Modified ultrafiltration protocols prior to (during rewarming) and following separation from bypass as permitted by reservoir volume is used

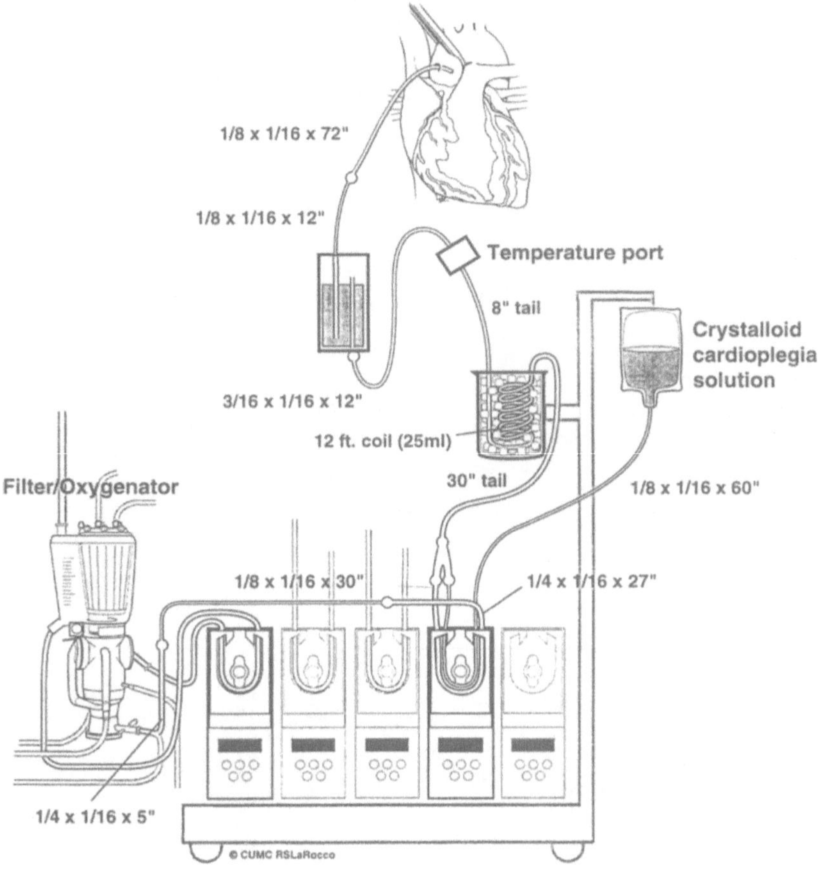

FIGURE 8.3. Cardiopulmonary bypass circuit demonstrating priming volumes, tubing loop length, and components used for typical pediatric patients under 10 kg.

for patients under 20 kg of body weight. More than 100 ml/kg of ultrafiltrate are removed in infants and children under 20 kg as a minimum, and frequently more. Heparin-coated circuits may be selectively employed when lengthy complex procedures are anticipated, such as reoperations.

Systemic administration of aprotinin is reserved for lengthy complex operations, reoperations, and patients with known preoperative coagulopathic states. When administered a low-dosage regimen consisting of a pre-bypass intravenous loading dose, a maintenance dose and a pump prime dose are employed. All other patients get a combination of pre-bypass epsilon amino caproic acid (100 mg/kg bolus) and/or post-bypass DDAVP (0.03 mmg/kg). We do not routinely use Amicar or DDAVP in patients receiving aprotinin.

No empiric use of component, platelet, or factor therapy is employed without evidence of bleeding or dramatic suppression of factor levels.

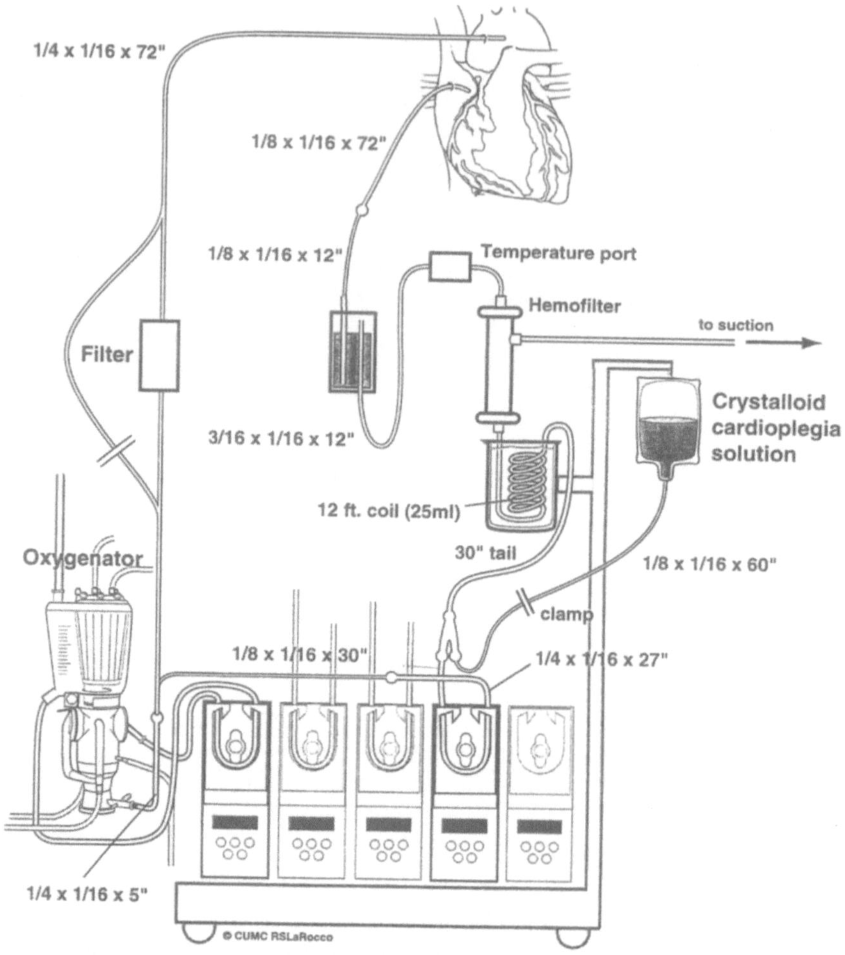

FIGURE 8.4. Miniaturized cardioplegia system employed at New York Hospital–Cornell Medical Center for infants and children.

Heparin is reversed routinely with protamine sulfate and every attempt made to normalize the ACT. Follow-up ACTs 4 to 6 hours following surgery are routinely performed to determine the need for subsequent doses of protamine sulfate.

Postoperative transfusion triggers are set consistent with the patient's hemodynamic status and underlying pathophysiology. Routine straightforward cases will have a transfusion trigger set at 22% to 23% hematocrit. Shed mediastinal blood is reinfused in all patients whose body weight exceeds 7 kg. All blood products used in neonates and infants are under 48 hours old and many of them are under 24 hours old. All of these products are leuko-reduced by the blood bank prior to transfusion and are also CMV negative. A single unit of fresh warm blood less than 4 hours old is made available for every patient under 10 kg body weight as well as every cyanotic patient undergoing reoperative surgery. Although not routinely transfused when needed, this very fresh warm blood seems to minimize the need for subsequent transfusion component therapy.

The above-described regimen appears to have successfully reduced the amount of blood products transfused in infants and children undergoing cardiac surgery at New York Hospital–Cornell Medical Center. We have gone to great lengths to selectively employ the most sophisticated, technologic, and pharmacologic protocols in all of our patients. We try very hard to do this on a case-by-case basis with preoperative planning conferences involving the surgical staff as well as the cardiology staff, critical care staff, hematology staff, parent, and patient when possible. Our perfusion staff as well as our cardiac anesthesia staff are always involved as well, as the roles they play are paramount in minimizing the use of blood products in these patients.

It is a never-ending challenge to push back the technical thresholds of cardiopulmonary bypass in order to further limit the requisite degrees of hemodilution associated with cardiac surgery in these highly complex and challenging patients. If one philosophically starts off attempting to prevent the wastage of every single milliliter of blood, the end result will be to dramatically minimize donor exposures to these patients. If one starts off with a philosophy that all infants and children undergoing cardiac surgery require blood products and they all have a moderate amount of postoperative blood loss, then that prophecy will certainly be self-fulfilling and one will continue to transfuse these patients indefinitely. By standing shoulder to shoulder with our colleagues performing adult cardiac surgery and our colleagues performing complex noncardiac surgery on infants and children, we can begin to attack the complex issues associated with blood conservation in this diverse and highly demanding group of patients.

References

1. Tsang VT, Mullaly RJ, Ragg PG, et al. Bloodless open-heart surgery in infants and children. *Perfusion* 1994(4):257–263.
2. Evans DA, Holder RL, Brawn WJ, et al. Post-operative blood loss following cardio-pulmonary bypass in children. *Eur J Cardiothorac Surg* 1994;8(1):25–29.
3. Maeda M, Koyama T, Murase M, et al. The indications and limitations of open heart surgery without homologous blood transfusion in children and infants. *Nippon Kyobu Geka Gakkai Zasshi* 1994;42(l):1–7.
4. Tasaki T, Ohto H, Noguchi M, et al. Autologous blood donation elective surgery in children. *Vox Sang* 1994;66(3):188.
5. Kharasch SJ, Millham F, Vinci RJ. The use of autotransfusion in pediatric chest trauma. *Pediatr Emerg Care* 1994;10(2):109–112.

6. Berniere J. Evolution of blood transfusion economy techniques in pediatric orthopedic surgery. *Arch Pediatr* 1995;2(2):108–110.
7. Budny PG, Regan PJ, Roberts AH. The estimation of blood loss during burns surgery. *Burns* 1993;19(2):134–137.
8. Carlier M, Van Obbergh LJ, Veyckemans F, et al. Hemostasis in children undergoing liver transplantation. *Somin Thromb Hemost* 1993;19(3):218–222.
9. Simpson MB, Georgopoulos G, Eilert RE. Intraoperative blood salvage in children and young adults undergoing spinal surgery with predeposited autologous blood: efficacy and cost effectiveness. *J Pediatr Orthop* 1993; 13(6):777–780.
10. Griffin TC, Buchanan GR. Elective surgery in children with sickle cell disease without preoperative blood transfusion. *J Pediatr Surg* 1993;28(5):681–685.
11. Aleksandrov AE, Lekmanov AU, Leont'ev AF, et al. Risk factors and their correction during shunt operation in children with extrahepatic portal hypertension. *Anestezio Reanimatol* 1994;3:8–10.
12. Presson RB Jr, Hillier SC. Perioperative fluid and transfusion management. *Semin Pediatr Surg* 1992;1(1);22–31.
13. Sobrinho AF, Baucia JA, Tranquitelle AM, et al. Pediatric heart surgery in a general hospital. Procedures and results in a 5 years' experience. *Arq Bras Cardiol* 1993;61(1):17–22.
14. Tsang VT, Mullaly RJ, Ragg PG, et al. Bloodless open-heart surgery in infants and children. *Perfusion* 1994;9(4):257-263.
15. Kawagicki M, Bergsland J, Subramanian S. Total bloodless open heart surgery in the pediatric age group. *Circulation* 1984;70(supp I):37.
16. Taylor KM. Perioperative approaches to coagulation defects. *Ann Thorac Surg* 1993;56(5 suppl):S78-S82.
17. Fleming RY, Herndon DN, Vaidya S, et al. The effect of erythropoietin in normal healthy volunteers and pediatric patients with bum injuries. *Surgery* 1992;112(2):424–431.
18. Hayshi J, Shinonaga M, Nakazawa S, et al. Does recombinant human erythropoietin accelerate erythropoiesis for predonation before cardiac surgery? *Jpn Circ J* 1993;57(6):475–479.
19. Schmoeckel M, Nollert G, Mempel M, et al. Effects of recombinant human erythropoietin on autologous blood donation before open heart surgery. *Thorac Cardiovasc Surg* 1993;41(6):364-368.
20. Seracini D, Pollini I, Lavoratti GC, et al. An echocardiographic study of the left ventricular functional indices in pediatric patients on hemodialysis and in treatment with recombinant human erythropoietin. *Pediatr Med Chir* 1994; 16(4):389–392.
21. Helm RE, Gold JP, Rosengart TK, et al. Erythropoietin in cardiac surgery. *J Cardiovasc Surg* 1993;8(5):579–606.
22. Horiba K, Itou Y, Terada H, et al. Experience of predeposit autologous blood transfusion and medication of recombinant human erythropoietin in pediatric open heart surgery. *Kyobu Geka* 1991;44(13):1146–1150.
23. Triulzi DJ, Gilmor, GD, Ness PM, et al. Efficacy of autologous fresh whole blood or platelet-rich plasma in adult cardiac surgery. *Transfusion* 1995; 35(8):67–634.
24. Kemmotsu H, Joe K, Nakamura H, et al. Predeposited autologous blood transfusion for surgery in infants and children. *J Pediatr Surg* 1995; 30(5):659–661.

25. Zanolli FA, Scremin A, Negri MG, et al. Predeposit hemodilution and intra- and post-operative blood salvage in the orthopaedic surgery of brain damaged children. *Int J Artif Organs* 1993;16(suppl 5):247–252.
26. Flynn JM, Cintron K, Canals RM. The use of autologous blood transfusions in pediatric orthopaedic surgery. *Bol Assoc Med P R* 1991;83(5):192.
27. Strauss RG, Wieland MR, Randels MJ, et al. Feasibility and success of a single-donor red cell program for pediatric elective surgery patients. *Transfusion* 1992;32(8):747–749.
28. Drinkwater DC, Laks H. Pediatric cardioplegic techniques. *Semin Thorac Cardiovasc Surg* 1993;5(2):168–175.
29. Milne AA, Murphy WG, Reading SJ, et al. Fibrin sealant reduces suture line bleeding during carotid endoarterectomy: a randomized trial. *Eur J Vasc Endovasc Surg* 1995;10(1):91–94.
30. Tabuchi N, deHoan J, van Oeveren W. Topical effect of aprotinin on the surgical wound in cardiac surgery. *J Thorac Cardiovasc Surg* 1995; 109(2):400–402.
31. O'Regan DJ, Giannopoulos N, Mediratta N, et al. Topical aprotinin in cardiac operations. *Ann Thorac Surg* 1994;58(3):778–781.
32. Cicek S, Tatar H, Demirkilic U, et al. Topical use of aprotinin in cardiac surgery. *J Thorac Cardiovasc Surg* 1995;110(2):568–569.
33. Gontijo B, Fantini FA, Alcocer EP, et al. Secondary sternotomy in pediatric heart surgery. *Arq Bras Cardiol* 1994;62(2):103–106.
34. Achauer BM, Miller SR, Lee TE, et al. The hemostatic effect of fibrin glue on graft donor sites. *J Burn Care Rehabil* 1994;15(1):24–28.
35. Beppu T, Imai Y, Fukui A. A computerized control system for cardiopulmonary bypass. *J Thorac Cardiovasc Surg* 1995;109(3):428–438.
36. Hill AG, Green RC, Abe BF, et al. Pediatric perfusion practice in North America. *Perfusion* 1993;8:29.
37. Friesen RH, Tornabene MA, Coleman SP. Blood conservation during pediatric cardiac surgery: ultrafiltration of the extracorporeal circuit volume after cardiopulmonary bypass. *Anesth Analg* 1993;77(4):702–707.
38. Yoshikawa Y, Niwaya K, Hasegawa J, et al. Effect of blood conservation in open-heart surgery: a comparison of 3 different methods. *Kyobu Geka* 1994;47(13):1059–1062.
39. Honek T, Horvath P, Kucera V, et al. Minimisation of priming volume and blood saving in paediatric cardiac surgery. *Eur J Cardiothorac Surg* 1992; 6(6):308–310.
40. Bilfinger TV, Moeller JR, Kurusz M, et al. Pediatric myocardial protection in the United States: a survey of current clinical practice. *Thorac Cardiovasc Surg* 1992;40(4):214–218.
41. Hirschi RB. Oxygen delivery in the pediatric surgical patient. *Curr Opin Pediatr* 1994;6(3):341–347.
42. Yau TM, Carson S, Weisel RD, et al. The effect of warm heart surgery on postoperative bleeding. *J Thorac Cardiovasc Surg* 1992;103(6):1155–1163.
43. van Iterson M, van der Waart FJ, Erdmann W, et al. Systemic haemodynamics and oxygenation during haemodilution in children. *Lancet* 1995;346(8983): 1127–1129.
44. Wajon PR, Walsh RG, Symons NL. A survey of cardiopulmonary bypass perfusion practices in Australia in 1992. *Anaesth Intens Care* 1993; 21(6):814–821.

45. Naik SK, Knight A, Elliott M. A prospective randomized study of a modified technique of ultrafiltration during pediatric open-heart surgery. *Circulation* 1991;84(5 suppl):442–431.
46. Nagatsu M, Harada Y, Takeuchi T. Initial ultrafiltration to the priming solution with preserved blood for cardiopulmonary bypass in infants. *Kyobu Geka* 1995;48(4):281–285.
47. Groom RC, Al BF, Albus RA, et al. Alternative method of ultrafiltration after cardiopulmonary bypass. *Ann Thorac Surg* 1994;58(2):573–574.
48. Elliott MJ. Ultrafiltration and modified ultrafiltration in pediatric open heart operations. *Ann Thorac Surg* 1993;56(6)1518–1522.
49. Millar AB, Armstrong L, van der Linden J, et al. Cytokine production and hemofiltration in children undergoing cardiopulmonary bypass. *Ann Thorac Surg* 1993;56(6):1499–1502.
50. Behr D, Hernvann A, Pouard P, et al. Interleukin-6 and C-reactive protein during pediatric cardiopulmonary bypass. *Clin Chem* 1995;41(3):467–469.
51. Journois D, Pouard P, Greeley WJ, et al. Hemofiltration during cardiopulmonary bypass in pediatric cardiac surgery. Effects on hemostasis, cytokines, and complement components. *Anesthesiology* 1994;81(5):1181–1189.
52. Withington DE, Man WK, Elliott MJ. Histamine release during paediatric cardiopulmonary bypass. *Can J Anaesth* 1993;40(4):334–339.
53. Kriesmer P, Payne NR, Tessmer J, et al. Activated clotting time tests with heparinase in the management of pediatric patients with cardiopulmonary bypass. *ASAIO J* 1993;39(4):942–945.
54. Hashimoto K, Yamagishi M, Sasaki T, et al. Heparin and antithrombin III levels during cardiopulmonary bypass: correlation with subclinical plasma coagulation. *Ann Thorac Surg* 1994;58(3):799–804.
55. Wang JS, Lin CY, Karp RB. Comparison of high-dose thrombin time with activated clotting time for monitoring of anticoagulant effects of heparin in cardiac surgical patients. *Anesth Analg* 1994;79(1):9–13.
56. Litin SC, Gastineau DA. Current concepts in anticoagulant therapy. *Mayo Clin Proc* 1995;70(3):266–272.
57. Martin P, Horkay F, Rajah SM, Walker DR. Monitoring of coagulation status using thrombelastography during paediatric open heart surgery. *Int J Clin Monit Comput* 1991;8(3)183–187.
58. Szalados JE, Ouriel Shapiro JR. Use of the activated coagulation time and heparin dose-response curve for the determination of protamine dosage in vascular surgery. *J Cardiothorac Vas Anesth* 1994;8(5):515–518.
59. Jobes DR, Aitken GL, Shaffer GW. Increased accuracy and precision of heparin and protamin dosing reduces blood loss and transfusion in patients undergoing primary cardiac operations. *J Thorac Cardiovasc Surg* 1995;110(1):36–45.
60. De Laria GA, Tyner JJ, Hayes CL, et al. Heparin-protamine mismatch. A controllable factor in bleeding after open heart surgery. *Arch Surg* 1994; 129(9):944–950.
61. Jon LC, Rees GM, Kovacs IB. Different anticoagulants and platelet reactivity in cardiac surgical patients. *Ann Thorac Surg* 1993;56(4):899–902.
62. Kondo NI, Maddi R, Ewenstein BM, et al. Anticoagulation and hemostasis in cardiac surgical patients. *J Cardiovasc Surg* 1994;9(4):443–461.
63. Del Re MR, Ayd JD, Schultheis LW, et al. Protamine and left ventricular function: a transesophageal echocardiography study. *Anesth Analg* 1993; 77(6):1098–1103.

64. Brister SJ, Ofosu FA, Buchanan MR. Thrombin generation during cardiac surgery: is heparin the ideal anticoagulant? *Thromb Haemost* 1993;70(2):259–262.
65. Reich DL, Yanakakis MJ, Vela-Cantos FP, et al. Comparison of bedside coagulation monitoring tests with standard laboratory tests in patients after cardiac surgery. *Anesth Analg* 1993;77(4):673–679.
66. Kam PC. Use of desmopressin (DDAVP) in controlling aspirin-induced coagulopathy after surgery. *Heart Lung* 1994;23(4):333–336.
67. Salzman EW, Weinstein MJ, Reilly D, et al. Adventures in hemostasis. Desmopressin in cardiac surgery. *Arch Surg* 1993;128(2):212–217.
68. Dilthey G, Dietrich W, Spannagl M, et al. Influence of desmopressin acetate on homologous blood requirements in cardiac surgical patients pretreated with aspirin. *J Cardiothorac Vasc Anesth* 1993;7(4):425–430.
69. Temeck BK, Bachenheimer LC, Katz NM, et al. Desmopressin acetate in cardiac surgery: a double-blind, randomized study. *South Med J* 1994; 87(6):611–615.
70. Reynolds LM, Nicholson SC, Jobes DR, et al. Desmopressin does not decrease bleeding after cardiac operation in young children. *J Thorac Cardiovasc Surg* 1993;106(6)954–958.
71. Sloan EM, Alyono D, Klein HG, et al. 1-Deamino-8-D-arginine vasopressin (DDAVP) increases platelet membrane expression of glycoprotein lb in patients with disorders of platelet function and after cardiopulmonary bypass. *Am J Hematol* 1994;46(3):199–207.
72. Temeck BK, Bachenheimer LC, Katz NM, et al. Desmopressin acetate in cardiac surgery: a double-blind, randomized study. *Soutb Med J* 1994; 87(6):611–615.
73. Cattaneo M, Pareti FI, Sighetti M, et al. Platelet aggregation at high shear is impaired in patients with congenital defects of platelet secretion and is corrected by DDAVP: correlation with the bleeding time. *J Lab Clin Med* 1995;125(4):540–547.
74. Sheridan DP, Card RT, Pinilla JC, et al. Use of desmopressin acetate to reduce blood transfusion requirements during cardiac surgery in patients with acetylsalicylic-acid-induced platelet dysfunction. *Can J Surg* 1994;37(l):33–36.
75. Rocha E, Hildago F, Llorens R, et al. Randomized study of aprotinin and DDAVP to reduce postoperative bleeding after cardiopulmonary bypass surgery. *Circulation* 1994;90:921–927.
76. Daily PO, Lamphere JA, Dembitsky WP, et al. Effect of prophylactic epsilon-aminocaproic acid on blood loss and transfusion requirements in patients undergoing first-time coronary artery bypass grafting. *J Thorac Cardiovasc Surg* 1994;108(1):99–108.
77. Djulbegovic B, Hannan MM, Bergman GE. Concomitant treatment with factor IX concentrates and antifibrinolytics in hemophilia B. *Acta Haematol* 1995;94(suppl 1):43–47.
78. Penta de Peppo A, Pierri MD, Scafuri A, et al. Intraoperative antifibrinolysis and blood-saving techniques in cardiac surgery. Prospective trial of 3 antifibrinolytic drugs. *Tex Heart Inst J* 1995;22(3):231–236.
79. Ranucci M, Como A, Pavesi M, et al. Renal effects of low dose aprotinin in pediatric cardiac surgery. *Minerva Anesthesiol* 1994;60(7–8):361–366.
80. Levy JH, Bailey JM, Salmenpera M. Pharmacokinetics of aprotinin in preoperative cardiac surgical patients. *Anesthesiology* 1994;80(5):1013–1018.
81. Davis R, Whittington R. Aprotinin. A review of its pharmacology and

therapeutic efficacy in reducing blood loss associated with cardiac surgery. *Drugs* 1995;49(6):954–983.
82. Elliot MJ, Allen A. Aprotinin in pediatric cardiac surgery. *Perfusion* 1990;5:73.
83. Dietrich W, Mossinger H, Spannagl M, et al. Hemostatic activation during cardiopulmonary bypass with different aprotinin dosages in pediatric patients having cardiac operations. *J Thorac Cardiovasc Surg* 1993; 105(4):712–720.
84. Bodt J, Zickmann B, Schindler E, et al. Influence of aprotinin on the thrombomodulin/protein C system in pediatric cardiac operations. *J Thorac Cardiovasc Surg* 1994;107(5):1215–1221.
85. Herynkopf F, Lucchese F, Pereira E, et al. Aprotinin in children undergoing correction of congenital heart defects. A double-blind pilot study. *J Thorac Cardiovasc Surg* 1994;108(3):517–521.
86. Edmunds LH Jr. Invited letter concerning: aprotinin use in pediatric cardiac operations. *J Thorac Cardiovasc Surg* 1993;105(4):705–711.
87. Dietrich W, Mossinger H, Spannagl M, et al. Hemostatic activation during cardiopulmonary bypass with different aprotinin dosages in pediatric patients having cardiac operations. *J Thorac Cardiovasc Surg* 1993;105(4):712–720.
88. Huang H, Ding W, Su Z, et al. Mechanism of the preserving effect of aprotinin in platelet function and its use in cardiac surgery. *J Thorac Cardiovasc Surg* 1993;106(l):11–18.
89. Karaski JM, Teasdale SJ, Norman P, et al. Prevention of bleeding after cardiopulmonary bypass with high-dose tranexamic acid. Double-blind, randomized clinical trial. *J Thorac Cardiovasc Surg* 1995;110(3):835–842.
90. Boughenou F, Madi-Jebara S, Massonet-Castel S, et al. Fibrinolytic inhibitors and prevention of bleeding in cardiac valve surgery. Comparison of tranexamic acid and high dose aprotinin. *Arch Mal Coeur Vais* 1995;88(3):363–370.
91. Corbeau JJ, Monrigal JP, Jacob JP, et al. Comparison of effects of aprotinin and tranexamic acid on blood loss in heart surgery. *Ann Fr Anesth Reanim* 1995;14(2):154–161.
92. Cofey, A, Pittman J, Halbrook H, et al. The use of tranexamic acid to reduce postoperative bleeding following cardiac surgery: a double-blind randomized trial. *Am Surg* 1995:61(7):566–568.
93. Arom KV, Emery RW. Decreased postoperative drainage with addition of epsilon-aminocaproic acid before cardiopulmonary bypass. *Ann Thorac Surg* 1994;57(5):1108–1112.
94. Haidet KK. Aminocaproic acid. *Neonatal Netw* 1995;14(3):75–77.
95. Delrossi AJ, Cernaianu AC, Botros S, et al. Prophylactic treatment of postperfusion bleeding using EACA. *Chest* 1989;96:27–30.
96. VanderSalm TJ, Ansell JE, Okike ON, et al. The role of epsilon-aminocaproic acid in reducing bleeding after cardiac operation: a double-blind randomized study. *J Thorac Cardiovasc Surg* 1988;95:538–540.
97. Wilson JM, Bower LK, Fackler JC, et al. Aminocaproic acid decreases in the incidence of intracranial hemorrhage and other hemorrhagic complications of ECMO. *J Pediatr Surg* 1993;28(4):536–540.
98. Contrearas M, Ala FA, Greaves M, et al. Guidelines for the use of fresh frozen plasma. British Committee for Standards in Haematology, Working Party of the Blood Transfusion Task Force. *Transfus Med* 1992;2(2):97–98.
99. Goodnough LT, Despotis GJ, Hogue CW Jr, et al. On the need for improved transfusion indicators in cardiac surgery. *Ann Thorac Surg* 1995;60(2):473–480.

100. Brown MM, Kemper KM. Control of postoperative bleeding in the cardiac surgery patient. *J Cardiovasc Nurs* 1993;7(4):59–70.
101. Speiss BD. Cardiac anesthesia risk management. Hemorrhage, coagulation and transfusion:a risk-benefit analysis. *J Cardiothorac Vasc Anesth* 1994;81(1 suppl 1):19–22.
102. Lefevre P. Which technique should be chosen to reuse blood loss intraoperatively? Does the type of surgery constitute any contraindication for reutilization (cancer, infection)? *Ann Fr Anesth Reamin* 1995;15(suppl 1):53–62.
103. Petaja J, Lunddstrom U, Leijala M, et al. Bleeding and use of blood products after heart operations in infants. *J Thorac Cardiovasc Surg* 1995; 109(3):524–529.
104. Atsumi N, Abe M, Sakakibara Y, et al. Influence of ionized calcium concentration during cardiopulmonary bypass on pediatric cardiac surgery. *Kyobu Geka* 1994;47(7):544–548.
105. Gunning KA, Sugru M, Sloane D, et al. Hypothermia and severe trauma. *Aust N Z J Surg* 1995;65(2):80–82.
106. Phillips GR 3rd, Kauder DR, Schwab CW. Massive blood loss in trauma patients. The benefits and dangers of transfusion therapy. *Postgrad Med* 1994;(4):61–62, 67–72.
107. Muntean W, Zenz W, Finding K, et al. Inhibitor to factor V after exposure to fibrin sealant during cardiac surgery in a two-year old child. *Acta Paediatr* 1994;83(1):84–87.
108. Matsuoka S. Screening for post-transfusion hepatitis C—importance of enrollment and recall of blood transfusion recipients. *Nippon Kosbu Eisei Zasshi* 1994;41(9):933–937.
109. Matsuoka S, Tatara K, Hayabuchi Y, et al. Post-transfusion chronic hepatitis C in children. *J Paediatr Child Health* 1994;30(6):544–546.
110. Ni YH, Chang MH, Lue HC, et al. Posttransfusion hepatitis C virus infection in children. *J Pediatr* 1994;125(5 pt 1):709–713.
111. Frederick T, Mascola L, Eller A, et al. Progression of human immunodeficiency virus disease among infants and children infected perinatally with human immunodeficiency virus or through neonatal blood transfusion. Los Angeles County Pediatric AIDS Consortium and the Los Angeles County-University of Southern California Medical Center and the University of Southern California School of Medicine. *Pediatr Infect Dis J* 1994; 13(2):1091–1097.
112. Bowden RA, Slichter SJ, Sayers M, et al. A comparison of filtered leukocyte-reduced and cytomegalovirus (CMV) seronegative blood products for the prevention of transfusion-associated CMV infection after marrow transplant. *Blood* 1995;86(9):3599–3603.
113. Bocsan IS, Neamtu A, Radulescu A, et al. The markers of hepatitis B, C and D viral infection in multiply transfused patients. *Bacteriol Virusol Parazitol Epidemiol* 1995;40(2):109–113.
114. Xu D, Yonetani M, Uetani Y, et al. Acquired cytomegalovirus infection and blood transfusion in preterm infants. *Acta Paediatr Jpn* 1995;37(4):444–449.
115. Delage G. Transfusion-transmitted infections in the newborn. *Transfus Med Rev* 1995;9(3):271–276.
116. Wright JG, McGeer AJ, Chyatte D, et al. Exposure rates to patients' blood for surgical personnel. 1993;114(5):897–901.

Part II
Intraoperative Decision Making in Cardiac Surgery

9
Hemostasis and the Effect of Cardiopulmonary Bypass on Hemostasis

Su-Pen Bobby Chang and Richard Stennet

Hemostasis

Hemostasis is a dynamic ongoing physiologic process. The body reacts to vascular injury by local vasoconstriction and the activation of a barrage of cellular and biochemical mediators/activators to repair the injury. Concurrently opposing mediators/inhibitors are activated to locally limit the repair process, thus protecting the essential fluidity of the circulation. The call to clot is always accompanied by the message to temper the action. During the seemingly quiescent phases, the hemostatic system is actively maintaining the blood in a fluid state. It is the perturbation of this intricate "homeostatic" hemostasis during cardiac surgery by synthetic or foreign nonvascular surfaces, exogenous pharmaceuticals, endogenous biochemical mediators, and surgical steel that results in post-bypass coagulopathy.

Hemostasis is characterized by several recurrent themes of regulation:

1. Co-dependency on the interactions and the regulatory interplay of the vascular, platelet, coagulation protein, fibrinolytic, and inflammatory systems. As soon as one system is activated, others are activated to participate and also to mediate the response.
2. Activators and inhibitors are activated concurrently and exist at every level providing checks and balances.
3. Fail-safe mechanism: cellular and biochemical mediators along with enzymatic and structural proteins exist in inactive or less active forms until activated to participate in coagulation.
4. The activation of a part of the system can set off "cascades" and "domino (catalytic) effects" to accelerate and decelerate the response.

Vascular System

The vascular system has been increasingly recognized as a metabolic and physiologically active organ, not as a mere "conduit" or container for the distribution of blood. The response to vascular injury is dependent on the interaction of the blood vessel walls with circulating cellular elements and proteins.[1-6]

The endothelial cells of the intima provide a physical barrier to blood movement across the vessel walls and also maintain the blood in a fluid state. The basement membrane, which is synthesized by the endothelium, provides a physical barrier to separate circulating blood from the thrombogenic components of the subendothelium. In addition, the electrical charges of endothelial membrane proteins repel circulating coagulation proteins. The endothelium also synthesizes antithrombotic cell surface components such as nitric oxide, prostacyclin, thrombomodulin, heparin-like glycosaminoglycan, tissue plasminogen activator, and adenosine triphosphatase (ADPase) (Fig. 9.1).

Nitric Oxide

Nitric oxide (NO) is a platelet inhibitor and is now recognized as the much searched for endothelium-derived relaxing factor. Nitric oxide is synthesized in the endothelial cytosol from 1-arginine by NO synthase with

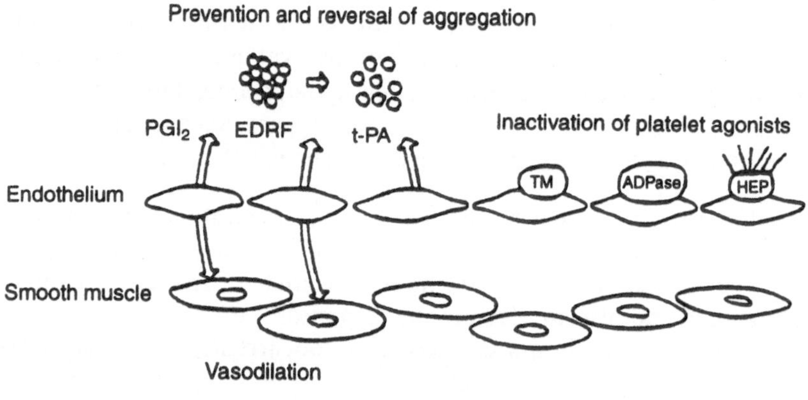

FIGURE 9.1. Vasoactive and antiaggregatory substances released by normal endothelium. Endothelial cells both retain and release into the blood many substances that are antiaggregatory and fibrinolytic. Among them, the soluble products include prostacyclin (PGI^2), endothelium-derived relaxing factor (EDRF), and tissue plasminogen activator (t-PA). Thrombomodulin (TM), ADPase, and the heparin-like glycosaminoglycan heparin sulfate (HEP) are located on the endothelial surface, where they degrade or otherwise interfere with thrombin and ADP, two potent platelet agonists. Some endothelium-derived antiplatelet substances, including prostacyclin and EDRF, also diffuse from endothelium to vascular smooth muscle to produce vasodilation. Endothelial cells also release many substances that do not affect aggregation, including endothelin. (From Ware and Heistad.[3])

nicotinamide adenine dinucleotide phosphate (NADP) as a cofactor. Nitric oxide diffuses from the endothelium into the vascular smooth muscle and vascular lumen. Nitric oxide stimulates guanylate cyclase in target cells, which increases the levels of cyclic guanosine monophosphate (cGMP). Cyclic GMP activates cGMP-dependent protein kinases, which in turn phosphorylates vasodilator-stimulated phosphoprotein (VASP). Phosphorylated VASP increases calcium reuptake resulting in lower cytoplasmic concentrations of calcium. The result is vascular smooth muscle relaxation and vasodilation. Nitric oxide synthase is active constitutively, thus nitric oxide likely modulates basal vascular tone. Lower cytoplasmic calcium levels also inhibit platelet adhesion, aggregation, granule release, and activation by agonists. NO is rapidly inactivated by hemoglobin. Since platelets are distributed more peripherally in flowing blood than the more central traveling erythrocytes, nitric oxide can diffuse from the endothelium and exert its action on platelets before being inactivated by hemoglobin.

Prostacyclin

Prostacyclin, a platelet inhibitor and vasodilator, is manufactured from endothelial membrane phospholipids through the sequential action of phospholipase A_2, cyclooxygenase, peroxidase, and prostacyclin synthetase enzymes. Prostacyclin can also be made through the endoperoxide shunt. Platelet-released thromboxane and platelet-derived precursors are converted into prostacyclin in the endothelial cell. Prostacyclin synthesis and release is induced by pulsatile pressure, platelet-derived mediators (serotonin, platelet-derived growth factor, interleukin-1, ADP, thromboxane), and endogenous plasma mediators (bradykinin, thrombin).

Prostacyclin is locally acting because of its short half-life of less than one circulation time. It is broken down rapidly in plasma to 6-keto prostaglandin $PGF_{1\alpha}$. Prostacyclin binds to a G-protein–containing receptor linked to adenylate cyclase. Adenosine triphosphate (ATP) is converted to cyclic adenosine monophosphate (cAMP). Cyclic AMP activates cAMP-dependent protein kinases, which in turn phosphorylate VASP. Calcium reuptake is increased, which results in decreased levels of cytoplasmic calcium. Smooth muscle is relaxed with resultant vasodilation. Platelets are inhibited by the increase in cyclic AMP.

Prostacyclin and NO, respectively through cAMP and cGMP, act synergistically to modulate vascular tone and to inhibit platelet activation. As mentioned above, nitric oxide is likely the basal mediator of vascular tone given the constitutive nature of nitric oxide synthase. Prostaglandins are produced in increased amounts after damage or perturbation of cell membranes. This suggests that the prostacyclin system exists to back up the nitric oxide system during states in which nitric oxide production is impaired, i.e., damaged endothelium.

Tissue Plasminogen Activator

Tissue plasminogen activator (t-Pa), which is synthesized by endothelial cells, catalyzes the formation of plasmin. t-Pa can have both activating and inhibiting effects on platelets. Initially t-Pa can activate platelets and cause aggregation in a turbulent system. If the platelets fail to aggregate, then they are not responsive to further stimulus. t-Pa can degrade platelet glycoprotein receptors, which are necessary for platelet activation by agonists.

Thrombomodulin

Thrombomodulin is an endothelial surface protein that avidly binds thrombin. Thrombin, a potent platelet activator, is removed from circulation. Thrombomodulin also activates protein C, which is an anticoagulant protein.

ADPase

ADPase is an endothelial surface-bound nucleotidase. ADPase dephosphorylates adenosine diphosphate (ADP) to adenosine monophosphate (AMP), adenosine, and inosine, thus limiting platelet activation by ADP. Adenosine also is a platelet inhibitor as it increases platelet cAMP levels.

Heparin-Like Glycosaminoglycan

Heparin-like glycosaminoglycans are integrated into the protein skeleton of the endothelial membrane. These heparins bind and accelerate local antithrombin III activity.

In contrast, the endothelium also synthesizes components necessary for clot formation such as factor V and VII, von Willebrand factor, tissue factor, platelet-activating factor, and plasminogen-activating inhibitor.

Factors V and VII

Factors V and VII are key proenzymes in the coagulation cascade.

von Willebrand Factor

von Willebrand factor (vWF) mediates the initial adhesion of platelets to vascular subendothelium. vWF is synthesized by both endothelial cells and platelets. The endothelium produces vWF constitutively but also increases production and release after stimulation by thrombin, histamine, cytokines, stretch, and shear stress.

Tissue Factor

Tissue factor is normally produced in small amounts by the endothelium; however, production is greatly increased after stimulation. Tissue factor, when complexed with factor VII, initiates the protein coagulation cascade.

Platelet-Activating Factor

Cytokine stimulation provokes the endothelial release of platelet-activating factor (PAF), an inflammatory mediator. PAF activates platelet aggregation and granule release. However, PAF can inhibit platelets by upregulating endothelial NO synthase with resultant increase in NO production.

Plasminogen-Activating Inhibitor

The endothelium also produces plasminogen-activating inhibitor (PAI), a serine protease, which binds and neutralizes tissue plasminogen activator. PAI is activated once it is bound to vitronectin in the subendothelium.[3]

Last, the endothelium also acts as a biochemical transducer for endogenous and exogenous substances through the synthesis of endothelium relaxation factor, which is now recognized as NO. In areas of endothelial disruption, vasodilators have no effect or can cause paradoxic vasoconstriction. In contrast, the endothelium also produces vasoconstrictor substances such as endothelin and angiotensin II.

The media is mainly composed of vascular smooth muscle and is responsible for the maintenance of vascular tone. Vascular smooth muscle cells synthesize structural proteins, which are highly thrombogenic, such as elastin, collagen, and complex polysaccharides such as glycosaminoglycan. The adventitia, the outermost layer of the blood vessel, is made up of fibroblasts and structural proteins such as collagen.

The initial response to vascular injury is vasoconstriction. This may be adequate for capillaries and small arterioles. However, breaks in larger vessels will require thrombus formation. The exposure of highly thrombogenic proteins and polysaccharides in the media and adventitia promotes coagulation. Larger disruptions require surgical repair.

Platelet System

Platelets play the central role in the repair of vascular injury.[1-3,5,7-11] Platelets adhere to the disrupted vascular surface, aggregate to form a platelet plug, secrete cofactors, provide an essential membrane surface for the coagulation cascade, generate fibrin/platelet plug, and induce fibrinolysis, inflammation, and local vascular change.

Platelets, like other components of the hemostatic system, circulate in a nonreactive state until activation is triggered by agonists. The rate and extent of platelet activation is dependent on the particular agonist, concentration of agonist, and continued presence of stimulus (Fig. 9.2).

Activation can be triggered by collagen and glycoprotein molecules found on nonendothelized surfaces, such as plaque, synthetic surfaces that absorb molecules, and subendothelial tissue at vascular injury sites. Platelet activation can also be initiated by ADP, thromboxane, and thrombin in the circulating blood. Platelet activation results in platelet adherence, aggregation, and secretion.

Adherence

Disruption of endothelium exposes circulating blood to subendothelial matrix, which contains collagen and large adhesive glycoproteins such as vWF, fibronectic, vitronectin, laminin, and thrombospondin. These proteins contain the RGD domain, which is a tripeptide sequence consisting of arginine-glycine-aspartic acid. The RGD domain is recognized by glycoprotein receptors (integrins) on the platelet surface membrane.

Initially, the GPIb glycoprotein receptor on the platelet membrane binds exposed von Willebrand factor. Another platelet receptor binds to fibronectin, which is also exposed in the vascular subendothelium. After this initial step in platelet adherence, other platelet glycoprotein receptors bind to matrix molecules such as laminin, collagen, thrombospondin, and vitronectin. Platelets then undergo a conformational shape change, which allows "spreading" of platelets to cover more of the exposed thrombogenic surface. Platelet spreading on collagen triggers platelet activation. Once activated, platelets change shape from smooth discoid to spherical with pseudopod extrusion. Concurrently a conformational change occurs in the platelet surface GP IIb/IIIa glycoprotein receptor, which exposes binding sites for fibrinogen, fibronectin, vitronectin, and vWF. This results in further spreading and allows for platelet aggregation.

Primary Aggregation

GP IIb/IIIa receptors bind fibrinogen very tightly. Several platelets can bind to a single fibrinogen molecule. Platelet-to-platelet binding by fibrinogen bridges from platelet aggregates and plugs. Conformational change of GP IIb/IIIa can be induced by:

1. collagen exposure, as above
2. ADP/thromboxane released by other activated platelets
3. thrombin generated by the coagulation cascade.

At this stage, platelet activation is still a reversible process. If stimulus for activation is not sufficient to continue, platelets can separate and conformationally revert back to their resting discoid shape.

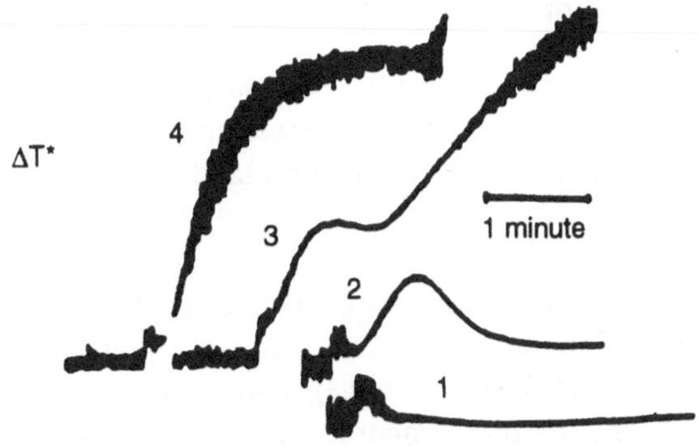

FIGURE 9.2. Platelet response occurs in a graded fashion, depending on type of stimulus, concentration of stimulus and persistence of stimulus. The graded response of platelets to increasing concentrations of a platelet agonist is depicted in four in vitro aggregation curves. The curves were obtained by combining turbid platelet-rich plasma (PRP) with increasing amounts of an agonist (thrombin) in a platelet aggregometer. The platelet aggregometer measures the extent of platelet aggregation, an observable manifestation of platelet activation. This photo-optical instrument measures light transmittance through samples of platelet-containing plasma. Platelet-rich plasma is normally turbid and transmits light poorly. When activating agonists are added, stimulating platelet activation and causing aggregation, the turbidity of the plasma decreases. Light transmittance through the plasma sample progressively increases with the formation of increasingly large platelet aggregates. The amount of light transmitted is then recorded and produces an aggregation curve. With increasing degrees of platelet aggregation, the reduction in turbidity and change in light transmittance are greater, and the corresponding curves show larger upward deflections from the baseline. In curve 1, PRP is combined with thrombin 0.05 units/ml. Platelet shape change indicated by narrowing of the baseline took place within a few seconds, but aggregation did not occur. Within 10 min, the baseline recovers its normal amplitude as platelet discoid shape is restored (not shown). In curve 2, where PRP is combined with thrombin 0.1 unit/ml, upward deflection of the tracing indicates that a change in light transmittance occurred after shape change had developed. The change in light transmission coincides with an initial wave of aggregation. Platelet clumps dispersed completely in this sample, as indicated by a decrease in light transmittance and a return of the recording to baseline. Platelet discoid shape is restored and the baseline recovers its normal amplitude within 10 min (not shown). Curve 3, recorded when PRP was exposed to thrombin 0.15 unit/ml, demonstrates that an initial phase of aggregation was followed by a brief period in which disaggregation began. The pause was followed by a rapid increase in light transmission as a second wave of aggregation took place. Initiation of secondary aggregation is entirely dependent on granule contents and TXA2 extruded from platelets. Curve 4 was obtained when PRP was treated with thrombin 0.18 unit/ml. The first and second waves of aggregation are fused together, obscuring the biphasic nature of the platelet response. This occurred because the high concentration of agonist caused acceleration of the platelet activation sequence and rapid development of secondary aggregation. (From Campbell and Edmunds.[1])

Secondary Aggregation

If the inciting stimulus is sufficient, secondary aggregation, which involves prostaglandin synthesis and granule secretion, can take place. Secondary aggregation is irreversible. The activated platelet can no longer revert back to a resting discoid form. Activated platelets synthesize arachidonic acid metabolites, primarily thromboxane, from platelet membrane phospholipids. Thromboxane, a powerful platelet activator and aggregant, is released into the milieu. Depending on the stimulus, platelets will secrete the contents of their cytoplasmic alpha granules, dense granules, and lysosomes. The contents of these vacuoles promote coagulation by activating other platelets and providing cofactors for the protein coagulation cascade (Table 9.1). The inflammation pathway is also promoted by released chemotactic factor, which attracts leukocytes, and by released permeability factor and hydrolases, which increase vascular permeability and damage. Thrombin and collagen are able to induce secretion from all three vacuole types. Epinephrine, ADP, and thromboxane induce secretion only from alpha and dense granules.

Platelet products of secondary aggregation also have vasoactive effect. ADP and serotonin released from platelet storage granules bind to endothelial P_{2y} purinoreceptors and serotoninergic receptors, respectively, and cause vasodilation. Thromboxane is a vasoconstrictor. However, thromboxane can also secondarily stimulate the endothelial formation of prostacyclin, a vasodilator, through the "endoperoxide shunt."

Regulation of Platelet Activation (Fig. 9.3)

Platelet glycoprotein receptors are coupled to guanine nucleotide-binding regulatory proteins known as G proteins. G proteins act on enzymes and ion channels to produce second messengers and mediate ion flow.

Platelet activation is thought to occur through G-protein activation of phospholipase C and phospholipase A_2. These two enzymes catalyze the formation of arachidonic acid from two platelet membrane phospholipids, phosphatidylinositol and phosphatidylcholine. Arachidonic acid in the platelet is converted to thromboxane A_2, through the mediation of cyclooxygenase and thromboxane synthetase. Thromboxane A_2 in turn increases phospholipase C activity and thus promotes further platelet activation. In addition to formation of arachidonic acid, phospholipase C also cleaves membrane protein phosphatidylinositol 4,5-biphosphate (PIP_2) to form diacyglycerol (DAG) and inositol triphosphate (IP_3). IP_3 increases the concentration of intracellular calcium through dense tubule and endoplasmic reticulum calcium release. Calcium along with calmodulin regulates the phosphorylation of myosin light chains. It is myosin's interaction with actin that produces platelet shape change and granule movement. DAG

TABLE 9.1. Contents of platelet secretory granules and their physiologic activities.

Secretory granules and contents	Physiologic activities
Alpha granules	
Coagulation factors	Cofactors for enzymatic cascade
Fibronogen	
Factor V	
High molecular weight kininogen (HMWK)	
Glycoproteins	Participate in cell adhesion and cell-to-cell interactions
von Willebrand factor	
Thrombospondin	
Fibronectin	
Platelet-specific proteins	
Platelet factor 4 (PF4)	PF4 potentiates ADP-induced platelet aggregation and has antiheparin activity
Low affinity (LA) platelet factor 4 (β-thromboglobulin)	LA-PF4 possesses antiheparin activity
Cationic proteins	
Mitogenic factor	Stimulates vascular smooth muscle growth
Permeability factor	Increases endothelial permeability
Chemotactic factor	Attracts leukocytes
Bactericidal factor	Promotes mild antimicrobial activity
Dense granules	
Adenine nucleotides (ADP,ATP)	ADP stimulates platelet aggregation and secretion
Guanosine nucleotides (GDP,GTP)	Function unknown
Pyrophosphate	No physiologic function
Calcium	Uncertain, promotes coagulation
Serotonin	Vasoconstriction, stimulates platelet aggregation and secretion in nonhuman species
Lysosomes	
Acid hydrolases	Hydrolytic activity in acid environments
Neutral proteases	Propagate vascular damage and promote vascular permeability

From Campbell and Edmunds.[1]

activates protein kinase C, which phosphorylates a 47-kd protein that controls platelet granule release.

To temper the platelet activation response, G proteins coupled to glycoprotein receptors are also linked to adenylate cyclase in the platelet membrane. Adenylate cyclase catalyzes the formation of cAMP from ATP. cAMP inhibits platelet function by:

1. calcium uptake, which lowers cytoplasmic calcium concentration
2. inhibiting phospholipase C, which results in less IP_3 and DAG
3. inhibiting phospholipase A_2 and cyclooxygenase, with resultant diminished prostaglandin synthesis.

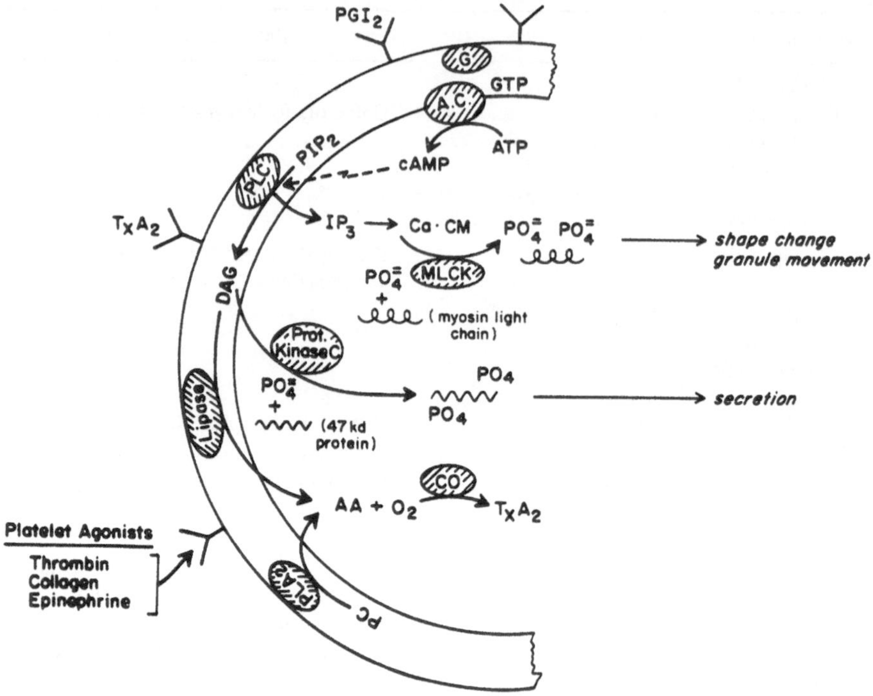

FIGURE 9.3. The biochemical basis of platelet activation and secretion. Binding of agonists such as thrombin, epinephrine, or collagen sets in motion a chain of events that hydrolyzes membrane phospholipids, inhibits adenylate cyclase, mobilizes intracellular calcium, and phosphorylates critical intracellular proteins. The net result is shape change, movement of granules to the canalicular system, generation of mediators like thromboxane A_2, and granule secretion. A.C., adenylate cyclase; G, guanine nucleotide binding protein; PIP_2, phosphatidylinositol 4,5-biphosphate; PLC, phospholipase C; DAG, diacylglycerol; PLA_2, phospholipase A_2; PC, phosphatidylcholine; AA, arachidonic acid; CO, cyclooxygenase; O_2, oxygen; IP_3, inositol triphosphate; cAMP, cyclic AMP; Ca-CM, calcium calmodulin complex; MLCK, myosin light chain kinase. (From Handin.[11])

Protein Coagulation System

The protein coagulation system is dynamically entwined with the platelet and vascular system in the formation of clot and linked with the fibrinolytic system in dissolution and limitation of clot.[2,6,9,12,13] In addition, the protein cascade participates in complement activation and the inflammatory response to injury. Due to tight physiologic control, coagulation does not extend beyond the area of vascular injury. The protein coagulation system has built in "fail-safe" mechanisms to limit clot formation:

1. Each protein exists as an inactive proenzyme until sequentially activated.

2. Components form complexes on membrane surfaces, which are available only in the region of vessel injury. Cells expressing these unique membranes must be triggered to adhere to the areas of tissue injury.

Platelet function and the coagulation cascade are enjoined. Four coagulation cofactors—fibrinogen, factor V, vWF, and high molecular weight kininogen (HMWK)—are manufactured and released from platelet alpha granules. Activated platelets have receptors for cofactors VIIIa and Va. The coagulation cascade complexes form and interact on platelet membrane surfaces. In addition, thrombin, which is formed by the coagulation cascade, is a potent platelet agonist.

Procoagulant Proteins (Fig. 9.4)

Procoagulant proteins are serine proteases and protein cofactors that circulate in the blood in inactive forms called zymogens. They are synthesized in the liver, except for FIII (tissue factor, present in subendothelium and expressed constitutively on nonvascular cells) and FVIII (synthesized by many organs). The cleavage of peptide bonds by a specific activated serine protease converts a zymogen to an active enzyme. The C-terminal halves bear the catalytic domain that expresses protease activity. The specific N-terminal halves give each protein its biospecificity. FII, VII, IX, and X have γ-carboxyglutamic acid that act to bind calcium and cell membranes. Vitamin K is required for the synthesis of these chains. Epidermal growth factor domains of factors VII, IX, X, and XII, and kringle domains of prothrombin and XII are required for the formation of protein complexes.

Factors V and VIII are structurally unrelated to the serine proteases. Factors V and VIII are pro-cofactors that both have three homologous A domains, a large B domain, and two C domains. Like the serine proenzymes, the pro-cofactors require the cleavage of a specific peptide bond for activation.

Tissue factor, factor III, unlike the other coagulation proteins, is a membrane protein rather than an enzyme. A hydrophobic transmembrane domain anchors the protein in the cell membrane. The extracellular domain is a receptor for FVII.

Anticoagulant Proteins

The activity of the procoagulant system is modulated by circulating anticoagulant proteins, which inhibit or slow the rate of activation of procoagulant proteins.

Protein C and protein S are vitamin K–dependent plasma proteins that have structures similar to the procoagulant serine proteases. Protein C inactivates cofactors V and VIII. Protein C is activated by the action of thrombin. Circulating thrombin promotes clotting; however, when

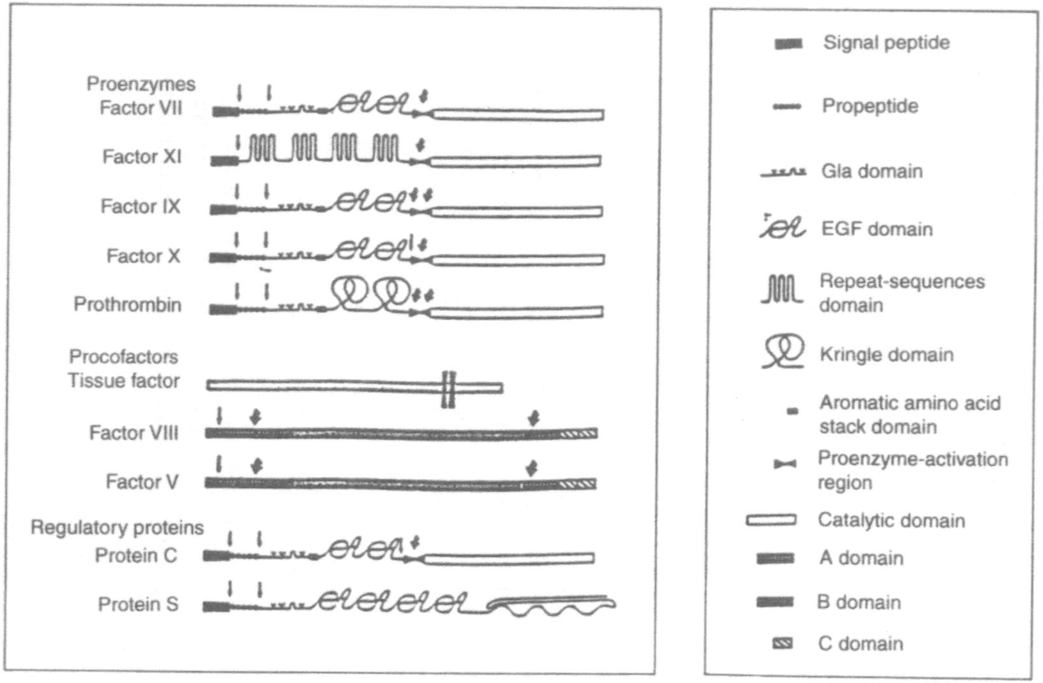

FIGURE 9.4. Domains of the enzymes, receptors, and cofactors involved in blood coagulation and regulation. The components of blood coagulation are proenzymes, procofactors, and regulatory proteins. The proenzymes, including protein C, contain a catalytic domain, an activation region, and a signal peptide. The vitamin K–dependent proteins include a propeptide and γ-carboxyglutamic acid (G1a) domain. Other important domains include the epidermal growth factor-like (EGF) domain, the kringle domain, and the repeat-sequence domain. Tissue factor is an integral membrane protein unrelated to other known proteins. Factors V and VIII have marked similarities in structure. Sites of intracellular peptide bonds cleaved during synthesis are indicated by straight arrows, and sites of peptide bonds cleaved during protein activation are indicated by curved thick arrows. The transmembrane domain of tissue factor is shown within the phospholipid bilayer. The domain closest to the C-terminal of protein S does not share sequence homology with the protease domains of other vitamin K–dependent proteins. (From Furie and Furie.[12])

thrombin binds to the endothelial membrane receptor thrombomodulin, this complex activates protein C to inhibit the clotting process. Protein S is a cofactor for protein C. Another inhibitor, called tissue factor pathway inhibitor, inactivates the extrinsic pathway by binding to tissue factor–factor VII complexes.

Antithrombin III (ATIII) is another circulating procoagulant protein inhibitor. ATIII scavenges thrombin and factors IXa and Xa that move away from the growing clot. The binding of ATIII to procoagulant proteases results in neutralized complexes. ATIII activity is accelerated 1000-fold by heparin molecules, which are located on endothelial membranes.

Coagulation Cascade

The coagulation cascade was classically described as two separate and distinct pathways, intrinsic and extrinsic, leading to factor X activation. The intrinsic pathway was activated by the contact of factor XII to nonvascular surfaces. This was followed by the sequential activation of factors XI, IX, and X. The extrinsic pathway was initiated by the formation of a complex between tissue factor and factor VII with resultant factor X activation. Once factor X was activated, both pathways shared the same sequential steps that resulted in the formation of thrombin and fibrin.

The two-pathway explanation is important for understanding in vitro clot formation and for interpretation of laboratory coagulation tests, prothrombin time (PT) and partial thromboplastin time (PTT). However, in vivo coagulation appears to function quite differently. In vivo, the two pathways are interdependent and less distinct (Fig. 9.5). Tissue factor is likely the key initiator of coagulation. The traditional two-pathway theory has been modified because of several clinical observations:

1. Patients with a hereditary deficiency of factor XII, prekallikrein, or HMWK, have abnormally prolonged partial thromboplastin times but no clinical problems with hemostasis. These factors likely are not as important in in vivo coagulation.
2. Patients with factor XI deficiency may or may not have bleeding difficulties.
3. Tissue factor seems to be the key initiator of in vivo coagulation activation.
4. Tissue factor/factor VIIa complex activates not only FX, but also FIX. Thus, FIX and FVIII, both traditionally part of the FXII (intrinsic) activation pathway, have central roles in the tissue factor activation pathway (extrinsic).

Coagulation requires the presence of membrane surfaces to accelerate the assembly of activated complexes. Tissue factor is found on the surface of nonvascular cells and stimulated monocytes. Platelet membranes provide the critical surface in vivo for the formation of coagulation protein

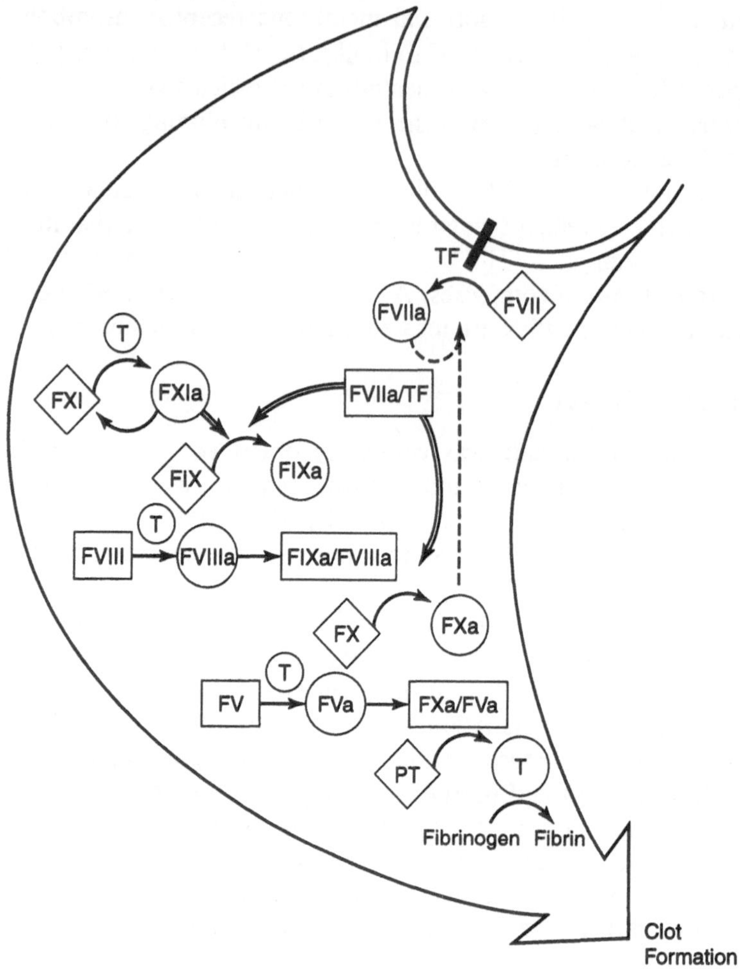

FIGURE 9.5. The following scheme is a closer model to in vivo blood coagulation. Blood coagulation is initiated by tissue factor (TF) expressed on the cell surface. When plasma comes in contact with tissue factor, factor VII (FVII) binds to this receptor. The complex of activated factor VIIa (FVIIa) and tissue factor activates factors IX (FIX) and X (FX). The proteolytic activation of factor VII to VIIa, factor XI (FXI) to XIa (FXIa), factor VIII (FVIII) to VIIIa (FVIIIa), and factor V (FV) to Va (FVa) through feedback mechanisms, such as the conversion of prothrombin (PT) to thrombin (T) or other enzymes (dashed arrows), greatly accelerates blood clotting. The process culminates with the generation of fibrin and its polymerization to form a fibrin clot. The open arrows indicate the action of enzymes on substrates, and the narrow solid arrows indicate the conversion of a protein from one functional state to another after the cleavage of one or more peptide bonds. (From Furie and Furie.[12])

complexes. Activated platelets express many receptors for factors VIIIa and Va, critical cofactors for the activation of protease complexes. Calcium is required for the binding of the α-carboxy-glutamic acid chains of vitamin K-dependent factors (II, VII, IX, X) to cell membranes:

1. The exposure of cell surfaces expressing tissue factor to plasma proteins leads to binding of factor VII in the initial step of coagulation. The factor VII/tissue factor complex has low coagulant activity. Factor VIIa/tissue factor complex is a stronger protease activator. The initial enzyme for factor VII activation has yet to be identified. However, once the cascade is initiated, later-formed activated enzymes, namely FXa and FVIIa have a positive feedback mechanism to activate FVII and thus accelerate the cascade.
2. Factor VIIa/tissue factor complex activates both FX and FIX.
3. Factor IXa in complex with cofactor Va converts prothrombin to thrombin.
4. Thrombin cleaves fibrinogen to fibrin, which can polymerize and cross-link with other fibrin molecules to form the fibrin clot.
5. Thrombin plays a central role by initially accelerating coagulation and then decelerating the coagulation cascade once coagulation is under way. Once thrombin is formed, it accelerates the activation of cofactors VIII and V. In addition, thrombin activates FXI to FXIa. Factor XIa can provide an additional mechanism for the activation of FIX, other than the initial TF/VIIa complex. Thrombin is also a potent platelet activator and recruits platelets to the fibrin clot. Thrombin also acts to limit the speed and extent of coagulation, thus preventing thrombosis beyond the area of endothelial damage. Thrombin causes endothelium to release prostacyclin (potent vasodilator and platelet inhibitor) and tissue plasminogen activator (promotes fibrinolysis). Thrombin also interacts with thrombomodulin on platelet surfaces to activate protein C. Protein C in turn inactivates the key cofactors V and VIII.

Fibrinolytic System

The fibrinolytic system limits thrombus formation to the hemorrhage region. As clotting is activated, its breakdown is simultaneously begun. The coagulation cascade and fibrinolytic system are dynamically linked and inseparable.[2,6,8,9,14]

Fibrinogen and Fibrin

Fibrinogen exists as two symmetric molecules joined by covalent disulfide bonds. Each of the two symmetric molecules is made up of three subunits with characteristic amino acid sequences (Fig. 9.6A). Thrombin activates fibrinogen to fibrin by binding to its central link. The result is the release of

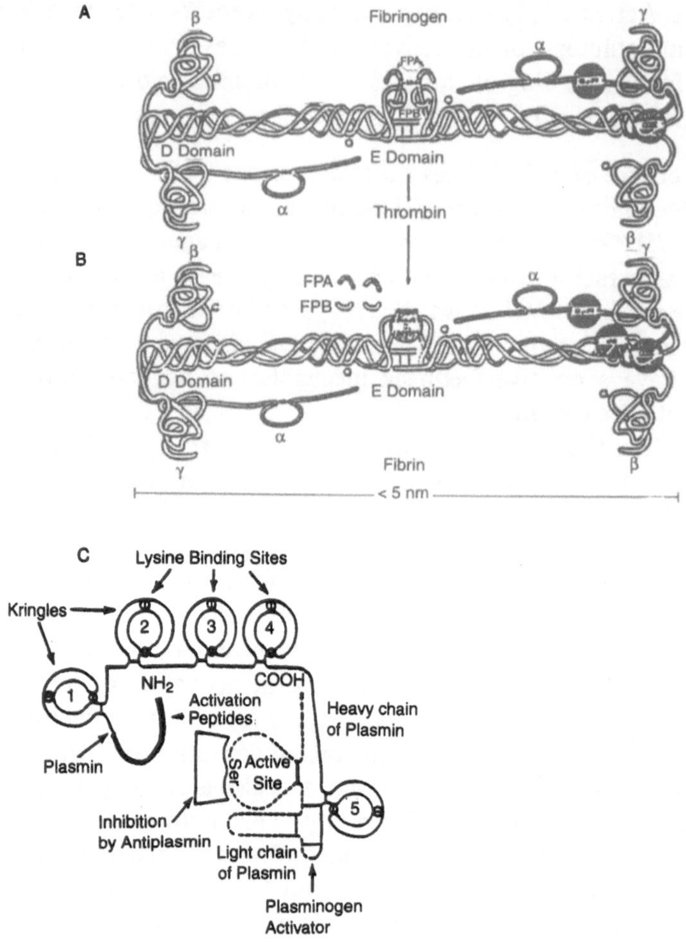

FIGURE 9.6. Fibrinogen and plasminogen. Diagram of fibrinogen (A) and fibrin (B). Each fibrinogen consists of three polypeptide chains attached with a mirror image molecule held together by disulfide bonds. Thrombin attacks the central region releasing fibrinopeptide A and B (α, PI) and allowing α_2-PI factor XIII and tPA. (C) A schematic diagram of the structure of plasminogen and plasmin. The five kringles are noted as are the regions interacting with antiplasm. (Adapted with permission from Spiess.[6])

fibrinopeptides A and B, which exposes central and peripheral binding sites for other activated fibrin molecules. Fibrin molecules cross-link and form a polymerized network. The conformational change also opens up binding sites for circulating regulatory molecules—factor XIII, α_2-plasminogen inhibitor, and tissue plasminogen activator (Fig. 9.6B).

α_2-Plasminogen Inhibitor

α_2-Plasminogen inhibitor (PI) in conjunction with factor XIII binds to the fibrin molecule at a lysine residue. α_2-Plasminogen inhibitor is a rapid inhibitor of plasmin and tissue plasminogen activator (Fig. 9.6A,B), thus promoting further fibrin polymerization. However, its inhibitory activity can be overcome by high levels of plasma.

Tissue Plasminogen Activator

Tissue plasminogen activator (t-Pa) is synthesized by vascular endothelium. As the primary activator of plasminogen, t-Pa is instrumental in the breakdown of the fibrin clot. t-Pa has much greater affinity and activity for formed fibrin than fibrinogen alone. It is only after fibrinogen is cleaved to fibrin that the necessary lysine residues are exposed for t-Pa binding (Fig. 9.6B). Thus fibrin, once formed, will trigger clot lysis.

Clot lysis, like clot formation, occurs by intrinsic and extrinsic pathways.[15] Figure 9.7 illustrates the fibrinolytic pathways and the by-products of fibrin formation and breakdown. With activation of the

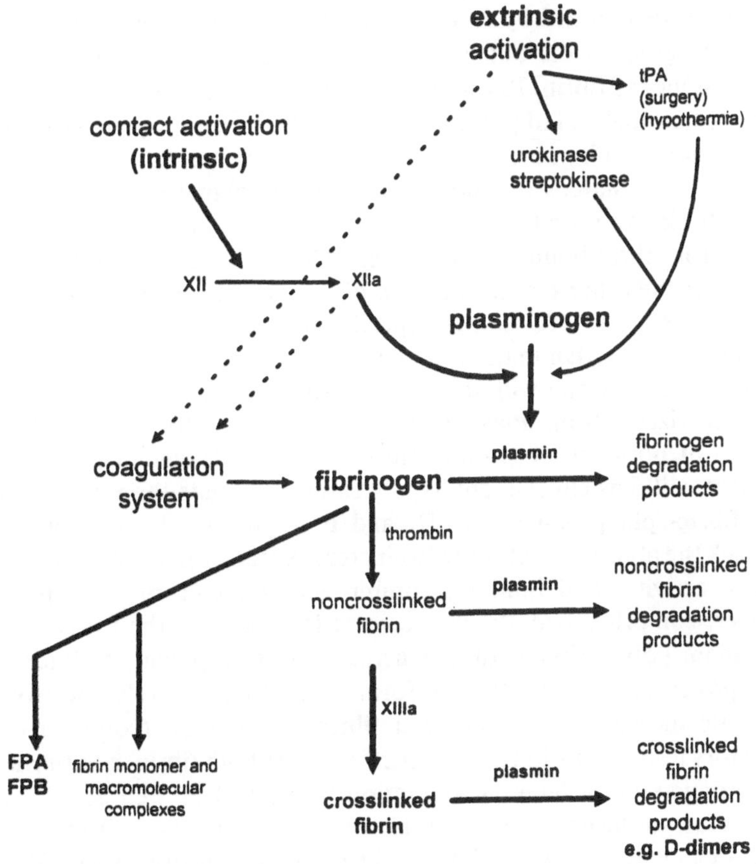

FIGURE 9.7. The fibrinolytic pathway and the by-products of fibrin formation and breakdown. FPA, fibrinopeptide A; FPB, fibrinopeptide B; tPA, tissue plasminogen activator.

extrinsic pathway, there is a release of plasminogen activators, tissue plasminogen activator (t-Pa) by endothelial cells, and urokinase plasminogen activator (u-Pa) by monocytes, macrophages, and fibroblasts.[15,16] In the case of *intrinsic* fibrinolysis, plasminogen is activated by factor XIIa formed during the contact phase of coagulation. The physiologic importance of this latter pathway has not been established but is believed to be the means by which fibrinolysis is initiated during cardiopulmonary bypass (CPB).[16] Plasminogen can also be activated by *exogenous* means, e.g., by streptokinase and staphylokinase. In either situation, plasminogen is cleaved to form plasmin by the respective serine proteases. Plasmin also facilitates further plasminogen activation via a positive feedback loop.[15]

Plasminogen and Plasmin (Fig. 9.6C)

Plasminogen, like the procoagulant serine enzymes, circulates as a zymogen requiring activation to form plasmin. Plasminogen is a polypeptide whose structure is determined by 24 disulfide bonds. Amino acid sequences form loops (kringles) on the outside of the molecule that are binding sites for lysine residues of fibrin. Plasmin is formed by the cleavage of peptide bonds on the N-terminal end of plasminogen. This leaves an exposed lysine residue on the end of plasmin. Plasminogen is activated by t-Pa, thrombin, kallikrein, urokinase, streptokinase, and staphylokinase. Streptokinase and urokinase cleaves both fibrin-bound and free plasminogen. t-Pa has greater affinity for fibrin-bound plasminogen. Clinically, t-Pa may be advantageous over the other kinases because of its specifity for fibrin clots.

Plasmin is a powerful and nonspecific endopeptidase that promotes the fibrinolytic and inflammation systems while inhibiting the protein coagulation system. Plasmin will attack either fibrinogen, unpolymerized fibrin, or polymerized fibrin. Plasmin cleaves fragments off each of the three subunits of both fibrinogen and fibrin. The first fragment formed, the x fragment, still has clotting ability. Plasmin then splits the x fragment into three fibrin-split products—Y, D, and E fragments. These products not only lack the ability to clot, but also increase vascular permeability, increase plasmin activity, and inhibit thrombin activity. One of these products, D-dimer, comprises two attached central D regions of the fibrin molecule and cannot polymerize. D-dimers actually act as a potent inhibitor of the serine proteases necessary for clot formation. D-dimer levels, therefore, are a specific measure of polymerized fibrin degradation (common clinical laboratory tests for fibrin-split products measure both fibrin- and fibrinogen-split products via a latex agglutination technique) as well as an indirect measure of antihemostatic potential. Plasmin interferes with the coagulation protein cascade by inactivating the essential cofactors V and VIII and factors IX and XI. Plasmin promotes the inflammatory response by activating FXII, complement C3, and kallikrein.

Various checks and balances exist to ensure that fibrinolysis is controlled and localized to form clot under normal conditions:

1. The actions of t-Pa are enhanced by fibrin so that fibrinolysis tends to occur close to thrombi.
2. A scavenging protein, α_2-antiplasmin, is typically present in the vicinity of this polymerized fibrin and essentially consumes any plasmin formed from localized fibrinolysis.
3. A circulating regulatory protein, α_2-plasminogen inhibitor (PI), acts as a rapid and effective inhibitor of t-Pa and plasmin that may have escaped local consumption.[17]

Inflammation System

The inflammation system is interlinked with blood coagulation. The hemostasis system can initiate or promote the inflammatory response to injury. Circulating Hageman's factor (FXII) can be activated to FXIIa by contact with negatively charged surfaces and artificial surfaces. FXIIa in turn can activate XI to promote coagulation, but also activates prekallikrein to kallikrein to promote inflammation. Kallikrein cleaves HMWK to produce bradykinin. FXIIa also initiates the classic pathway of the complement system. Feedback control exists as cofactors for FXII activation: prekallikrein, HMWK, and FXI. Neutrophils are activated by complement, kallikrein, and FXIIa. Activated platelets also promote inflammation by secreting products that increase vascular permeability and leukocyte chemotactic factors. The fibrinolytic system activates inflammation through plasmin- and fibrin-split products. Plasmin activates complement C3 and kallikrein. Fibrin-split products increase vascular permeability. Leukotrienes and prostaglandins that are formed during the hemostatic process can play a large role in inflammation.[18,19]

Conversely, coagulation can be promoted by the inflammatory response. Complement and oxygen radicals formed during the inflammatory response can damage endothelium, thus exposing thrombogenic collagen matrix. In addition, leukocytes and platelets called in to participate in inflammation can provide membrane surfaces and tissue factor (particularly activated monocytes) for coagulation.[18,19]

Alteration of Hemostasis Associated with Cardiopulmonary Bypass

The coagulation defect associated with cardiopulmonary bypass is multifactorial in origin. Given the web of interdependence and interplay spun by the vascular system, the platelet system, the protein coagulation system, the fibrinolytic system, and the inflammation system during normal hemostasis, it is not surprising that no single defect predominates. Consequently, the search for therapy and especially for prophylaxis for post-bypass coagulopathies proves to be difficult. Single-armed approaches directed at individual systems have not proven to be successful, neither in the research for the etiology of coagulation defects nor in clinical treatment.

Interactions with Nonendothelialized Surfaces

The coagulopathy for cardiopulmonary bypass starts with the contact of blood with nonendothelial surfaces: the synthetic surface of the extracorporeal circuit, blood-air interfaces, or exposed subendothelial surfaces after surgically induced vascular injury. In addition, blood is subjected to mechanical trauma and shear stress forces. The result is the activation and amplification of the vascular, platelet, coagulation, fibrinolytic, and inflammation systems.

Synthetic Surface of the Extracorporeal Circuit

Plasma proteins are adsorbed or deposited onto synthetic surfaces almost immediately when heparinized blood makes contact. This protein layer forms a coating of 100 to 200 Å.[20] The makeup of this layer is not reflective of the plasma protein composition of the blood,[21] but is dependent on the surface characteristics of the synthetic material. Fibrinogen, factor XII, vWF, fibrinectin, thrombospondin, immunoglobulin G, and albumin are adsorbed in varying and unpredictable amounts depending on the surface material.[1,22]

Initially, the adsorbed protein layer consists primarily of fibrinogen. Surfaces that are hydrophobic tend to adsorb more fibrinogen than those that are hydrophilic.[23] The binding of adsorbed fibrinogen by GPIIb/IIIa receptors (fibrinogen receptors) on activated platelets results in platelet aggregation and further platelet activation.

The character of the adsorbed protein layer changes over time with resultant changes in surface thrombogenicity.[24] Fibrinogen is displaced by HMWK, albumin, factor XII and other proteins.[1,24] This protein flux is not very well understood, and the search for a nonthrombogenic, noninflammation-activating surface has been difficult. Either the adsorbed fibrinogen changes conformation (whereby it is no longer recognizable by platelet receptors), fibrinogen becomes deadsorbed, or platelet fibrinogen receptors are altered. Over time, some platelets detach and return to the circulation. The synthetic surface becomes "passivated" or less thrombogenic. Platelets are initially activated by either thrombin, ADP from damaged erythrocytes and activated platelets, circulating epinephrine, or release products from platelets and leukocytes.

Despite large amounts of administered heparin, the protein coagulation cascade is activated during cardiopulmonary bypass. Thrombin is formed and the fibrinolytic platelet, and complement systems are activated. By binding to antithrombin III, heparin causes a conformational change in ATIII that accelerates thrombin inhibition. Heparin-ATIII complexes inhibit multiple serine proteases of the coagulation cascade, including factor Xa and IXa. However, heparin-ATIII does not inhibit factor VIIa, nor is it a major inhibitor of contact factors XIIa, XIa, or kallikrein.[25,26] Thus, heparin inhibits the later segments of the intrinsic and common pathways, but cannot prevent the initial steps of activation of the extrinsic or intrinsic pathways. Heparin also fails to be a complete anticoagulant, because once thrombin is bound to fibrin, thrombin is protected against the actions of the heparin-ATIII complex. Heparin sensitivity varies widely in individuals and commercial preparations differ in activity.

Contact activation of the intrinsic pathway during cardiopulmonary bypass had been previously accepted as the mechanism of thrombin generation on bypass. Factor XII in the presence of prekallikrein and HMWK is activated when blood contacts a negatively charged surface. Factor XII is adsorbed onto the protein layer that covers the surface of synthetic materials and is activated by the negative charges of some of the other adsorbed proteins. In turn, factor XIIa with its cofactor, HMWK, activates factor XI, kallikrein, complement, and neutrophils. Factor XIa activates the rest of the intrinsic pathway. Kallikrein can activate kinin, the fibrinolytic system, the complement system, and factor XII (positive feedback).[24,25]

As mentioned previously, the new view of the coagulation cascade is one of greater integration of both intrinsic and extrinsic pathways (Fig. 9.5). It is now recognized that tissue factor/factor VII activation is the predominant in vivo initiator of the protein coagulation system. Factor VIIa/TF can activate both the former separate intrinsic and extrinsic paths by activating FIX and FX, respectively.[26] Recently, the prevailing belief that contact activation of FXII-initiated thrombin formation on bypass has been brought into question. The development of new assays to measure coagulation factor levels and activation products has led investigators to suggest that tissue factor/factor VII activation is the main trigger for thrombin formation during extracorporeal circulation. This is more in line with the view of normal in vivo coagulation.

Boisclair and colleagues[28] measured perioperative levels of FXIIa, FIX activation peptide (AP), and prothrombin fragment F_{1+2} in eight patients undergoing coronary artery bypass grafting (CABG). FIX AP is the peptide released when FIX is cleaved by FXIa or TF/VIIa. F_{1+2} is the fragment released during the activation of prothrombin to thrombin by FXa. The investigators found that F_{1+2} levels rose moderately after chest opening, and then increased dramatically on bypass. FIX AP levels remained indistinguishable from controls until rising 20 min before separation from bypass and peaking 20 min after separation from bypass. FXIIa levels increased slightly after chest opening but subsequent levels were statistically not significantly changed. There was no correlation between FXIIa levels and F_{1+2} levels. A significant correlation was found between FIX AP and F_{1+2} levels, and investigators observed that FIX AP levels rose later in the procedure than F_{1+2} levels. Investigators suggested that the TF/VIIa pathway provides the major procoagulant trigger during CPB surgery, rather than the contact activation of FXII. They also suggest that since FX activation and thrombin formation preceded that of FIX activation, perhaps (1) thrombin mediated the activation of FXI, and (2) TF/VIIa activates FX preferentially to FIX. One must keep in mind that FVII/TF levels were not measured (no reliable assay was available at the time), the number of patients was small and the number of time measurements was limited, and the fact that FXIIa is adsorbed onto the surface of synthetic membranes and may be difficult to assay accurately.[27]

Other investigators have questioned the predominance of FXII contact activation through case reports of patients with severe factor XII deficiencies who have successfully undergone cardiac surgery with cardiopulmonary bypass. Burman et al[29] reported increases in F_{1+2} and thrombin-antithrombin complexes during extracorporeal circulation in a 12-year-old with severe FXII deficiency undergoing atrial septal defect and patent ductus arteriosus repair. These increases were comparable to those found in normal patients. As with Boisclair et al's[28] patients, there was no rise in FIX AP levels.

Regardless of the inciting event, there is agreement concerning the persistence of thrombin formation despite heparin anticoagulation. Investigators measuring fibrinopeptide A,[29] fibrin monomers,[30] F_{1+2},[27,28] and thrombin-antithrombin complexes[28,31] have shown the inability of heparin to totally prevent thrombin formation.[32] Thrombin formation plays a central role in the activation of the multiple systems of hemostasis and in the coagulopathy of extracorporeal bypass.

Blood-Air Interfaces

In the late 1970s, the bubble oxygenator was recognized as a source of platelet damage and has since fallen out of favor for use during CPB. Animal studies, as well as some carefully controlled clinical studies have demonstrated clear decrements in platelet function and, to a lesser extent, platelet number with the use of bubble oxygenators versus membrane oxygenators.[33,34] Platelet damage, in this instance, is caused mainly by direct blood-gas interfaces created within the bubble oxygenators. Another interface for blood-gas interaction that remains prevalent in open-heart surgery requiring CPB is at the sucker tip and in the suction lines of the cardiotomy suction apparatus.[35,36] At such interfaces, turbulence and high shear stresses of up to 300 N/m^2 are induced, which result in platelet damage and destruction. In addition, plasma proteins, including coagulation factors may undergo significant denaturation.[15] Platelet adherence and activation also occurs at blood-air interfaces as each bubble presents a new nonendothelialized surface and plasma protein films containing fibrinogen. Contact activation of the fibrinolytic and inflammatory pathways may also be enhanced. Indeed, Boonstra and colleagues[36] have demonstrated that a technique using "controlled" cardiotomy suction can result in improved ADP-induced platelet aggregation and shorter postoperative bleeding times. This translated into significant reductions in postoperative blood loss in cases where perfusion times were 3 hours or more and when the total volume of cardiotomy suction exceeded 65 L. It has also been suggested that the theoretical advantage of membrane oxygenators is clinically eliminated by the creation of blood-gas interfaces during vigorous suctioning.[37,38]

Exposure of Subendothelial Tissue

Disruptions in the endothelium created during surgery will expose subendothelial proteins. As described earlier, the platelet, coagulation protein, fibrinolytic, and inflammation systems are activated to promote hemostasis.

Effect of Cardiopulmonary Bypass on the Platelet System

Platelet dysfunction has been most commonly cited as the primary coagulation defect induced by cardiopulmonary bypass. However, not all investigators have arrived at this conclusion. Given the interdependency of the multiple systems involved with coagulation and hemostasis, it is accurate only to state that platelet dysfunction plays a major role in the coagulation defect induced by cardiopulmonary bypass.

Evidence for Platelet Defect

1. Thrombocytopenia in excess to degree of hemodilution
2. Increased template bleeding time
3. Decrease in platelet force development
4. Dysfunction in shear-induced pathway of platelet function
5. Decreased platelet aggregation.

Proposed Etiology of Platelet Defect

1. Platelet activation and degranulation resulting in partial depletion of granule stores and impotent platelets
2. Alteration or damage of platelet membrane glycoprotein receptors

3. Circulating platelet inhibitor—heparin, plasmin
4. Hypothermia.

The literature on the effect of extracorporeal bypass on platelets is characterized by a lack of concurrence. Definitive conclusions have not been possible. Conflicting and disparate data arise due to:

1. In vivo vs in vitro studies. In vivo studies have the advantage of greater clinical significance; however, results between studies are varied due to differences in patient population, surgical technique, preoperative medications (particularly antiplatelet medications and anticoagulants), anesthetic medications and techniques, heparin doses and target levels, transfusion thresholds, intraoperative hypothermia, differing time frames and frequency of measurements, continually evolving technology in circuit and oxygenator composition, surface area and prime composition. In addition, very few clinical studies have actually correlated specific platelet defects with significant differences in clinical bleeding. In deference to investigators, one must recognize the difficulties in accurately measuring intra- and postoperative bleeding. Also, at times it is impossible to distinguish what percentage of blood loss is due to surgical reasons versus coagulopathy.

   In vitro studies have the advantage of being able to study coagulation and bypass without patient or physician variables. In addition, variables such as platelet sequestration, metabolism, and clearance are eliminated. Bypass circuitry and constituents can be controlled. However, conclusions as to whether found abnormalities are of clinical import or actually contribute to bleeding are impossible.
2. Platelet aggregation tests performed by different investigators differ in technique and equipment with resultant differences in sensitivity and specificity.
3. Preparation, fixation, storage, and anticoagulation of blood samples vary from study to study. For instance, some investigators centrifuge and separate blood samples into platelet-rich plasma and platelet-poor plasma, while others investigate whole blood samples. Some investigators add citrate or ethylenediaminetetra acetate (EDTA) or heparin to the samples to prevent clot formation from occurring during the sampling and study process. It is unlikely that the mechanical and chemical processing of blood samples does not influence the outcome of platelet aggregation, platelet product, or platelet receptor studies.
4. Monoclonal antibodies to receptors used during these studies vary from investigation to investigation as new ones are developed. Does the decrease in binding of monoclonal antibodies to the receptors in these studies represent decreased receptor binding of in vivo agonists or decrease in receptors, or just a loss of recognizable epitope for the monoclonal antibody alone?

5. Laboratory assays and techniques have increased in sensitivity and specificity as new technology is developed. In addition, patient population, preoperative medical treatment, and surgical and bypass techniques are ever changing and improving. Can studies from different years be realistically compared?

Thus, it is understandable why there is such a lack of agreement and inconclusiveness in the search for the elusive platelet defect of cardiopulmonary bypass. Aside from technological and experimental problems, the "platelet defect" is likely multifactorial and exists in varied degrees from case to case.

Evidence for Platelet Defect

Thrombocytopenia

Thrombocytopenia occurs during cardiopulmonary bypass in varying degrees. Most authors report a decrease to 30% to 50% of pre-bypass levels.[10,39] This decline is due to a combination of factors:

1. Hemodilution from non–blood circuit prime
2. Platelet adherence and aggregation induced by contact with synthetic surface (particularly oxygenators and filters), protamine, protamine-heparin complexes, circulating catecholamines, and ADP released from hemolyzed red blood cells (RBCs)[10]
3. Platelet destruction at blood-gas interfaces, notably from bubble oxygenators and cardiotomy suction devices.

In Vitro Studies. In vitro studies show a different pattern of thrombocytopenia during perfusion with a membrane versus a bubble oxygenator. The largest surface area by far in the extracorporeal circuit is the oxygenator. Addonizio and coinvestigators[40,41] demonstrated in an in vitro circuit with a membrane oxygenator that the circulation of human blood resulted in a decrease to 18% of initial levels within 15 minutes of circulation. Over time, the platelet count rose steadily to reach a stable value of 55% of initial levels after 2 hours of circulation. Over the following 4 hours, platelet count rose slightly but not significantly.[40] Analysis of platelet morphology using electron microscopy revealed varying degrees of granule and tubular loss; platelet aggregates and almost all platelets had lost their discoid shape.[41] The increase in platelet count over time is presumed due to passivasation of the foreign surface. As the protein layers change and the amount of exposed fibrinogen decreases, previously adhered platelets return to the circulation and platelet aggregates disjoin.[10] Further evidence that platelet alterations in in vitro membrane oxygenator circuits arise from platelet activation due to synthetic surface contact, rather than mechanical damage, comes from studies with albumin and prostacyclin. Albumin conformationally alters fibrinogen binding to the synthetic surfaces and thus decreases synthetic surface affinity for platelets. Prostacyclin, a potent platelet inhibitor, reduces platelet adherence and aggregation. Priming of the extracorporeal circuit with 2.5% albumin preserved platelet counts to 90% to 95% of initial levels throughout 6-hour experiments.[40] Similar results were obtained with the addition of PGE_1 ranging from concentrations of 0.1 to 10 μM. Platelet counts fell within 15 minutes to 78% of initial levels, but rose within 1 hour to 87%. Platelet counts subsequently remained stable for the duration of the 6 hour studies.[42] In both studies electron microscopy revealed preservation of subcellular architecture and preservation of organelles. However, most platelets had undergone some degree of shape change.[40,41]

Addonizio and colleagues[42] also looked at the relative contribution of blood flow rate and circuit surface area on platelet loss during in vitro circulation. Three circuits were used, one with a 0.3 M^2 surface area without an oxygenator, and two with membrane oxygenators giving a surface area of 0.3 M^2 and 0.9 M^2. In the two circuits with oxygenators, the difference in surface area was solely due to the different size of the membrane oxygenator. Blood was circulated at two rates, 300 ml/min and 1000 ml/min. The main difference in platelet loss depended on the presence and size of the oxygenator. Low versus high flow rates made a significant difference only in the smaller oxygenator where platelets decreased less at the lower flow rates. Removal of the oxygenator preserved platelet counts at 95% even at high flow rates. However, at high flow rates, platelet loss between the small and large oxygenator groups was similar. Platelet loss during use of a membrane oxygenator circuit is due in large part to its large surface area, but is also due to the resultant changes in the geometry of blood flow. The efficiency of gas transport is dependent on secondary flows that promote mixing of gas and blood in passages within the oxygenator. Platelet aggregate formation has been shown in regions of separated flow and at shunt vortexes. Thus, the necessary geometry of blood flow obscures the benefit of reduced surface areas, particularly at high blood flows.[43]

In vitro experiments with circuits containing bubble oxygenators show a more gradual decline in platelet numbers during circulation. In addition, there is no evidence for return of platelets to the circulation. Addonizio and colleagues[43] showed a decrease within 2 minutes to 73% of initial counts and then a gradual decline to 29% at 2 hours. The more gradual decline in platelets is due to the decreased surface area of the bubble oxygenator. However, platelets do adhere to fibrinogen-containing plasma protein films at air-blood interfaces and also at required blood filters. There is lack of return to the circulation because blood-gas interfaces are known to denature plasma proteins and mechanically destroy platelets.[1,10] In vitro methods to preserve platelet count by preventing platelet adhesion and aggregation such as albumin priming and addition of prostacyclin were only partially effective. Albumin priming could only preserve platelet counts to 58% after 2 hours.[40] Higher concentrations of prostacyclin were required in bubble oxygenators versus membrane oxygenators for platelet preservation.[43] This is further evidence of a direct mechanical platelet injury in addition to platelet surface activation.[1]

In Vivo Studies. In in vivo studies, thrombocytopenia is largely due to hemodilution, although some authors have found a decrease in platelet count further than the hemodilution correction. Platelet decreases due to adhesion and aggregation are masked in in vivo studies due to the large decrease caused by hemodilution, recruitment of new platelets, and the possible counting of platelet fragments. Also differences between membrane and bubble oxygenator perfusion are masked by the use of field suctioning, which creates air-blood interfaces and damages platelets.[37]

Harker et al[44] found that platelet count in in vivo, correlated with a bubble oxygenator, fell by 50% of baseline during cardiopulmonary bypass, which correlated with the degree of hemodilution from electrolyte priming solution. Throughout bypass, platelet count showed little further decrease.

Edmunds et al[45] found in CABG patients perfused with a membrane oxygenator that platelet counts when corrected for dilution did not decrease significantly at 45 min into the bypass nor at 1 hour after protamine. Platelet counts actually increased slightly, but significantly in a bubble oxygenator pump. Authors theorize that the increase in the bubble oxygenator group may be due to counting of platelet fragments along with the recruitment of additional platelets. Recruitment of new platelets is masked in the membrane oxygenator system because of large initial losses.

Zilla et al[46] found in patients undergoing bypass with a bubble oxygenator that dilution-corrected platelet counts dropped to 85% after sternotomy, and to 69% during the first 8 minutes of bypass. After this early decrease, no major changes in platelet counts were encountered during surgery.

Van den Dungen et al[37] found in CABG patients that platelet count decreased by 25% in the pre-bypass period, and after 5 minutes of bypass platelet count decreased to about 50% in both membrane and bubble oxygenators. This could not be accounted for by hemodilution alone. After 30 minutes, platelet counts improved in the membrane oxygenator group but decreased in the bubble oxygenator group, although this was not statistically significant.

The decline in platelet numbers usually is not enough alone to cause a coagulopathy. Most authors report platelet counts greater than 100,000 during and after bypass. Studies by Schmidt and Pike failed to find correlation between postoperative bleeding and degree of thrombocytopenia.[39] The circulating platelets exist in a spectrum of activated states, from new bone marrow–released platelets to unactivated discoid platelets to partially activated to completely degranulated to destroyed platelet ghosts and membrane fragments. It is not the low number of platelets but the heterogenicity and dysfunctional states of these circulating platelets that contribute to post-bypass coagulopathy.[10]

Bleeding Time

Several investigators have found that template bleeding time becomes prolonged during cardiopulmonary bypass and remains prolonged in the postoperative period.[39,44,45,47]

Khuri et al[48] studied 85 patients who underwent cardiac surgery with membrane or bubble oxygenators. They found that bleeding times increased from a preanesthetic value of 7.7 minutes to 12.9 minutes at 2 hours post-bypass. By 24 hours the mean bleeding time improved to 10.5 min and then gradually decreased to 9.5 min at 72 hours. The 2-hour post-CPB bleeding time related by univariate analysis to preoperative bleeding time, total CPB time, D-dimer level, and 4-hour post-bypass blood loss. Using univariate and multivariate analysis, predictors of extended bleeding time at 2 hours were duration of CPB, low temperature, D-dimer levels, and 4-hour post-bypass blood loss.

Harker et al[44] found that template bleeding time was predictive of patients at risk of severe bleeding. Thirty-one patients perfused with bubble oxygenators undergoing mainly CABG procedures were studied. These patients had normal bleeding times prior to heparinization and after heparinization before bypass. With the onset of bypass, bleeding time increased to 19 minutes despite maintenance of platelet count at 151,000. Bleeding times progressively increased and correlated with duration of bypass. By 2 hours of bypass, no patient had a bleeding time less than 30 min, although platelet counts remained stable. Plasma platelet factor 4 and B-thromboglobulin increased progressively along with increases in bleeding time. Bleeding times post-bypass were significantly different when the patients were divided into two groups. Ten patients had severe bleeding that required greater than 10 units of transfused blood. These patients were analyzed separately as group 2, the others as group 1. Bleeding times in group 1 decreased to 15.2 min at 20 min after protamine and normalization of bleeding time occurred within 2 to 4 hours after protamine. However, in group 2, bleeding times remained elevated at 23 and 29 min, respectively, at 2 to 4 hours and 6 to 8 hours post-bypass. Analysis also revealed that bleeding time correlated with the amount of blood transfused and duration of bypass. Also, estimated blood loss correlated with amount of whole blood transfused.

Reduction in Platelet-Mediated Force Development

Greilich and colleagues[48] demonstrated that platelet-mediated force development is significantly reduced by cardiopulmonary bypass. Platelet force development is physiologically important in the control of microvascular bleeding: to increase the tensile strength of the platelet plug to withstand the shear stress of turbulent blood flow and to reapproximate interruptions in vascular integrity. Platelets not only have to adhere and aggregate at sites of vascular injury, but also need to have sufficient cytoplasmic activity to generate a cytoskeleton capable of retraction. Platelet force development is dependent on both platelet concentration and function. Blood samples were adjusted to platelet counts of 200,000 for all measurements by dilution of platelet-rich plasma with platelet-poor plasma.

Investigators used a Hemodyne clot retractormeter, which measures the platelet force development within a clot formed between a thermostated cup and a parallel upper plate that is coupled to a displacement transducer. As the clot is formed, platelets pull fibrin strands, which have become attached to the cup and upper plate, inward, thus transmitting force through the platelet fibrin network.[26] Patients undergoing elective CABG were studied; all were receiving aspirin and nitroglycerin, half were receiving intravenous heparin. Mean activated clotting time (ACT), aPTT, and platelet force development did not differ preoperatively in those who received heparin and those who had not. Post-bypass ACT returned to baseline after protamine; however, aPTT remained significantly increased. Platelet force development was abolished during CPB. After bypass and protamine, platelet force development recovered but median recovery was only 55% of pre-bypass levels. The percent recovery inversely correlated with tube thoracostomy drainage at 12 and 24 hours. Heparin inhibition of thrombin formation is likely the reason for abolishment of platelet force development during bypass. The incomplete recovery after protamine suggests that CPB induces platelet dysfunction. Although ACT was normalized, aPTT remained elevated post-bypass in this study. Investigators do acknowledge that residual heparin could in part have contributed to the decrease in force development.[48]

Dysfunction of Shear-Induced Pathway of Platelet Function

High-velocity blood flow and reactive vascular spasm in arterioles induce "shear stress" at sites of vascular disruption. Hemostasis requires platelets to respond to shear stress with activation and induction. Tabuchi and colleagues,[49,50] using a novel shear-inducing technique, the in vitro bleeding test (Thrombostat 4000), demonstrated dysfunction of the shear-induced pathway of platelet function in patients undergoing CABG with a membrane oxygenator. Blood samples were aspirated under a constant pressure of 40 mm Hg through a Teflon capillary that ended in an aperture with a cellulose acetate filter covered with collagen type I and soaked with ADP or collagen. Bleeding volume was recorded until a platelet plug occluded the aperture. Investigators found that bleeding volume through the artificial capillary increased abruptly after the start of cardiopulmonary bypass. Bleeding volume increased throughout the bypass period. After bypass, bleeding volume decreased but remained more than double that recorded pre-bypass. In a second study, patients were given 325 mg of aspirin preoperatively. In comparison with patients not given aspirin, aspirin-treated platelets were not affected differently before bypass, but had 30% more bleeding volume through the artificial capillary post-bypass. In a third study, blood loss from chest tubes was measured for 24 hours post-bypass. Investigators found that bleeding volume through the in vitro bleeding test correlated with blood loss. Platelet count, ACT, and hematocrit did not correlate with blood loss.[50]

Decreased Platelet Aggregation

Most but not all investigators have reported defects in platelet aggregation associated with cardiopulmonary bypass. It is very difficult to compare studies due to differences in sample processing technique, lack of standardization, and semiquantitative nature of aggregation tests. Most studies concur that cardiopulmonary bypass results in a decreased response of platelets to aggregating stimuli; however, data actually correlating decreased aggregation to blood loss is sparse.

Wachtfogel and colleagues[51] examined platelet aggregation to epinephrine in an in vitro–simulated bypass circuit with a spiral coil membrane oxygenator. In five experiments with citrated centrifuged samples of platelet-rich plasma, investigators determined the threshold doses of epinephrine required to produce biphasic aggregation of >57%. Mean threshold concentration of epinephrine increased from 0.4 μmol/L before recirculation to 9.4 μmol/L after just 2 min of circulation. After 2 hours, even 100 μmol/L of epinephrine was insufficient to induce platelet aggregation. Addonizio and colleagues,[41] looking at aggregation thresholds in in vitro experiments with simulated recirculation with membrane and bubble oxygenators, had similar results. Platelets become insensitive to aggregating agents ADP and epinephrine within 1 hour.

Harker et al[44] investigated platelet aggregation induced by ADP or collagen using platelet-rich plasma anticoagulated with 3.2 trisodium citrate. Study patients underwent mainly CABG procedures and were perfused with a bubble oxygenator. Platelet concentration in samples was adjusted to 300,000. Aggregation before and during bypass was assessed by comparing the concentration of ADP or collagen required to produce a 50% change in optical transmission. There was no change in aggregation after heparin administration before the onset of bypass. Aggregometry revealed a greatly reduced platelet response to ADP and collagen beginning with bypass and persisting for 3 hours after bypass.

McKenna and colleagues[39] studied 13 patients undergoing valve replacement with perfusion using a bubble or disk oxygenator. Blood samples with platelet concentration of 150,000 were prepared by centrifuging citrated whole blood followed by mixing platelet-rich plasma with platelet-poor plasma. Maximum aggregation and rate of aggregation were determined by change and rate of change of light transmission through blood samples after ADP, collagen, or epinephrine was added. With low-dose ADP, 1×10^{-6} M, mean maximal aggregation and rate of aggregation decreased from 32.6% pre-bypass to 14.6% at the end of bypass. Aggregation recovered somewhat to 27% at 1 to 2 hours after protamine. Pattern of change was similar with a high dose of ADP, 3×10^{-6} M. Aggregation to collagen and epinephrine also showed reduction at the end of bypass followed by improvement 1 to 2 hours post-protamine (patients with abnormal aggregation prior to bypass were excluded). The investigators found no correlation between preoperative aggregation abnormalities and blood replacement or bleeding times. Noting that the aggregation defect to ADP was more marked than that to collagen or epinephrine, the investigators proposed that perhaps platelets became refractory to ADP because of continued ADP exposure through ADP release from hemolyzed red cells.

Edmunds and colleagues[45] investigated aggregation to ADP by measuring minimal threshold concentrations of ADP that achieved complete aggregation (second-wave aggregation). Platelet-rich plasma from centrifuged samples of citrated blood were studied from 35 patients undergoing CABG with bubble or membrane oxygenators. Threshold ADP concentration increased significantly during bypass in both oxygenator groups. One hour after protamine, ADP threshold remained significantly elevated in patients perfused with membrane oxygenators, while ADP threshold decreased and recovered to slightly above pre-bypass levels in the bubble oxygenator group. Authors rejected the hypothesis that membrane oxygenator systems cause less trauma to platelets. Other studies have shown that cardiotomy suctioning, which creates air-blood interfaces, decreases the theoretical advantage of membrane oxygenators over bubble oxygenators.

Zilla and colleagues[46] studied ADP- and collagen-induced aggregability in 18 patients undergoing CABG with bubble oxygenators. Aggregation to ADP and collagen was assessed in citrated, centrifuged plasma by percent light transmission. Prior to bypass, platelet aggregation to ADP was reduced to 92% and to collagen was reduced to 62% of initial values. After 15 min of bypass, ADP-induced aggregability decreased further to 74% and collagen responsiveness decreased to 47%. Aggregation decreased further and reached a nadir after protamine administration. One hour later, ADP aggregability remained low at 28% and collagen aggregability recovered slightly to 23%. Twenty-four hours postoperation, aggregability to ADP improved to 68%, but collagen aggregability improved only to 40%.

Rinder and colleagues[52] studied platelet aggregation in 36 patients undergoing CABG and five patients undergoing aortic valve replacements with membrane oxygenator perfusion. Whole blood samples were analyzed by flow cytometry for identification of platelet aggregates. Aggregation response to 10 μmol of ADP decreased significantly after 10 minutes of bypass and decreased further by the end of bypass. Whole blood samples have the theoretical advantage over centrifuged samples of less chance of inducing platelet activation during sample processing. Nadir response to ADP occurred at 1 to 4 hours post-bypass and returned to baseline levels 18 hours after bypass. However, no correlation was found between degree of aggregation defect and chest tube drainage after 24 hours.

Mammen and colleagues[53] also studied platelet aggregation using whole blood aggregometry. Thirty patients undergoing primarily CABG procedures with bubble oxygenators were studied. Platelet aggregation to ADP decreased significantly after initiation of bypass and remained low during bypass. ADP aggregation decreased further after the administration of protamine. After 24 hours, ADP aggregation improved but was still significantly less than before bypass. Aggregation to collagen decreased after heparin administration, initiation of bypass, and remained low until the end of bypass. There was no further decrease after protamine. Collagen aggregation was normal after 24 hours. Ristocetin aggregation was unchanged until the administration of protamine and this effect persisted at 24 hours post-bypass. The authors concluded that aggregability was impaired by bypass as it relates to the release reaction (ADP and collagen), but not in response to surface contact alone (ristocetin). Also the reduction in aggregation to ADP and ristocetin after protamine suggests that protamine or heparin-protamine complex changed the platelet surface or alternatively caused the disappearance of larger platelets. The investigators found no relationship between pump time and thrombocytopenia and impaired aggregation.

Data Not Supporting Decreased Platelet Aggregation

Wenger and colleagues,[54] in contrast did not find a significant change in platelet aggregability to ADP. Platelet-rich plasma from 12 patients undergoing CABG or valve surgery with bubble oxygenators was sampled preoperation and 30 min after start of bypass. Threshold dose of ADP required to produce second wave aggregation did not change significantly.

Kestin and colleagues[55] studied platelet reactivity to agonists not by aggregometry but by whole blood flow cytometry assay for membrane markers of activation after the addition of agonists: phorbol myristate acetate, thromboxane A_2 analogue, and ADP with epinephrine. Twenty patients undergoing CABG (one with concurrent valve replacement) with a membrane oxygenator were studied. Investigators found that platelet reactivity to added agonists as evidenced by upregulation of platelet surface P-selectin and GPIIb/IIIa complex and downregulation of GPIb/IX complex was not altered by cardiopulmonary bypass. Kestin et al found that administration of heparin-augmented PMA induced upregulation of P-selectin and downregulation of GPIB/IX complex. This activation effect was reversed by protamine. Kestin also found that cardiopulmonary bypass did not inhibit thrombin-induced activation when samples were washed free of heparin.

However, platelets with the administered heparin were unreactive to thrombin at time points of 5 min after heparin, initiation of bypass, beginning of maximal hypothermia on bypass, and 45 min after start of bypass.

Kestin et al[55] postulated that there was no intrinsic defect induced by cardiopulmonary bypass; rather the platelet defect was due to a lack of in vivo agonists as a result of bypass. Kestin et al suggested that heparin inhibition of thrombin, "the preeminent platelet activator," played a major role. However, one must note that the investigators used more heparin than in other studies or in common clinical practice. Patients received an initial bolus of 4 mg/kg, which was followed by additional doses as needed to keep an ACT of ≥999 seconds.

Etiology of Platelet Defect

Most investigators agree that platelet dysfunction contributes to the coagulation deficiency observed after cardiopulmonary bypass. However, agreement on the etiology of the platelet defect incurred during cardiopulmonary bypass has been lacking. The only conclusion that can be made is that separate evidence for platelet degranulation, defects in glycoprotein platelet receptors, and extrinsic factors, such as heparin, hypothermia, and products of fibrinolysis have been found to account for platelet dysfunction. The lack of concurrence leads these authors to hypothesize that there is no single defect, but rather a combination of multiple defects, which occur in varying degrees during differing clinical circumstances.

Platelet Degranulation

Evidence for Platelet Degranulation. Platelets undergoing cardiopulmonary bypass and cardiac surgery are exposed to stimulation from encounters with foreign surfaces, thrombin formed by the coagulation cascade, ADP from hemolyzed erythrocytes and activated platelets, and subendothelial proteins exposed by vascular trauma. Once platelets are activated and undergo release of their granule contents, they are no longer effective participants of hemostasis. As mentioned earlier, photomicrographs have revealed that platelets are heterogeneous after cardiopulmonary bypass, ranging from newly released granule-rich platelets, to shape-changed but granule-intact platelets, to platelets with partial granule depletion, to platelets with total granule depletion, to platelet fragments. In vivo studies in general have shown a smaller percentage of altered platelets than in vitro studies. This is perhaps due to the partial clearance of altered platelets in vivo and also the recruitment of new platelets into the circulation. Circulation of granule-deficient platelets is hypothesized as the reason for platelet dysfunction after cardiopulmonary bypass.

Beurling-Harbury and Galvan[56] studied citrated, centrifuged, platelet-rich plasma samples from 88 patients undergoing cardiac surgery with perfusion through a bubble oxygenator. Investigators measured total and releasable ADP and ATP in pre-bypass and post-bypass plasma samples exposed to the potent platelet activator thrombin. A decrease of about 30% in releasable ADP and ATP and total ADP was found after cardiopulmonary bypass. Whether this was due to platelets having undergone dense granule release during bypass or whether hemostatically reactive granule-rich platelets were selectively removed during bypass cannot be elucidated from this study. In any event, the circulation of a platelet population with less secretory ADP and ATP after bypass would be less hemostatically responsive. In addition, the authors reported that nucleotide depletion of ≥ 0.5 nmol/10^8 platelets of releasable ADP was significantly associated with chest tube drainage above 400 cc; however, this correlation was not absolute. Releasable ADP depletion ≥ 1 nmol/10^8 platelets correlated with a bypass time greater than 90 min. However, bypass time did not correlate with blood loss or red cell transfusion requirement. Twelve patients who received platelets intraoperatively were excluded in the platelet analysis. Conclusions from these data must be made with the caveat that results may or may not have been different if these 12 patients had been included.

Harker and colleagues[44] reported evidence of alpha granule release by measuring platelet factor IV and B-thromboglobulin (B-TG) in 31 patients undergoing surgery with cardiopulmonary bypass and bubble oxygenator perfusion. Blood samples were centrifuged to separate platelets from plasma. Plasma PFIV rose sharply after heparin, while B-TG rose acutely after the onset of bypass. Both PFIV and B-TG increased progressively throughout bypass reaching peak levels at the end of bypass. Platelet content of PF4 was reduced from pre-bypass levels of 1.32×10^{-6} ng/fl platelet volume to 0.96×10^{-6} ng/fl platelet volume. Photomicrographs (two patients only) revealed that circulating platelets were partially depleted of alpha granules. Three hours after protamine, B-TG and PFIV decreased from peak levels by 86% and 60%, respectively. Twelve hours after bypass, B-TG and PFIV returned to preoperative levels. A direct relationship was found between bleeding time, plasma levels of PF4 and B-TG and duration of bypass. Harker et al concluded that the progressive platelet dysfunction was a consequence of platelet activation and paralleled the release and partial depletion of alpha granule content. Mammen and colleagues[58] also found a similar pattern and time course of plasma PF4 and B-TG in five patients studied. Harker et al, in contrast to Beurling-Harbury and Galvan, did not find evidence of dense granule release. However, the investigators chose to study only small subsets of the 31 patients for evidence of dense granule release. Here are their findings.

1. Platelet content of dense granule constituent ATP and ADP did not change significantly during bypass in the four patients studied.

2. Photomicrographs of two patients did not show any significant change in number of dense bodies per platelet cross section.
3. In six patients studied, the ratio of ^{14}C-serotonin/^{15}Cr did not decrease during bypass or postoperative day 1, suggesting that dense granules were not released.[44]

In in vitro–simulated circulation, Addonizio and colleagues[42] found that plasma levels of the alpha granule product, low-affinity platelet factor 4, rose within 2 min of recirculation and continued to rise throughout the 6-hour studies. The investigators found no significant difference in LAPF4 release between low (300 ml/min) and high (1000 ml/min) flow rates or between circuits containing membrane oxygenators with small versus large surface areas (0.3 M^2 vs 0.9 M^2 surface circuit area). Removal of the membrane oxygenator and replacement with an equivalent surface area of tubing resulted in significantly less platelet secretion. It is hypothesized that the altered flow patterns produced by the oxygenator resulted in greater platelet activation and secretion. In further experiments, Addonizio and colleagues[40,43,57] found that inhibition of platelet activation with PGI_2 or precoating of circuits with albumin resulted in significantly decreased levels of secreted LAPF4 in in vitro and in vivo (rhesus monkeys) circulation with membrane and bubble oxygenators. In the above studies, all samples were centrifuged to separate platelet-rich plasma from platelet-poor plasma.

Rinder and colleagues[52] used flow cytometry and IE3, a monoclonal antibody directed against granule membrane protein-140, to assess the percentage of circulating activated platelets in whole blood samples in 41 patients undergoing bypass. Alpha granule release is marked by fusion of the granule membrane with platelet surface membrane. GMP-140, an alpha granule membrane protein, is expressed on the platelet membrane. Monoclonal antibody binding to GMP-140 increased steadily throughout bypass from a pre-bypass percentage of 7% to a peak of 29% just before termination of bypass. By 2 to 4 hours post-bypass, activated platelets decreased to 19% and approached baseline at 18 hours. Peak levels of activation did not correlate with duration of bypass or chest tube drainage. As mentioned earlier, Rinder et al also found an aggregation defect to ADP. However, the peak decrease of aggregation response occurred 2 to 4 hours post-bypass. The platelet aggregation defect was temporally and qualitatively different from platelet activation. Rinder et al concluded that "cardiopulmonary bypass causes a complex constellation of platelet defects, which include alpha granule release, prolonged circulation of activated, 'spent' platelets, and impaired platelet aggregation."[52]

Nieuwenhuis and colleagues[58] used a monoclonal antibody 2.28 directed against a protein antigen localized to lysosomes that is exposed on the surface of thrombin-activated platelets. Using flow cytometry, in paraformaldehydefixed and then washed samples from 10 patients undergoing cardiopulmonary bypass with bubble oxygenators, the investigators found that the percentage of 2.28 positive platelets in circulation increased from 5.5% before bypass to 24.6% 20 min after bypass.

Evidence Against Significant Platelet Degranulation. Zilla and colleagues[46] investigated platelet activation in 15 patients undergoing CABG with bubble oxygenator perfusion by examining platelet morphology and ultrastructure. Activation was also assessed by measurement of platelet-dense granule content of adenine nucleotides and serotonin, plasma levels of released alpha granule constituents PF4 and B-TG, plasma levels of dense granule constituent serotonin, and plasma levels of platelet-synthesized thromboxane B_2. During the first 15 min of bypass, scanning electron microscopy revealed that 43% of platelets had undergone shape change indicative of early activation or primary aggregation. However, only 6% had progressed to irreversible secondary aggregation. Transmission electron microscopy revealed centralization of granules and mitochondria, but only occasional evidence of granule exocytosis. Granule content and plasma levels of release products did not change significantly. After 15 min of bypass, platelets began to show evidence of recovery. By late bypass, 80% of platelets were in an unactivated smooth discocyte form. During bypass, platelet aggregation to ADP was diminished. Plasma platelet factor 4 and B-thromboglobulin levels did rise by the end of bypass, but the absolute levels were small. Only 3.4% of total platelet factor 4 was reported in the plasma. Since secondary aggregation results in release of 98.4% of platelet factor 4, only a negligible percentage of platelets in this study had undergone alpha granule release. In addition, parameters of cellular lysis, free hemoglobin, and lactic dehydrogenase, had concomitantly increased. Platelet lysis could have contributed to the elevated levels of PF4 and B-TG. The authors concluded that platelet stimulation during bypass occurred early and that stimulus is enough to produce primary aggregation, but not enough to produce significant secondary aggregation and granule release. Platelets seem to recover during the course of bypass, possibly because of replacement by new platelets but more likely because of decreased sensitivity and aggregability due to reasons other than granule depletion (i.e., receptor alteration or circulating inhibitory factor).

In Kestin and colleagues'[55] aforementioned study, the investigators also examined alpha granule release. Using whole blood flow cytometry technique, they investigated binding of monoclonal antibody S12 toward P-selectin (also known as GMP-140). Cardiopulmonary bypass did not result in any significant increase in P-selectin expression on circulating platelets. There was only a minimum increase in percentage of P-selectin positive platelets from 2% preoperation to 3.1% at 45 min of bypass, and 2.9% at completion of bypass. Using whole blood methods, George and colleagues[58] and Abrams and colleagues[60] also demonstrated that cardiopulmonary bypass did not significantly increase the expression of P-selectin.

Dechavanne and colleagues[61] also used flow cytometry but on centrifuged platelet-rich plasma on seven patients undergoing CABG or mitral valve replacement (MVR) with perfusion through bubble oxygenators. Alpha granule secretion was elevated by monoclonal antibody binding of LYP8 directed against thrombospondin (an alpha granule protein that rebinds to platelet membrane after granule release) and LYP7 directed against an alpha granule glycoprotein present on platelet surfaces only after secretion. LYP8 and LYP7 binding remained unchanged before and after bypass. In addition, Dechavanne et al measured mean alpha granule number per platelet cross section in five patients by electron microscopy and found no change after bypass.

Kestin et al[55] speculated that reported evidence of increased plasma PF4 and B-TG from CPB-induced alpha granule secretion may result from either degranulated platelets that are rapidly cleared from circulation, noncirculating degranulated platelets adherent to synthetic surfaces and vessel walls, platelet lysis in vivo or in vitro, or artifactual in vitro degranulation and secretion from platelet activation during laboratory preparation of assays, particularly as a result of platelet and plasma separation.

Alteration of Platelet Glycoprotein Receptors

Several investigators have found that monoclonal antibody binding specific to platelet glycoprotein receptors, GPIb (von Willebrand factor receptor), GPIIb/IIIa (fibrinogen receptor), and α_2-adrenergic receptor (ADP receptor) is reduced during and after cardiopulmonary bypass. The alteration of these receptors has been postulated to be one reason for platelet dysfunction caused by extracorporeal circulation. Postulated theories include:

1. After platelet receptors negotiate adherence and aggregation to synthetic surfaces, platelet membranes are resealed and receptors are altered. Platelets then return to circulation but without functional receptors.
2. After initial adherence and aggregation, platelet membrane fragments with receptors remain on the synthetic surface after platelet detachment. Platelet fragments and damaged platelets with fewer receptors then return to circulation.
3. Mechanical trauma from shear stress, turbulence, and surface contact results in platelet fragmentation and membrane shedding.
4. Platelets rich in receptors preferentially adhere and aggregate on synthetic surfaces. Left behind in the circulation are platelets poor in receptors that don't adhere and aggregate.[62]
5. Cleavage of receptors by plasmin or complement.[63]

Evidence for Platelet Receptor Abnormalities. Musial and colleagues[62] investigated the effect of in vitro extracorporeal circulation with a membrane oxygenator. The investigators stimulated the exposure of fibrinogen receptors with ADP stimulation and with the proteolytic enzyme chymotrypsin. Prior studies had demonstrated that the fibrinogen receptor exposed by either method was identical. Blood samples were centrifuged and then washed. Fibrinogen receptors were assessed through ^{125}I fibrinogen binding and also by B59.2, a monoclonal antibody, directed against the GPIIb/IIIa complex. After 2 hours of circulation ^{125}I fibrinogen binding decreased significantly in chymotrypsin-treated platelets (from 41,370 to 13,230), and decreased, although not statistically significant in ADP stimulated platelets (from 55,750 to 35,100). Binding constant of fibrinogen to platelets remained unchanged during circulation. B59.2 antigenic binding sites were reduced by approximately 40% after 2 hours of circulation in both an ADP and a non-ADP-stimulated group. Investigators also found that the addition of PGE_2 preserved the number of B59.2 antigenic sites. Authors conclude that recirculation causes a partial loss of fibrinogen receptors and molecules of the GPIIb/IIIa complex.

Wachtfogel and colleagues[51] studied platelet α_2-adrenergic receptors during simulated in vitro extracorporeal circulation containing a membrane oxygenator. Investigators found a 10-fold decrease in platelet aggregation sensitivity to epinephrine after 2 min of circulation and >100-fold decrease after 2 hours. Paralleling the decrease in sensitivity was a decrease in α_2-adrenergic binding sites from a mean of 235 sites to 139 sites per platelet, without a change in dissociation constant, after just 2 min of circulation. After 2 hours, binding was so weak that neither the number of sites nor the dissociation constant could be determined.

In clinical studies, George et al[59] and Rinder et al,[68] both using monoclonal antibody binding, whole blood samples, and membrane oxygenators, demonstrated decreases in platelet surface concentrations of GPIb and GPIIb/IIIa. Rinder et al analyzed 24 patients undergoing CABG or aortic valve replacement (AVR). In the 8 patients studied for GPIb, GPIb decreased to 84% by the end of CPB and decreased further to 72% at 2 to 4 hours after bypass. Levels returned to baseline by 18 hours. In the 16 patients studied for GPIIb/IIIa, GPIIb/IIIa levels decreased to 79% at the end of bypass and remained at this level 2 to 4 hours post-bypass. The GPIIb/IIIa receptor loss was less, because during platelet activation this receptor normally increases. When platelets were divided into activated and nonactivated subsets, GPIIb/IIIa was reduced by 47% in activated platelets and 63% in nonactivated platelets. Receptor loss did not correlate with duration of bypass or chest tube drainage.[63] George et al found in 10 patients undergoing cardiopulmonary bypass surgery significant decreases in both GPIB and GPIIb/IIIa concentration, although values were all within the normal range. The two studies differed in that Rinder et al found platelet activation and granule release to be temporally linked with receptor loss, while George et al found less evidence of granule release. Rinder et al's study had a longer bypass time (average of 110 vs 74 minutes), which may account for the greater incidence of platelet activation. George et al also measured membrane particles in serum and plasma and found an increase in GPIIb molecules in membrane microparticles after bypass, suggesting that the increased turbulence and shear stress of bypass may have damaged platelets and receptors.

Wenger and colleagues[54] also found evidence of receptor loss in a study of 12 patients undergoing CABG or valve replacement surgery with cardiopulmonary bypass through a bubble oxygenator. In centrifuged samples, they found that platelet fibrinogen receptors, as measured by ^{125}I fibrinogen binding after ADP incubation, decreased by 59% 1 hour after bypass. There was no change in binding affinity. Platelet GPIIIa, determined by antibody binding, also decreased significantly to 70% of pre-bypass levels. Analysis of detergent (Triton X-100) washings from the perfusion circuit after bypass in five patients revealed significant amounts of platelet membrane GPIIIa antigen while no antigen was detected after saline rinses. Authors concluded that surface-adhered platelets become detached as bypass continues, however, leaving behind membrane fragments containing fibrinogen receptors. Dechavanne and colleagues[61] also found a reduction in GPIIb/IIIa receptors after bypass in seven patients undergoing CABG or MVR. Like Wenger et al, Dechavanne et al used monoclonal antibody binding, washed and centrifuged platelet samples, and bubble oxygenator perfusion. The number of LYP18 (monoclonal antibody directed against GPIIb/IIIa) binding sites decreased from a pre-bypass number of 72,671 to 49,775 at the end of bypass. Using fluorescence analysis, the percentage of fluorescent platelets after LYP18 incubation decreased from 75% to 66% after bypass; however, the mean fluorescence intensity was unchanged. The authors concluded that there is a reduction in GPIIb/IIIa receptor complex after bypass; however, not all platelets are affected.

Evidence Not Supporting Platelet Receptor Abnormalities. Not all studies showed membrane glycoprotein receptor abnormalities after bypass. Metzelaar and colleagues,[64] using monoclonal antibody binding, flow cytometry, and washed centrifuged samples, studied 17 patients undergoing CABG or valve replacement with perfusion through a membrane oxygenator. Investigators found a significant increase of plasma membrane expression of GPIIIa when comparing samples 15 min after bypass to pre-bypass. Plasma membrane expression of GPIb was unchanged.

Abrams and colleagues,[60] using flow cytometry and monoclonal antibodies on whole blood samples (no centrifugation or washing), studied nine patients undergoing CABG with perfusion with a membrane or bubble oxygenator. After 60 min of bypass, platelets exhibited a threefold increase in PAC1 binding (PAC1 antibody binds specifically to activated GPIIb/IIIa antigen). However, the fluorescence profile was broad, indicating that some platelets expressed more fibrinogen receptors than others. Using two other antibodies, the investigators found a small but statistically insignificant decrease in the number of GPIIB and GPIIIa molecules on intact platelets.

Kestin and colleagues,[55] in the aforementioned study, also looked at monoclonal antibody binding to platelet receptors in 20 patients undergoing CABG (one patient also had concomitant valve replacement) with perfusion through a membrane oxygenator. Whole blood assays revealed no significant change in platelet surface expression of GPIb-IX or GPIIb/IIIa expression before, during, and after cardiopulmonary bypass. Using a panel of monoclonal antibodies, the investigators found that CPB did not result in significant change or alteration in receptor expression, irrespective of whether the monoclonal antibody used was directed against the von Willebrand factor binding site of GPIb, the thrombin binding site of GPIB, the GPIb/IX complex, three different epitopes near the fibrinogen-binding site on the GPIIb/IIIa complex, or GPIIIa. Also there was no change in ristocetin-induced binding of von Willebrand factor, plasma glycocalicin (proteolytic product of GPIb), nor binding of exogenous fibrinogen to platelets activated in vitro with ADP.

Extrinsic Factors Causing Platelet Defect

Heparin Inhibition of Thrombin. Kestin et al's[55] study mentioned above postulated that cardiopulmonary bypass did not affect intrinsic platelet function.

Presented supporting data included:

1. normal platelet reactivity in vitro to platelet agonists
2. no loss of platelet surface GPIb and GPIIb/IIIa receptors
3. minimal increase of circulating degranulated platelets.

In contrast, Kestin et al found that platelet reactivity in vivo was depressed after heparinization and during bypass, and recovered at 2 to 24 hours post-bypass. Reduced platelet reactivity was noted by increased bleeding time and also by lack of thromboxane TX B_2 (stable metabolite of thromboxane) generation and lack of upregulation of platelet surface P selectin (component of alpha granule membrane) in shed blood from the bleeding time wound. In addition, platelet reactivity to thrombin in whole blood samples were unreactive after heparinization, while platelet reactivity to thrombin was normal when platelets were washed free of heparin. Kestin et al concluded that intrinsic platelet function is not affected by bypass, but that platelet dysfunction of bypass is due to extrinsic factors, namely heparin suppression of thrombin, the "preeminent agonist." It must be noted that Kestin et al's patients received larger doses of heparin than patients in other studies. The more complete suppression of thrombin along with the analysis of undisturbed whole blood samples likely resulted in less platelet activation. This may account for their findings, which differ from most other studies. These patients received 4 mg/kg heparin load and then supplemental doses to keep the ACT >999 seconds.

Hypothermia. Transient-platelet dysfunction occurs at low temperatures. Valeri and colleagues[65] studied the effect of temperature on platelet function in 37 patients undergoing CPB by differentially cooling and warming both upper extremities. Each patient had the temperature in one arm increased with a water-filled blanket set at 40°C, while the other arm was either allowed to equilibrate with the environment or was cooled with ice. The temperature difference between the extremities averaged 7.3°C with a range from 27.1°C to 35.1°C during CPB. There was found to be an increase in bleeding time and a reduction in the level of thromboxane (TXB_2) produced by platelets at the bleeding site. This group had shown in another study a significant correlation between bleeding time and postoperative nonsurgical blood loss.[66] It appears that local hypothermia may have reduced the enzymatic activity of thromboxane synthetase. Other evidence of hypothermia-induced platelet dysfunction includes alterations in platelet morphology, enhanced platelet adhesiveness, and inhibition of ADP-induced platelet aggregation.[15,67]

Animal studies have implicated platelet sequestration by the splanchnic circulation during periods of hypothermia as another cause of impaired hemostasis.[68] There is no clear evidence that this occurs in humans, however, as significant thrombocytopenia has not been consistently documented during or after CPB.

Plasmin and Products of Fibrinolysis. As part of the checks and balances control of hemostasis, to limit the propagation of clot to area of injury, plasmin and fibrin degradation products inhibit platelet activity. However, if fibrinolytic activity is excessively activated during cardiopulmonary bypass, plasmin-induced platelet dysfunction can add to the coagulopathy. In in vitro studies, investigators have demonstrated a dose- and time-dependent plasmin inhibition of platelet aggregation in response to platelet agonists, thrombin,[69,70] ionophore A23187,[69] collagen,[69] and ADP.[70] Schafer[71] and Adelman[72] found that plasmin, also in a dose-dependent manner, inhibited thrombin, ionophore, and collagen-stimulated thromboxane B_2 formation. Schafer et al[71] further demonstrated that prostacyclin and plasmin caused a synergistic inhibition of thrombin- and ADP-induced aggregation and synergistic inhibition of thrombin-stimulated rise in platelet cytosolic calcium.

Multiple mechanisms of plasmin-induced platelet dysfunction have been proposed:

1. Proteolysis of platelet glycoprotein receptors: Adelman et al[72] demonstrated that plasmin in concentrations of 0.05 to 1.0 CU/ml produced progressive loss of GPIb with a simultaneous increase in released glycocalicin (a proteolytic fragment of GPIb). Stricker et al[70] showed that incubation of pharmacologic doses of tissue plasminogen activator and plasminogen with platelets resulted in degradation of GPIb and GPIIb/IIIa receptors and appearance of glycocalicin. Consequently, plasmin inhibited ristocetin-mediated agglutination, which is dependent on vWF and GPIb.[70,72]
2. Increase in platelet cyclic AMP: Adnot et al[14] demonstrated that plasmin, through proteolysis, caused an increase in adenylate cyclase activity in in vitro intact platelet and platelet membrane preparations. As discussed earlier, platelet aggregation is inhibited by adenylate cyclase activity and the formation of cyclic AMP. Plasmin also suppresses the effect of adrenergic agonists on platelets by inactivating the guanosine triphosphate (GTP)-dependent inhibition of cyclic AMP.
3. Impairment of prostaglandin mobilization: Schafer and Adelman[69] proposed that plasmin inhibits platelet function in part by blocking the mobilization of arachidonic acid. Plasmin did not affect arachidonate-induced platelet aggregation or thromboxane formation. Plasmin did block thrombin-induced release of arachidonic acid from platelet membrane phospholipids.
4. Activation of protein kinase C: Schafer and Adelman[69–72] also noted that plasmin activates platelet protein kinase C. Protein kinase C activation results in platelet granule release, but this kinase also has a feedback control role and inhibits further extracellular signal transduction in response to thrombin and other agonists.
5. Reduction in available fibrinogen: Plasmin degradation of fibrinogen reduces available agonists for GPIIb/IIIa receptors, thus impairing platelet-to-platelet aggregation.
6. Increase in products of fibrin and fibrinogen degradation: Products of fibrin and fibrinogen degradation also inhibit platelet aggregation. These degradation products bind to fibrinogen and/or GPIIb/IIIa receptors, thus interfering with platelet-fibrinogen-platelet linking.[73]

Effect of Cardiopulmonary Bypass on the Coagulation Protein System

Coagulation proteins are affected by dilution, denaturation, consumption, inhibition, and hypothermia during cardiopulmonary bypass.

Extracorporeal prime, cardioplegia, and administered fluids will dilute coagulation factors to 50% to 80% of preoperative levels. Normal hemostasis requires only 20% to 40% of normal coagulation protein.[2,25] Factor V, being more labile, decreases further than the other coagulation factors; however, levels remain above 15%, which is above the threshold level needed for normal factor V activity. Factors VIII:c and vWF are released in greater quantities in response to stress. Levels of these factors remain normal or increase despite hemodilution. Dilution of coagulation factors is usually not enough to cause a coagulopathy except in children or very small adults, in whom the prime to patient blood volume can be significant. Coagulation proteins normally return to baseline levels within 12 hours after bypass.[25]

The additive effects of consumption, denaturation, and hypothermia in addition to the lower levels resulting from dilution, however, can at times produce a coagulopathy requiring transfusion of additional coagulation proteins. Coagulation proteins are consumed by the activation of the intrinsic and extrinsic coagulation pathways and also by deposition onto synthetic surfaces. Turbulent flow and exposure to air-blood interfaces through oxygenators and cardiotomy suction devices can denature coagulation proteins. Fibrin degradation products generated by fibrinolysis during cardiopulmonary bypass can act as circulating inhibitors of coagulation proteins. Hypothermia affects coagulation factors, in addition to its effects on platelets. At low body temperatures, enzymatic cleavage is known to slow[74,75] and a heparin-like inhibitor of factor Xa may be activated.[76] Enzymatic reactions attenuate 7% for each 1°C.[13] As shown by Reed et al,[74] prolongation of clotting times during mild to severe hypothermia is independent of clotting factor levels in vitro. These coagulation defects may be more pronounced if rewarming is inadequate. Note that clotting times measured in vitro at 37°C will not be prolonged. In other words, normal values returned from the hospital laboratory will not confirm hypothermia-induced coagulopathy and should not reduce the urgency for rewarming the bleeding patient.

Effect of Cardiopulmonary Bypass on the Fibrinolytic System

Fibrinolysis is a normal hematologic activity accompanying normal coagulation. It is usually controlled and confined to the vicinity of formed clot, thus serving to remodel the clot and, eventually, remove thrombus once the damaged endothelium is restored. On the other hand, fibrinolysis has also been determined to occur in nonphysiologic circumstances such as during and after cardiopulmonary bypass (CPB). Indeed, CPB can be shown to activate a number of plasma protein cascades, as well as blood cells, to produce powerful proteolytic enzymes. These enzymes mediate not only the bleeding complications of CPB but the thrombotic and inflammatory complications as well.[19] This occurs to some degree in all patients undergoing cardiopulmonary bypass surgery.

Fibrinolysis Induced by Cardiopulmonary Bypass

Numerous studies have led us to conclude that CPB activates the fibrinolytic pathway[16,77–81] (Fig. 9.8). Various fibrin-split products have been identified during and immediately following CPB or use of other extracorporeal circuits.[77,82,83] More recently, investigators not only have documented specific increased levels of plasma D-dimer produced by the lysis of

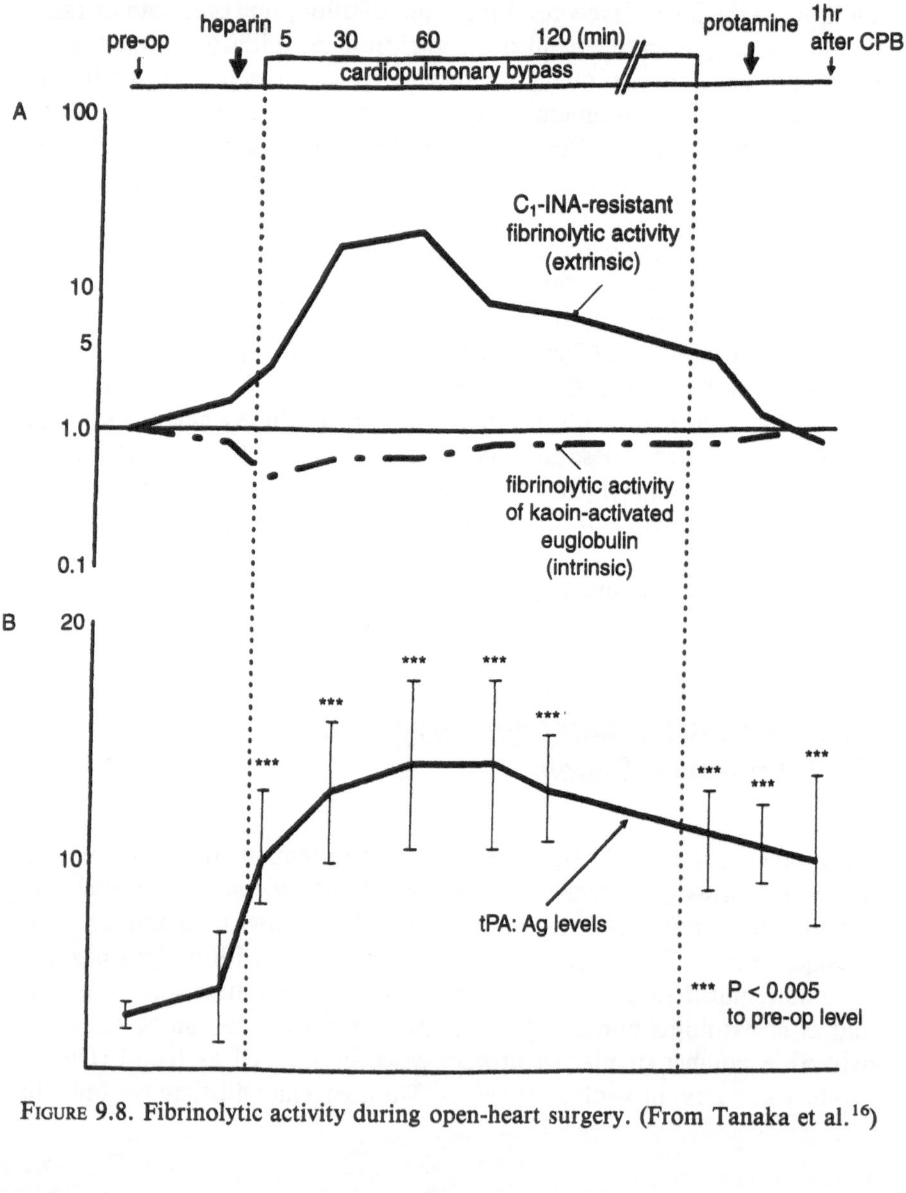

FIGURE 9.8. Fibrinolytic activity during open-heart surgery. (From Tanaka et al.[16])

fibrin, but also have shown these levels to increase progressively during CPB.[84] Plasminogen activator concentrations have also been shown to rise during CPB (Fig. 9.8B), while levels of the naturally occurring circulating plasmin inhibitor, PAI-1, remain unchanged or decrease.[16,81] In addition, plasminogen concentrations measured on blood samples taken from patients undergoing CPB reveal marked decreases in plasminogen levels that cannot be attributed to dilution. Increased free protease activity has also been documented during CPB and shown to be further stimulated by neutralization of heparin with protamine; it appears that these plasminogen and protease levels do not return to normal for 3 to 6 days.[85]

The mechanism by which the fibrinolytic system is activated by CPB and by other extracorporeal circuits is not totally understood. It does appear that the intrinsic system is stimulated initially (Fig. 9.8A).[16] As it turns out, heparin is not an ideal anticoagulant. It acts primarily at the end of the coagulation cascade and not at the beginning.[86] Despite clinically adequate doses of heparin, factor XII and the intrinsic fibrinolytic pathway are activated by contact with the extracorporeal circuit, which contains a large surface of thrombogenic material. Factor XIIa, in turn, is a strong stimulator for the formation of kallikrein and eventually the formation of free plasmin.[77] Tanaka et al[16] and others[15] have indeed documented the formation of fibrinopeptide fragments (FPA and FPB) and thrombin-antithrombin complexes[80,86] during CPB as evidence of continued thrombin activity. Once initiated, the ongoing cause of fibrinolysis appears to be extrinsic in nature, through release of tissue plasminogen activator by endothelial cells and urokinase plasminogen activator by monocytes, macrophages, and fibroblasts. As shown in Figure 9.8, C1-INA–resistant fibrinolytic activity, which is reflective of extrinsic fibrinolytic activity, increases and peaks during CPB.[16]

t-Pa is consequently released from the vascular endothelium. Extrinsic fibrinolysis is predominant for much of the duration and is, perhaps, the main source of the "hyperfibrinolysis" often observed during CPB.[81,87–89] The mechanism of t-Pa release is unknown but may be connected to "ever present levels of thrombin stimulation, humoral mechanisms, the function of protein C, or an action of heparin."[77] In effect, as with coagulation, the intrinsic and extrinsic pathways of fibrinolysis are most likely highly interrelated and interactive as to constitute a single pathway once initiated.

Hypothermia induced during cardiopulmonary bypass accentuates fibrinolysis. This appears to be a direct effect on enzymatic activity, but may also be due to cold-induced thromboplastin release from the vascular endothelium.[15,90]

Clinical Implications

The most important clinical consequence of ongoing fibrinolysis is hemorrhage, and in many cases the moderate fibrinolytic state manifested during CPB resolves spontaneously with inconsequential clinical impact. Fibrinolysis accompanying CPB may lead to a breakdown of clot after operation. In addition, some fibrin degradation products inhibit essential coagulant enzymes and intercalate between sheets of fibrin monomers to prevent cross-linking. Fibrin degradation products may also inhibit platelet function directly. Sustained fibrinolysis, therefore, effectively inhibits physiologic hemostasis. So long as plasminogen is activated only in the vicinity of fibrin formation, presumably in the extracorporeal circuit, "a systemic fibrinolytic state should not ensue." However, should the checks and balances noted above to ensure localized fibrinolysis be inundated by unrestrained plasmin generation, systemic manifestations may develop.[15] This possibility is thought to be less likely with current generations of oxygenators, the use of less thrombogenic bypass circuits, and careful monitoring of anticoagulation status during CPB. Nevertheless, even fibrin degradation products formed extracorporeally might be expected to mar hemostasis. Journois et al[84] have shown serum D-dimer levels to remain elevated long past the termination of CPB.

The presence (and levels) of fibrin degradation products alone does not correlate with a patient's likelihood to experience significant postoperative blood loss.[77,80] Certainly, with normal hepatic function, fibrin degradation products are rapidly cleared after the cessation of CPB. Nevertheless, the incidence of significant ongoing fibrinolysis post-CPB may be as high as 10% in patients having open-heart surgery.[83,91] The best evidence to date that fibrinolysis is an important cause of post-bypass bleeding, however, is the fact that antifibrinolytics such as aprotinin, and e-amino caproic acid (EACA) and its analogues reduce postoperative bleeding after CPB.[19,92]

In addition to the potential hemorrhagic complications, activation of the coagulation cascade and fibrinolytic system may also activate the complement cascades and the inflammatory response to CPB.

Effect of Cardiopulmonary Bypass on the Inflammation System

Blood coming into contact with the negatively charged artificial surfaces of the bypass machine facilitates a so-called whole body inflammatory response."[19] Complement pathways and leukocytes[18,93,94,95] are activated by factor XIIa, the enzyme derived from contact activation of factor XII. As noted before, coagulation and fibrinolytic and kallikrein cascades are similarly and simultaneously activated in this manner. Anaphylatoxins C3a and C5a are potent inflammatory mediators generated with complement activation via the alternative pathways (contact activation) within minutes of the onset of CPB (Fig. 9.9).[93] The classic pathway, in turn, is activated at blood-air interfaces and also by heparin-protamine complexes. This is recognized by the formation of C4. C3a is also formed with plasmin and

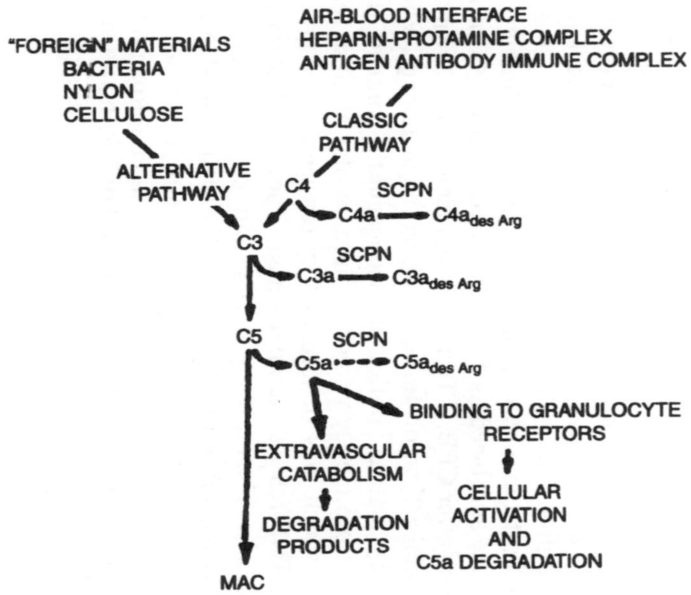

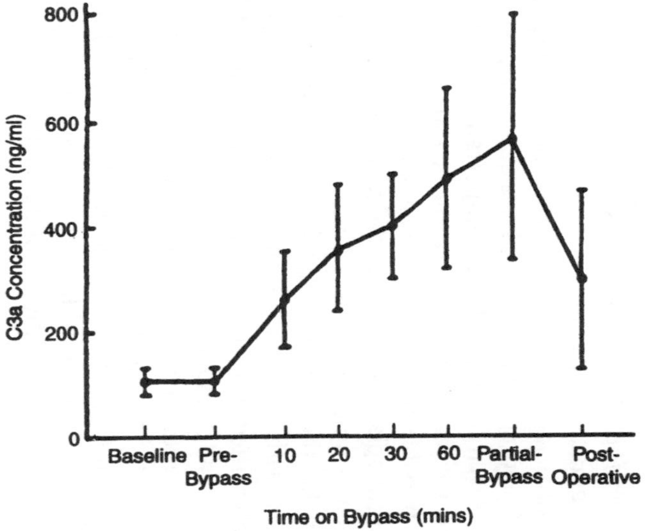

FIGURE 9.9. (A) Complement activation during cardiopulmonary bypass. (B) Plasma levels of C3a in patients undergoing cardiopulmonary bypass. (Reproduced with permission from Chenoweth et al.[93])

kallikrein activation but in less significant amounts. Note that the alternate and classic pathways converge to generate terminal cleavage products (C5b-9), which form a cell membrane attack complex capable of cell destruction.

In addition, Wachtfogel et al[96] have shown that purified plasma factor XIIa aggregates human neutrophils and causes exocytosis of elastase. Kallikrein may also induce leukocyte chemotaxis, aggregation, and degranulation.[18] Such neutrophil-derived elastases, glycoproteins (e.g., lactoferrin), and oxygen free radicals have important roles in inflammation and host immunologic responses. More recent investigations have focused, however, on the possible role of endotoxins and cytokines during CPB. Hypoperfusion of the splanchnic beds by the reduced peak arterial pressure associated with the nonpulsatile flow of the pump may cause release of plasma endotoxin by the intestinal mucosa.[97] Endotoxin levels do rise during CPB, peak with removal of the aortic clamp, and have been correlated with intensified oxygen free radical formation.[18,97] Monocytes, on the other hand, and presumably under the influence of complement activation and increased circulating endotoxins, may release cytokines including (but not limited to) tumor necrosis factor-α (TNF), interleukin-1β (IL-1), and interleukin-6 (IL-6).[97–99] The whole body inflammatory response to CPB is, therefore, considerably complex. It is not completely understood nor, in fact, is it completely deciphered.

Clinical Implications

It is generally believed that systemic inflammatory mediators contribute to the morbidity associated with CPB and other extracorporeal circuits.[18] Anaphylatoxins are vasoactive, resulting in vasoconstriction and increased vascular permeability. They also induce histamine release and modulate portions of the host immune response. Cardiac and pulmonary dysfunction, renal failure, and bleeding tendencies have, indeed, been related to C3a levels 3 hours after CPB.[94] Terminal complement cleavage may further augment neutrophil activation and cause direct tissue damage. With respect to the pulmonary system, Butler and colleagues[18] contend that tissue damage may be more closely related to intraalveolar elastase release, the defenses against which may be impaired by oxygen-derived free radicals. Endotoxin and TNF release are intertwined. These are known important mediators in sepsis. Their effects during and post-CPB are less clear. However, as Jansen et al[97] note, TNF is a mediator of general inflammation and induces fever, tachycardia, and hypotension, which are commonly observed post-CPB. In addition, it is possible that endotoxin release could lead to disseminated intravascular coagulation (DIC) with attendant thrombocytopenia, enhanced fibrinolysis, and significant nonsurgical bleeding as is prone to occur in severe sepsis.

References

1. Campbell F, Edmunds LH. Platelet function and cardiopulmonary bypass. In: Gravlee G, Davis R, Utley J, eds. *Cardiopulmonary Bypass, Principles and Practice.* Baltimore: Williams & Wilkins, 1993;407–435.
2. Spiess B, Chang SP. Intraoperative coagulation disorders. In: Thomas S, Kramer J, eds. *Manual of Cardiac Anesthesia.* 2nd ed. New York: Churchill Livingstone, 1993;517–552.
3. Ware J, Heistad D. Platelet-endothelium interactions. *N Engl J Med* 1993; 328(9):628–635.
4. Vane J, Anggard E, Botting R. Regulatory functions of the vascular endothelium. *N Engl J Med* 1990;323(1):27–36.
5. Body S. Platelet activation and interactions with the microvasculature. *J Cardiovasc Pharmacol* 1996;27(suppl 1):S13–S25.
6. Spiess B. The contribution of fibrinolysis to postbypass bleeding. *J Cardiothoracic Vasc Anesth* 1991;5(6)(suppl 1):13–17.
7. Campbell F, Addonizio V. *Platelet Function Alterations During Cardiac Surgery.* pp. 85–109.
8. Collier B. Platelets and thrombolytic therapy. *N Engl J Med* 1990;322(1):33–42.
9. Spiess B. Perioperative coagulation concerns: function, monitoring, and therapy. *Clin Anesthesia Updates* 1993;4(3):1–16.
10. Campbell F. The contribution of platelet dysfunction to postbypass bleeding. *J Cardiothorac Anesth* 1991;5(6)(suppl 1):8–12.
11. Handin R. Bleeding and thrombosis. In: Braunwald E, Isselbacker K, Petersdorf R, et al, eds. *Harrison's Principles of Internal Medicine.* 11th ed. New York: McGraw-Hill, 1987;266–272.
12. Furie B, Furie B. Molecular and cellular biology of blood coagulation. *N Engl J Med* 1992;326(12):800–806.
13. Horrow J. Management of coagulopathy associated with cardiopulmonary bypass. In: Gravlee G, Davis R, Utley J, eds. *Cardiopulmonary Bypass, Principles and Practice.* Baltimore: Williams & Wilkins, 1993;436–466.
14. Adnot S, Feffy J, Hanoune J, et al. Plasmin: a possible physiological modulator of the human platelet adenylate cyclase system. *Clin Sci* 1987;72:467–473.
15. Horrow J. Management of coagulation and bleeding disorders. In: Kaplan J, ed. *Cardiac Anesthesia.* 3rd ed. Philadelphia: WB Saunders, 1993;951–994.
16. Tanaka K, Motoshi T, Isao Y, et al. Alterations in coagulation and fibrinolysis associated with cardiopulmonary bypass during open heart surgery. *J Cardiothorac Anesth* 1989;3:181–188.
17. Tamaki T, Aoki N. Cross-linking of a_2-plasmin inhibitor catalyzed by activated fibrin stabilizing factor. *J Biol Chem* 1982;257:767–772.
18. Butler J, Rocker GM, Westaby S. Inflammatory response to cardiopulmonary bypass. *Ann Thorac Surg* 1993;55:552–559.
19. Gorman JH III, Edmunds LH Jr. Blood anethesia for cardiopulmonary bypass. *J Cardiovasc Surg* 1995;10:270–279.
20. Baier RE, Dutton RC. Initial events in interactions of blood with a foreign surface. *J Biomed Mater Res* 1969;3:191–206.
21. Uniyal S, Brash JL. Patterns of absorption of proteins from human plasma onto foreign surfaces. *Thromb Haemost* 1982;47:285–290.
22. Ziats MP, Pankowsky DA, Tierney BP, et al. Absorption of Hageman factor

(factor XII) and other human plasma proteins to biomedical polymers. *J Lab Clin Med* 1990;115:687–696.
23. Lindon JN, McManama G, Kushner L, et al. Does the conformation of absorbed fibrinogen dictate platelet interactions with artificial surfaces? *Blood* 1986;68:355–362.
24. Gorman J, Edmunds L. Blood anesthesia for cardiopulmonary bypass. *J Cardiovasc Surg* 1995;10:270–279.
25. Salempera M, Levy J, Harker L. Hemostasis and cardiopulmonary bypass. In: Mora C, ed. *Cardiopulmonary Bypass, Principles and Techniques of Extracorporeal Circulation.* New York: Springer-Verlag, 1995;88–113.
26. Dietrich W. Reducing thrombin formation during cardiopulmonary bypass: is there a benefit of the additional anticoagulant action of aprotinin. *J Cardiovasc Pharmacol* 1996;27(suppl 1):S50–S57.
27. Boisclair M, Lane D, et al. Mechanism of thrombin generation during surgery and cardiopulmonary bypass. *Blood* 1993;82(11):3350–3357.
28. Burman J, Chung H, et al. Role of factor XII in thrombin generation and fibrinolysis during cardiopulmonary bypass. *Lancet* 1994;344:1192–1193.
29. Tanaka K, Takao M, Yada I, et al. Alterations in coagulation and fibrinolysis associated with cardiopulmonary bypass during open heart surgery. *J Cardiothorac Anesth* 1989;3:181–188.
30. Young J, Kisker C, Doty D. Adequate anticoagulation during cardiopulmonary bypass determined by activated clotting time. *Ann Thorac Surg* 1978;26:231–240.
31. Tanaka K, Wada K, Morimoto T, Shomura S, et al. The role of the protein C-thrombomodulin system in the physiologic anticoagulation during cardiopulmonary bypass. *Trans Am Soc Artif Int Organs* 1979;35:373–375.
32. Journois D, Mauriat P, Pouard P, et al. Assessment of coagulation factor activation during cardiopulmonary bypass with a new monoclonal antibody. *J Cardiothorac Anesth* 1994;8(2):157–161.
33. Peirce EC II. The membrane versus bubble oxygenator controversy (editorial). *Ann Thorac Surg* 1980;29:497–499.
34. van den Dungen JJAM, Karliczek GF, Brenken U, et al. Clinical study of blood trauma during perfusion with membrane and bubble oxygenators. *J Thorac Cardiovasc Surg* 1982;83:108–116.
35. de Jong JC, Duis JH, Sibinga CT, et al. Hematologic aspects of cardiotomy suction in cardiac operations. *J Thorac Cardiovasc Surg* 1980;79:227–236.
36. Boonstra PW, van Imhoff GW, Eysman L, et al. Reduced platelet activation and improved hemostasis after controlled cardiotomy suction during clinical membrane oxygenator perfusions. *J Thorac Cardiovasc Surg* 1985;89:900–906.
37. van den Dungen JJ, Karliczek GF, Brenken U, et al. Clinical study of blood trauma during perfusion with membrane and bubble oxygenators. *J Thorac Cardiovasc Surg* 1982;83:108–116.
38. Ten Duis H, De Jong J, Van Asseldong A, et al. Improved hemocompatibility in open heart surgery. *Trans Am Soc Artif Intern Organs* 1978;24:656.
39. McKenna R, Bachmann F, Whittaker B, et al. The hemostatic mechanism after open heart surgery. *J Thorac Cardiovasc Surg* 1975;70(2):298–308.
40. Addonizio V, Macarak E, Nicolaou K, et al. Effects of prostacyclin and albumin on platelet loss during in vitro simulation of extracorporeal circulation. *Blood* 1979;53(6):1033–1042.
41. Addonizio V, Macarak E, Niewiarowski S, et al. Preservation of human

platelets with prostaglandin E1 during in vitro simulation of cardiopulmonary bypass. *Circ Res* 1979;44(3):350–357.
42. Addonizio V, Colman RW, Edmunds LH. The effect of blood flow rate and circuit surface area on platelet loss during extracorporeal circulation. *Trans Am Soc Artif Intern Organs* 1978;24:650–655.
43. Addonizio V, Strauss J, Colman R, Edmunds L. Effects of prostaglandin E1 on platelet loss during in vivo and in vitro extracorporeal circulation with a bubble oxygenator. *J Thorac Cardiovasc Surg* 1979;77(1):119–126.
44. Harker L, Malpass T, Branson H. Mechanisms of abnormal bleeding in patients undergoing cardiopulmonary bypass: acquired transient platelet dysfunction associated with selective alpha-granule release. *Blood* 1980;56(5):824–834.
45. Edmunds L, Ellison N, Colman R, et al. Platelet function during cardiac operation: comparison of membrane and bubble oxygenators. *J Thorac Cardiovasc Surg* 1982;83:805–812.
46. Zilla P, Fasol R, Groscurth P, et al. Blood platelets in cardiopulmonary bypass operations: recovery occurs after initial stimulation, rather than continual activation. *J Thorac Cardiovasc Surg* 1989;97:379–388.
47. Khuri S, Wolfe J, Josa M, et al. Hematologic changes during and after cardiopulmonary bypass and their relationship to the bleeding time and nonsurgical blood loss. *Thorac Cardiovasc Surg* 1992;1:94–107.
48. Greilich P, Carr M, Carr S, Chang A. Reductions in platelet force development by cardiopulmonary bypass are associated with hemorrhage. *Anesth Analg* 1995;80:459–465.
49. Tabuchi N, deHaan J, van Oeveren W. Rapid recovery of platelet function after cardiopulmonary bypass. *Blood* 1993;82:2930–2931.
50. Tabuchi N, Tigchelaar I, van Oeveren W. Shear-induced pathway of platelet function in cardiac surgery. *Semin Thromb Hemost* 1995;2(suppl 2):66–70.
51. Wachtfogel Y, Musial J, Juenkin B, et al. Loss of platelet α2-adrenergic receptors during simulated extracorporeal circulation: prevention with prostaglandin E1. *J Lab Clin Med* 1985;105(5):601–607.
52. Rinder C, Bohnert J, Rinder M, et al. Platelet activation and aggregation during cardiopulmonary bypass. *Anesthesiology* 1991;75:388–393.
53. Mammen E, Koets M, Washington B, et al. Hemostasis changes during cardiopulmonary bypass surgery. *Semin Thromb Hemost* 1985;11(3):281–282.
54. Wenger R, Lukasiewicz H, Mikuta B, et al. Loss of platelet fibrinogen receptors during clinical cardiopulmonary bypass. *J Thorac Cardiovasc Surg* 1989; 97:235–239.
55. Kestin A, Valeri C, Khuri S, et al. The platelet function defect of cardiopulmonary bypass. *Blood* 1993;82(1):107–117.
56. Beurling-Harbury C, Galvan C. Acquired decrease in platelet secretory ADP associated with increased postoperative bleeding in post-cardiopulmonary bypass patients and in patients with severe valvular heart disease. *Blood* 1978;52(1);13–22.
57. Addonizio V, Strauss J, Macarak E, et al. Preservation of platelet number and function with prostaglandin E1 during total cardiopulmonary bypass in rhesus monkeys. *Surgery* 1978;83:619–625.
58. Nieuwenhuis H, van Oosterhout J, Rozemuller E, et al. Studies with a monoclonal antibody against activated platelets: evidence that a secreted 53000-molecular weight lysosome-like granule protein is exposed on the surface of activated platelets in the circulation. *Blood* 1987;70:838–845.

59. George J, Pickett E, Saucerman S, et al. Platelet surface glycoproteins. Studies on resting and activated platelets and platelet membrane microparticles in normal subjects, and observations in patients during adult respiratory distress syndrome and cardiac surgery. *J Clin Invest* 1986;78:340–348.
60. Abrams C, Ellison N, Budzynski A, Shattil S. Direct detection of activated platelets and platelet-derived microparticles in humans. *Blood* 1990; 75(1):128–138.
61. Dechavanne M, French M, Pages J, et al. Significant reduction in the binding of a monoclonal antibody (LYP 18) directed against the IIb/IIIa glycoprotein complex to platelets of patients having undergone extracorporeal circulation. *Thromb Haemost* 1987;57(1):106–109.
62. Musial J, Niewiarowski S, Hershock D, et al. Loss of fibrinogen receptors from the platelet surface during simulated extracorporeal circulation. *J Lab Clin Med* 1985;105:514–522.
63. Rinder C, Mathew J, Rinder H, et al. Modulation of platelet surface adhesion receptors during cardiopulmonary bypass. *Anesthesiology* 1991;75:563–570.
64. Metzelaar M, Korteweg J, Sixma J, et al. Comparison of platelet membrane markers for the detection of platelet activation in vitro and during platelet storage and cardiopulmonary bypass surgery. *J Lab Clin Med* 1993;121(4):579–587.
65. Valeri RC, Khabbaz K, Khuri SF, et al. Effect of skin temperature on platelet function in patients undergoing extracorporeal bypass. *J Thorac Cardiovasc Surg* 1992;104:108–116.
66. Khuri SF, Wolfe JA, Josa M, et al. Hematologic changes during and after cardiopulmonary bypass and their relationship to the bleeding time and nonsurgical blood loss. *J Thorac Cardiovasc Surg* 1992;104:94–107.
67. Feingold HM, Pivacek LE, Melaragno AJ, et al. Coagulation assays and platelet aggregation patterns in human, baboon and dog blood. *Am J Vet Res* 1986;47:2197–2199.
68. Villalobos TJ, Aderson E, Barila TG. Hematologic changes in hypothermic dogs. *Proc Soc Exp Biol Med* 1985;89:192–198.
69. Schafer A, Adelman B. Plasmin inhibition of platelet function and of arachidonic acid metabolism. *J Clin Invest* 1985;75:456–461.
70. Stricker R, Wong D, Shiu D, et al. Activation of plasminogen by tissue plasminogen activator on normal and thrombasthenic platelets: effects on surface proteins and platelet aggregation. *Blood* 1986;68(1):275–280.
71. Schafer A, Zavoico G, et al. Synergistic inhibition of platelet activation by plasmin and prostaglandin I_2. *Blood* 1987;69(5):1504–1507.
72. Adelman B, Michelson A, Loscalzo J, et al. Plasmin effect on platelet glycoprotein Ib-von Willebrand factor interactions. *Blood* 1985;65(1):32–40.
73. de Haan J, Shonberger J, Haan J, et al. Tissue-type plasminogen activator and fibrin monomers synergistically cause platelet dysfunction during retransfusion of shed blood after cardiopulmonary bypass. *J Thorac Cardiovasc Surg* 1993;106(6):1017–1023.
74. Reed RL II, Bracey AW, Hudson JD, et al. Hypothermia and blood coagulation: dissociation between enzyme activity and clotting factor levels. *Circ Shock* 1990;32:141–152.
75. Staab DB, Sorenson VJ, Fath JJ, et al. Coagulation defects resulting from ambient temperature-induced hypothermia. *J Trauma* 1994;36:634–638.
76. Cornillon B, Mazzorana M, Durea G, et al. Characterization of a heparin-like

activity released in dogs during deep hypothermia. *Eur J Clin Invest* 1988; 18:460–464.

77. Spiess BD. The contribution of fibrinolysis to postbypass bleeding. *J Cardiothorac Vasc Anesth* 1991;5(suppl):13–17.
78. Andersen MN, Mendelow M. Fibrinolysis during and after extracorporeal circulation. *Surgery* 1963;84:649–657.
79. Giuliani R, Swarcer E, Martinez-A E, et al. Fibrin-dependent fibrinolytic activity during extracorporeal circulation. *Thromb Res* 1991;61:369–373.
80. Marengo-Rowe AJ, Levenson JE. Fibrinolysis: a frequent cause of bleeding. In: Ellison N, Jobes DR, eds. *Effective Hemostasis in Cardiac Surgery.* Philadelphia: WB Saunders, 1988;41–55.
81. Baños G, de la Peña A, Izaguirre R. The vascular plasminogen activator as source of the fibrinolytic potential observed during cardiopulmonary bypass. *Thromb Res* 1992;67:579–588.
82. Mammen E, Kocts MH, Washington B, et al. Hemostasis changes during cardiopulmonary bypass surgery. *Semin Thromb Hemost* 1985;11:281–292.
83. Bick R. Hemostasis defects associated with cardiac surgery, prosthetic devices and other extracorporeal circuits. *Semin Thromb Hemost* 1985;11:249–280.
84. Journois D, Mauriat P, Pouard P, et al. Assessment of coagulation factor activation during cardiopulmonary bypass with a new monoclonal antibody. *J Cardiothorac Vasc Anesth* 1994;8:157–161.
85. Holloway SD, Summaria L, Sandessara J, et al. Decreased platelet number and function and increased fibrinolysis contribute to postoperative bleeding in cardiopulmonary bypass patients. *Thromb Hemost* 1988;59:62–67.
86. Brister SJ, Ofosu FA, Buchanan MR. Thrombin generation during cardiac surgery: Is heparin the ideal coagulant? *Thromb Haemost* 1993;70:259–262.
87. Teufelsbauer H, Proidi S, Havel M, et al. Early activation of hemostasis during cardiopulmonary bypass: evidence for thrombin mediated hyperfibrinolysis. *Thromb Haemost* 1992;68:250–252.
88. Kucuk O, Kwaan HC, Frederickson J, et al. Increased fibrinolytic activity in patients undergoing cardiopulmonary bypass operation. *Am J Hematol* 1986; 23:223–229.
89. Paramo JA, Rifon J, Llorens R, et al. Intra- and postoperative fibrinolysis in patients undergoing cardiopulmonary bypass surgery. *Haemostasis* 1991; 21:58–65.
90. Yoshihara H, Yamamoto T, Mihara H. Changes in coagulation and fibrinolysis occurring in dogs during hypothermia. *Thromb Res* 1985;37:503–512.
91. Spiess BD, Tuman KJ, McCarthy RJ, et al. Thrombelastographic diagnosis of coagulopathies in patients undergoing cardiopulmonary bypass. *Anesth Analg* 1989;68:S273.
92. Blauhut B, Klima U, Bettelheim P, et al. Comparison of the effects of aprotinin and tranexamic acid on blood loss and related variables following cardiopulmonary bypass. *J Thorac Cardiovasc Surg* 1994;108:1083–1091.
93. Chenoweth DE, Cooper SW, Hugli TE, et al. Complement activation during cardiopulmonary bypass: evidence for generation of C3a and C5a anaphylatoxins. *N Engl J Med* 1981;304:497–503.
94. Kirklin JK, Westaby S, Blackstone EH. Complement and the damaging effects of cardiopulmonary bypass. *J Thorac Cardiovasc Surg* 1983;86:845–857.
95. Chenoweth DE. Complement activation during cardiopulmonary bypass. In:

Utley J, ed. *Pathophysiology of Cardiopulmonary Bypass*. Baltimore: Williams & Wilkins, 1983;49–60.
96. Wachtfogel YT, Pixley RA, Kucich U, et al. Purified plasma factor XIIa aggregates human neutrophils and causes degranulation. *Blood* 1986; 67:1731–1737.
97. Jansen NJG, van Oeveren W, Gu YJ, et al. Endotoxin release and tumor necrosis factor formation during cardiopulmonary bypass. *Ann Thorac Surg* 1992;54:744–748.
98. Haeffner-Cavaillon N, Roussellier N, Ponzio O, et al. Induction of interleukin-1 production in patients undergoing cardiopulmonary bypass. *J Thorac Cardiovasc Surg* 1989;98:1100–1106.
99. Cruickshank A, Fraser WD, Burns HJG, et al. Response of serum interleukin-6 in patients undergoing elective surgery of varying severity. *Clin Sci* 1990; 79:161–165.

10
Monitoring of Coagulation: Management of Heparin and Protamine

STEPHEN J. LAHEY

Conventional cardiac surgery performed in medical centers throughout the world would be impossible without the use of cardiopulmonary bypass. This technology diverts a patient's circulating blood volume as it enters the right atrium and effectively supplants the functions of both the heart and lungs. During this process, blood is exposed to thrombogenic surfaces in the oxygenator and pump tubing before returning to the patient. A safe and reliable method of anticoagulation followed by reversal of anticoagulation is, therefore, crucial to the performance of cardiopulmonary bypass and the completion of complex cardiac surgical procedures. Presently, the most effective means of providing temporary anticoagulation is with heparin.

Heparin, a glycosaminoglycan derived from mast cells throughout the body, was originally isolated from the liver in 1916. Today most heparin is commercially extracted from bovine lung or porcine intestinal mucosa. In 1938 Chargaff and Olsen[1] isolated the polypeptide protamine, which was found to effectively block heparin and reverse anticoagulation. The following year, Gibbon[2] reported heparin anticoagulation and cardiopulmonary bypass in animal models. However, it was not until 1953 that Gibbon[3] first used heparin anticoagulation clinically with cardiopulmonary bypass and heparin reversal with protamine to repair an atrial septal defect in a young woman.

Pharmacology

Although much is known of the pharmacokinetics of heparin when used as an anticoagulant, surprisingly little is known of the role of heparin as it occurs in nature. Its role as an in vivo anticoagulant is, in all likelihood, quite minor compared with that of hepar*an*, a related glycosaminoglycan expressed on endothelial cell surfaces. It is the activation of antithrombin III (AT III) by endothelial heparan rather than by heparin that maintains normal physiologic anticoagulation.[4]

Clinical anticoagulation is accomplished when commercially prepared, exogenously administered heparin binds to circulating AT III. The resulting stoichiometric change in the AT III molecule dramatically enhances its ability to bind and inactivate thrombin. As this happens, there is less and less thrombin available to convert fibrinogen to fibrin. In addition, factor VIII of the intrinsic pathway and factor V of the common coagulation pathway are activated by thrombin. Fibrin clot formation is retarded as circulating thrombin levels are progressively depleted by the activated heparin–AT III complex. Several other cofactors of the clotting cascade are directly inhibited by AT III. Again, this inhibition is greatly enhanced by the AT III–heparin complex.[5] Several indirect effects of heparin also promote or enhance anticoagulation. Platelet functions, such as aggregation and adhesiveness, are thought to be adversely affected by heparin.

The clearance of heparin–AT III complexes, as well as that of the thrombin-heparin–AT III complexes, most likely occurs in the reticuloendothelial system and follows standard first-order kinetics. However, the conventionally measured half-life of heparin is dose related, with longer (and different) half-life degradation curves seen with higher doses.[6] In general, the half-life of an intravenous 100-U/kg bolus is approximately 1 hour.

Monitoring Heparin Therapy During Cardiopulmonary Bypass

Direct Heparin Concentration Assays

Several methods for directly measuring heparin concentrations are currently available. These techniques are conceptually appealing because they necessarily avoid the many variabilities noted in measuring the anticoagulant effect of heparin during cardiopulmonary bypass. Nevertheless, disadvantages also exist. Most of the commercially available assays of heparin concentration require plasma samples making routine intraoperative use cumbersome. A protamine titration assay can be used with whole blood samples. By careful successive dilution, a measurement of the approximate protamine concentration needed to neutralize all of the heparin in a given sample can be made. If the precise ratio of protamine to heparin needed to allow clot formation is known, the heparin concentration can be accurately derived.

Additionally, several commercially available assays of direct heparin concentration utilizing colorimetry are used but, as with fluorogenic assays, patient-to-patient accuracy is inconsistent. Further research, emphasizing intraoperative reproducibility of data, is warranted.

Indirect Heparin Assays

Several laboratory tests—the thrombin time (TT) and activated partial thromboplastin time (aPTT), and the activated clotting time (ACT)—are commonly used in clinical medicine to indirectly measure plasma heparin concentration. The time required for a given blood or plasma sample to clot can be prolonged by increasing concentrations of added heparin. However, heparin exerts its inhibitory effect at multiple locations in the intrinsic, extrinsic, and common pathways of the clotting cascade. Several important coagulation factors including thrombin, factor VIII, factor V, and factor IX are serine proteases (active enzymatic site contains a serine residue). The biologic activity of AT III is as a serine protease inhibitor. When complexed with heparin, AT III becomes a far more potent inhibitor, thereby inhibiting multiple coagulation factors. This inhibition is most potent against thrombin. As a result, most of these assays are exquisitely sensitive at heparin concentrations well below that used clinically for cardiopulmonary bypass. This, therefore, limits their usefulness as assays for heparin dosing during cardiac surgery.

The thrombin time (TT), for example, measures the conversion of fibrinogen to fibrin, one of the final steps in clot formation. This enzymatic reaction is mediated by thrombin, which, in turn, is naturally inhibited by its interaction with AT III. Even the smallest concentrations of heparin greatly enhances this inhibitory effect of AT III on thrombin. The delay in conversion of fibrogen to fibrin is an indirect measure of the exogenously administered heparin concentration. However, even the smallest concentrations of heparin enhance inactivation of thrombin by AT III. As a result, the TT is prolonged by minimal doses of heparin and cannot be used to guide heparin administration during cardiac surgery. Although less sensitive to heparin than TT, aPPT has limited use during cardiopulmonary bypass surgery because of heparin's broad effect on the clotting cascade and because the dose required to produce safe anticoagulation prolongs the aPTT indefinitely.

The critical importance of obtaining frequent, reliable, and reproducible measures of heparin anticoagulation during cardiopulmonary bypass is obvious. In 1975 Bull et al[7] attempted to establish a heparin dose-response curve during extracorporeal circulation utilizing an efficient, automated method of measuring the activated whole blood clotting time (ACT). With this method, which is almost universally used in clinical cardiac surgery today, levels of anticoagulation can be monitored quickly and easily. A timer begins when 2 ml of whole blood are placed in specialized test tubes containing diatomaceous earth (celite), which activates clotting. A small magnetic flange is located in the bottom of the test tubes, which are then placed in a heated measuring unit (e.g., the International Technidyne Hemochron ACT). The magnetic flange begins to move, matching the one revolution per minute of the sample test tube while in the measuring unit. This begins as fibrin formation occurs. As the flange moves from the "6 o'clock" to the "9 o'clock" position a small microswitch is tripped, stopping the timer.

Bull and his colleagues felt that a target ACT, i.e., the time required before noticeable clot develops in the celite-activated whole blood sample, should be between 400 and 600 seconds with a theoretical ideal of 480 seconds.[8] An ACT level in this range would ensure safe anticoagulation during cardiopulmonary bypass. The so-called Bull curve (Fig. 10.1) is constructed with ACT (in seconds) on the x-axis versus. heparin dose (mg/kg) on the y-axis. A preoperative ACT (point A) is determined on celite-activated whole blood samples from each patient. Patients are then treated with heparin (2 mg/kg). Five minutes after the heparin dose is administered, a second ACT (point B) is determined. The resulting line plotted between points A and B allows for the extrapolation to point C,

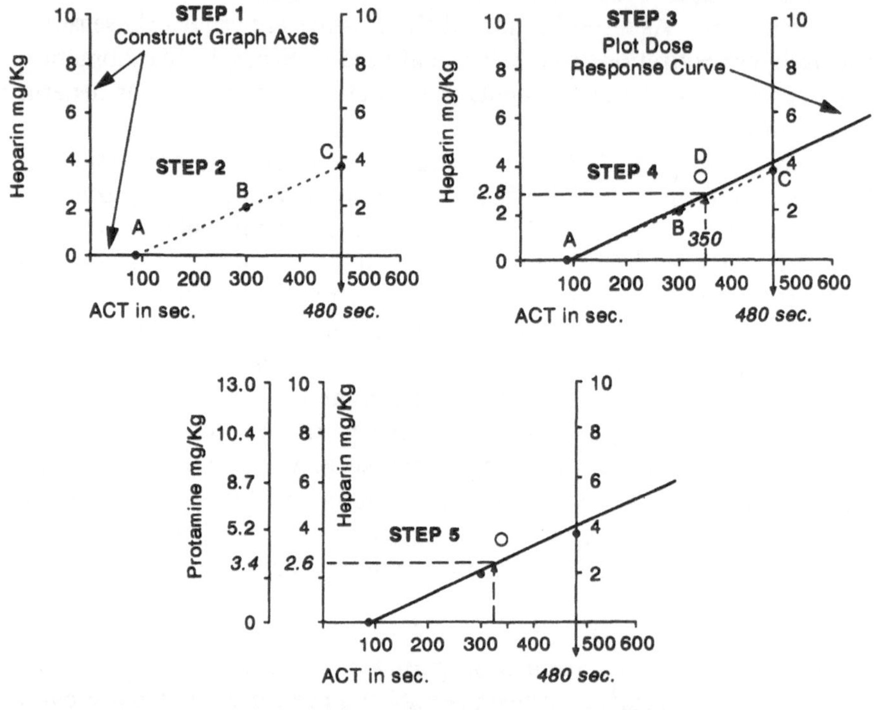

FIGURE 10.1. The Bull curve. Step 1: Construct graph with "ACT in seconds" on the x-axis and "Heparin mg/kg" on the y-axis. Determine initial ACT (point A). Step 2: Determine initial ACT (A) and administer 2 mg/kg heparin, then measure ACT (B) and plot both values. Extrapolate an imaginary line through A and B to intersect with 480-second line to find point C. Example: 3.5 mg/kg heparin is needed to produce 480-second ACT or 1.5 mg/kg in addition to the 2 mg/kg heparin already given. Step 3: After required heparin has been given, measure ACT. Plot point D. If point D does not superimpose on point C then a dose-response curve is drawn from A to a point midway between C and D. Step 4: After 60 minutes, measure the ACT. Determine amount of heparin in patient's circulation from the dose response curve. Example: Assume an ACT of 350 seconds. The heparin level would be 2.8 mg/kg. To return to 480 seconds, 1.2 mg/kg of heparin is needed. Step 5: To reverse anticoagulation, circulating heparin level is determined as in step 4. The neutralizing dose of protamine is heparin level (mg/kg) × 1.3. Example: ACT of 325 seconds is measured. Heparin level is 2.6 mg/kg, and 3.4 mg/kg protamine is required. (From Bull SW with permission[8]).

which predicts the amount of additional heparin needed to prolong the ACT to a safe level for cardiopulmonary bypass. Additional samples are drawn on an hourly basis during the surgery to maintain safe anticoagulation. Additionally, Bull et al assumed that the same linear relationship could be exploited when determining the appropriate protamine dose for complete reversal of heparin at the conclusion of cardiopulmonary bypass, since the authors noted that 1.3 mg of protamine will effectively neutralize 1 mg of heparin.

While this report by Bull and his colleagues was truly a landmark study and is almost universally used in cardiac surgery today, it should be remembered that many factors (hypothermia, platelet inhibition and destruction, hemodilution, and the administration of aprotinin) have varying effects on the ACT. These factors influence the assumed linear relationship between heparin dose and the measured ACT. However, if sufficiently high ACT levels are maintained throughout cardiopulmonary bypass, the Bull algorithm can provide a safe method of predicting adequate anticoagulation.

It was the opinion of Bull and his associates that safe anticoagulation during cardiopulmonary bypass could be ensured when frequent heparin dose supplementation was used to maintain the ACT at a theoretically ideal level of 480 seconds. The authors also suggested that ACT levels at or below 300 seconds would be associated with catastrophic clotting in the extracorporeal membrane and circuit. Conversely, it was felt that increased bleeding would be seen with ACT levels in excess of 600 seconds. Since that time, the scientific literature has been flooded with studies recommending higher or sometimes lower minimum ACT levels for the safe conduct of cardiopulmonary bypass. These reports have heightened the confusion over this issue. Unfortunately, many studies have been based on historical controls and others have studied limited numbers of patients, compromising their statistical accuracy. Additional confusion has been created by the failure of some studies to establish a clear distinction between intraoperative and postoperative bleeding and by the lack of uniform criteria used to initiate transfusion therapy. Even the methods used to document the failure of anticoagulation in published studies has varied enormously (e.g., no visible clot seen on the membrane oxygenator vs. exquisitely sensitive bioassays of plasma fibrinopeptide A).

Currently, at our institution, we recommend an initial dose of 3 mg/kg. If the patient has been on intravenous heparin for longer than 24 hours prior to surgery, indicating the development of possible heparin resistance, the heparin dose is increased to 5 mg/kg. *The ACT is monitored every 30 minutes to ensure ACT levels in excess of 480 seconds during cardiopulmonary bypass.*

Heparin Resistance

The requirement for unusually large (3 mg/kg) doses of heparin to push the ACT into safe levels for cardiopulmonary bypass is, by definition, heparin resistance. The occurrence of heparin resistance is rare, but it will be increased if the clinician establishes a "minimum safe ACT" that is inappropriately high. Nevertheless, several clinical situations exist that promote a heparin resistance state. Septic shock or severe thrombocytosis, for example, alter the anticoagulation response curve to heparin.

Acquired Antithrombin III Deficiency

The most common etiology of heparin resistance, is prolonged heparin therapy in the preoperative period. During heparin administration, AT III complexes with the heparin molecule and is cleared by the reticuloendothelial system. This depletes the patient's stores of AT III. AT III, as mentioned above, complexes with heparin, increasing heparin anticoagulation properties. Not surprisingly, patients with impaired hepatic synthesis, who may have deficient levels of AT III, are also more prone to develop acquired AT III resistance while receiving preoperative heparin. The diagnosis of acquired AT III deficiency is most often made in the operating room when an ACT $\geq$ 300 seconds is not achieved despite heparin doses in excess of 600 U/kg. Additional doses of heparin can be administered, but if the ACT remains below 300, exogenous AT III provided by fresh frozen plasma should be given. The clinician in these situations must weigh the risk of hepatitis exposure associated with the administration of fresh frozen plasma against the risk of a low ACT during cardiopulmonary bypass. Currently, clinical experience with purified preparations of AT III concentrate is limited.[9] Less common etiologies of acquired AT III deficiency are seen in Table 10.1.

Table 10.1. Etiologies of acquired antithrombin III deficiency.

Decreased synthesis from liver cirrhosis
Drug induced
L-asparaginase
Estrogens
Heparin
Increased excretion
Protein-losing enteropathy
Inflammatory bowel disease
Nephrotic syndrome
Accelerated consumption
Disseminated intravascular coagulation
Surgery
Dilutional
Cardiopulmonary bypass
Autologous blood withdrawal

From Gravlee.[4]

Congenital Antithrombin III Deficiency

Premature infants and some neonates are found to have lower than expected levels of circulating AT III. This accounts for the occasional need to use higher than normal doses of heparin during cardiopulmonary bypass in this patient population. This relative deficiency improves as hepatic function in the neonate matures. A distinct autosomal dominant disease is rarely seen in adults, which is associated with decreased production of AT III. Varying phenotypic expression of the disease is seen. However, some of these patients will present with spontaneous pathologic coagulation problems such as pulmonary embolus and arterial thrombosis. Treatment of AT III deficiency status will depend on the relative degree of AT III deficiency. Most patients will only require additional heparin to achieve adequate anticoagulation for cardiopulmonary bypass. Some, however, will require routine administration of exogenous AT III.

Complications of Heparin Therapy and Heparin Rebound

Heparin's effect on hemostasis and coagulation is profound, and the most common adverse outcome associated with heparin is excessive bleeding. In addition to heparin effects on plasma coagulation, heparin releases tissue plasminogen activator, which stimulates fibrinolysis. Heparin is known to bind to platelets directly decreasing their effect in clot formation and further exacerbating the bleeding diathesis. Other rare adverse reactions associated with heparin administration include hypotension secondary to a precipitous decrease in systemic vascular resistance, anaphylactoid reactions, and disseminated intravascular coagulation.

Although a multiplicity of factors contribute to the incidence of this complication, bleeding following cardiopulmonary bypass is a source of significant postoperative morbidity. In addition to the deleterious effects of hypothermia and hemodilution, excessive bleeding can occur when insufficient doses of protamine are administered to reverse the anticoagulation effects of heparin. This may also be associated with the "heparin rebound" phenomenon. This phenomenon has been explained by the sudden loss of the procoagulant effect of administered protamine because the half-life of heparin is substantially longer than that of protamine, allowing for a reactivation of heparin's anticoagulant effect. This explanation has been challenged recently because, based on traditional theory, heparin rebound should occur in every cardiac surgical case using cardiopulmonary bypass. A more plausible explanation offered by Soloway and Christiansen[9] states that patients with depressed levels of AT III (secondary to prolonged preoperative heparin therapy) are hemodiluted, further lowering AT III levels, and massively heparinized to achieve a safe ACT level for cardiopulmonary bypass. However, clinical anticoagulation is not achieved by heparin per se, but rather by the heparin–AT III complex. The larger doses of heparin used to achieve the minimum safe ACT result in huge amounts of free unbound heparin that remains in the circulation. If, after the patient returns to the intensive care unit, he or she is given an infusion of fresh frozen plasma (FFP), this infusion provides an exogenous source of free AT III that can now complex with the free unbound heparin, causing reanticoagulation. Note that, according to this explanation, heparin rebound would not be observed if FFP were not transfused.

Heparin-Induced Thrombocytopenia

In rare instances, the use of heparin can be associated with the production of heparin-specific antibodies that affect the pathologic aggregation of platelets.[10] This process can result in clinical thrombocytopenia (platelet count $<100{,}000\ mm^3$) in the absence of disseminated intravascular coagulation or sepsis as well as sporadic arterial and venous thrombosis in multiple end organs. The true incidence of heparin-induced thrombocytopenia (HIT) is unknown. Cardiac surgeons, however, can expect to see this life-threatening syndrome more frequently with the widespread use of heparin in patients undergoing percutaneous transluminal coronary angioplasty (PTCA)/atherectomy prior to coronary bypass surgery or in patients treated with intravenous heparin to control unstable angina.

HIT syndrome presents in two distinct forms. Type I occurs soon after exposure to heparin (within 5 days) and rarely causes clinically evident thrombosis. Type II has its onset anywhere from 5 to 22 days after the initial heparin exposure and is associated with a more profound thrombocytopenia and may include intravascular thrombosis (arterial and venous). Widespread end-organ damage may result in clinical evidence of a cardiovascular accident (CVA), myocardial infarction, pulmonary embolus, gastrointestinal tract bleeding and infarction, renal failure, and multiple areas of skin necrosis. These patients usually do not exhibit the fever, microangiopathic hemolytic anemia, and renal and neurologic dysfunction that are pathognomonic of thrombotic thrombocytopenic purpura (TTP). Similarly, disseminated intravascular coagulation must be ruled out by the usual screening tests.

It should be noted that the occurrence of the syndrome does not seem to be dose related. HIT has been reported with the use of only subcutaneous heparin.[11] Similarly, the syndrome was recently reported in 12 patients whose only exposure to heparin was heparin-coated pulmonary catheters.[12]

The diagnosis of HIT is usually made by clinical presentation since laboratory testing is inconsistent and lacks sufficient sensitivity. It should be suspected any time unexplained arterial or venous obstruction occurs in the postoperative setting. A precipitous and unexplained decline in platelet count in excess of 30% is an early warning sign and should prompt immediate cessation of all heparin exposure. If this has occurred prior to planned cardiac surgery, the clinician may be forced to consider alternative (and less well documented) methods of anticoagulation while on cardiopulmonary bypass.

Protamine

Protamine, a strongly cationic protein derived from salmon sperm, has been used for over 30 years to neutralize the highly negatively charged heparin and reverse its anticoagulant effect. Once bound to protamine, heparin can no longer complex with AT III, preventing coagulation. Thrombin function returns and the clotting cascade returns to normal. However, accurate reversal of anticoagulation following cardiopulmonary bypass is difficult for several reasons including the lack of homogeneous purity in commercial preparations of heparin, patient-to-patient differences in the rate of heparin metabolism, and varying clinical effectiveness of different protamine preparations. Confounding this issue is the direct effect of protamine on platelet function, which may result in poor clot formation. Several authors, including Ellison et al,[13] have demonstrated decreased platelet aggregation in response to adenosine diphosphate (ADP) and collagen when exposed to the heparin-protamine complex.

Protocols for protamine administration vary based on the method of measuring heparin dosage. The most commonly used strategy for heparin reversal is that proposed by Bull et al[7] (Fig. 10.1). Based on a final ACT, measured at the conclusion of cardiopulmonary bypass, the amount of heparin needed to be neutralized can be extrapolated from the dose-response curve. Likewise, the protamine dose can be extrapolated, since the authors contend that a constant dose relationship exists between heparin and protamine: 1 mg of protamine neutralizes approximately 1 mg of heparin. In clinical practice, the *authors suggest that 1.3 mg of protamine be used for every 1 mg of heparin* to minimize lot-to-lot variability of the protamine and to provide excess protamine when anticipating heparin rebound. This technique of protamine administration is routinely used at the Deaconess Hospital in Boston, Massachusetts.

Adverse Effects of Protamine

The administration of protamine at the conclusion of cardiopulmonary bypass may be associated with a variety of protamine reactions. The precise nature of these reactions, as well as the different degrees of severity observed, is poorly described and poorly understood.

The most feared protamine reaction is a rare but catastrophic event that can occur after minimal exposure to protamine. Profound arterial hypotension occurs secondary to intense pulmonary vascular constriction, severe bronchospasm, pulmonary artery hypertension, and right ventricular failure.

The reaction is reported to be the expression of two differing immunologic etiologies. Both are associated with the activation of complement (as measured by elevated C3a and C5a levels) and the resultant outpouring of thromboxane B_2, a potent vasoconstrictor. The release of thromboxane appears to be concentrated in the pulmonary vasculature, thus initiating this dreaded reaction.

A true anaphylactic reaction to protamine is even more rare and is an immunoglobulin E (IgE)-mediated event that occurs in the absence of heparin. The IgE antibody is directed against protamine itself and therefore requires prior exposure to protamine in some form. It has been observed that many of the patients who have had documented IgE-mediated (i.e., true anaphylactic) protamine reactions have been diabetics whose prior exposure to protamine was in the form of neutral protamine Hagedorn (NPH) or protamine-zinc insulin. Other patients thought to be at risk for having preformed antiprotamine IgE antibodies are those patients with documented fish allergies. Since commercial preparations of protamine are extracted from salmon sperm, these patients may be at risk of having preformed "anti-fish" antibodies that would cross-react with exogenously administered protamine. Whether male patients who have had vasectomies are at risk of having antisperm antibodies that would cross-react with salmon sperm–derived protamine is unknown.

A similar clinical presentation of pulmonary vascular vasoconstriction and profound loss of systemic vascular resistance can be seen in an IgG-associated reaction to the intact protamine-heparin complex. This reaction represents the so-called anaphylactoid reactions since it does not represent a classic immunologic response. Unlike the IgE-mediated reaction, the IgG-mediated reaction requires the participation of not only protamine but heparin as well. The presence of a circulating antiprotamine IgG antibody, specifically directed against the protamine of the intact protamine-heparin complex, suggests prior exposure to protamine. Since this form of the reaction is not exclusive to diabetics, the exposure presumably occurred in the cardiac catheterization laboratory or at some point in the past. The extent to which antigen-IgG immune complexes activate complement, kinins, and other vasoactive substances will dictate the severity of the reaction.

A very rare reaction to protamine may present as a massive pulmonary alveolar capillary leak occurring more than 1 hour after the uneventful administration of protamine. Depending on the severity of the reaction, profound hypoxia due to massive shunting and critical decreases in lung compliance can be seen.

The most commonly observed adverse reaction to protamine is a systemic

TABLE 10.2. Classification of adverse protamine reactions.

Type I:	Hypotension due to rapid administration
Type II:	Anaphylactoid responses
	A: Antibody-mediated anaphylaxis
	B: Immediate anaphylactoid responses without antibody involvement
	C: Delayed anaphylactoid response (noncardiac pulmonary edema)
Type III:	Catastrophic pulmonary vasoconstriction

From Horrow.[15]

hypotension that appears to be related to the speed with which the protamine is injected.[14] This usually mild reaction is thought to be secondary to the sudden degranulation of peripheral mast cells, causing a pathologic systemic histamine release. The sudden rise in pulmonary venous thromboxane levels, as well as activation of complement as measured by elevated C5a levels, is not seen with this milder reaction. The abrupt but non–life-threatening hypotension can be modified by pretreating patients with H1 and H2 receptor blockers. Such pretreatment, however, will have little, if any, effect on either the IgE-mediated anaphylactic reaction, or the IgG-associated anaphylactoid reaction. Whether the histamine release is less profound when protamine is injected into the left atrium is unclear and still debated in the literature.

In an attempt to consolidate and categorize the different clinical presentations of adverse protamine reactions, Horrow[15] has offered the classification shown in Table 10.2.

Protamine Reactions: Treatment

Preoperative screening of all cardiac surgical patients for antibodies to protamine at the present time is impractical and expensive. However, any patient with a prior history of possible adverse reaction to protamine should warrant special care and attention. While the prophylactic administration of H1 and H2 receptor blockers may theoretically lessen hypotension caused by histamine release, the most efficient method of treatment of protamine reactions should be to stop the infusion of protamine. Systolic hypotension and mild elevations in pulmonary artery pressures usually return to normal quickly with minimum support. The protamine infusion can then be resumed but at a slower rate.

The severe pulmonary vasoconstrictive reaction is a dramatic and catastrophic situation with a plummeting arterial pressure and a rising pulmonary artery pressure. Treatment must be initiated promptly and decisively. A scenario of progressive interventions of increasing clinical import should be initiated beginning with cessation of the protamine infusion. $CaCl_2$ and epinephrine are administered to support systemic pressure while pulmonary vasodilators (e.g., nitroglycerin or isoproterenol) are used to lower pulmonary hypertension and ameliorate the acute right ventricular failure. Studies using the potent pulmonary vascular smooth muscle relaxant nitric oxide are promising but lack the statistical support of numerous clinical trials. Massive steroid infusion may be helpful.

The patient will not survive unless this acutely deteriorating cycle is interrupted. If pharmacologic interventions prove unsuccessful, the surgeon may be forced to reheparinize the patient and return to cardiopulmonary bypass. Whether patients improve because of total right and left heart support or because of the transient nature of most anaphylactic reaction is arguable. Interestingly, even after this intense anaphylactic-type reaction has occurred, protamine infusion has successfully been resumed at a very slow rate.

Protamine Alternatives

Great effort has been made to find a protamine substitute. In the early days of cardiopulmonary bypass, hexadimethrine bromide, or polybrene, was used successfully to reverse heparin. However, polybrene was associated with similar pulmonary vasoconstrictive reactions and significant nephrotoxicity.[16] Toluidine blue and methylene blue have also been investigated as possible alternatives to protamine in reversing the anticoagulation effect of heparin.

The most promising agent under investigation is platelet factor 4 (PF4). This substance, purified from the alpha granules of human platelets that are available in recombinant form, appears to be as effective as protamine in reversing heparin.[17] Increased release of naturally occurring PF4 may explain why patients with extreme thrombocytosis appear to be heparin resistant. Further clinical trials of the recombinant form of PF4 are eagerly awaited.

References

1. Chargaff E, Olsen KB. Studies on the chemistry of blood coagulation, VI. Studies of the action of heparin and other anticoagulants. The influence of protamine on the anticoagulant effect in vivo. *J Biol Chem* 1938;125:671–676.
2. Gibbon JH Jr. The maintenance of life during experimental occlusion of the pulmonary artery followed by survival. *Surg Gynecol Obstet* 1939;69:602–614.
3. Gibbon JH Jr. Application of a mechanical heart and lung apparatus to cardiac surgery. *Minn Med* 1954;37:171–185.
4. Gravlee GP. Anticoagulation for cardiopulmonary bypass. In: Gravlee GP, Davis RF, Utley JR, eds. *Cardiopulmonary Bypass Principles and Procedures.* Baltimore: Williams & Wilkins, 1993;340–380.
5. Bjork I, Olson ST, Shore JD. Molecular mechanisms of the accelerating effect of heparin on the reactions between antithrombin and clotting proteinases. In: Lane DA, Lindahl U, eds. *Heparin Chemical and Biological Properties, Clinical Applications.* Boca Raton, FL: CRC Press, 1989;229–255.

6. Tollefsen DM, Blinder MA. Heparin. In: Hoffman R, Benz EJ, Shattil SJ, Furie B, Cohen HJ, Silberstein LE, eds. *Hematology: Basic Principles and Practice*. 2nd ed. New York: Churchill 1995;1807.
7. Bull SW, Huse WM, Brauer FS, Korpman RA. Heparin therapy during extracorporeal circulation, II. The use of a dose response curve to individualize heparin and protamine dosage. *J Thorac Cardiovasc Surg* 1975;69:685–689.
8. Hoffman DL. Purification and large scale preparation of antithrombin III. *Am J Med* 1989;87(suppl 3B):23s–26s.
9. Soloway HB, Christiansen TW. Heparin anticoagulation during cardiopulmonary bypass in an antithrombin III deficient patient. Implications relative to the etiology of heparin rebound. *Am J Clin Path* 1980;73:723–725.
10. Phillips DE, Payne DK, Mills GM. Heparin induced thrombotic thrombocytopenia. *Ann Pharmacother* 1994;28:43–46.
11. Bell WR, Royall RM. Heparin-associated thrombocytopenia: a comparison of three heparin preparations. *N Engl J Med* 1980;303:902–907.
12. Laser JL, Nichols WK, Silver D. Thrombocytopenia associated with heparin-associated antiplatelet antibodies. *Arch Intern Med* 1989;149:2285–2287.
13. Ellison N, Edmunds LH, Coleman RW. Platelet aggregation following heparin and protamine administration. *Anesthesiology* 1978;48:65–68.
14. Stoelting RK, Henry DP, Verbur KM, et al. Haemodynamic changes and circulating histamine concentrations following protamine administration to patients and dogs. *Can Anesth Soc J* 1984;31:534–540.
15. Horrow JC. Protamine: A review of its toxicity. *J Anesth Analg* 1985; 64:348–361.
16. Haller JA, Ransdell HT, Stowens D, Rubel WF. Renal toxicity of polybrene in open-heart surgery. *J Thorac Cardiovasc Surg* 1962;44:486–491.
17. Zucker MS, Katz IR. Platelet factor 4: production, structure, and physiologic and immunologic action. *Proc Soc Exp Biol Med* 1991;198:693–702.

11 Intraoperative Autologous Blood Donation Practices

ROBERT E. HELM AND KARL H. KRIEGER

Three general strategies are available for the procurement of autologous blood prior to cardiopulmonary bypass: (1) *preoperative* autologous donation of whole blood, (2) *intraoperative* autologous donation of whole blood, and (3) intraoperative platelet plasmapheresis. The first of these, preoperative autologous donation (PAD), was reviewed in Chapter 3. There it was seen that PAD can effectively reduce homologous blood use by allowing a simple unit-for-unit autologous-for-homologous blood substitution. Its role in cardiac surgery today, however, is necessarily limited by the changing characteristics of the patient pool, and the decreased preoperative time available to allow for appropriate red cell mass regeneration. Issues of cost-effectiveness, logistical complexity, administrative burden, and resource allocation in the rapidly adjusting health care environment place additional constraints on more widespread application of PAD. This trend will likely continue in the future.[1]

Intraoperative autologous donation (IAD) of whole blood avoids the pitfalls encountered by preoperative donation: it does not require a delay in surgery, it is technically and administratively simple, and it can be performed efficiently and with minimal additional cost. In addition, the blood product obtained by IAD is superior to that obtained by PAD. The maximum storage life of platelets is 5 days, and coagulation factors V and VIII rapidly upgrade (within 24 to 48 hours) in refrigerated whole blood.[2,3] Therefore, unless component separation is performed (and typically it is not), preoperatively donated whole blood stored for more than 5 days contains nonfunctional platelets and is lacking in coagulation factor activity. It is useful only for its red cell fraction. In direct contrast, because intraoperatively donated blood is reinfused within 2 to 3 hours following withdrawal, it contains the full complement of red cells, platelets, and coagulation factors. It is therefore able to improve oxygen-carrying capacity, but in addition it provides a volume of fresh platelets and coagulation factors for reinfusion post–cardiopulmonary bypass to help combat coagulopathic bleeding. While it will be seen that its efficacy in this latter regard is currently questionable, the "pan preservation" of blood is an important attribute of IAD.

The third option for the procurement of autologous blood prior to cardiopulmonary bypass—platelet-rich plasmapheresis (PRP)—is a relatively new addition to the blood conservation armamentarium. Its use is based on the assumption that coagulopathic bleeding that accompanies the use of the heart-lung apparatus is primarily attributable to platelet dysfunction, and therefore that the selective preservation of a portion of platelets can serve to attenuate the magnitude of the coagulopathy that develops. Despite initial excitement, PRP has not received widespread acceptance because, although it does not require the prolonged preoperative time allotment of PAD, it otherwise encounters the same obstacles with respect to cost-effectiveness, technical and administrative complexity, and resource allocation. In addition, the actual effectiveness of PRP as a blood conservation measure has come to be questioned.

This chapter begins by reviewing the literature relating the development and application of the techniques of intraoperative autologous donation of whole blood and platelet plasmapheresis in cardiac surgery. The relative merits of IAD and PRP are analyzed, and the rationale underlying the general acceptance of whole blood IAD over PRP are presented. The next section focuses on the mechanism behind the effectiveness of whole blood IAD, and on using this knowledge to optimize its application and maximize its benefit. The third and final section provides a practical guide for the use of this optimized version of IAD as part of a comprehensive blood conservation program.

History and Development

Intraoperative Autologous Donation of Whole Blood

In 1957 Dodrill et al[4] described a technique in which a large portion of a patient's blood volume was removed before cardiopulmonary bypass, and then reinfused following separation from the heart-lung apparatus. This early form of intraoperative autologous donation was performed in an effort to decrease the magnitude of the insult of CPB, and the large volume homologous transfusion that accompanied the use of CPB at that time.

A significant portion of the detrimental effects of CPB were thought to be due to the use of rather massive amounts of homologous blood. In the late 1950s at our institution, for example, it was typical to transfuse 15 to 20 units of homologous whole blood per case.[5] Because blood conservation techniques that would eventually allow a reduction in the volume of blood required were not yet available, early investigators sought methods to increase the quality of the blood that was transfused. The first attempts at improving the quality of the blood product transfused involved the use of only fresh banked blood. Such fresh donor blood for open-heart procedures was typically obtained on the morning of surgery from logistically difficult prearranged donations. Yet despite these efforts at obtaining fresh blood, severe coagulopathic bleeding continued to accompany the use of the CPB circuit. Dodrill et al advanced the use of fresh blood one step further, by exchange transfusing fresh donor blood for fresh autologous blood before the start of CPB, and then preserving this removed autologous blood for reinfusion post-CPB. Protected from destruction and degradation by the CPB circuit, post-bypass reinfusion of this fresh autologous blood presumably served to help normalize the structure and function of blood, and therefore to decrease coagulopathic bleeding. The value of this procedure was very clear to Dodrill et al at the time. In their words: "The advantages of this exchange transfusion are so great and so protean that time and space do not permit a complete statement of its advantages—suffice it to say that the advantages are great, and that the possibilities for good have not been completely utilized."[4(p62)] While *preoperative* procedurement of autologous blood had been a recognized technique in surgery for over 50 years, Dodrill et al's was the first attempt to purposely remove a portion of a patient's blood volume *intraoperatively* for the express purpose of preserving the structure and function of that patient's own blood.

By the mid-1960s, the growing blood conservation movement, sparked by the enormous growth of cardiac surgery and its drain on the national blood supply and by the growing concern over the infectious and immunologic risks of homologous blood, and encouraged by the successful introduction of non-blood prime and normovolemic hemodilution, was eager to explore new avenues for blood conservation. In this setting, in 1968 Hardesty et al[7] rejuvenated interest in intraoperative preservation of whole blood (IAD) by analyzing its effects on platelet number and function in a prospective study of 14 patients. They found that platelet number and adhesiveness were well preserved in the blood bags during the time of storage, and that reinfusion of the IAD blood—a volume equivalent to 25% of the effective blood volume (EBV)—at the end of bypass resulted in an improvement in overall postoperative platelet adhesiveness, and an increase in platelet number. While in comparison to a group of retrospective controls postoperative bleeding was *not* decreased, the improvement in platelet function, coupled with the intuitive appeal of the technique, began a 25-year period of investigation into the merit of IAD in cardiac surgical blood conservation.

The 1970s saw several additions to the whole-blood IAD literature as groups began to try to further characterize and quantitate its effects. In 1972 Hallowel et al[8] performed a prospective randomized controlled study withdrawing an average of 1250 ml of blood from 25 patients, with 25 others serving as controls. They found that homologous transfusion requirement was decreased by 25% in those patients who had undergone IAD (2540 ml vs 3400 ml), but that postoperative blood loss and platelet count were unaffected. That same year, Wagstaffe et al[9] reported on a prospective randomized controlled study that evaluated two IAD techniques—drawing from the arterial line before heparin administration, and drawing the donated blood from the venous return cannula after heparinization. They found that compared with controls, these two techniques resulted in a significant decrease in postoperative bleeding (57.8% and 36.0%, respectively). Effects on platelet number and function and overall homologous transfusion requirement were not discussed. A third study in 1973 by Ochsner et al[10] evaluated the use of 800 to 1200 cc of IAD in 300 patients in a randomized prospective controlled study. They found a decrease in homologous transfusion requirement of 49% (3331 cc to 1688 cc), a reduction in postoperative bleeding of 20%, and a mean platelet count increase of 28,000 after IAD reinfusion. Important to note in this study is that the authors utilized an aggressively low transfusion trigger on CPB (approximately 15%) and that this may help to account for the very significant benefit of IAD which they found. In 1974 Zubiate et al[11] reviewed their experience during a 1-year period in which 477 patients were operated on for coronary artery disease. They found that combining non-blood prime with whole blood IAD of 1000 to 1500 cc enabled them to avoid transfusion in 71% of these patients without any untoward side effects. While impressive, especially at this early stage of blood conservation (intraoperative salvage had not yet been introduced), it is difficult to draw conclusions as to the contribution made by hemodilution as no control group was provided. In 1975 Cohn et al[12] published a retrospective review of 400 consecutive cardiopulmonary bypass cases in which 44% had whole blood IAD—either 500 or 1000 ml—performed. They found that if 500 cc was removed, transfusion requirement was decreased from 5.0 to 4.3 units, and that if 1000 cc was removed there was a further decrease to 3.9 units—both significant improvements. This study is important because it is the only study in the literature until very recently that attempted to analyze the potential *volume dependency* of the benefit that IAD provides. However, the results obtained by this study must be interpreted with caution as this was a nonrandomized study, and those patients with low hematocrits or those who were judged unable to donate likely did not undergo IAD, or had the smaller volume removed. That same year, Silver[13] performed a prospective randomized controlled trial of IAD versus control using a mean IAD volume of two units, and found that homologous transfusion requirement was decreased by two units (20%) per patient in the 20 patients per group studied. Data as to transfusion guidelines and hematocrits were unavailable, and so any possible transfusion bias is difficult to assess.

It was a study in 1975 by Pliam et al[14] that first questioned the efficacy of IAD as a blood conservation measure. In a prospective randomized controlled study of 122 patients undergoing cardiopulmonary bypass, the authors found no clear benefit with the use of an average of 1200 cc IAD. Although their results are difficult to interpret, they appear to indicate that while post-CPB intraoperative banked blood requirement was decreased, total intraoperative banked blood requirement was actually increased. In other words, more banked blood was likely given in the IAD group to maintain an acceptable hematocrit on bypass. What this study does not reveal is what the transfusion trigger on bypass was. If it was not sufficiently low, as in Ochsner et al's[10] study, then removal of autologous blood would have to have been accompanied by infusion of banked blood. In effect, the use of IAD may have led to a paradoxical increase in homologous transfusion, entirely defeating the original purpose. IAD can only be fully effective if removal of the IAD volume is not coupled with homologous blood replacement, and this can only occur if the transfusion trigger used during CPB in conjunction with IAD is sufficiently low. So what Pliam et al's study may indicate is not that IAD is not an effective blood conservation measure, but that whole blood IAD must be performed in an overall context that will allow it to work. Nevertheless, the study by Pliam's group cast the first doubt on the utility of IAD, doubt that has helped hinder universal acceptance of the technique to this day. A second negative study appeared in the literature the same year. Sherman et al[15] performed a prospective study using matched historical controls. They found that withdrawing two units of blood pre-bypass had no effect on decreasing homologous transfusion requirement or postoperative bleeding. Characteristics of this study that may or may not have affected outcome are (1) that one unit of homologous blood was transfused before IAD so that the IAD blood contained a mixture of both banked and fresh autologous blood, and (2) that the IAD volume was both heparinized and stored in citrate-phosphate dextrose (CPD). This latter factor may have played a role in the rather noticeable postoperative (i.e., post-IAD reinfusion) transfusion requirement seen in the IAD group. The nonrandomized format, small sample size, and lack of standardized transfusion guidelines are characteristics of this study that should also be noted.

The 1970s were rounded out by a series of studies again supporting the benefit of whole blood IAD. In 1977 Kaplan et al[16] experimented with different methods of withdrawing the IAD volume, and found that platelet number was best preserved by withdrawing heparinized blood from the venous return cannula immediately prior to bypass (compared with drawing from the arterial line or the central venous line). They were able to demonstrate an 18% reduction in overall homologous blood product requirement with the use of IAD in this prospective randomized controlled study. In 1977 Lilleaasen[17] evaluated the use of IAD in aortic valvular surgery. Thirty patients were randomized to undergo either moderate or extreme hemodilution during CPB. Extreme hemodilution was achieved with both total crystalloid circuit prime and an average of 855 ml IAD. The author found a 71% decrease in homologous blood product use and a 47% decrease in postoperative bleeding with the use of IAD and extreme hemodilution. The following year in a retrospective review of 240 cardiac procedures, Yeh[18] was able to demonstrate a 25% decrease in homologous transfusion requirement with whole blood IAD. Lack of randomization resulted in a higher preoperative hemoglobin in the IAD group, likely skewing results in favor of IAD, however. Finally, in 1978 Cosgrove et al[19] reported on a series of 50 patients in whom a comprehensive blood conservation program, which included the use of a mean of 675 ml IAD, was applied. They found that 94% of these patients were able to be operated on without the need for homologous blood, although the limited nature of this study must be kept in mind.

The 1980s brought important advances to the blood conservation field. Intraoperative salvage with Cell Saver-type apparatus was introduced and accepted as an essential blood conservation measure, and numerous pharmacologic interventions were tested and deployed. A new form of IAD in which platelets were selectively removed and preserved from the heart-lung machine (platelet-rich plasmapheresis, PRP) was introduced to cardiac surgery, helping to spark renewed interest in the intraoperative autologous preservation techniques in general. Several studies related to the use of whole blood IAD appeared in the literature during this time.

In 1981 Utley et al[20] published a review of whole blood IAD that firmly supported its use. This was followed in 1987 by a similar positive review by Martin et al.[21] That same year, Szecsi's group[22] performed a prospective randomized controlled trial comparing the combined use of three autologous transfusion techniques versus not using any of these techniques. The three blood conservation measures included whole blood IAD, intraoperative salvage, and postoperative shed blood reinfusion. The authors found a 50% reduction in homologous blood product use with this combined approach. However, as with several other IAD studies presented in this review, it is difficult to assess the contribution of IAD to these savings, as multiple blood conservation techniques were combined. A small 15-patient prospective randomized study performed in 1987 by Dale et al[23] showed a marked improvement in platelet count and platelet function with an average of 850 ml of whole blood IAD, and also served to illustrate the importance of allowing hemodilution to proceed to low (but physiologically and clinically acceptable) levels. By allowing "extreme" hemodilution on bypass, they were able to demonstrate a decrease in transfusion requirement of 70%, and yet at the same time show improvement in platelet count and postoperative bleeding. A prospective randomized controlled study of relatively small volume whole blood IAD (10 ml/kg) by Deitrich et al[24] in 1989 showed that the addition of IAD to a set of blood conservation measures decreased homologous blood requirement by 40%. Postoperative bleeding, platelet counts, and platelet function were not discussed.

In the 1990s with all of the basic mechanical blood conservation measures in place, attention turned to pharmacologic interventions aimed at decreasing the coagulopathy of CPB. Despite the number of studies performed on IAD in the previous three decades, studies assessing the effectiveness of IAD in blood conservation continued to appear in the literature, indicating that previous investigators had not been able to unequivocally demonstrate its benefit (or lack thereof).

In 1991 Ovrum et al[25] published a review of 121 patients undergoing coronary artery bypass graft (CABG) procedures utilizing a simple blood conservation program that included an average of 815 ml of whole blood IAD. None of the patients required homologous transfusion. As in previous review format studies, however, the benefit of IAD can only be surmised. Later that year, Ovrum's group[26] published a second review in which 98.6% of 500 patients undergoing elective CABG did not require homologous transfusion. Again, whole blood IAD was utilized as part of their simple program, but also again, its actual contribution to the benefit found can only be conjectured because of the study design utilized. An interesting 1991 study by Ness et al[27] compared the effects of whole blood IAD and preoperative autologous donation on homologous blood exposure and transfusion requirement in major urologic surgery. They found that whole blood IAD had the equivalent effect of two to three units of preoperatively donated blood. The following year, Scott et al's[28] retrospective analysis of efficacy and cost of various blood conservation measures concluded, after stepwise linear regression analysis, that the performance of whole blood IAD (mean 575 ± 140 cc) was the single strongest negative predictor of homologous blood requirement. A study by Hudson et al,[29] also using a relatively small volume of IAD (10% of blood volume or approximately 450 cc), showed a suggestive but not statistically significant benefit with respect to homologous blood requirement, but no effect on postoperative bleeding or coagulation. The relative small volume used may have affected these results. Gilmer, in a preliminary report of a prospective randomized study, found that whole blood IAD (17% of EBV, or approximately two units of whole blood) resulted in a suggestive but not statistically significant decrease in transfusion requirement and postoperative bleeding. In 1993 Schonberger et al[30] evaluated IAD using a retrospective matched control format in 100 patients undergoing internal mammary artery (IMA) grafting. The two groups were well matched for risk factors for bleeding and transfusion. The authors found that 800 ml IAD (withdrawn through the venous cannula after heparinization) served to significantly increase postoperative platelet count and hemoglobin concentration, while at the same time decrease postoperative bleeding and transfusion for both red cells and coagulation factors. Despite the limitations of the retrospective format, this study is notable because of the degree to which the groups were matched, and the constancy of other study variables possibly affecting outcome, such as the use of a set of strict transfusion guidelines. In 1993 we undertook a prospective randomized controlled study of IAD in 70 patients (35 IAD, 35 control) in which a calculated maximum volume of blood was removed in an effort to magnify the effects of the technique.[31] We found that relative to controls, patients in the IAD group (who had a mean of 1549 ml of whole blood removed and reinfused) had a decreased requirement for red cell transfusion. There was, however, no decrease in postoperative bleeding, nor in platelet or coagulation factor transfusion requirement. Finally, Petry et al[32] retrospectively evaluated 90 patients undergoing CABG surgery. In the nonrandomized IAD group 500 to 1000 ml of IAD was removed via the venous cannula after heparin administration. The authors found that red cell transfusion requirements were significantly decreased in patients who had IAD performed. This study had several limitations, however, including probable inadequate group matching (it was likely that it was the healthier patients with higher pre-CPB hematocrits who became candidates for blood removal), and lack of measurement of important outcome variables such as postoperative bleeding and platelet count.

Intraoperative Platelet Plasmapheresis

Platelet plasmapheresis—a continuous centrifugation technique that allows the selective removal of platelets from circulating whole blood—was introduced to the field of hematology by Tullis et al[33] in 1968. An important advance, with many hematologic applications, it found its way into the cardiac surgery arena in the late 1970s as a means of platelet preservation. Cardiopulmonary bypass circuit-induced platelet dysfunction had long been thought to be the primary lesion underlying postoperative coagulopathic bleeding,[34] and multiple studies had served to confirm and help characterize this dysfunction.[35,36] The simple rationale for use of intraoperative PRP in cardiac surgery was that selective removal and preservation of a significant percentage of a patient's platelets from degradation and destruction by the heart bypass circuit would serve to improve overall postoperative platelet function, and lead to a decrease in postoperative bleeding and homologous transfusion requirement. It had the theoretical benefit over IAD that improvement in platelet number and function and amelioration of bleeding could be accomplished without a decrease in oxygen carrying capacity. Thus it was particularly attractive in those patients with low preoperative red blood cell mass and/or hematocrits, or to those surgeons who preferred (albeit unnecessarily) to maintain high hematocrits during CPB.[37]

First used in cardiac surgery outside the United States by Harke et al[38] in 1977 and Ferrari et al[39] in 1987, the first American blood conservation study utilizing intraoperative PRP was performed in 1988 by Giordano et al.[40] They found that the removal of 1000 to 1200 cc of platelet-rich plasma pre-bypass (with post-bypass reinfusion) resulted in a significant decrease in the intraoperative and postoperative use of plasma, platelets, and packed red blood cells (PRBCs). Furthermore, the authors found that the percentage of patients receiving no homologous blood exposure nearly doubled. Despite significant limitations, including the use of different surgeons for each of the study groups (PRP and control), and therefore a nonrandomized format, this initial study sparked a significant amount of interest in the technique of PRP. In 1989 Giordano et al[41] published a report comparing 387 consecutive cardiac surgical patients in whom PRP was performed to 147 retrospective controls. While the authors found a significant decrease in homologous blood use (12.91 vs 5.31 units per patient), the rather high overall blood usage as well as the limited retrospective study format should be noted. In 1990 Jones et al[42] performed a prospective randomized controlled nonblinded study of PRP (up to 1000 ml) versus control that clearly supported the benefit of intraoperative PRP. The use of PRP was found to lead to a decrease in intraoperative red cell mass loss, a reduction in homologous blood requirement (from 1.8 to 0.67 units per patient), and a doubling of the number of patients spared exposure to homologous blood (66% vs 32%). That same year, Del Rossi et al[43] performed a prospective randomized nonblinded trial of PRP vs control. They were able to demonstrate a rather remarkable benefit, despite the very small volume of PRP that was utilized (220 ml), and despite a very small sample size (18 patients, 9 per group). Postoperative bleeding decreased 25%, and transfusion requirement decreased from 9750 ml of homologous products in controls to 3500 ml in the PRP group. It is very important to note, however, that the transfusion difference between groups was isolated to FFP use (24 FFP units in the nine control patients vs 4 FFP units in the nine PRP patients). This amounts to the use of an average of approximately two units of FFP per patient in the control group, an unusually high amount. Closer analysis reveals that the transfusion of this product was based on the results of an isolated laboratory test—elevation of the postoperative partial thromboplastin time (PTT)—not on the rate of postoperative bleeding. In most centers the treatment of an isolated laboratory abnormality would not be viewed as appropriate. Also of concern is the use of the PTT to guide the use of FFP. In our institution we have found elevation of the PTT to be rare.[31] If such elevations are present, they are typically due to residual heparin effect, and are appropriately and easily corrected with an additional dose of protamine. Postoperative prothrombin times are conversely frequently elevated in the post-bypass period,[31] although these elevations are typically not associated with clinically significant bleeding and do not require treatment. It is an elevated prothrombin time, in the presence of clinically significant bleeding—not an isolated PTT—that would be expected to respond to the use of FFP. The design and, in turn, the results of this study must therefore be placed in question.[44]

An interesting study performed in 1990 by Boldt et al[45] examined the effects of different types of plasmapheresis. Pheresis technique can be adjusted to obtain specific blood fractions. Boldt's group used this ability to obtain two different types of plasmapheresis product—platelet-poor plasma (the noncellular plasma fraction of blood) and platelet-rich plasma (platelets and variable amounts of other cellular elements). Forty-five patients were prospectively randomized to three groups: platelet-poor plasma, platelet-rich plasma, and control in which no pheresis was performed. Approximately 800 cc of plasmapheresis product was obtained in the two pheresis groups. The results were in accordance with what might be intuitively expected. The platelet-poor group, in which primarily plasma and plasma proteins were preserved, had the highest postoperative levels of plasma coagulation-related proteins (fibrinogen, antithrombin III). The platelet-rich group, in which platelets and other cellular elements such as white cells were preserved, showed the highest platelet counts and the lowest levels of polymorphonuclear (PMN) elastase, a marker of white blood cell activation and damage. PMN elastase levels were highest in the control group, suggesting that withdrawal of part of the white cell fraction in the platelet-rich group may have been important in reducing the overall inflammatory response to CPB. Consistent with this finding was the significant decrease in chest tube output seen between the PRP and control groups (500 ± 170 ml vs 696 ± 130 ml). In a second study using the same prospective three-group model with 12 patients per group, Boldt et al[46] looked at the effects of the two types of plasmapheresis on platelet function. Using standard aggregometry—response to adenosine diphosphate (ADP), epinephrine, and collagen—the authors found that compared to control and platelet-poor plasma, platelet-rich plasma produced the highest postoperative platelet counts, and best preserved platelet aggregation measured at 45 minutes post-CPB. These numerical and functional improvements correlated with a suggestive but not statistically significant decrease in postoperative bleeding in the PRP group versus the control group.

In 1991 Jones et al[49] studied PRP of up to 1000 ml in a retrospective review of 300 patients. They found that addition of PRP to their blood conservation program decreased the rate of homologous transfusion from 68% to 36%. The nonprospective nature of this study must be kept in mind, however. An important finding of their study is that lowering the transfusion trigger on bypass from 21% to 15% resulted in further dropping homologous exposure from 36% to 18% (it will be seen that a basic tenet of this chapter is that allowing a sufficiently low transfusion trigger on bypass, particularly after whole blood IAD, is necessary to realize the full benefit of intraoperative autologous donation techniques—Jones et al's study serves to nicely illustrate this point). In 1992 Davies et al[48] removed 857 ml of platelet- *and* leukocyte-rich plasma from 35 consecutive patients undergoing coronary bypass procedures, and compared the results to those found with 35 randomly selected retrospective controls. The modified PRP technique used by the authors, which removed as much as 30% of circulating leukocytes, was found to decrease postoperative bleeding by 40%, and homologous blood exposure by over 50% (from 3.9 units to 1.6 units). In a second study using the same technique, and in which similar results were obtained, the authors stressed the importance of removing white cells as well as platelets, and of removing as much of each of these components as possible.[49] They cite their average 51% harvesting of circulating platelets, and 27% of circulating white cells, and compare this to the 9%, 15%, and 30% of platelet yields obtained by Del Rossi et al,[43] Giordano et al,[41] and Jones et al[42] in the studies discussed previously. In the authors' words: "The physiologic trespass of CPB is due to massive activation of platelets, leukocytes, and the inflammatory and coagulation cascades. The success of the technique (PRP) depends on the extent of depletion of cellular elements from the bloodstream prior to the initiation of CPB."[49] It should be noted, however, that the authors' high-yield technique required an 11.5-F temporary hemodialysis catheter to be placed in the internal jugular vein in order to obtain adequate flow, and an average of 9.9 full blood volume pheresis cycles. Obvious are the additional risk and effort involved in executing their optimized PRP collection process. Nevertheless, the findings of Davies et al[48] and Wells et al[49] extend those of Boldt et al[49] (who found decreased markers of white cell damage/activation in conjunction with the use of PRP) and provide further support for the role that preservation of white cells and platelets may play in reducing the inflammatory response to CPB, and in decreasing postoperative coagulopathic bleeding. The last study in the literature to support the use of PRP in cardiac surgery was performed by Ferraris et al,[50] who evaluated the use of PRP in two separate patient groups: those at high risk for postoperative blood transfusion, and those at low risk for postoperative blood transfusion (as determined by the ratio of the preoperative bleeding time to the preoperative red blood cell volume). The authors found that the removal of 700 to 800 ml of PRP (an estimated 10% to 15% of circulating platelets) resulted in an improvement in transfusion requirement relative to control (8.1 vs 2.9 units per patient) only in the high-risk group, suggesting that specifically targeting this patient group is more resource- and cost-efficient. No difference was found between any of the groups with respect to postoperative bleeding.

Despite the positive results found in the initial PRP literature, by the late 1980s other investigators had come forward with results that began to cast doubt on the general utility of selectively preserving platelets through platelet-rich plasmapheresis. The first data questioning the routine preservation of platelets appeared in the form of two prospective randomized trials examining the effect of prophylactic administration of banked platelets following CPB. In 1975 Harding et al[51] randomized 60 patients paired for age and procedure type to receive or not receive four units of homologous platelets following separation from CPB. They found no difference between groups with respect to the time required for hemostasis post-bypass. Unfortunately, data regarding postoperative bleeding were not provided. In 1984 Simon et al[52] performed a similar prospective randomized controlled trial in 28 patients. They found that while the prophylactic reinfusion of four units of homologous platelets post-CPB prevented the bleeding time prolongation that was seen in the control group, there was no decrease in postoperative bleeding (as measured by chest tube output). The lack of effect of the postoperative reinfusion of platelets on decreasing postoperative bleeding received further support from a series of investigations that utilized electron microscopically measured platelet aggregation to assess post-CPB platelet function.[53–57] The first of these studies was reported by Mohr et al[53] in 1988. They found that one unit of fresh (drawn within 24 hours of surgery) whole homologous blood raised the platelet count post-bypass the same as four units of fresh homologous platelets. They also found that one unit of whole blood was able to return postoperative bleeding to normal, whereas it took eight units of fresh platelets to do this. In addition, platelet thromboxane formation and aggregation were higher with one unit of fresh whole blood than with ten units of platelet concentrate. A suggestive but not statistically significant decrease in postoperative bleeding was seen in the whole blood group. Mohr et al postulated that multiple factors could account for the superiority of whole blood versus platelet concentrates, including platelet damage during PRP processing, the maintenance of important red cell–plasma-platelet interactions in whole blood, and the fact that larger, more active platelets are probably not well preserved by PRP. The latter can be understood by realizing that PRP only sequesters 60% to 70% of platelets from a given processed blood volume, and so 20% to 30% are immediately returned to the patient in the red cell fraction. The platelets that sediment with the red cell fraction are larger, younger, and probably functionally more active.[58–61] Thus PRP fails to preserve an important group of platelets from the detrimental effects of the bypass circuit. In support of the importance of larger platelets in post-bypass hemostasis is Mohr et al's[54] 1992 finding that patients with clinically significant postoperative bleeding had lower mean platelet volumes than those who did not bleed. Lavee et al[55] also found evidence that one of the reasons for the superior effect of whole blood versus platelet concentrates is that whole blood better preserves platelet volume. These results of Mohr and Lavee were confirmed by Martinowitz et al[56] in 1990, who found that the reinfusion of fresh whole homologous blood was superior to the reinfusion of fresh plasma concentrates in the postoperative period with respect to restoring postoperative platelet aggregation. In 1993 these authors confirmed the findings of their previous 7 years of investigation in a prospective randomized study of the reinfusion of autologous whole blood (whole blood IAD) versus autologous platelet concentrates (intraoperative PRP) following cardiopulmonary bypass.[57] Twenty-five patients undergoing cardiac surgery were randomized to receive either whole blood IAD (volume not specified) or 600 to 700 ml intraoperative PRP. Interestingly, the yield of platelets in the withdrawn PRP volume was not found to be significantly higher than in the whole blood IAD volume. Following PRP/IAD reinfusion, a significant improvement in platelet aggregation was seen in the whole blood IAD group relative to the PRP group. No difference in chest tube output was seen between the two groups, but there was a suggestion of a decreased need for homologous transfusion in the whole blood IAD group. Based on these findings, the authors felt justified in questioning the need for selective platelet preservation versus the simple, easy, and far less expensive use of fresh whole autologous blood.

Other groups of investigators began to question the utility of PRP as well. A 1992 prospective randomized placebo-controlled and blinded study by Castro in repeat valvular surgery patients found no benefit to performing PRP with respect to overall transfusion requirement. While the volume of PRP sequestered was not recorded, nor was the effect on postoperative blood loss reported, the blinding of the anesthesiologist in charge of all post-CPB decision making lends credence to these findings. A second prospective randomized trial that year by Shore-Lesserson et al[62] looked at the effect of PRP on post-CPB thromboelastographically measured coagulability in patients undergoing reoperative cardiac procedures. Relative to control patients the authors found no measurable benefit from the sequestration and reinfusion of 15 ml/kg of PRP. A study by Gilmer randomized patients to undergo either whole blood IAD (17% of EBV), PRP (20% of plasma volume), or neither technique (control). They found a suggestive decrease in postoperative bleeding and transfusion requirement in both the whole blood IAD and PRP groups versus the control group, but these differences did not reach statistical significance. There was no difference seen between the whole blood and PRP groups at the time of this preliminary report. An important prospective randomized blinded study was performed in 1993 by Tobe et al.[63] After randomization, 51 patients undergoing primary coronary artery bypass grafting had 8 to 10 ml/kg of platelet-rich plasma removed. In the group randomized to not receive PRP this plasma was returned *prior to* CPB. In the PRP group the sequestered plasma was returned *following* CPB. The authors found that although prothrombin times were significantly lower in the PRP group following PRP reinfusion, there was no difference in the surgeons' subjective measure of excessive bleeding, chest tube output, transfusion requirement, or other measures of abnormal coagulation (thromboelastography, partial thromboplastin time, activated clotting time, fibrinogen, or platelet count). This study is notable both for its unique design and for the use of specific transfusion guidelines. In a third prospective randomized and blinded study, Ereth et al[64] randomized 56 patients to receive either PRP or sham PRP (performed by simulating PRP behind a visual barrier) in conjunction with repeat valvular surgery. The authors found that the removal of 15% to 20% of the plasma volume (600 to 700 ml) had no effect on intraoperative or postoperative bleeding, nor did it serve to decrease homologous transfusion requirement. The last study to appear in the literature was a prospective randomized study of 40 patients undergoing primary cardiac surgery performed in 1994 by Wong et al.[65] The authors removed 30% of the plasma volume as PRP, and compared the effects to control patients in whom no PRP was performed. They found no difference in several postoperative coagulation parameters (platelet count, PT, PTT, ACT, thromboelastography), postoperative chest tube drainage, or transfusion requirement.

The Value of PRP in Cardiac Surgical Blood Conservation

In response to the conflicting results of the many studies of PRP to date, several letters and editorials have appeared discussing the utility and cost-effectiveness of the technique, as well as its overall applicability to the cardiac surgical setting.[44,61–68] In a 1993 editorial titled "Autologous Platelet-Rich Plasma in Cardiac Surgery: Aesthetics Versus Virtue," Gravlee[44] addressed several of these issues. At a time when the clearly negative prospective randomized and blinded studies of de Castro, Tobe, and Erech had not yet been performed, Gravlee concluded that the evidence in favor of the use of PRP in cardiac surgery was not convincing, and that "those who choose not to use autologous platelet-rich plasma in cardiac surgery should do so without guilt." He based this conclusion on the fact that (1) routine prophylactic homologous platelet transfusion has never been shown to be of benefit, and is considered by most to be inappropriate,[51,52,69] (2) a majority of the prospective randomized controlled trials of PRP have shown no significant reduction in postoperative bleeding, and (3) a majority of the prospective randomized controlled trials of PRP have demonstrated no significant decrease in the need for homologous transfusion. In addition, none of the blinded studies of PRP have shown *any* significant clinical benefit.

We would add to this several additional points against the routine use of PRP in cardiac surgery. First, the value of selective platelet preservation in general can be questioned. As Gravlee pointed out, studies of prophylactic homologous platelet transfusion have never shown these to be of clinical benefit.[51,52] In addition, while higher platelet counts were seen in several of the studies in which this parameter was discussed, sufficient correlation between decreased platelet count and increased postoperative blood loss has also never been clearly demonstrated.[31,52] Similarly, measures of platelet function, such as surface expression of activation antigens or aggregation response to agonists, generally have not been clearly linked to worse bleeding or transfusion outcome.[52,70,71] The routine use of PRP therefore cannot be justified on the basis of improved platelet parameters alone. It also is important to recognize that even when PRP is appropriately adjusted and optimally applied,[48,67] it selectively removes primarily smaller platelets, returning to the patient a majority of the pool of larger platelets (which sediment with the red cell fraction). It has been well documented, however, that larger platelets are younger and functionally superior.[58-61] The most important pool of platelets is therefore not preserved by PRP, undergoing not only full exposure to the CPB circuit, but also experiencing the added processing of the pheresis procedure itself (which may lead to its own degree of hematologic dysfunction).[72-74] We have recently shown that the reinfusion of three to four units of fresh *whole* autologous blood following CPB had no significant effect on postoperative bleeding.[75] This blood volume would be expected to contain approximately one quarter to one third of the patient's platelets—a number that compares favorably with the percentage of platelets removed by many of the PRP studies. In addition this blood would contain both large and small platelets, as well as red cells, white cells, and the full complement of plasma proteins. If nonselective preservation of this large volume of whole blood did not decrease postoperative blood loss, then it becomes difficult to accept the ability of PRP to achieve this result.

A second general argument against the use of PRP is that it is labor intensive, and adds significant complexity to the overall management of the patient. An operating room staff member (e.g., perfusionist, blood bank technician, or anesthesiologist) must be dedicated to the task of performing PRP, and this person and the PRP equipment must be imposed on an already often crowded operating theater, adding to the complexity of set-up, increasing the number of concurrent patient interventions, and likely making emergent interactions more confusing and difficult. In the report by Davis et al[48] (*proponents* of the use of PRP), the authors discuss the increase in patient monitoring and pharmacologic and fluid manipulation that is often required: "It is important to realize that PP (PRP) is a procedure that must be directly controlled by the anesthesiologist. This technique cannot be abrogated to a technician or perfusionist for fear of cardiovascular instability. Platelet pheresis in this context is a complex medical procedure demanding added vigilance, additional central venous access, and even for routine cases, far greater pharmacologic intervention by the anesthesiologist. The potential risks include hypovolemia, hypothermia, and citrate-induced toxicity." In their platelet-leukocyte plasmapheresis paper, Davis et al report routinely using an 11.5-F hemodialysis catheter in the internal jugular position and performing a mean of 9.9 full blood volume pheresis cycles. Obviously these maneuvers are not without additional patient risk, particularly during the pre-CPB period when significant cardiovascular disease has not yet been corrected. Alternatively, less invasive means for platelet preservation have become available. These include the use of less reactive biocompatible CPB circuitry, as well as pharmacologic preservation agents such as aprotinin and the antifibrinolytics.[78-83] The use of these newer options is simple, involves the use of little or no additional labor, and is likely more cost-effective than PRP when all costs are considered. In addition, several of these interventions have the important attribute of proven clinical efficacy.

Issues of cost and resource allocation also argue against the routine use of

PRP in cardiac surgery. While Davies et al[68] recently stated that PRP actually helped reduce their overall hospitalization costs from $38,746 to $31,996, the retrospective control group used for this analysis makes these results more difficult to interpret than the authors suggest, as a wide range of cost-reducing measures were likely to have been progressively introduced during the time period addressed. The cost of PRP must take into consideration the original outlay for the pheresis machines, the costs for the disposable tubing and other components used for each pheresis, maintenance contracts, the salary and benefits of the additional persons required to run the pheresis machines in each of the operating rooms, and the cost of complications that might arise from the pheresis process (equipment malfunction, citrate toxicity, large-bore access site bleeding or misadventure, etc.). At Gravlee's institution in 1993 the charge for PRP was $1000. At our institution this sum would pay for six units of platelets, two units of FFP, and one unit of PRBCs. In a recent study of patients undergoing elective and urgent CABG procedures, we found that patients required a mean of 0.28 unit of homologous red cell units, 0.66 unit of homologous platelets, and 0.35 unit of homologous FFP. Converting these transfusion requirements to dollars (one RBC unit = $220, one platelet unit = $120, one FFP unit = $55) would lead to an approximate total transfusion cost per patient at our institution of $160.05 per patient. The routine use of PRP at our institution for CABG patients would, therefore, lead to a net loss of $839.95 per patient.

Whole Blood IAD Versus Platelet Plasmapheresis

The final and perhaps most convincing argument against the use of PRP is that its use precludes the use of whole blood IAD—a simple and inexpensive blood conservation measure that, when optimally performed, clearly *is* of clinical benefit. The superiority of whole blood IAD arises from its simple attribute of preserving *all* of the elements of whole blood from loss and degradation during CPB. Whole blood IAD, when optimally applied, therefore, does all that PRP does—and significantly more. It not only removes and preserves a portion of platelets and plasma, but in addition preserves what can be regarded as the primary component of blood—the red cell.

Autologous red cell losses that occur in the cardiac surgical patient can be divided into two categories with respect to intraoperative autologous donation practices (whole blood IAD and PRP): (1) those that occur intraoperatively, while the donated blood is outside the body, and (2) those that occur postoperatively following autologous blood reinfusion. PRP seeks to decrease the need for homologous red cell transfusion by addressing only the latter of these types of blood loss. What PRP does not at all address is the former source of autologous red cell loss—that which occurs during the entire intraoperative period preceding protamine reversal of heparin. These intraoperative red cell losses occur prior to CPB during chest opening and vein graft harvesting, during CPB as a result of mechanical loss and destruction by the CPB and intraoperative salvage apparatus, and immediately following CPB during the brief time before protamine is administered and any withdrawn autologous blood products are reinfused. Obligatory and constant, these losses can amount to 25% to 40% of the patient's original red cell volume in the typical cardiac surgical case, as indicated by the typical drop in hematocrit that is seen to occur by the time that the patient has arrived in the ICU. It is these intraoperative losses that provide the background for the need for transfusion—the presence or absence of postoperative bleeding simply helps to "put the patient over the edge." Whole blood IAD lies in distinct contrast to PRP by addressing both types of autologous red cell loss—intraoperative and postoperative. It not only preserves platelets and plasma from direct loss, postoperative bleeding, but it also preserves red cells, white cells, and all other elements of whole blood from loss and degradation during CPB. In a recent study of whole blood IAD we were able to quantitate the red cell-preserving effects of removing a calculated maximum volume of whole blood.[75] We found that the removal of three to four units of fresh whole blood resulted in a red cell savings of approximately one unit per patient. This red cell savings was attributable to decreased intraoperative losses only, as postoperative bleeding was entirely unaffected. Whether the lack of benefit of fresh autologous and homologous platelet and coagulation factor infusion post-CPB was due to inferior quality of the reinfused product, or to an overwhelming of the reinfused blood by the "activated" blood that remained in the patient during CPB, remains to be determined.[75] It stands, however, that large-volume IAD served to significantly decrease homologous transfusion requirement through a direct volume-dependent prevention of the loss of red cells during this intraoperative period. This red cell-preserving attribute of whole blood IAD is entirely lacking in PRP.

In addition to its red cell-preserving effects, whole blood IAD is comparatively simple to perform, does not require additional personnel or equipment, and costs only the price of the standard citrate phosphate dextrose Adsol-1 (CPDA-1) blood collection bags utilized for blood collection ($2.90/bag).*

During the pre-CPB period the surgeon or anesthesiologist can utilize only one autologous blood preservation technique—either whole blood IAD or PRP—but not both. For the majority of patients with adequate preoperative red cell mass and hematocrit, this choice becomes straightforward. Whole blood IAD is simpler, less expensive, less invasive, involves far

*Estimated cost based on the 48-bag/case hospital cost. (Standard screening, testing, administrative, and nursing costs that add significantly to the cost of homologous blood are not required for IAD blood.)

less pharmacologic and technical manipulation, and preserves the only portion of blood—the red cell fraction—that actually benefits from intraoperative donation as currently practiced. In the less common case of low hematocrit/red cell mass, where removal of additional red cell mass through IAD is not possible because of further compromise in oxygen carrying capacity, the choice becomes whether or not to apply PRP to selectively preserve autologous platelets and plasma. While some institutions may have the funds to keep this rather expensive intraoperative pheresis capability on reserve for when such circumstances arise, such funding will become less and less available as health care continues to evolve, particularly when PRP has been shown not to provide significant benefit. Alternative pharmacologic and technical measures aimed at the prevention and treatment of the coagulopathy of CPB will likely eliminate the theoretical need for selective mechanical platelet preservation in even these cases. It is therefore difficult to foresee a future for the use of PRP in cardiac surgery. Because of its intraoperative red cell saving effect, however, whole blood IAD will continue to have an important role in cardiac surgical blood conservation. The following section discusses the ways in which the technique of whole blood IAD can be optimized to yield maximum blood savings.

Optimal Application of Whole Blood IAD

It can be seen from the preceding review that, in contrast to PRP, a majority of the studies of whole blood IAD in some way support its benefit as a blood conservation measure. Evident, however, is the striking inconsistency in results, particularly with respect to postoperative bleeding and transfusion requirement. The findings of all of the controlled studies (either retrospective or prospective) are seen in Table 11.1. By analyzing and understanding the results of these previous studies of IAD, valuable insight can be gained toward achieving improved results. Such an assessment reveals three basic factors that underlie the suboptimal results—and therefore the inconsistent findings—obtained by a majority of prior studies of whole blood IAD: (1) changes and advances in the field of cardiac surgery that have served to alter the relative effects achieved by IAD, (2) the inconsistent and often inadequate design of previous IAD studies, and most importantly (3) the use of suboptimal IAD technique. It is only through the use of an optimized version of whole blood IAD that maximum blood conservation benefit can be expected. It is only through appropriate prospective randomized study of this optimized version of IAD, in the context of cardiac surgery and blood conservation as currently practiced, that an accurate evaluation of this benefit can be obtained.

TABLE 11.1. Previous controlled IAD studies: blood volumes withdrawn and results.

Study	IAD volume	Results				
		Bleeding	Transfusion	Hematocrit	Platelet count	Platelet/coag function
Schonberger JP, et al (1993)	800 ml	+	+	+	+	o
Szecsi J, et al (1989)	844 ml	+	+	o	o	o
Hardesty et al (1968)	25% EBV (1000 ml)	o	nm	nm	+	+
Cohn L, et al (1975)	500 or 1000 ml	nm	+	nm	nm	nm
Hallowel P, et al (1972)	1252 ml	o	+	o	o	nm
Silver H (1975)	2 units	nm	+	nm	nm	nm
Wagstaffe JG, et al (1972)	840 or 1040 ml	+	nm	nm	+	nm
Dale J, et al (1987)	850 ml	+	+	nm	+	+
Kaplan, JA, et al (1977)	685–768 ml	o	+	nm	+	o
Scott WJ, et al (1992)	575 ml	nm	+	nm	nm	nm
Deitrich W, et al (1989)	725 ml	–	+	o	nm	nm
Ochsner JL, et al (1973)	20% EBV (900 ml)	+	+	nm	+	nm
Cosgrove DM, et al (1979)	625 ml	nm	nm	nm	nm	nm
Ovrum E, et al (1991)	799 ml	nm	nm	nm	nm	nm
Lilleaasen P (1977)	605 ml	+	+	nm	+	nm
Zubiate P, et al (1974)	1000 ml	nm	nm	nm	nm	nm
Sherman et al (1975)	2 units (900 ml)	o	o	nm	nm	nm
Pliam et al (1975)	1270 ml	–	–	nm	nm	nm
Hudson et al (1992)	10% EBV (400 ml)	–	–	nm	nm	nm
Gilmer GD, et al (1992)	17% EBV (650 ml)	–	–	nm	nm	nm

+, benefit obtained from using IAD; o, no benefit from using IAD; –, worse outcome with the use of IAD; nm, not measured.

The Evolving Nature of Cardiac Surgery

The set of circumstances—the blood conservation "background"—upon which whole blood IAD is performed has progressively changed since 1957. At the time of the original IAD study by Dodrill et al,[4] the transfusion requirement was typically between 20 and 30 units of whole donor blood per patient. Two of the major advances in blood conservation—bloodless circuit priming and intraoperative salvage—had not yet been achieved. The CPB circuit itself was relatively crude, with large foreign surface areas and employing the more traumatic bubble oxygenator. In addition, because the safety of hemodilution was not yet accepted, when Dodrill et al removed IAD blood, it was immediately replaced by banked blood (i.e., exchange transfusion). This set of circumstances is far different from that found in practice today. Bloodless circuit prime and intraoperative salvage have become the norm. The CPB circuit has been refined, with decreased volume and surface area, the option of more biocompatible surfaces, less traumatic and lower volume membrane oxygenators, and less traumatic centrifugal pumps. The safety of intraoperative and postoperative hemodilution has been accepted. Pharmacologic agents allowing the manipulation of perioperative red cell mass, and protection of blood from the inflammatory and coagulopathic response to CPB ("blood anesthesia"[82]) are now available. Because of these changes that have occurred in the basic way in which cardiopulmonary bypass and blood conservation are performed, the effects of IAD on bleeding and transfusion requirement in 1995 would be expected to be quite different from those in 1957, and from those in 1975, when only partial progress had been made. Results of studies during these various times therefore must be appropriately interpreted. While the findings of the past yield important information, the efficacy of IAD can only be judged by its performance in conjunction with and in relation to currently practiced blood conservation measures.

The Importance of Study Design

Also underlying the inconsistent findings of previous studies of IAD is a general inadequacy in study design. In a 1994 editorial Lemmer[83] discussed several criteria that must be met by any blood conservation study so that its results can be meaningfully interpreted. If a study is not randomized, then appropriate demographic data must be given to assure uniform distribution of risk factors for bleeding and transfusion. The criteria used for transfusion ("transfusion triggers") must be uniformly applied to each group. The hemoglobin or hematocrit used as the trigger for each transfusion should be recorded to help ensure that there was in fact uniform application of the stated criteria. Recording of the timing of transfusions (e.g., on CPB) is useful in assessing the effects of an intervention. The set of adjuvant therapies should be listed and be similar in the two groups. Data should be recorded as both the percent of patients transfused as well as the average number of units transfused per patient per group. Finally, the use of red cells should be separated from the use of platelets, FFP, and cryoprecipitate, as the former are used to treat low oxygen carrying capacity, the latter postoperative bleeding. Table 11.1 lists the controlled studies of whole blood IAD presented in this section. Evident is the paucity of prospective randomized trials. Analysis also reveals a general lack of appropriate study group matching or controlling for bleeding and transfusion risk factors. The set of transfusion guidelines used was generally not listed, and data allowing assessment of the uniformity of transfusion were generally not available (hematocrits for red cell transfusion; postoperative bleeding for platelet and coagulation factor use). The net result of this general inadequacy in study design is a true difficulty in objectively determining the effectiveness of IAD as a blood conservation measure.

The Importance of IAD Technique

The third and the most important factor underlying the inconsistent findings of previous studies of IAD is the wide variation in IAD technique employed. Only by applying the most effective form of IAD can its true value be revealed and its benefit accurately judged. Analysis of prior IAD studies, and particularly those with negative findings, such as those by Plian[15] and Sherman,[16] reveals that optimization of three general aspects of IAD are important to its becoming a maximally effective blood conservation measure: (1) removal, preservation, and reinfusion of a *calculated safe maximum volume* of autologous blood, (2) use of the *lowest safe level of anemia* as the trigger for red cell transfusion during CPB, and (3) reinfusion of *IAD blood before banked blood* during CPB if withdrawal of IAD leads to hematocrits lower than the identified lowest safe level of anemia. These elements are inexorably linked to one another. Only by identifying the lowest safe level of anemia can the maximum volume of autologous whole blood be removed. Only by using the lowest safe level of anemia to trigger red cell transfusion during CPB can the maximum portion of this withdrawn blood be kept from premature reinfusion during CPB. Only by reinfusing portions or all of this withdrawn blood (and any other available autologous blood) before turning to banked blood can the potential for causing an iatrogenic increase in homologous red cell use be avoided. Put most simply, in order to optimize IAD one must remove and preserve as much blood as is safely possible, and use banked blood only absolutely when necessary.

The Calculated Safe Maximum IAD Volume

As demonstrated in Table 11.1, a majority of studies of IAD have removed relatively small IAD blood volumes.[16,17,19,24,25,28–30] Logic would suggest, however, that if the removal of blood for the purposes of preserving it from harm is good, then the removal of as much blood as possible should provide for the greatest good. While the few studies that removed larger volumes of blood have generally yielded improved results, only two published studies have directly addressed the probable volume-dependent nature of IAD. Cohn et al[12] retrospectively reviewed their experience in 400 consecutive CABG patients and found that patients with 1000 ml of IAD blood removed had a 3.9 unit per patient transfusion requirement versus 4.5 units per patient when 500 ml was removed. We recently prospectively evaluated the volume dependency of IAD's benefit.[75] Patients ($n = 90$) were randomized to three groups: (1) calculated "maximum" volume of IAD blood removed, (2) calculated "small" volume of IAD blood removed (based on target hematocrit on CPB of 23%), and (3) control (no IAD blood removed). A mean of 1607 cc (the equivalent of 32% of the EBV, 22 ml/kg body weight, and 3.4 whole blood units) of whole blood was removed in the large volume group, and 798 cc in the small volume group. The effects of IAD on the red cell and platelet/coagulation compartments of the blood were separately assessed. It was found that while there was a suggestive decrease in red cell transfusion requirement in the small volume group versus the control group (in both the percentage of patients transfused as well as in the mean number of units transfused per patient per group), the decrease in transfusion requirement only became statistically significant when the large volume of IAD blood was removed. Interestingly, no improvement in postoperative bleeding, platelet and coagulation function, or platelet and coagulation factor transfusion requirement was found, indicating that the benefit of IAD was limited to red cell preservation. The volume-dependent reduction in red cell transfusion requirement seen with IAD can be explained by three mechanisms. First, when one third of a patient's blood volume is removed, this portion of blood does not suffer the percentage loss (from hemorrhage and hemolysis) that it would suffer if left in the body and extracorporeal circuit.[84–86] Second, because the remaining two thirds of the patient's red cell mass that does remain in the body is redistributed in the full blood volume, when blood losses do occur into lap pads and discard suckers, the number of the red cells lost per milliliter of blood lost is decreased. Third, during the critical period immediately following separation from CPB, when increases in both blood volume and oxygen carrying capacity are desirable, the simple availability of IAD blood serves to decrease the need for homologous red cell transfusion by allowing for a direct autologous for homologous blood substitution. Immediately after separation from CPB the hematocrit of the patient is approximately what it was at the end of the bypass run—typically 18% to 24%. At this time point patients are typically in need of volume, which at first can be met with residual circuit volume infusion through the arterial line. This unprocessed circuit blood would not be expected to raise the patient's hematocrit, however. Once this initial early source of red cells is depleted, the surgeon or anesthesiologist must turn to crystalloid or colloid support, which serves to lower rather than raise the patient's hematocrit. At this critical time, and particularly if the patient is having difficulty remaining separated from CPB, a decrease in hematocrit is not desirable. Often, therefore, the physician will elect to administer homologous red cells, even though these cells are only temporally necessary (i.e., in the longer run, once the remainder of the residual circuit blood volume has been reinfused and the patient has had time to diurese extra intravascular fluid volume, these transfused red cells will have provided an unnecessary net increase in red cell mass). If fresh whole IAD blood is available at this critical immediate post-CPB time point, however, it can be used to directly replace these homologous red cell transfusions, and in addition provide excellent colloid support. This availability of IAD blood in the immediate post-CPB period is a subtle but essential component of the benefit that it provides.

Because IAD serves to decrease red cell requirements in a volume-dependent manner, when seeking to optimize blood conservation efforts, the maximum amount of blood should be removed from each individual patient. This can be accomplished by calculating the volume of blood to be removed using individual patient parameters (initial hematocrit in the operating room, estimated blood volume), the additional "blood volume" added by the CPB circuit, and by using as a target for this calculation the lowest hematocrit level that can be safely tolerated under conditions of heart-lung bypass (the equations at our institution, as well as details of their clinical application are presented in more depth below). Through calculation and removal of a calculated maximum IAD volume as much blood as possible is spared from operative losses and from degradation and destruction by the CPB apparatus, and maximum red cell savings can be obtained.

The Lowest Safe Level of Anemia

The maximum volume IAD calculation must take into account the two distinct stages of hemodilution that occur when IAD is performed in the setting of cardiopulmonary bypass. The first stage of hemodilution occurs in conjunction with the acute removal of IAD blood prior to CPB, and the drop in hematocrit that occurs is directly related to the amount of fluid replacement that is administered. The "drier" that a patient is kept, the less the drop in hematocrit that is seen. The second level of hemodilution occurs when the patient is placed on the heart-lung apparatus. The initiation of bypass causes a redistribution of the patient's remaining red cell mass in a new blood volume—that consisting of the plasma volume filling the patient's blood vessels combined with the priming solution volume filling the components of the CPB apparatus (i.e., tubing, oxygenator). The two-step hemodilution that occurs with use of IAD and CPB necessarily leads to more advanced degrees of anemia than typically experienced in other forms of surgery. While deep anesthesia, hypothermia, and cardiac protection enable an increased tolerance to low oxygen carrying capacity, there nevertheless exists a physiological lowest safe level of hemodilution and anemia that should not be transcended. In order for the technique of IAD to be optimized in respect to the volume of blood removed, it is therefore paramount that the lowest safe level of anemia be identified.

Chapter 16 discusses indications for red cell transfusion and reviews the laboratory and clinical data delineating the lowest safe level of anemia both prior to and during CPB. In the non-CPB setting optimal oxygen delivery from a rheologic standpoint has been shown to occur at a hematocrit of 30%,[87–89] but several studies suggest that hematocrits lower than this number are well tolerated,[90,91] and may even be protective in the setting of ischemia.[92] Nevertheless, 30% can be used as an appropriate number for the hematocrit that should not be transgressed during the preoperative period when performing IAD. In fact, with appropriate but judicious administration of fluid, the hematocrit is seldom found to drop below the 30% mark. In a prospective study of large volume hemodilution versus control we found that even with removal of an average of 1549 ml of whole blood from patients with an average preoperative hematocrit of 39% and a mean body weight of 79 kg, our average pre-CPB hematocrit was 33 ± 3%, only 3% lower than patients in the control group.[75] Only two patients experienced post-IAD, pre-CPB hematocrits of less than 30% (lowest = 26.9%), and these patients did not demonstrate any adverse sequelae.

Clinical data regarding tolerance to anemia during CPB are largely anecdotal,[10,93] but points to a lower acceptance hematocrit level of 15%. Because the heart is relatively protected during CPB, other organs such as the brain serve as better markers of the adequacy of oxygen delivery. Recent data suggest that a hematocrit of at least 15% is adequate to maintain cerebral oxygen delivery under conditions of moderate hypothermia.[94] Laboratory data support the safety of a 15% transfusion trigger during CPB.[95] It has been our own clinical experience that a hematocrit during CPB of 15% is well tolerated, and we use this number both as the trigger for red cell transfusion during CPB, and as the basis for establishing the "target" hematocrit on CPB of 18% that is used in our calculation of the maximum IAD volume (see below).[31]

Reinfusion of IAD Blood Before Banked Blood

The goal of IAD is to decrease homologous transfusion requirement by preserving a maximum amount of the patient's own blood from the destructive effects of the heart-lung apparatus. As discussed above, this maximum amount of blood can be obtained by removing a volume that is calculated with respect to individual patient blood volume and CPB circuit parameters, as well as to the lowest safe hematocrit during CPB. However, the final goal of reducing transfusion requirement through maximum autologous preservation can only be met if the removed IAD volume is actually kept from the CPB circuit, and if this preservation does not somehow paradoxically lead to an increase in homologous blood use. These two stipulations can be met, and the final goal achieved, by adhering to two basic guidelines regarding the use of blood during CPB. First, all transfusions given during CPB must be administered only if the hematocrit falls below the safe level of anemia. Second, when the patient's hematocrit does drop to or below the lowest safe level of anemia, IAD blood must be reinfused before banked blood.

A majority of previous studies have returned only banked blood during CPB, preferring to preserve the IAD blood for reinfusion post-CPB. It was thought that the IAD blood contained fresh platelets and clotting factors, and that these should be saved to help to correct the relative coagulopathy that accompanies use of the heart-lung apparatus. This logic has two pitfalls, however. First, it assumes that IAD and reinfusion of relatively fresh whole blood post-CPB decreases coagulopathic bleeding. This has never been clearly demonstrated in the past (Table 11.1), a past with a noted paucity of prospective randomized controlled trials. In a recent prospective study of 90 patients undergoing CABG surgery, half of whom were randomized to have a mean IAD volume of 1589 ml removed, we clearly demonstrated a complete lack of benefit with respect to decreasing postoperative bleeding.[75] In fact, even when the 13 patients in the large volume IAD group who had 1800 cc or more of fresh whole blood reinfused were analyzed separately, no improvement in postoperative bleeding was seen. Withholding IAD blood for reinfusion post-CPB therefore cannot be justified on this basis. The second conceptual difficulty with reinfusing banked red cells before IAD blood during CPB is the very real potential for paradoxically increasing homologous red use, particularly when large volume IAD is utilized. Removal of such large volumes necessarily decreases the hematocrit during CPB. If a sufficiently low transfusion trigger is not utilized, the chances of reaching hematocrits below the trigger are markedly increased by performing IAD. If banked blood is utilized for these breaches, patients with very adequate *overall* autologous red cell mass (the IAD volume plus the volume remaining in the patient) have the very real chance of being transfused simply because their hematocrit was transiently and iatrogenically lowered during CPB by the IAD process.[14] Following reinfusion of IAD blood post-CPB, patients who are transfused with banked blood in such a way typically have unnecessarily high hematocrits, indicating that the homologous transfusion during CPB was in fact unnecessary. We chose in our above study to reinfuse all IAD blood before banked in order to eliminate the possibility of unnecessary red cell transfusion.[75] By adopting this strategy 5 of the 11 patients in the IAD group who required return of part or all of their IAD blood during CPB were spared unnecessary homologous red cell transfusion, as postoperatively, following reinfusion of the remaining IAD blood, no additional homologous red cells or other blood products were required.

Clinical Application of Maximum Volume IAD

In the previous section the findings and shortcomings of previous IAD studies were discussed, and this information was used to outline the fundamentals for optimally performing whole blood IAD. Concisely stated, the general concept is that the maximum amount of autologous blood must be preserved without causing patient injury or a paradoxical increase in homologous blood requirement. This section presents the step-by-step details of how this is done at New York Hospital–Cornell Medical Center.

Patient Selection

A majority of cardiac surgical patients are eligible to have IAD performed. Two general factors must be assessed in judging the both the suitability of a patient to undergo IAD and the amount of blood that can be withdrawn: (1) disease status, and (2) starting hematocrit and red cell mass in the operating room.

A traditional contraindication to *preoperative* autologous donation and blood donation in general—advanced cardiac disease—cannot be applied to the cardiac surgical patient undergoing IAD, as it is a severe cardiac disease that has brought the patient to the operating room.[96] Obviously the traditional blood donation criteria must be modified. In fact, only one disease situation precludes the use of IAD in the cardiac surgical patient, and only a handful more limit the amount of blood that should be withdrawn. The only absolute contraindication to the use of IAD is ongoing bacteremia or septicemia.[97] The difficulty in this situation (e.g., septic endocarditis) lies in the withdrawal of microorganisms into the IAD bags along with the patient's blood. The typical 2- to 3-hour room temperature storage period theoretically would allow for unencountered organism growth, and therefore for the potential of a very deleterious reinfusion of microorganisms following termination of CPB.

While not directly contraindicating the use of IAD, several other disease states do serve to limit the amount of blood that should be withdrawn, primarily by requiring that oxygen delivery not be compromised during the pre-CPB period. These states include active ischemia (emergent revascularization procedures), severe left main coronary artery disease, and severe cerebrovascular disease. In these states stenoses that critically limit flow require that the hematocrit not drop significantly below 30%—the level that for rheologic considerations provides for optimal oxygen delivery under these conditions.[87,88] For these same reasons it is critical to maintain sufficient volume status in these patients by adequately replacing withdrawn blood with crystalloid.[98] This ensures adequate cardiac output and helps to maintain perfusion pressure. While we have found that in most cardiac surgical patients a 1.8:1 ratio of fluid to blood removed is sufficient to maintain hemodynamic stability, in patients with critical vascular stenoses more liberal and "traditional" replacement of 2.5–3:1 should be utilized. This full volume resuscitation necessarily leads to more rapid and advanced hemodilution prior to the initiation of CPB, and so less blood is able to be withdrawn. In these patients we typically remove blood more slowly, giving liberal replacement as needed according to systemic blood pressure, filling pressures, and cardiac index. Because patients respond differently, a hematocrit is checked after the first bag. An additional bag is withdrawn if the hematocrit is above 33% to 35%, depending on the patient's size. Usually no more than two IAD bags (approximately 1000 ml) are withdrawn from these patients.

While the patients with critical coronary vascular stenoses are largely protected from their lesions during and presumably following CPB, patients with cerebrovascular disease are less protected, particularly during normothermic perfusion and during times of low pressure/flow. In patients with a history of stroke or severe cerebrovascular or peripheral vascular disease, in addition to maintaining the pre-CPB hematocrit above 30%, we prefer to maintain the hematocrit at 18% or above during CPB. In this specific subgroup of patients we therefore modify the maximum volume IAD calculation (see the following section) to include a higher target hematocrit during CPB, and only allow the hematocrit to decrease to 18% during CPB before reinfusing withdrawn IAD blood.

Concern has traditionally been voiced against the withdrawal of blood from patients with critical aortic stenoses. More recent studies in the preoperative autologous donation literature, however, have provided clear evidence that with appropriate monitoring and adequate fluid replacement, donation in these patients can be safely and successfully performed.[99-102] Analysis of the physiology of aortic stenosis reveals that it is not low hematocrit itself that places these patients in a compromised position, but hemodynamic alterations that are often associated with low hematocrit that serve to alter either stroke volume or increase heart rate—namely, hypovolemia and or tachycardia. Therefore, while IAD is not contraindicated in aortic stenosis (in fact in no other situation are hemodynamics more intensely monitored and controlled by a more highly trained specialists than in the operating room), care should be taken to appropriately and fully replace withdrawn blood with crystalloid to maintain ventricular filling and stroke volume, and to avoid diastolic perfusion limiting reflex tachycardia.

The second factor that must be used to guide patient eligibility for IAD is the hematocrit and red cell mass of the patient. This is for strictly mathematical reasons: If the patient does not have enough red cell mass to yield a hematocrit on CPB of 15% or greater (18% or greater if severe cerebrovascular or peripheral vascular disease is present), then IAD cannot be performed. The IAD calculation discussed in the following section can be used to determine who these patients are. Eligibility according to this criterion will necessarily vary among institutions depending on such factors

$$HCT_{pre\ CPB} = HCT_{Target} \times (EBV + 1400) / EBV$$
$$IAD\ VOLUME = EBV\ (HT_{Initial} - HCT_{Pre\ CPB}) / HCT_{Initial}$$

$HCT_{Pre\ CPB}$ = hematocrit post-IAD withdrawal, immediately prior to initiation of CPB.
HCT_{Target} = hematocrit desired during CPB (we utilize a value of 18%).
EBV = patient's estimated blood volume based on a height-weight-sex normogram.
1400 ml = CPB circiut prime volume.
$HCT_{Initial}$ = hematocrit value obtained in the operating room prior to IAD blood withdrawal.

FIGURE 11.1. Equations used to calculate the maximum volume of autologous blood that can be safely removed from any given patient during the intraoperateive pre-CPB period.

as the amount of crystalloid administered prior to and during CPB, and the CPB circuit volume.

Calculating the Volume of Blood to Be Withdrawn

Based on this simple concept of serial hemodilution, and using 15% as the lowest safe level of anemia, we have developed two equations that allow the maximum volume IAD calculation to be easily performed (Fig. 11.1). Similar equations have been put forth by others.[30,103–106] The first equation uses the patient's estimated blood volume and the circuit prime volume to back-calculate what hematocrit just prior to CPB would yield a target hematocrit on CPB of 18% (18% is used as the target hematocrit in the IAD calculation to allow a one-unit safety margin against overwithdrawal of blood, and to allow for a 2 to 3 percentage point drift downward to the lowest safe 15% hematocrit level that typically occurs during CPB). The result of this first equation is the hematocrit that when present immediately prior to CPB will yield a hematocrit of 18% on CPB.*

The patient's estimated blood volume can be easily calculated based on patient weight, or a more accurate estimate can be made using a gender-specific height-weight nomogram. We have found the height-weight sex tables generated by Albert[107] (using the Hidalgo et al[108] equation) to be particularly useful. The CPB circuit volume can vary greatly between institutions. Chapter 12 stresses the importance of using the smallest possible CPB circuit, and consequently the lowest possible circuit prime

*This post-IAD hematocrit is a hypothetical number based on the theoretical assumption that full intravascular volume replacement is administered. We have found this to be unnecessary, however, and we typically administer only 50% to 60% of the traditional 3:1 crystalloid (to blood removed) volume. Intravascular equilibration therefore does not typically occur when using IAD, and the hematocrit measured following IAD blood removal but prior to CPB is typically 3 to 5 percentage points higher than the number predicted by the equation.

volume, as it is the volume of crystalloid and new synthetic vascular space (the tubing, reservoir, and filters) into which the patient's red cells must spread that determines the drop in hematocrit that will occur with initiation of CPB. Until 1993 our institution utilized a CPB circuit with a prime volume of 2200 ml. With adjustments in tubing size and length and a change to a smaller volume oxygenator, this volume has been decreased by 45% to 1200 ml, and the volume of IAD blood that can be safely withdrawn has increased proportionately. Further decrease in the CPB circuit crystalloid prime volume can be achieved with the technique of anterograde-retrograde autologous prime, by which the patient's blood is used to replace the prime solution in the CPB immediately prior to CPB by draining blood both retrograde from the aortic root cannulae and anterograde through the venous cannulae (Chapter 12). The cumulative effect of combining the use of a low prime circuit with autologous blood circuit priming is impressive. In a recent review of our perfusion experience, all patients undergoing CABG procedures during 1993, prior to the introduction of the low prime circuit and autologous blood circuit priming, were compared to all patients undergoing CABG during 1994, after the introduction of these two circuit and circuit prime volume limiting techniques.[109] It was found that despite an increase in the amount of total IAD blood withdrawn prior to CPB (1.6 units vs 0.8 unit), and a 50% decrease in the number of homologous PRBC units transfused during CPB, the mean low hematocrit was 20% higher during CPB (20% vs 18%) in the minimum prime group. Risk-adjusted outcomes such as length of hospital stay, postoperative complications, and mortality were not different between the two groups, suggesting overall safety as well as efficacy.

The hematocrit derived from the first equation is used in the second equation to calculate, based on the patient's starting hematocrit in the operating room and estimated blood volume, the volume of blood that must be removed from the patient in order to achieve the target CPB hematocrit of 18%. The patient's starting hematocrit is typically determined on arrival in the operating room following arterial line insertion. It is important to use this number, and not the preoperative value, as hematocrit changes often occur during the night prior to surgery while the patient is NPO, and during anesthetic induction when significant volumes of fluid may be infused. In addition, the device used to measure the hematocrit in the operating theater is often different from the one used at other times. In our institution a Coulter counter is used to measure hematocrits in the ICU and on the patient floor, while a blood gas machine (Instrumentation Laboratories) is used in the operating room. These machines measure hematocrit by different methodologies, and we have found hematocrits to be approximately 1 to 2 percentage points lower when using the blood gas apparatus.

The IAD calculation typically yields a value in the range of 1200 to 2000 ml. A 70-kg 5′10″ male with a starting hematocrit in the operating room of 40%, and using a CPB circuit with a total prime volume of 2000 ml, would lead to a calculated IAD volume of 1819 ml. A similarly sized female patient with the same starting hematocrit would have a calculated volume of 1575 ml. These values are meant as guides only. While it is not recommended that more than this calculated volume be removed, it may be desirable to remove less than this volume depending on the patient's clinical status, as well as on the way in which the patient's intraoperative pre-CPB course unfolds.

Method of Blood Withdrawal

As soon as the first hematocrit in the operating room has been drawn (typically following arterial line insertion) and the cordis introducer and Swan-Ganz catheter are placed, the donation process can be initiated. In a majority of cases we remove the blood from a 9.0-F cordis introducer (Arrow International, Inc., Reading, PA) that has a special large bore side port and high-flow stopcock. Previous to the introduction of this larger catheter in 1993, we had used the side port of an 8.5-F cordis introducer for blood withdrawal, and found that often, because of low flow rates, it was difficult to obtain the full IAD volume. The inability to obtain the required blood volume rarely occurs with the new wide bore cordis, even with a 5-lumen Swan-Ganz catheter in place. Alternatively, a separate 14-G internal or external jugular vein line can be inserted. This is occasionally done at our institution when a patient is on multiple medications and has poor peripheral access.

The blood bags used for IAD collection are identical to those used for standard donor blood collection. We use bags containing CPDA-1 anticoagulant* (Baxter Healthcare Corp., Deerfield, IL).[110] The bags are labeled with the patient's name, history number, and date prior to the initiation of collection. The needle of the blood collection line is inserted into a rubberized adapter port attached to an in-line stopcock. We have found that it is helpful to collect the blood with the blood bags placed on a special rocker scale that both weighs and continuously agitates the blood bags during collection (Donormatic DM-S Automatic Donor Scale, Lifeline Instruments, San Jose, CA). We began using these scales when we realized that the occasional clots that were encountered in the IAD bags were consistently attributable to two causes: (1) inadequate CPD-blood mixing, and (2) low blood flow rates, which allowed stasis and coagulation in the collection line as the blood was being collected. The use of the rocker scale

*CPDA-1 anticoagulant contains 26.3 g/L trisodium citrate, 3.27 g/L citric acid, 31.9 g/L dextrose, 22 g/L monobasic sodium phosphate, and 0.275 g/L adenine. Citrate is used to bind most of the ionized calcium and therefore prevent activation of the calcium-dependent steps of the coagulation cascade. Additionally, it acts to retard glycolysis. Dextrose and adenine are used to support continued adenosine triphosphate (ATP) generation by stored red cells, which remain active even at the recommended blood bank storage temperature of 1° to 6°C. Sodium phosphate is used as a buffer to maintain pH during storage.

ensures adequate CPD-blood mixing, while at the same time allowing the rate of bag filling to be monitored. If the rate is seen to slow, the position of the cordis/neck is adjusted. If the rate remains slow, a 10- to 20-ml syringe is attached in line to the cordis side port from which the blood is being drawn, and 10 to 15 ml of blood is drawn from the patient. This blood is then directed into the blood bag. Typically this flushing maneuver will reestablish flow, and can be repeated as necessary. When a bag is filled to the recommended volume of 450 to 500 ml, the needle is withdrawn from the port, several occluding knots are tied in the collection line, and the needle is severed and placed in an appropriate "sharps" container. The bag is numbered and the weight of the bag is recorded on the perfusion and anesthesia flow sheets. The filled bags are placed in a designated area in the operating room until the time of reinfusion.

Minor debate exists in the literature over when and from what line the IAD blood should be withdrawn. The most commonly applied methods utilize blood withdrawal from the venous side of the circulation, either through the central venous catheter,[12,13,27,111] as practiced at our institution, or through the venous cannulae of the CPB circuit as CPB is initiated.[7,9,21,24] Less commonly, blood is drawn from the arterial circulation, either through the radial arterial line during the pre-CPB period,[9,10,111] or from the aortic cannulae immediately prior to CPB.[97] Withdrawal through the radial arterial line is least commonly practiced and not recommended as patient blood pressure monitoring is lost during the time that blood is being removed. When removing large volumes of IAD blood, this lost monitoring time can constitute much of the pre-CPB period, a period of time during which adequate monitoring of blood pressure is crucial, particularly when large volumes of blood are being drained. Removal of blood immediately prior to bypass either through the arterial or venous cannulae is simple and easy to perform, but it has at least four relative drawbacks. First, the blood removed in this manner is fully heparinized, theoretically compromising platelet function, and necessitating additional protamine titration following IAD reinfusion. Heparinization is no longer recognized by the American Association of Blood Banks (AABB) as an appropriate form for long-term (>48 hours) *homologous* blood storage, and is recommended that blood not be stored in heparin for longer than 8 hours.[112] Heparin is an activator of the complement system,[113,114] and has been shown to have detrimental effects on platelet function.[115–118] In addition, because dextrose and adenine substrates are lacking when blood is stored in heparin, no preservative function is provided. This may become particularly important at the room temperatures in which IAD blood is typically stored. Conversely, citrate storage is the AABB recommended form of storage for virtually all blood.[110] Citrate is an inhibitor of complement; it inhibits unwanted red cell glycolysis and metabolism during storage, and provides substrate and buffering capacity to support the metabolism that does occur.[110] Although comparison of the results obtained by the IAD studies using heparin[7,9,14–16,25] and citrate[8–10,12,13,15,16,19,21] storage reveals no clear difference in respect to reduction in postoperative bleeding, the removal of blood into bags containing citrate anticoagulant prior to heparinization is theoretically preferable.

The second drawback to blood removal through the CPB circuit lines at the time of initiation of CPB is that it typically does not allow the removal of as much blood as possible (i.e., the "maximum" calculated volume). The importance of the removal of the maximum possible volume of IAD blood has been emphasized throughout this chapter, and is supported both clinically[12,31,75] as well as theoretically.[106] With appropriate patient monitoring and fluid supplementation, it is relatively simple over the full 45- to 90-minute pre-CPB period to slowly remove 1200 to 1800 ml of whole blood from a typical cardiac surgical patient. The acute and rapid removal of this same volume might be expected to cause significant hemodynamic derangement, particularly when superimposed on the already significant and obligatory physiologic insult of initiating CPB.

The third argument against the acute withdrawal of the IAD volume at the time of bypass initiation is that it does not provide protection (against red cell mass loss) during the entire pre-CPB period while chest opening, mammary artery preparation, and saphenous vein harvesting are taking place. It is during this time that significant blood losses occur into lap pads, sponges, and discard suckers. The one third of the patient's blood that could have been protected from such loss is not, and the blood that is lost has a higher concentration of autologous components. If IAD is performed at the onset of CPB, significant, unnecessary, and irreplaceable red cell losses have already occurred, and an important component of the benefit that IAD provides is therefore lost.

Fourth and finally, the acute removal of the IAD volume as bypass is begun precludes the use of complementary blood conservation techniques such as anteroretrograde autologous blood priming of the CPB circuit. By withdrawing IAD blood slowly over time prior to CPB the patient is allowed to maintain relatively stable hemodynamic and volume status. This allows the perfusionist to minimize the hemodilution that occurs at the initiation of bypass by acutely draining most of the crystalloid from the circuit and replacing it with autologous blood from the patient. Autologous blood is drained anterograde from the patient through the venous cannulae to displace the venous side prime, and retrograde through the aortic cannulae to displace the prime filling the arterial side of the CPB circuit. This is performed immediately prior to and during the initiation of CPB. It is difficult to imagine this technique being applied concurrently with and in addition to acute IAD at the initiation of CPB, without causing acute and severe intravascular depletion. Conversely, the withdrawal of IAD through the central venous cordis is simple, allows for appropriate patient monitoring and fluid resuscitation, and allows the maximum amount of blood to be safely and successfully removed and preserved for post-CPB reinfusion.

During IAD withdrawal, patient monitoring needs are altered only in that additional attention must be paid to the patient's systemic blood pressure, in conjunction with their filling pressures and cardiac index. As stated previously, a crystalloid replacement to IAD blood removed ratio of 1.5–2:1 is typically adequate to maintain hemodynamic stability while at the same time minimizing hemodilution. Patients with ongoing ischemia, poor ventricular function, or other significantly compromising cardiac or vascular lesions should be more fully volume resuscitated as required on an individual basis.

Method of Preservation

The optimal way in which to preserve withdrawn IAD blood during the 2- to 3-hour period that it is outside the body has yet to be determined. Several issues remain unresolved, primarily because IAD is such a specialized procedure typically left in the hands of anesthesiologists and surgeons whose primary concern is the operation at hand. These preservation issues include (1) the type of anticoagulant, (2) the importance of agitation, and (3) storage temperature.

The type of anticoagulant-preservative solution optimal for IAD storage remains to be determined. As discussed in the previous section, while the use of citrate-based storage solutions is theoretically preferable to simple heparinization, IAD studies to date have not shown one or the other of these two methods of anticoagulation to be superior. Because, for the reasons stated in the previous section, we prefer to draw blood throughout the pre-CPB period, and because of the preservation benefits provided by the dextrose, adenine, and phosphate contained in CPDA-1, we utilize this method of anticoagulation-preservation.

Several additive solutions are Food and Drug Administration (FDA) approved and available to enhance RBC survival in homologous and autologous blood stored for blood bank utilization. These include AS-1 (Adsol), AS-3 (Nutrical), and AS-5 (Optisol).[119,120] Each is a 100-ml mixture of additional glucose, adenine, and other nutrients that is contained in a satellite bag that is introduced to the primary citrate whole blood mixture immediately following collection. Although the use of these additive solutions is theoretically appealing in the perioperative setting, particularly when blood is stored for longer periods or at higher operating room temperatures, their use for intraoperative purposes has not yet been investigated.

Other potential solutions for enhancement of blood survival have been investigated in the blood banking literature as well. Of particular note are investigations concerning the use of aprotinin to enhance platelet and coagulation factor preservation in stored blood. The effectiveness of aprotinin in ameliorating the inflammatory coagulopathy of CPB is well established. Less well known are investigations of the use of aprotinin to enhance platelet and coagulation factor preservation in blood collection bags.[121-123] For example, Bode and Norris[124] recently investigated the effects of a wide range of inhibitors of platelet activation and protease activity on stored platelet concentrates. It is interesting to note that of the wide range of inhibitors tested by these authors, both alone and in combination, aprotinin yielded the most significant improvement in platelet numerical, morphologic, and functional preservation. Because aprotinin is becoming more widely used in the cardiopulmonary bypass setting, and because its infusion is typically started prior to or during IAD collection, similar blood levels to those achieved in the body are achieved in the IAD bags. The presence of aprotinin in these bags may help to improve short-term platelet and coagulation factor preservation, and limit the inflammatory response that occurs during preservation. Although our recent studies with large maximum volume IAD have clearly demonstrated that whole blood reinfusion post-CPB does not decrease coagulopathic bleeding,[31,75] perhaps aprotinin-enhanced preservation of this maximum volume of platelets and coagulation factors would allow IAD to provide this benefit. Our studies in the Jehovah's Witness population, in whom both maximum volume IAD and aprotinin were utilized as part of an overall comprehensive blood conservation approach, support this possibility.[125] Despite their very high risk for excessive bleeding, these patients were found to bleed exceptionally small amounts following their open-heart procedures. Although the chest tube drainage volumes were significantly less when compared to patients receiving large volume IAD only, the absence of a control group receiving full-strength aprotinin only does not allow the possible benefits to be formally assessed and statistically validated. A study assessing the combined use of aprotinin and large volume IAD is currently under way at our institution.

A second issue of importance with respect to the optimal storage of IAD blood during the time that it is outside the body is optimal storage temperature. Two competing forces must be considered: (1) the reduction in metabolism and protein activation and consumption afforded by hypothermia, and (2) the derangements in platelet and coagulation factor function caused by hypothermia. Fortunately, typical operating room temperature serves to strike a balance between the two. While the AABB recommends storage of red cells at 1° to 6°C, it allows up to 8 hours of room temperature temporary storage until the time of separation into components (enough nutrient substrate is available in the CPDA-1 bags to support an 8-hour room temperature storage period).[2] Because ambient operating room temperature is typically relatively hypothermic (22°–24°C) in comparison to "normal" room temperature, the relatively short-term IAD storage time at these temperatures would be expected to provide for a healthy red cell population. While hypothermia is desirable for red cell storage, hypothermia is at least transiently detrimental to platelet function. Moderate hypothermia during CPB (26°–32°C) has been shown to decrease platelet thromboxane A_2 synthesis,[126] inhibit in vitro aggregation,[127] and prolong in vivo bleeding time.[127,128] The AABB, however, recommends platelet storage at 20° to 24°C (what the cardiac surgeon or anesthesiologist would consider moderate to severe hypothermia).[129] Operating room temperatures at our institution are typically in the range of 22° to 24°C, which approximates this AABB target temperature. The function of platelets contained in IAD blood stored at room temperature would therefore not be expected to be compromised relative to donor platelets on the basis of operating room hypothermia alone. Room temperature IAD storage appears to provide for an appropriate balance between the needs of the blood platelets and red cell populations.

An issue that has arisen in our own application of IAD, and that has been discussed previously, is the importance of IAD bag agitation during collection and storage. Agitation during collection allows for continuous and complete mixing of blood with anticoagulant-preservative. We have found a combined rocker-scale device to be particularly useful for the collection of IAD blood. The scale is useful to ensure filling to the AABB recommended 450 ± 10% ml blood volume for the standard collection bags.[110] Actual calculated IAD volumes should be rounded to the nearest multiple of 400 to 500 ml so that this ratio is maintained in all bags.

Method of Reinfusion

Withdrawn IAD blood can be returned either during CPB or following CPB, with the goal being the latter. Blood is only returned during CPB if the transfusion trigger being utilized (15% at our institution) is breached. An ordered protocol for red cell transfusion is used for these breaches in an effort to maximize the volume of IAD blood kept from reinfusion during CPB, and to minimize the use of homologous red cells. When the hematocrit decreases to 15% or less, the first maneuver is to immediately process and reinfuse all available salvaged blood from the Cell Saver reservoir. If excess cardiotomy reservoir volume is available, this can be transferred to the Cell Saver for processing and reinfusion as well. If this volume is judged to be insufficient, either by volume estimate or a rechecking of the hematocrit, or if no Cell Saver is available, then one unit of IAD blood is immediately reinfused into the CPB circuit through a 40-U filter. The hematocrit is then rechecked, and additional units of IAD blood are reinfused as required. Only after all IAD blood has been returned to the patient are banked red cells utilized.

Reinfusion of the IAD blood is initiated following termination of CPB. Ideally, reinfusion should be started after protamine reversal of heparin. This decreases exposure of the preserved blood to the detrimental effects of

TABLE 11.2. Order of blood product reinfusion during and following cardiopulmonary bypass.

A. During CPB
1. Preoperatively donated autologous blood (PAD)
2. Intraoperatively donated autologous blood (IAD)
3. Allogeneic (banked) packed red cells (platelets, FFP, and cryoprecipitate not indicated)
B. Following CPB
1. IAD blood
2. Cell Saver/Residual circuit blood
3. PAD blood
4. Allogeneic blood

heparin, and in addition allows time for immediate post-CPB bleeding attributable to heparin anticoagulation to subside, preventing what would otherwise be immediate and unnecessary loss of part of the preserved IAD blood. While it is therefore optimal to wait until after protamine reversal to reinfuse the IAD blood, the gains are modest and must be weighed against the need for adequate oxygen carrying capacity in this immediate post-CPB period. We therefore base the timing of IAD reinfusion on the last (weaning) hematocrit measured during CPB. If this hematocrit is less than 20% (19% or less), then we initiate IAD reinfusion immediately upon termination of CPB, not waiting for protamine reversal. If the hematocrit is 20% or greater, then reinfusion is initiated after the initial protamine dose is given. The IAD blood is reinfused as rapidly as possible, and always through a blood warming device. Typically two to three units of IAD blood can be reinfused over a 20- to 40-minute period post-CPB, as most patients are in need of volume during this period. All blood is returned to the patient; units that are not able to be infused in the operating room (a relatively rare occurrence) are reinfused in the postoperative intensive care unit. IAD blood reinfusion is followed by reinfusion of all available Cell Saver or otherwise processed residual CPB apparatus blood. The IAD reinfusion protocol utilized at the New York Hospital–Cornell Medical Center is summarized in Table 11.2.

Use in Combination with Other Blood Conservation Measures

The use of IAD in conjunction with other blood conservation measures is both unavoidable and essential. References to such interactions have been made throughout this chapter. IAD can be used in addition to preoperative autologous donation. Ideally, PAD should be performed at least 3 weeks in advance of surgery to allow for sufficient red cell mass regeneration by the time of surgery, so that IAD can be performed as well. When withdrawing

IAD blood, crystalloid administration should be minimized in order to limit the degree of unnecessary hemodilution that occurs. A minimum volume CPB oxygenator and circuit should be used, and retrograde autologous circuit priming should be performed to further minimize the hemodilution that occurs with the combined use of IAD and CPB. The lowest safe level of anemia should be pursued and allowed during CPB, so that maximum IAD blood can be preserved from loss and destruction. Intraoperative cell salvage should be used skin to skin (with appropriate washing using a Cell Saver–type apparatus) to minimize autologous red cell losses, but also to provide red cells for use as a buffer against the need for IAD reinfusion during CPB. Following CPB, IAD reinfusion should be completed as rapidly as clinically possible in order to restore oxygen carrying capacity. This is followed by residual CPB circuit blood reinfusion, and then by shed mediastinal blood reinfusion in the ICU. Newer adjuvant pharmacologic blood conservation therapies such as aprotinin may work in concert with IAD to improve its effectiveness in combating the coagulopathy of CPB. Although IAD as currently practiced does not by itself decrease postoperative coagulopathic bleeding, it does provide mechanical protection of one quarter to one third of a patient's platelets and plasma. Methods to suppress the inflammatory response to CPB such as aprotinin and the use of biocompatible CPB circuits may improve the hemostatic effectiveness of these preserved platelets and factors. This may be achieved not only by decreasing the inflammatory coagulopathy in the two thirds of patient's blood that remains in the circuit and into which the IAD blood must be reinfused post-CPB, but also through a direct improvement in IAD preservation. As discussed previously, because aprotinin is started prior to IAD collection during the pre-CPB period, the same aprotinin concentration that is achieved in the body is achieved in the IAD bags. There is evidence in the blood banking literature that the presence of aprotinin in blood bags may improve platelet preservation in these bags.[124] This potential for aprotinin to improve the quality of the IAD product is currently under investigation at our institution.

Special Situations: The Jehovah's Witness Population

The Jehovah's Witness faith does not allow the use of homologous blood. It also typically does not allow the use of autologous blood once this blood has been separated from the body. The use of the heart-lung machine is allowed, however, because the column of blood circulating in the CPB circuit remains in continuous contact with the body's own circulation (a "continuous closed circuit") at all times. This same principle can be used to construct a specialized IAD circuit so that the intraoperative collection, preservation, and reinfusion of autologous blood can be performed in adherence to Jehovah's Witness Church doctrine. The existence of this key "loophole" allows heart surgery to be performed in this population with much greater safety and efficacy than previously possible, for it is this group of patients more than any other that requires maximum red cell preservation.

The circuit developed at the New York Hospital–Cornell Medical Center for use in the Jehovah's Witness population utilized a closed loop originating and ending at a series of stopcocks attached to the 9.0-F wide-bore cordis introducer. The blood bag is spiked with a preprimed reinfusion line prior to blood collection. This reinfusion line and the blood bag collection line are then both attached to the cordis stopcocks, thereby establishing a closed circuit prior to opening of the stopcock and blood collection. Blood collection and reinfusion are thereby able to be performed through a continuous closed circuit that remains connected to the patient at all times. We have collected up to five bags of IAD blood from a single patient using this method.

Summary

Intraoperative autologous blood donation practices serve to preserve a portion of the cardiac surgical patient's blood from intraoperative loss and destruction. While the relatively expensive and labor intensive selective preservation of platelets has demonstrated little clinical benefit, intraoperative removal of whole blood clearly provides an important mechanism for preserving autologous red cell mass. When striving to achieve optimal blood conservation results using whole blood IAD, attention to details that help to maximize its effectiveness is essential. Central is the removal and preservation of a maximum volume of autologous blood from each individual patient. However, this removal must be accomplished in a procedural context that allows for full expression of the benefit of IAD, while at the same time ensuring patient safety. Future improvements in IAD storage technique, and in blood anesthesia in general, may ultimately unlock the potential of whole blood IAD to improve postoperative platelet and coagulation factor function and to decrease postoperative bleeding.

References

1. Etchason J, Petz L, Keeler E, et al. The cost effectiveness of preoperative autologous blood donation. *N Engl J Med* 1995;332:719–724.
2. Walker RH, ed. *American Association of Blood Banks Technical Manual.* 11th ed. Bethesda, MD: American Association of Blood Banks, 1993;66.
3. Walker RH, ed. *American Association of Blood Banks Technical Manual.* 11th ed. Bethesda, MD: American Association of Blood Banks, 1993;61.
4. Dodrill FD, Marshall N, Nyboer J, et al. The use of the heart-lung apparatus in human cardiac surgery. *J Thorac Surg* 1957;33(1):60–73.
5. Internal Memo. The New York Hospital–Cornell Medical Center Blood Bank records/archives. 1958.

6. Grant FC. Autotransfusion. *Ann Surg* 1921;74:253–254.
7. Hardesty RL, Bayer WL, Bahnson HT. Technique for the use of autologous fresh blood during open-heart surgery. *J Thorac Cardiovasc Surg* 1968; 56(5):683–688.
8. Hallowel P, Bland MB, Buckley M, et al. Transfusion of fresh autologous blood in open-heart surgery. *J Thorac Cardiovasc Surg* 1972;64(6):941–948.
9. Wagstaffe JG, Clarke AD, Jackson PW. Reduction of blood loss by restoration of platelet levels using fresh autologous blood after cardiopulmonary bypass. *Thorax* 1972;27:410–414.
10. Ochsner JL, Mills NL, Leonard GL, et al. Fresh autologous blood transfusions with extracorporeal circulation. *Ann Surg* 1973;177(6):811–817.
11. Zubiate P, Kay JH, Mendez AH, et al. Coronary artery surgery. A new technique with use of little blood if any. *J Thorac Cardiovasc Surg* 1974; 68(2):104–109.
12. Cohn LH, Fosberg AM, Anderson WP, et al. The effects of phlebotomy, hemodilution, and autologous transfusion on systemic oxygenation and whole blood utilization in open-heart surgery. *Chest* 1975;68(3):283–287.
13. Silver H. Banked and fresh autologous blood in cardiopulmonary bypass surgery. *Transfusion* 1975;15(6):600–603.
14. Pliam MB, McGoon DC, Tarhan. Failure of transfusion of autologous whole blood to reduce banked-blood requirements in open-heart surgical patients. *J Thorac Cardiovasc Surg* 1975;70:338–343.
15. Sherman MM, Dobnik, Dennis RC, et al. Autologous blood transfusion during cardiopulmonary bypass. *Chest* 1975;70(5):592–595.
16. Kaplan JA, Cannarella C, Jones EL, et al. Autologous blood transfusion during cardiac surgery. A reevaluation of three methods. *J Thorac Cardiovasc Surg* 1977;74(1):4–10.
17. Lilleaasen P. Moderate and extreme hemodilution in open-heart surgery. *Scand J Thorac Cardiovasc Surg* 1977;11:97–103.
18. Yeh T, Shelton L. Blood loss and blood bank requirement in coronary artery bypass surgery. *Ann Thorac Surg* 1978;26(1):11–16.
19. Cosgrove DM, Thurer RL, Lytle BW, et al. Blood conservation during myocardial revascularization. *Ann Thorac Surg* 1979;28(2):184–188.
20. Utley JR, Moores WY, Stephens DB. Blood conservation techniques. *Ann Thorac Surg* 1981;31(5):482–489.
21. Martin E, Hansen E, Peter K. Acute limited normovolemic hemodilution: a method for avoiding homologous transfusion. *World J Surg* 1987;11:53–59.
22. Szecsi J, Batonyi E, Liptay P, et al. Early clinical experience with a simple method for authotransfusion in cardiac surgery. *Scand J Thorac Cardiovasc Surg* 1989;23:51–56.
23. Dale J, Lilleaasen P, Erikssen. Hemostasis after heart surgery with extreme or moderate hemodilution. *Eur Surg Res* 1987;19:339–347.
24. Deitrich W, Barankay A, Dilthey G, et al. Reduction of blood utilization during myocardial revascularization. *J Thorac Cardiovasc Surg* 1989; 97:213–219.
25. Ovrum E, Holen EA, Lindstein-Ringdal MA. Elective coronary artery bypass surgery without homologous blood transfusion. *Scand J Thorac Cardiovasc Surg* 1991;25:13–18.
26. Ovrum E, Holen EA, Abdenoor M, Oystese R, et al. Conventional blood

conservation techniques in 500 consecutive coronary artery bypass operations. *Ann Thorac Surg* 1991;52:500–505.

27. Ness PM, Bourke DL, Walsh PC. A randomized trial of perioperative hemodilution versus transfusion of preoperatively deposited autologous blood in elective surgery. *Transfusion* 1991;31:226–230.
28. Scott WJ, Rode R, Castlemain B, et al. Efficacy, complications, and cost of a comprehensive blood conservation program for cardiac operations. *J Thorac Cardiovasc Surg* 1992;103:1001–1007.
29. Hudson R, Zoellner PA, Williams CM, et al. Isovolemic hemodilution in cardiac bypass surgery. The Society for Cardiovascular Anesthesiology meeting, April 1992.
30. Schonberger JP, Bredee JJ, Tijan D, et al. Intraoperative predonation contributes to blood saving. *Ann Thorac Surg* 1993;56:893–898.
31. Helm RE, Klemperer JD, Rosengart T, et al. Intraoperative autologous donation: volume-dependent red cell preservation. *Surg Forum* 1994; 45:249–252.
32. Petry AF, Jost T, Sievers H. Reduction of homologous blood requirements by blood-pooling at the onset of cardiopulmonary bypass. *J Thorac Cardiovasc Surg* 1994;107:1210–1214.
33. Tullis JL, Eberle WG, Baudanza P, Tinch R. Platelet-pheresis: description of a new technic. *Transfusion* 1968;8(4):154–164.
34. Harker LA, Malpass TW, Branson HE, et al. Mechanism of abnormal bleeding in patients undergoing cardiopulmonary bypass: acquired transient platelet dysfunction associated with selective α granule release. *Blood* 1980; 56(5):824–834.
35. Mammen EF, Koets MH, Washington BC, et al. Hemostasis changes during cardiopulmonary bypass surgery. *Semin Thromb Hemost* 1985;11(3):281–292.
36. Campbell FW, Edmunds LH. Platelet function and cardiopulmonary bypass. In: Gravlee GP, Davis RF, Utley JR, eds. *Cardiopulmonary Bypass Principles and Practice.* Baltimore: Williams & Wilkins, 1993;407–435.
37. Boldt J, Kling D, Zickman B, et al. Acute preoperative plasmapheresis and established blood conservation techniques. *Ann Thorac Surg* 1990;50:62–68.
38. Harke H, Tanger D, Furst-Denzer S, et al. Effect of a preoperative separation of platelets on the postoperative blood loss subsequent to extracorporeal circulation in open-heart surgery. *Anesthesist* 1977;26:64–71.
39. Ferrari M, Zia S, Valbonesi M, et al. A new technique for hemodilution, preparation of platelet-rich plasma, and intraoperative blood salvage in cardiac surgery. *Int J Artif Organs* 1987;10:47–50.
40. Giordano GF, Rivers SL, Chung GKT, et al. Autologous platelet-rich plasma in cardiac surgery: effect on intraoperative and postoperative transfusion requirements. 1988;46:416–419.
41. Giordano GF, Rivers SL, et al. Determinants of homologous blood usage utilizing autologous platelet-rich plasma in cardiac operations. *Ann Thorac Surg* 1989;47:897–902.
42. Jones JW, McCoy TA, Rawitscher RE, et al. Effects of intraoperative plasmapheresis on blood loss in cardiac surgery. *Ann Thorac Surg* 1990; 49:585–590.
43. Del Rossi A, Cernaianu AC, Vertress RA, et al. Platelet-rich plasma reduces postoperative blood loss after cardiopulmonary bypass. *J Thorac Cardiovasc Surg* 1990;100:231–236.

44. Gravlee GP. Autologous platelet-rich plasma in cardiac surgery: aesthetics versus virtue. *J Cardiovasc Thorac Anesth* 1993;7(1):1–3.
45. Boldt J, von Bormann B, Kling D, et al. Preoperative plasmapheresis in patients undergoing cardiac surgery procedures. *Anesthesiology* 1990; 72:282–288.
46. Boldt J, Zickman B, Ballesteros M, et al. Influence of acute preoperative plasmapheresis on platelet function in cardiac surgery. *J Cardiothorac Vasc Anesth* 1993;7(1):4–9.
47. Jones JW, Rawitscher RE, McLean TR, et al. Benefit from combining blood conservation measures in cardiac operations. *Ann Thorac Surg* 1991; 51:541–546.
48. Davis GG, Wells DG, Mabee TM, et al. Platelet-leukocyte plasmapheresis attenuates the deleterious effects of cardiopulmonary bypass. *Ann Thorac Surg* 1992;53:274–277.
49. Wells DG, Davies GG. Platelet salvage in cardiac surgery. *J Cardiothorac Vasc Anesth* 1993;7(4):448–451.
50. Ferraris VA, Berry WR, Klingman RR. Comparison of blood reinfusion techniques used during coronary artery bypass operations. *Ann Thorac Surg* 1993;56:433–440.
51. Harding SA, Shakoor MA, Grindon AJ. Platelet support for cardiopulmonary bypass surgery. *J Thorac Cardiovasc Surg* 1975;70(3):350–353.
52. Simon TL, Bechara FA, Murphy W. Controlled trial of routine administration of platelet concentrates in cardiopulmonary bypass surgery. *Ann Thorac Surg* 1984;37(5):359–364.
53. Mohr R, Martinowitz U, Lavee J, et al. The hemostatic effect of transfusing fresh whole blood versus platelet concentrates after cardiac operations. *J Thorac Cardiovasc Surg* 1988;96:530–534.
54. Mohr R, Goor DA, Yellin A, et al. Fresh blood units contain large potent platelets that improve hemostasis after open heart surgery. *Ann Thorac Surg* 1992;53:650–654.
55. Lavee J, Martinowitz U, Mohr R, et al. The effect of transfusion of fresh whole blood versus platelet concentrates after cardiac operations. *J Thorac Cardiovasc Surg* 1989;97:204–212.
56. Martinowitz U, Goor DA, Ramot B, Mohr R. Is transfusion of fresh plasma after cardiac operations indicated? *J Thorac Cardiovasc Surg* 1990; 100:92–98.
57. Mohr R, Sagi B, Lavee J, et al. The hemostatic effect of autologous platelet-rich plasma versus autologous whole blood after cardiac operations: is platelet separation really necessary? *J Thorac Cardiovasc Surg* 1993; 105:371–372.
58. Boldt J, Zickman B, Benson M, et al. Does platelet size correlate with function in patients undergoing cardiac surgery? *Intensive Care Med* 1993;19:44–47.
59. Kraytman M. Platelet size in thrombocytopenias and thrombocytosis of various origin. *Blood* 1973;41(4):587–598.
60. Karpatkin S, Charmatz A. Heterogeneity of human platelets. I. Metabolic and kinetic evidence suggestive of young and old platelets. *J Clin Invest* 1969; 48:1073–1082.
61. Karpatkin S. Heterogeneity of human platelets. II. Functional evidence suggestive of young and old platelets. *J Clin Invest* 1969;48:1083–1087.
62. Shore-Lesserson L, Reich DL, DePerio M, Silvay G. Thromboelastographic

assessment of platelet-rich plasmapheresis during cardiac reoperations. *Anesthesiology* 1992;77(3a):abstract A137.
63. Tobe CE, Vocelka C, Sepulvada R, et al. Infusion of autologous platelet rich plasma does not reduce blood loss and product use after coronary artery bypass. *J Thorac Cardiovasc Surg* 1993;105:1007–1014.
64. Ereth MH, Oliver WC, Beynen FMK, et al. Autologous platelet-rich plasma does not reduce transfusion of homologous blood products in patients undergoing repeat valvular surgery. *Anesthesiology* 1993;79(3):540–547.
65. Wong CA, Franklin ML, Wade LD. Coagulation tests, blood loss, and transfusion requirements in platelet-rich plasmapheresed versus nonpheresed cardiac surgery patients. *Anesth Analg* 1994;78:29–36.
66. Whitten CW. Why is acute preoperative plasmapheresis not uniformly effective at decreasing bleeding following cardiac surgery? *J Cardiothorac Vasc Anesth* 1993;7(6):766–770.
67. Stover EP, Seigel LC. Platelet-rich plasmapheresis in cardiac surgery: efficacy may yet be demonstrated. *J Thorac Cardiovasc Surg* 1994;108(6):1148–1149.
68. Davies GC, Wells DG, Mabee TM, et al. Plateletpheresis and the cost of heart operations. *Ann Thorac Surg* 1992;53:943–944.
69. Consensus Conference. Platelet transfusion therapy. *JAMA* 1987;257:1777–1780.
70. Rinder CS, Bohnert J, Rinder HM, et al. Platelet activation and aggregation during cardiopulmonary bypass. *Anesthesiology* 1991;75:388–393.
71. Kestin AS, Valeri CR, Khuri SF, et al. The platelet function defect of cardiopulmonary bypass. *Blood* 1993;82(1):107–117.
72. Wun T, Paglieroni T, Holland P. Prolonged circulation of activated platelets following plasmapheresis. *J Clin Apheresis* 1994;9:10–16.
73. Boldt J, Kling D, Zickman B, et al. Acute preoperative plasmapheresis and established blood conservation techniques. *Ann Thorac Surg* 1990;50:62–68.
74. Wickey GS, Keifer JC, Larach DR, et al. Heparin resistance after intraoperative platelet-rich plasma harvesting. *J Thorac Cardiovasc Surg* 1992;103:1172–1176.
75. Helm RE, Klemperer JD, Rosengart TK, et al. Intraoperative autologous donation preserves red cell mass but does not decrease postoperative bleeding. *Ann Thorac Surg* 1996;62(5):1431–1441.
76. Videm V, Svennevig JL, Fosse E, et al. Reduced complement activation with heparin coated oxygenator and tubings in coronary bypass operations. *J Thorac Cardiovasc Surg* 1992;103:806–813.
77. Wagner WR, Johnson PC, Thompson KA, et al. Heparin-coated cardiopulmonary bypass circuits: hemostatic alterations and postoperative blood loss. *Ann Thorac Surg* 1994;58:734–741.
78. Bidstrup BP, Royston D, Sapsford RN, et al. Reduction in blood loss and blood use after cardiopulmonary bypass with high dose aprotinin (trasylol). *J Thorac Cardiovasc Surg* 1989;97:364–372.
79. Lemmer JH, Stanford W, Bonney SL, et al. Aprotinin for coronary bypass operations: efficacy, safety, and influence on early saphenous vein graft patency. *J Thorac Cardiovasc Surg* 1994;107:543–553.
80. Murkin JM, Lux J, Shannon NA, et al. Aprotinin significantly decreases bleeding and transfusion requirements in patients receiving aspirin and undergoing cardiac operations. *J Thorac Cardiovasc Surg* 1994;107:554–561.
81. Wachtfogel YT, Kuchich U, Hack CE, et al. Aprotinin inhibits the contact,

neutrophil, and platelet activation systems during simulated extracorporeal perfusion. *J Thorac Cardiovasc Surg* 1993;106:1–10.

82. Gorman JH, Edmunds LH. Blood anesthesia for cardiopulmonary bypass. *J Cardiovasc Surg* 1995;10:270–279.
83. Lemmer JH. Reporting the results of blood conservation studies: the need for uniform and comprehensive methods. *Ann Thorac Surg* 1994;58:1305–1306.
84. Salama A, Hugo F, Heinrich, et al. Deposition of terminal C5b-9 complement complexes on erythrocytes and leukocytes during cardiopulmonary bypass. *N Engl J Med* 1988;318:408–414.
85. Szymanski IO, Dean HM, Valeri CR, et al. Measurement of erythrocyte survival during open heart surgery. *Transfusion* 1970;10(4):163–170.
86. Hirayama T, Yamaguchi H, Allers H, et al. Evaluation of red cell damage during cardiopulmonary bypass. *Scand J Thorac Cardiovasc Surg* 1985; 19:263–265.
87. Hint H. The pharmacology of dextran and the physiological background for the use of rhemacrodex and macrodex. *Acta Anesth Belg* 1968;2:119–138.
88. Crowell JW, Smith EE. Determinations of the optimal hematocrit. *J Appl Physiol* 1967;22:501–504.
89. Spahn DR, Smith R, Schell RM, et al. Importance of severity of coronary artery disease for the tolerance to normovolemic hemodilution. Comparison of single versus multivessel stenoses in a canine model. *J Thorac Cardiovasc Surg* 1994;108:231–239.
90. Spahn DR, Smith R, McRae RL, et al. Effects of isovolemic hemodilution and anesthesia on regional function in left ventricular myocardium with compromised coronary flow. *Acta Anesth Scand* 1992;36:628–636.
91. Premaratne S, Harada RN, Chun P, et al. Effects of perfluorocarbon exchange transfusion on reducing myocardial infarct size in a primate model of ischemia reperfusion injury: a prospective randomized study. *Surgery* 1995;117: 670–676.
92. Cosgrove DM, Loop FD, Lytle BW, et al. Determinants of blood utilization during myocardial revascularization. *Ann Thorac Surg* 1985;40:380–384.
93. Newman MF, Leone BJ, White WD, et al. The effect of hemoglobin on cerebral oxygen delivery during hypothermic cardiopulmonary bypass and rewarming. *Circulation* 1993;88(4)(part 2):I-246(abstract 1327).
94. Kawata H, Shimizaki Y, Miyomoto H, et al. Limits of hemodilution in total bloodless hypothermic cardiopulmonary bypass. *Circulation* 1994;90(4)(part 2):I-48(abstract 249).
95. Walker RH, ed. *American Association of Blood Banks Technical Manual.* 11th ed. Bethesda, MD: American Association of Blood Banks, 1993;499.
96. Kruskall MS. Autologous blood collection and transfusion in a tertiary care center. In: Taswell HF, Pineda AA, eds. *Autologous Transfusion and Hemotherapy*. Boston: Blackwell Scientific, 1991;60–61.
97. Spahn DR, Leone BJ, Reves JG, et al. Cardiovascular and coronary physiology of acute isovolemic hemodilution: a review of non-oxygen and oxygen carrying solutions. *Anesth Analg* 1994;78:1000–1021.
98. Dzik WH, Fleisher AG, Ciavarella D, et al. Safety and efficacy of autologous blood donation before elective aortic valve operation. *Ann Thorac Surg* 1992;54:1177–1181.
99. Britton LW, Eastlund DT, Dziuban SW, et al. Predonated autologous blood use in elective cardiac surgery. *Ann Thorac Surg* 1989;47:529–532.

100. Mann M, Sacks HJ, Goldfinger D. Safety of autologous blood donation prior to elective surgery for a variety of potentially "high risk" patients. *Transfusion* 1983;23:229–232.
101. Love TR, Hendren WG, O'Keefe DD, Daggett WM. Transfusion of predonated blood in elective cardiac surgery. *Ann Thorac Surg* 1987;43:508–512.
102. Utley JR, Moores WY, Stephens DB. Blood conservation techniques. *Ann Thorac Surg* 1981;31:482–489.
103. Orr MD. Perioperative hemodilution. In: Taswell HF, Pineda AA, eds. *Autologous Transfusion and Hemotherapy.* Boston: Blackwell Scientific, 1991;106.
104. Cooper MM, Elliot MJ. Haemodilution. In: Jonas RA, Elliot MJ, eds. *Cardiopulmonary Bypass in Neonates, Infants, and Young Children.* Boston: Butterworth-Heinemann, 1994;98.
105. Adhoute BG. *Autotransfusion. Using Your Own Blood.* New York: Springer-Verlag, 1991;19–27.
106. Feldman JM, Roth JV, Bjoraker DG. Maximum blood savings by acute normovolemic hemodilution. *Anesth Analg* 1995;80:108–113.
107. Albert SN, ed. *Blood Volume and Extracellular Fluid Volume.* Springfield, IL: Charles C Thomas, 1971;281–282.
108. Hidalgo JU, Nadler SB, Bloch T. *J Nucl Med* 1962;3:92.
109. Rosengart TK, DeBoisw J, Helm RE, et al. Retrograde autologous priming (RAP) for cardiopulmonary bypass: a safe and effective means of decreasing hemodilution and transfusion requirements. *Circulation* 1995;92(8):Supp I-763.
110. Walker RH, ed. *American Association of Blood Banks Technical Manual.* 11th ed. Bethesda, MD: American Association of Blood Banks, 1993;51–52.
111. Laks H, Handin RI, Pilon RN, et al. The effects of acute normovolemic hemodilution on coagulation and blood utilization in major surgery. *J Surg Res* 1976;20:225–230.
112. Walker RH, ed. *American Association of Blood Banks Technical Manual.* 11th ed. Bethesda, MD: American Association of Blood Banks, 1993;55.
113. Orr MD. Perioperative hemodilution. In: Taswell HF, Pineda AA, eds. *Autologous Transfusion and Hemotherapy.* Boston: Blackwell Scientific, 1991;117.
114. Kirklin JK, Chenoweth DE, Naftel DC, et al. Effects of protamine administration after cardiopulmonary bypass on complement, blood elements, and the hemodynamic state. *Ann Thorac Surg* 1986;41:193–199.
115. Ellison N, Edmunds LH, Colman RW. Platelet aggregation following heparin and protamine administration. *Anesthesiology* 1978;48:65–68.
116. Sobel M, McNeill PM, Carlson PL, et al. Heparin inhibition of von Willebrand factor-dependent platelet function in vitro and in vivo. *J Clin Invest* 1991; 87:1787–1798.
117. Kappa JR, Fisher CA, Addonizio VP. Heparin-induced platelet activation: the role of thromboxane A2 synthesis and extent of platelet granule release in two patients. *J Vasc Surg* 1989;9:574–579.
118. John LCH, Rees GM, Kovacs IB. Inhibition of platelet function by heparin. An etiologic factor in post bypass hemorrhage. *J Thorac Cardiovasc Surg* 1993;105:816–822.
119. Beutler E. Preservation of liquid cells. In: Rossi EC, Simon TL, Moss GS, eds.

Principles of Transfusion Medicine. Baltimore: Williams & Wilkins, 1991; 47–56.

120. Simon TL, Marcus CS, Myhre BA, et al. Effects of AS-3 nutrient-additive solution on 42 and 49 day storage of red blood cells. *Transfusion* 1987; 27:178–182.
121. Bode AP, Miller DT. The use of thrombin inhibitors and aprotinin in the preservation of platelets stored for transfusion. *J Lab Clin Med* 1989; 113:753–758.
122. Harke H, Steinen G, Rahman S, et al. Aprotinin-ACD-blood: the effect of aprotinin on the release of cellular mediators and enzymes in banked blood. *Anaesthesist* 1982;31:165–171.
123. Lundsgaard-Hansen P. Is there a rationale for using a protease inhibitor as a standard additive to stored blood? *Vox Sang* 1983;45:1–5.
124. Bode AP, Norris HT. The use of inhibitors of platelet activation or protease activity in platelet concentrates stored for transfusion. *Blood Cells* 1992; 18:361–380.
125. Rosengart TK, Helm RE, Klemperer JD, et al. Combined aprotinin and erythropoietin use for blood conservation: results with Jehovah's Witnesses. *Ann Thorac Surg* 1994;58:1397–1403.
126. Valeri CR, Cassidy G, Khuri S, Feingold H, et al. Hypothermia-induced reversible platelet dysfunction. *Ann Surg* 1987;205:175–181.
127. Harker LA, Malpass TW, Branson HE, et al. Mechanism of abnormal bleeding in patients undergoing cardiopulmonary bypass: acquired transient platelet dysfunction associated with selective α-granule release. *Blood* 1980;-56(5):824–834.
128. Woodman RC, Harker LA. Bleeding complications associated with cardiopulmonary bypass. *Blood* 1990;76:1680–1697.
129. Walker RH, ed. *American Association of Blood Banks Technical Manual*. 11th ed. Bethesda, MD: American Association of Blood Banks, 1993;66.

12
The Influence of Oxygenator Type and Priming Volume on Blood Requirements

William DeBois and Karl H. Krieger

When cardiopulmonary bypass was introduced in clinical cardiac surgery, the pump oxygenator was primed with homologous blood. Despite Melrose's[1] discovery in 1953 that a dextrose and saline bloodless prime was safe for cardiopulmonary bypass, clinicians used fresh blood for the pump prime. Early cardiovascular surgeons and researchers felt that physiologic parameters must be kept as close to normal as possible. The first steps toward blood conservation, in the form of asanguineous priming were reported in the early 1960s.[2,3] This advancement in perfusion technique resulted in an immediate decrease in the use of homologous blood products. Interestingly, 30 years later few improvements have been made in the composition of pump prime.

New technology offers cardiac surgical programs several options that reduce homologous blood exposures. Presently perfusionists have available to them pump components that require lower prime volume, heparin-coated circuitry, and techniques that increase the use of intraoperative autologous blood. Additionally, improved anesthetic techniques and the acceptance of lower transfusion triggers while on bypass have helped to decrease total homologous blood exposure.

At the New York Hospital–Cornell Medical Center we have devised a perfusion circuit and accompanying techniques that help minimize blood usage. We hoped to aggressively identify techniques that reduce pump prime while keeping the circuit safe and simple. In addition, we felt that these changes had to be adaptable so that the perfusionist could safely apply them in the operating room. Dr. Denton Cooley, a cardiothoracic surgeon with over 60,000 bypass procedures to his credit, recommends that any prerequisite for improvement must employ the tenets of "modification, simplification, and application."[4] We also hoped that the simple design of the cardiopulmonary bypass circuit would not only reduce the chance of patient injury during routine and crisis bypass situations, but also simultaneously limit our liability.

This chapter reviews the subjects of pump prime, cardiopulmonary bypass componentry, pump modifications that reduce priming volume, our uses of heparin-coated circuitry, and our results with low prime perfusion. Perfusion techniques that safely decrease priming volume result in a significant reduction in the use of homologous blood and play a major role in a multimodality blood conservation program.

Bloodless Prime – A Historical Concern

Present efforts toward blood conservation have been prompted by a limited and potentially contaminated blood supply and an institutional goal to limit total homologous exposures throughout the hospital stay. While these same fears existed 40 years ago, earlier emphasis was on reducing the amount of blood used to *prime* the cardiopulmonary bypass circuit. It is worthwhile to review those early attempts at blood conservation since some of the problems observed then still exist today.

In 1960 Panico and Neptune[5] described a method of eliminating donor blood prime from the cardiopulmonary bypass circuit. Initially, the cardiopulmonary bypass circuit was primed with 1 L of physiologic saline. After arterial cannulation, a portion of the patient's blood was drained retrograde into the cardiopulmonary bypass circuit. Upon venous cannulation the patient's blood volume would be routed into a reservoir located in the oxygenator. In a series of more than 25 patients, Panico's group demonstrated that the use of bloodless prime was successful in reducing blood usage. As discussed later in this chapter, we have modified this technique and incorporated it into the New York Hospital (NYH) blood conservation program.

During the early stages of open-heart surgery, significant volumes of homologously donated blood were required to both prime the pump and correct postoperative bleeding. As cardiac programs expanded, blood banks were severely challenged with the need to gather donors, collect, process, store, and cross-match large amounts of homologous blood. Depending on the type of extracorporeal circuit used, volumes of blood equal to the patient's blood volume were consumed.

In 1962 Gadboys et al[6] described a syndrome of mild to severe arterial hypotension, fluid and electrolyte shift from the intravascular space, venous desaturation, and a decrease in the buffer base. In what they described as homologous blood syndrome, a sequestration of a significant volume of blood occurred that could not be measured in the circulating blood volume. Additionally, significant pulmonary complications appeared 1 to 2 days postperfusion. These phenomena appeared to be influenced by both the volume and rapidity of homologous blood displaced at the onset of cardiopulmonary bypass. Hypotheses included protein complex abnormalities resulting from air-fluid interfacing in the oxygenator system, leukocyte allergies, and platelet alterations. A solution, the group concluded, would be to eliminate homologous blood prime.

Even after previously mentioned studies, it was still believed that blood prime was necessary to prevent the problems associated with dilutional clotting factor deficiency. In early trials it was typical to use several units of homologous blood for the pump prime. While groups continued to use blood prime, Cooley et al[7] reported the use of a bloodless prime and disposable equipment in a series of 100 patients. In this 1962 report, Cooley et al used a technique that was initially reserved for emergency situations. Prior to this Cooley had demonstrated that animals woke up sooner and recovered faster when 5% dextrose crystalloid prime was used rather than homologous blood. The clinical technique involved the use of 5% dextrose prime (20 ml/kg) and one of two disposable bubble oxygenators (adult and pediatric use). The perfusions were conducted at normothermic temperatures. Utilizing gravity drainage, flow rates of approximately 80 ml/kg/min were obtained. Cooley et al reported significant advantages for cardiovascular patients with this technique (Table 12.1).

While earlier efforts were directed toward eliminating homologous blood from the prime, today's efforts hope to completely eliminate blood transfusion in cardiac surgery. Other chapters describe both pharmacologic and autologous methods of blood conservation. This chapter discusses how the cardiopulmonary bypass circuit influences blood usage and what modifications can be introduced to decrease total blood utilization. Intraoperatively, efforts should be made to recover blood lost, reduce usage of crystalloid volume pre-bypass, reduce prime volume, and return contents of cardiopulmonary bypass circuit post-bypass (Table 12.2).

Components of the Cardiopulmonary Bypass Circuit

Manufacturers' efforts to meet the demands of both cardiac groups and patient requirements have led to a multitude of cardiopulmonary bypass

TABLE 12.1. Advantages of disposable oxygenator, 5% dextrose prime, and normothermia.

Eliminates need for fresh donor blood
Increases availability of cardiopulmonary bypass as an emergency procedure
Provides economy in both personnel and equipment
Enhances adequate venous return during perfusion, facilitating venous drainage
Reduces postoperative bleeding and prevents postoperative cerebral, renal, and pulmonary complications
Permits the use of disposable equipment
Prevents hematologic complications including incompatibility, hepatitis, and thrombocytopenia
Conserves patient's own blood volume
Permits safer operation on infants
Permits operation on patients with religious opposition to blood transfusion

From Cooley et al.[7]

TABLE 12.2. Steps to reduce intraoperative hemodilution.

Use red cell scavenger system to recover blood loss precardiopulmonary bypass
Reduce crystalloid volume transfused precardiopulmonary bypass with the use of vasoconstrictors
Safely reduce circuit prime volume
Retrograde autologous priming (RAP)
Return contents of the pump postcardiopulmonary bypass directly, or by hemoconcentrating via hemofiltration or cell scavenger system

circuit variations. As a result there are as many different circuits as there are cardiac programs. Further understanding of these components can aid perfusionists in designing and perhaps simplifying the bypass circuit. Although the bypass circuit varies from program to program it does have a basic structure. The basic circuit consists of six components: (1) patient, (2) arterial-venous loop, (3) oxygenator, (4) arterial pump, (5) arterial line filter, and (6) a cardioplegia delivery system (Fig. 12.1). Optimal selection of each component is key to a comprehensive blood conservation program.

The Patient

Of primary importance in blood conservation is the patient's size and preoperative red cell volume. Review of our database revealed that patients weighing less than 70 kg were at highest risk of homologous transfusion. This patient group, while representing only 35% of our caseload, accounted for almost 60% of the homologous blood usage on cardiopulmonary bypass. In addition, these patients tended to have lower preoperative hematocrits, approximately 35%. These results appear to be supported by previous reports such as Cosgrove et al's[8] and Utley et al's,[9] in demonstrating the influence of patient weight and red cell volume on blood requirements.

Tables 12.2 and 12.4 demonstrate the effect of prime volume on varying patient weight and preoperative hematocrit. The problem is further complicated during the pre-bypass phase if patients require large amounts of intravenous crystalloid solution to maintain an adequate cardiac output.

Steps Taken to Minimize Hemodilution

Identify small patients (<70 kg), who have highest transfusion requirements.
Consider a low prime setup, $\frac{3}{8}$ venous line.
Avoid hemodilution pre-bypass.

The Arterial-Venous Loop

The arterial-venous (A-V) loop provides drainage of the patient's blood into the venous reservoir via a venous line and return of oxygenated blood via

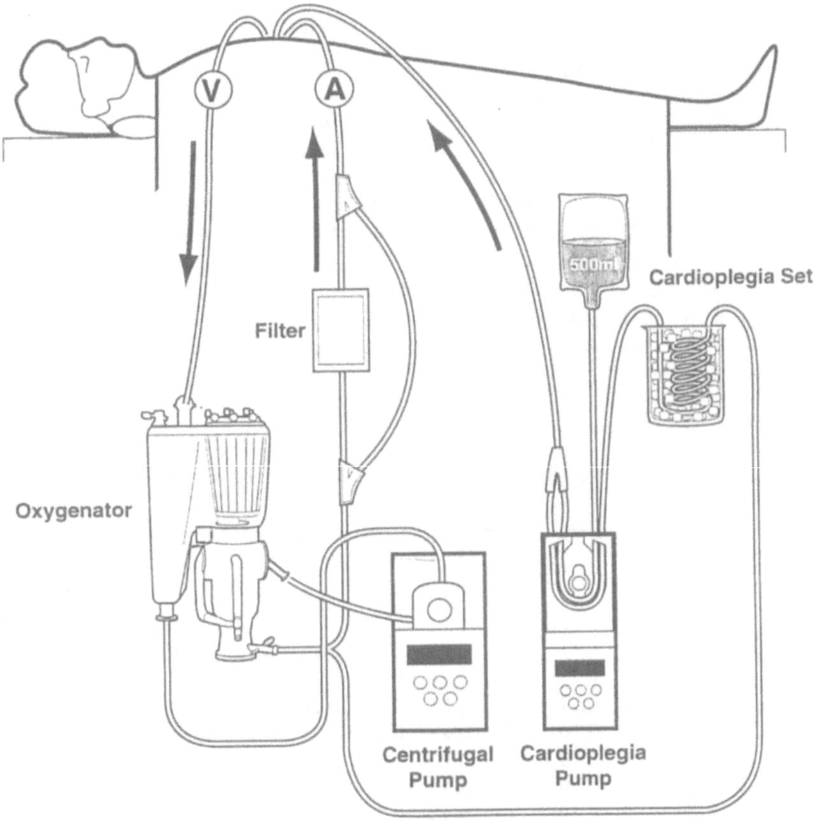

FIGURE 12.1. Simple cardiopulmonary bypass circuit.

the arterial line. A commonly used A-V loop for adult patients consists of a $\frac{1}{2}$-inch venous line and a $\frac{3}{8}$-inch arterial line. With this configuration we have successfully achieved flows of 6 L per minute. In smaller patients (less than 70 kg), this setup is unnecessary. A $\frac{1}{2}$-inch venous line can (1) decrease venous return, due to excessive negative pressure and resultant venous collapse, and (2) lead to excessive hemodilution. Our experience with Jehovah's Witness patients demonstrated that a $\frac{3}{8}$-inch venous line could be used on patients 70 kg or less. In this instance the entire A-V loop is $\frac{3}{8}$ inch. Initial concerns related to a $\frac{3}{8}$-inch-diameter venous line about decreased drainage were unfounded. The small patient requires flow rates less than 5 L (40 to 60 ml/kg/min) and this is achieved with a $\frac{3}{8}$-inch venous line.

We were concerned that the increased resistance of the smaller diameter tubing might impede venous drainage, leading to myocardial distention. As stated in Poiseuille's law, drainage (F) through the venous line will be indirectly related to the length of a tube (venous line) and directly influenced the radius of this tube:

TABLE 12.3. Estimated CPB hematocrit based on weight and prime volume.

	Patient weight (kg)											
Prime vol.	40	45	50	55	60	65	70	75	80	85	90	95
500	0.23	0.24	0.25	0.25	0.26	0.26	0.27	0.27	0.28	0.28	0.28	0.29
750	0.22	0.23	0.23	0.24	0.25	0.25	0.26	0.26	0.27	0.27	0.27	0.28
1000	0.20	0.21	0.22	0.23	0.24	0.24	0.25	0.25	0.26	0.26	0.27	0.27
1250	0.19	0.20	0.21	0.22	0.23	0.23	0.24	0.25	0.25	0.25	0.26	0.26
1500	0.18	0.20	0.20	0.21	0.22	0.23	0.23	0.24	0.24	0.25	0.25	0.25
1750	0.18	0.19	0.20	0.20	0.21	0.22	0.22	0.23	0.23	0.24	0.24	0.25
2000	0.17	0.18	0.19	0.20	0.20	0.21	0.22	0.22	0.23	0.23	0.24	0.24
2250	0.16	0.17	0.18	0.19	0.20	0.20	0.21	0.22	0.22	0.23	0.23	0.24
2500	0.16	0.17	0.18	0.18	0.19	0.20	0.20	0.21	0.22	0.22	0.23	0.23

HCT = 35%.
Anesth vol = 1000 cc.

TABLE 12.4. Estimated on CPB hematocrit based on 70 kg and varying prime volume.

	Preoperative hematocrit											
Prime vol.	25	27	29	31	33	35	37	39	41	43	45	47
500	0.19	0.21	0.22	0.24	0.25	0.27	0.28	0.30	0.31	0.33	0.34	0.36
750	0.18	0.20	0.21	0.23	0.24	0.26	0.27	0.29	0.30	0.32	0.33	0.35
1000	0.18	0.19	0.21	0.22	0.23	0.25	0.26	0.28	0.29	0.31	0.32	0.33
1250	0.17	0.19	0.20	0.21	0.23	0.24	0.25	0.27	0.28	0.29	0.31	0.32
1500	0.17	0.18	0.19	0.21	0.22	0.23	0.25	0.26	0.27	0.28	0.30	0.31
1750	0.16	0.17	0.19	0.20	0.21	0.22	0.24	0.25	0.26	0.28	0.29	0.30
2000	0.16	0.17	0.18	0.19	0.20	0.22	0.23	0.24	0.25	0.27	0.28	0.29
2250	0.15	0.16	0.17	0.19	0.20	0.21	0.22	0.23	0.25	0.26	0.27	0.28
2500	0.15	0.16	0.17	0.18	0.19	0.20	0.22	0.23	0.24	0.25	0.26	0.27

Weight = 70 kg.
Anesth vol = 1000 cc.

$$\mathrm{F} = \frac{\mathrm{IIR}^4 \Delta P}{8L\ V}$$

where F = flow
ΔP = pressure drop
R = radius of tube
L = length of tube
V = viscosity

or

$$\mathrm{F} = \frac{\Delta P}{R}$$

When the operating room table is 60 cm above the venous reservoir, a sufficient pressure gradient is developed to allow for adequate drainage. To

TABLE 12.5. Volume of fluid per foot of tubing.

Tubing size (inches)	Tubing volume per foot (ml)
$\frac{3}{16}$	5.43
$\frac{1}{4}$	9.65
$\frac{3}{8}$	21.74
$\frac{1}{2}$	38.64
$\frac{5}{8}$	60.33

Calculation based on Volume (ml) = II × radius (cm^2) × length (cm).

further assure adequate drainage we initiate bypass slowly, allowing for slow decompression of the heart. At the time of cannulation, the venous and arterial lines are trimmed to minimize length. Table 12.5 describes the priming volume of various sized tubing from $\frac{3}{16}$ inch to $\frac{5}{8}$ inch.

The length and diameter of the arterial and venous lines impacts on the prime volume of the cardiopulmonary bypass circuit (Table 12.6). For example, if the venous line were constructed of a 10-foot length of $\frac{1}{2}$-inch tubing and the arterial line is an 8-foot length of $\frac{3}{8}$-inch tubing, the total prime for the loop would be:

$$\begin{aligned} \text{Venous Line} &= 10 \text{ foot} \times 38.64\text{cc/foot} \\ \text{Arterial Line} &= 8 \times 21.74 \text{ cc/foot} \\ \text{Total Volume (ml)} &= 560.32 \text{ ml} \end{aligned}$$

Alternatively, in the smaller patient where flow is not expected to be greater than 5000 ml/min the length and diameter of the circuit tubing can be reduced:

$$\begin{aligned} \text{Venous Line} &= 7 \text{ foot} \times 21.74 \text{ cc/foot} \\ \text{Arterial Line} &= 5 \times 21.74 \text{ cc/foot} \\ \text{Total Volume (ml)} &= 260.88 \text{ ml} \end{aligned}$$

TABLE 12.6. Recommended cannula and arterial-venous loop.

Procedure	Patient weight	Arterial cannula	Arterial line diameter, length	Venous line diameter, length
CABG and adult	70 kg or greater	20 F	$\frac{3}{8}$ inch, 72 inch	$\frac{1}{2}$ inch, 100 inch
valves	Less than 70 kg	16–20 F	$\frac{3}{8}$ inch, 60 inch	$\frac{3}{8}$ inch, 84 inch
Pediatric	>13–35 kg	10–16 F	$\frac{3}{8}$ inch, 60 inch	$\frac{3}{8}$ inch, 84 inch
Infant	>7–13 kg	8–10 F	$\frac{1}{4}$ inch, 60 inch	$\frac{3}{8}$ inch, 84 inch
Neonates	7 kg or less	8 F	$\frac{1}{4}$ inch, 60 inch	$\frac{1}{4}$ inch, 84 inch

These simple modifications reduce the circuit prime by almost 300 ml. The use of a low prime oxygenator (Table 12.7) can further reduce total circuit prime an additional 500 ml.

Steps Taken to Reduce Hemodilution with the Arterial-Venous Loop

Situate pump console in a way that safely reduces the need for excessive tubing lengths.
Tailor the circuit to the size of your patient.

Oxygenator Selection

Oxygenators have evolved from what are known as bubble oxygenators, which were described as early as 1882, to film oxygenators and lastly membrane oxygenators.[10] Bubble-type oxygenators require a direct gas-blood interface, where oxygen and carbon dioxide–oxygen are bubbled directly into the blood. Membrane oxygenators involve diffusion of gas through permeable membrane that separates the blood and gas compartments. Film oxygenators utilized a large blood-gas interface by spreading out a blood film on a surface in an oxygen enriched environment. The most common type of film oxygenator were the rotating disk type, used clinically until the 1970s. Some disadvantages associated with disk oxygenators were large priming volumes and significant labor requirements for cleaning and assembly. The latter disadvantage actually caused the delay and cancellation of some open-heart procedures.

Debate in the 1980s centered on the issue of bubbler versus membranes as the oxygenators of choice for cardiopulmonary bypass. During the 1970s and 1980s bubbler oxygenators were popular because they were inexpensive and easy to use compared with the more physiologic membrane oxygenators. In one comparison of 80 patients undergoing cardiopulmonary bypass, Williams et al[11] found no clinical, hematologic, metabolic, or hemodynamic differences between patients with microporous Teflon membrane or bubble-film hybrid oxygenators. The only differences noted were those related to cost and complexity of use. The bubble oxygenators were less expensive and required less time to set up.

Membrane versus bubbler comparisons continued to appear in the cardiac literature in the 1980s. Liddicoat et al,[12] in a comparison of 91 patients, measured hemodynamic parameters, fluid balance, and arterial blood gases. They found these measurements to be more physiologic in the membrane oxygenator group at varying times of cardiopulmonary bypass. One advantage of membrane oxygenator systems is that they use a blender for oxygen and air mixing as a ventilating gas source, much like a classic ventilator. In contrast, bubbler systems require the use of a carbon dioxide–oxygen mixture, in addition to 100% oxygen, which is forced directly into the blood path. This difference allows the perfusionist to

TABLE 12.7. Available membrane (open) membrane oxygenators.

Company	Oxygenator name	Membrane configuration	Membrane material	Membrane surface area (M^2)	Flow rating (LPM)	Oxygenator and heat exchanger volume (ml)	System Prime @ minimum operating level (open system)	Pressure drop @ 4.5 LPM	VO_2 @ 4 LPM	VCO_2 @ 4 LPM	Heat exchanger performance	Heat exchanger material	Heat exchanger
Cobe	EXCEL	Flat sheet	Microporous polyproylene	3.0	.5–8.0	500	1022	130	246	228	0.55	Stainless steel	Convoluted tubing
	OPTIMA	Mat, fiber, flow outside	Microporous polyproylene hollow fibers	1.7	.5–8.0	260	632	101	240	220	0.74	Stainless steel	Brazed and textured sheet
Terumo	CAPIOX SX	Single fiber, flow outside	Microporous polyproylene hollow fibers	1.8	2–7.0	270	655	98	253	231	0.67	Stainless steel	840 tubes
Sorin	MONOLYTH	Mat fiber, flow outside	Microporous polyproylene hollow fibers	2.2	1–8.0	300	800	50	300	180	0.74	Epoxy coated stainless steel	Pleated and grooved sheet
Avecor	AFFINITY	Single fiber, flow outside	Microporous polyproylene hollow fibers	2.5	1–7.0	270	860	53	270	240	0.55	Stainless steel	Bellows
Sarns	TURBO	Mat fiber, flow outside	Microporous polyproylene hollow fibers	1.9	1–7.0	280	740	183	285	260	0.67	Stainless steel	Bellows
Bentley	UNIVOX	Radial cross-flow over fiber ribbon, flow outside	Microporous polyproylene hollow fibers	1.8	1–7.0	220	720	56	240	228	0.68	Stainless steel	Bellows

The first three oxygenators represent units currently being evaluated at NYH. In our comparison the Cobe Excel was compared to the two lowest prime oxygenators on the market. Our results clearly demonstrate that a significant reduction in prime volume, from 2200 to 1400 ml, decreases blood usage.

maintain arterial blood gases as more physiologic levels with membrane oxygenator systems.

In short bypass runs there are relatively few data that suggest benefits of membrane oxygenators over bubblers. A European study demonstrated that with bypass times less than 90 minutes, no functional differences could be noted, particularly with regard to hemolysis.[12] This group recommended the membrane oxygenator for complex procedures. Additionally, Clark et al[14] found that membranes offered no biochemical or hematologic advantages over bubblers when bypass times were kept below 2 hours. In longer perfusions (>2 hours), though, the membrane group had lower plasma hemoglobin levels, smaller losses of immunoglobulin (Ig)G, IgM, and C3, and fewer transfusions. Still further studies, such as those by Hicks et al[15] and Hessel et al,[16] demonstrated no significant clinical improvements using membrane oxygenators during routine cardiopulmonary bypass. Drawbacks to the membrane system were increased setup time and cost.

It is of interest that a majority of the studies performed involved the Travenol microporous polyproylene membrane oxygenator. In this system, which is well described by Beall et al,[17] the benefits of no direct blood-gas interface, separate control of oxygen and carbon dioxide, and elimination of antifoaming agents are clearly described. One unique characteristic of this system, however, was the requirement for two pumps for the arterial and venous pumping. In this design venous blood enters a venous bag and is pumped (venous pump) through the oxygenator and heat exchanger into the arterial reservoir. Blood is then pumped from the arterial reservoir (arterial pump) back to the patient. With two pumps this system increases complexity and blood trauma. With the introduction of a new Travenol membrane, which required only a single arterial pump, this system was simplified.[18]

Comparing newer single pump flat sheet membrane oxygenators to bubblers, Taylor's group[19] discusses the occurrence of microembolic ischemia during cardiopulmonary bypass. In this membrane-bubbler comparison, retinal ischemia was quantified via digital image analysis of fluorescein angiography. Of the 64 patients studied, the 30 patients in the membrane group appeared to be better protected against microembolic ischemia.

Although clear differences were noticed only during extended perfusion runs, the membrane-bubbler controversy ended as membrane oxygenators became less complex and less costly to manufacture. With increased usage (two thirds of all procedures in North America by 1987) suppliers were able to improve their manufacturing processes, which allowed for both a more reliable and affordable oxygenator. Zadeh et al[20] examined several biocompatibility and adaptability indices in a comparison of three types of oxygenators (bubbler, hollow fiber membrane, and flat sheet membrane). The flat sheet membrane group experienced significant advantages in red blood cell usage, and in white blood cell and platelet counts. The authors

TABLE 12.8. Benefits of open-reservoir membrane systems.

Category	Bubbler	Closed system
Biocompatibility	Less biocompatible	Similar to open systems
Ease of use	Similar setup	Requires more connections
Safety	Increased risk of massive air embolism	Possibly lower risk of air embolism, due to collapsible bag reservoir
Venous line air management	Similar to open-reservoir membrane, except sudden venous reservoir emptying could result in massive air embolism	Most difficult, requires the use of an extra source to help evacuate air in the reservoir bag

concluded that while the bubbler system was considered most "user friendly," the open reservoir flat sheet membrane with an integral cardiotomy reservoir offered comparable ease of use while retaining improved biocompatible properties.

We recommend the use of an open membrane oxygenator system over bubbler and closed membrane systems for several reasons. The greatest danger of a bubbler system is the lack of protection in the event of loss of venous return. Air immediately enters the arterial side of the pump oxygenator circuit and is more likely to reach the patient. In membrane systems large amounts of air can be dispersed across the membrane surface before reaching the patient. Additionally, the oxygenator itself can act as a reservoir for up to 500 ml of blood (Table 12.8).

Steps Taken to Minimize Hemodilution with Oxygenators

Use high-efficiency, low-prime oxygenators.
Initiate bypass with minimal volume in the venous reservoir.
Hemoconcentrate while on bypass.
Situate oxygenator to minimize tubing length.

Blood Pumps

The primary pump of the heart-lung console is the arterial pump, with the most common examples being the roller pump and centrifugal pumps. Even though centrifugal systems have significantly higher costs, current surveys estimate use is evenly divided. Centrifugal pumps are classified as nonocclusive kinetic pumps. As described by Galletti and Brecher[44], kinetic pumps such as the Biomedicus, Delphin, and Aries impact kinetic energy to the fluid through the forced rotation of cones or impellers. The level of potential energy, or pressure, is thereby increased resulting in flow. Output of kinetic pumps is directly related to inlet pressure and inversely related to outlet pressure, making these pumps both preload and afterload sensitive.

The nonocclusive characteristic has become one of the positive features of this type of pump for routine and long-term circulatory support. As expected, inlet and outlet pressures are limited. Due to the nonocclusive characteristic, though, there is a potential to exsanguinate patients via the arterial line. For this reason the perfusionist must always clamp the arterial line when the pump is off or at very low speed. Kolff et al[21] describe the use of a valve that prevents retrograde flow. During retrograde flow, air could be potentially aspirated around the arterial cannula purse strings. Perfusion diligence, manufacturers' alarms, and low-flow limiters protect against this event. Centrifugal pumps generate limited pressure on both the positive (outlet) and negative (inlet) sides. In the event of an accidental occlusion, system pressures reach no higher than 400 mm Hg.

In contrast, due to their occlusive nature, roller pumps are capable of generating unlimited pressure. This can lead to tubing rupture and tissue damage. Another safety advantage of centrifugal arterial pumps is a decreased risk of massive air embolism, due to the depriming feature of these pumps. Although controversial, some researchers have demonstrated benefits related to platelet preservation, decreased complement activation, and patient outcome.[22–25] Our experience at NYH has been positive in regard to safety and patient outcome. We presently use centrifugal pumps for a majority of our routine procedures, and almost exclusively when extended perfusion times are anticipated.

Steps Taken to Minimize Hemodilution with Pump SetupSituate pumps in a way to minimize tubing length.

Situate pumps in a way to minimize tubing length.
Flow arterial pumps at rates that do not exceed patient's metabolic requirements.
Consider the use of centrifugal pumps.

Arterial Line Filters

Several filters exist in the cardiopulmonary bypass circuit, but only the arterial line filter adds to the total circuit prime volume. Examples of these filters are the cardiotomy filter, pre-bypass filter, cardioplegia filter, gas filters, and the blood filters used for transfusions. The arterial filter, used by between 85% and 99% of cardiac centers, adds 200 to 250 ml of fluid to the total prime volume.[26]

The primary function of the arterial filter is the removal of fat and air emboli, denatured proteins, platelet-leukocyte aggregates, and fibrin material.[27] In the adult, arterial filters should facilitate flow rates of 6 L per minute without any hemolysis. Of the two types of filters, depth and screen, the screen filter is the most common type used for cardiopulmonary bypass. The average pore size is between 20 and 40 μm, and typically a 40-μm arterial filter will remove 95% of the emboli.

Although widely used, there is still debate about the efficacy of arterial filtration.[28] Questions exist about the role of arterial filtration in gaseous emboli production, hemolysis, complement activation, and platelet loss. There is no debate that arterial filters provide a significant advantage in the event of arterial air embolism. Functioning primarily as a bubble trap, arterial filters are an important safety device in the prevention of massive air embolism.

Cardioplegia Systems

Blood cardioplegia and crystalloid cardioplegia constitute two popular methods of providing myocardial protection. Comparative studies have demonstrated that blood cardioplegia significantly reduces the hemodilution and may improve protection.[10,29,30] Although crystalloid cardioplegia systems do not directly add to the circuit prime volume, use of these systems can increase hemodilution by several liters. Several centers deal with this problem by hemoconcentrating the circuit during and post-bypass. In contrast, blood cardioplegia systems add approximately 200 to 300 ml to the total pump priming volume, thereby limiting hemodilution.

The standard blood cardioplegia system consists of a roller pump, tubing, and a heat exchanger. Via the pump, blood is drawn from an oxygenator port via a $\frac{1}{4}$-inch line. The potassium solution is drawn with the same pump through a smaller $\frac{1}{8}$-inch line. The differential in tubing diameter results in a 4:1 ratio of blood to crystalloid solution. Two methods of cooling are (1) a heat exchanger coil submerged in ice water and (2) an integral heat exchanger fed with pumped ice water from a heater cooler. We have found that both of these methods achieve similar results. Temperatures of the cardioplegia solution are 4° to 10° and the myocardium cools to less than 15°. The submerged coil-type system is less expensive and has become our system of choice. When expected cardioplegia flow rates are less than 200 ml/min we use a cardioplegia system constructed with $\frac{1}{8}$-inch tubing throughout. This system has a prime volume of 80 ml and slightly higher line pressure.[31]

Steps That Minimize Hemodilution with the Cardioplegia System

Use blood cardioplegia (4:1 ratio) rather than crystalloid.
Scavenge to Cell Saver, the asanguineous cardioplegia solution circulated at the commencement of bypass.
Limit dose injections to 10 to 15 ml/kg every 15 to 30 minutes.
Augment protection with topical hypothermia.

Modifications to the Cardiopulmonary Circuit That Reduce Priming Volume

It is difficult to estimate the average cardiopulmonary bypass circuit prime volume, but a 1987 survey report estimated the median prime volume to be

2000 ml with a range from 1400 to 2500 ml.[32] Although such a wide range of prime volume should have an impact on blood requirements, little comparative adult data have been published. Kaneko et al[33] demonstrated in 36 adult patients that the use of autologous blood, hemoconcentration, and a low prime oxygenator could limit homologous exposure. We have utilized this concept in our program but have found limits related to the oxygenator size, venous reservoir capacity, and oxygen transfer. Several options exist for reducing the blood requirements (Table 12.9) on cardiopulmonary bypass. They include (1) pumpless heart surgery, (2) retrograde autologous priming (RAP) at commencement of cardiopulmonary bypass, (3) closed-circuit venous pumping, and (4) low-prime perfusion.

TABLE 12.9. Techniques that potentially reduce blood requirements for open-heart surgery patients.

Technique	Advantages	Disadvantages
Pumpless heart surgery	Reduces transfusion requirements; no hemodilution and reduces bleeding disorders related to trauma of cardiopulmonary bypass	Questionable early and long-term risks; may require pump standby; potentially increase ischemic incidents during manipulation of heart
Retrograde autologous priming (RAP) at commencement of CPB	Reduces transfusion requirements; reduces hemodilution; maintains normal hemoglobin levels; no extra disposables, inexpensive; allows for increased collection of intraoperative autologous donation (IAD)	Technically difficult; requires careful monitoring of patient's hemodynamic status pre-bypass; requires increased IAD in order to limit excessively high hematocrits during hypothermic bypass
Closed-circuit venous pumping	Can significantly reduce circuit prime volume	Closed circuit; any air entrained into venous line can be introduced to arterial system; increased difficulty in venting heart; techically more difficult than gravity drainage
Low-prime perfusion circuitry	Reduces transfusion requirements; reduces excessive hemodilution; technically simple; decreases circuit volume, allowing for increased venous reservoir volume, thereby increasing safety; increases amount of intraoperative autologous donation	Beneficial on smaller patients primarily; circuit modification can add to costs; must have patient information, i.e., weight, prior to setup

Pumpless Heart Surgery

Cardiopulmonary bypass results in a coagulopathy that can cause bleeding that may require homologous transfusion. Interestingly, Carrel[34] envisioned cardiac surgery performed without the use of a pump oxygenator as early as 1910. Review of our database demonstrated less than 5% of the cases could be done "off pump." Others suggest that utilization of this technique could reduce blood requirements as well as the expenditure on disposable equipment. Fanning et al[35] demonstrated in a series of 59 patients that reoperative coronary artery bypass grafting could be safely performed without cardiopulmonary bypass. The operative mortality was 3.4% and 40 out of the 59 (68%) patients required blood product transfusion. The average transfusion requirement for the 40 patients was 1.2 units. Questioning the advantages of coronary reoperation without the pump Cosgrove[36] reported that in 1500 consecutive reoperations mortality was also 3.4% with a mean transfusion requirement of two units. The benefits of both decreased blood product usage and bleeding complications were not apparent. In 1991 Benetti et al[37] reported a series of 700 patients undergoing coronary bypass grafting without cardiopulmonary bypass. Significant findings indicated only 10% of these patients required transfusion, and hospital costs were appreciably reduced. While these trials demonstrate some attractive advantages in terms of blood conservation, the increased risks and limited applications prevent widespread use. As Cosgrove stated in his editorial on this topic, in the *Annals of Thoracic Surgery*, the procedure is recommended only for patients with isolated circumflex disease or for patients with isolated right or left anterior descending disease or a combination of the two. Furthermore, it is not recommended for patients with a vessel size of less than 2 mm or for patients requiring grafting of the posterior descending branch of the right coronary artery. While appealing, this procedure is limited to a small subset of the operative population.

Retrograde Autologous Priming of the Cardiopulmonary Bypass Circuit (RAP)

As previously mentioned, Panico and Neptune[5] developed a method for autologously priming the cardiopulmonary bypass circuit. In 1990 Schill[38] further described a method of autologously priming the bypass circuit. In this procedure a standard pump circuit was used. At the initiation of cardiopulmonary bypass the crystalloid volume used to prime the circuit is displaced into an intravenous bag or container, while the patient's blood volume drains into the venous reservoir. After the venous line is blood primed, the arterial line is allowed to drain retrograde into the oxygenator, thereby further displacing crystalloid fluid out of the circuit. Depending on the patient and circuit size this maneuver takes 10 to 15 seconds. There is a resultant arterial pressure drop of 20 to 55 mm Hg but, usually this rapidly resolves with the initiation of cardiopulmonary bypass. Although seemingly difficult, this approach greatly reduces the impact of hemodilution associated with bypass. Schill states that the surgical group has used procedure in over 2000 cases. The 100 patients studied averaged only a 4.3 volume percent drop in hematocrit during cardiopulmonary bypass. If dangerously high hematocrit level are anticipated on bypass, autologous blood volume is removed prior to initiation of bypass and stored in Adsol transfusion bags for later reinfusion.

In a less aggressive approach DeBell[39] employed a modification of the recirculation line for either removing crystalloid prime at the initiation of bypass or for sequestering excessive blood during cardiopulmonary bypass. This circuit technique provides several advantages. First, there is no need to cut into the circuit, reducing the chance of contamination. Second, his design potentially provides a method to store pump prime for later use. This advantage is of significant consequence if expensive products such as albumin or aprotinin are used as additives. However, this technique is not without disadvantages. The addition of extra circuitry and clamps increases the risk of misapplication, resulting in overpressurization and line rupture or exsanguination and ischemia. As DeBell warns, drainage from the arterial line can cause air entrainment into either the aortic cannula or oxygenator. To avoid this problem, (1) the drainage site should be maintained above the level of the heart and (2) during aortic cannulation a "stretch-dilation, double purse string" should be used.

We are presently utilizing a modification of this technique in conjunction with a low-prime circuit (Fig. 12.2). We routinely place the RAP drainage bag on the pump console IV pole. In this position the bag is at a higher level than the heart and eliminates the chance of entraining air into the aorta. The RAP technique is accomplished in three sites:

1. *Drain arterial line.* Retrogradely prime the arterial line and filter back to the oxygenator outlet. Aided by the patient's blood pressure, this fluid is routed into the recirculation bag. During this maneuver arterial pressure usually remains constant as the 300 ml removed decreases afterload, resulting in an increase in cardiac output.
2. *Drain venous reservoir and oxygenator.* With arterial line clamped proximal to the filter, the arterial filter purge line and recirculation line are opened. While the purge line drains, the arterial pump is turned on at 200 ml/min. This blood primes the reservoir, oxygenator, and centrifugal pump. At this point 800 ml have been removed from the circuit.
3. *Drain venous line and initiate full bypass.* Simultaneously turn off the arterial pump, and close, purge, and clamp recirculation line. Unclamp the arterial line and drain venous line into RAP bag. When venous line becomes sanguineous, clamp the RAP bag and initiate full bypass.

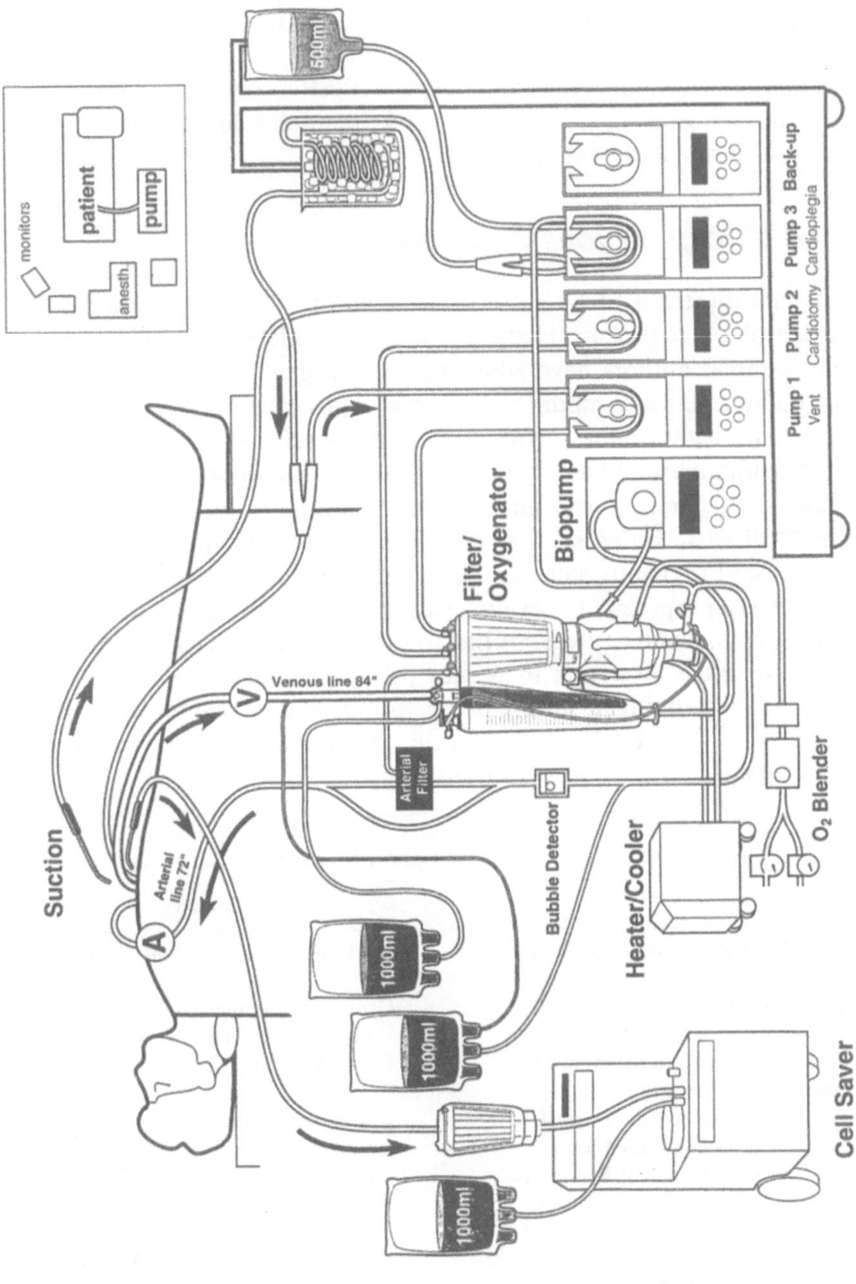

FIGURE 12.2. The NYH low-prime circuit.

This procedure is begun after heparin is given and the arterial cannula is inserted. To avoid any hemodynamic instability, patients must be normovolemic prior to "RAPPINING." The anesthesiologist may elect to give doses of phenylephrine (200 μg) to maintain the systolic blood pressure above 100 mm Hg. The entire process of removing approximately 1200 ml of pump prime takes approximately 5 minutes. This reduces the risk of hemodynamic instability that others have noticed when removing volume too rapidly. Our results indicate that the RAP procedure significantly reduces homologous blood exposure and maintains higher hemoglobin levels both during and post-bypass.[40]

Closed-Circuit Venous Pumping

Circuit modifications that reduce prime volume offer the advantages of decreased blood requirements and reduced synthetic surface exposure. In recent examples authors have addressed "low-prime" circuits by reducing tubing diameters, setup modifications, and replacement of gravity venous drainage with active pump suction.[41–43] In a majority of the original work on cardiopulmonary bypass, active suction was incorporated for venous drainage via a pump or vacuum suction.[44] Conceptually, as Galletti and Brecher[44] discuss, active suction drainage and gravity drainage worked equally as well if venous collapse is avoided. A major drawback to active drainage was a propensity to develop excess negative pressure causing either the atria, femoral vein, or venous line to collapse. Active venous drainage, has been revisited in efforts to reduce priming volume, and to improve femoral venous drainage during reoperations and percutaneous bypass procedures.[42,45,46] Table 12.10 reviews the advantages and disadvantages of both active and gravity types of drainage.

TABLE 12.10. Active suction versus gravity siphon for venous drainage.

Active suction	Gravity
Requires additional equipment such as pump or vacuum source	Does not require additional equipment
Increased hemolysis	Gentle suction, maximum pressure is approximately negative 50 cm H_2O
Potential to entrain air in the event of decreased venous return	Does not entrain air
Increases priming volume of circuit if large-size venous line is used; can decrease priming volume if low-volume tubing used; newer methods utilizing centrifugal pumping have demonstrated significant reductions in priming volumes; technically more difficult and entails increased cost due to extra pump	Currently the most common method of venous drainage; technically easy, no extra cost

In recent work centrifugal pumps have been promoted for use as both the venous and arterial pump. This has been demonstrated in systems such as percutaneous bypass used for emergency support in catheter lab procedures. Criticisms of this system are the lack of cardiotomy suction, the inability to vent, and the venting, in addition to lacking a venous reservoir for volume storage. Some investigators have addressed these concerns in both the laboratory and clinical setting. In both settings, groups have constructed circuits consisting of a single centrifugal pump, venous and arterial lines, an arterial filter, and an oxygenator with an integral heat exchanger. The total prime volume is reduced to 800 to 900 ml, which is 50% less than the average circuit. Although these circuits appear to be quite desirable in terms of blood conservation, no comparative data are available regarding blood usage. Additionally, the potential for air embolism appears to be increased. Due to the direct communication between the venous and arterial lines, air entrained on the venous side is capable of passing into the arterial side. In a system used clinically, a bubble trap may be placed in the venous line. Furthermore, entrained air can then be removed via suction out of the system (Fig. 12.3). The circuit was used clinically on 25 patients without incident. One major problem in this type of system is that the venous line or cardiotomy reservoir must be open when the arterial pump is on. Otherwise air can be entrained across the membrane oxygenator.

Low-Prime Perfusion

At NYH, low-prime perfusion involves the use of the low-prime circuitry and retrograde autologous priming. These maneuvers result in decreased surface contact activation, improved venous reservoir volume, and decreased levels of hemodilution.[40,47] Although prime reduction is most beneficial in patients weighing less than 70 kg, it allows us to remove additional amounts of intraoperative autologous blood pre-bypass in large patients as well. Reductions in prime volume are achieved with the use of a low prime hollow fiber oxygenator (Terumo Corporation), smaller caliber A-V loops ($\frac{3}{8}$-inch diameter) and components such as the arterial filter and cardioplegia delivery system. The use of $\frac{1}{8}$ inch versus $\frac{1}{4}$ inch in the cardioplegia circuit reduced prime volume by 155 ml.[31]

Another important advantage of low-prime setups is the increased amount of intraoperative autologous donation (IAD) that can be removed pre-bypass. In smaller patients (<70 kg) up to two units of IAD blood are removed pre-bypass. In larger patients up to four units of IAD blood are removed. It was found that in larger patients this maneuver was necessary in order to avoid excessively high hematocrits (>30%) during hypothermic cardiopulmonary bypass, especially if RAP is employed. If the hematocrit on pump is higher than 30%, up to 1L of blood volume is collected in a storage bag for transfusion post-bypass.

Our group has demonstrated that a 40% reduction in the bypass prime

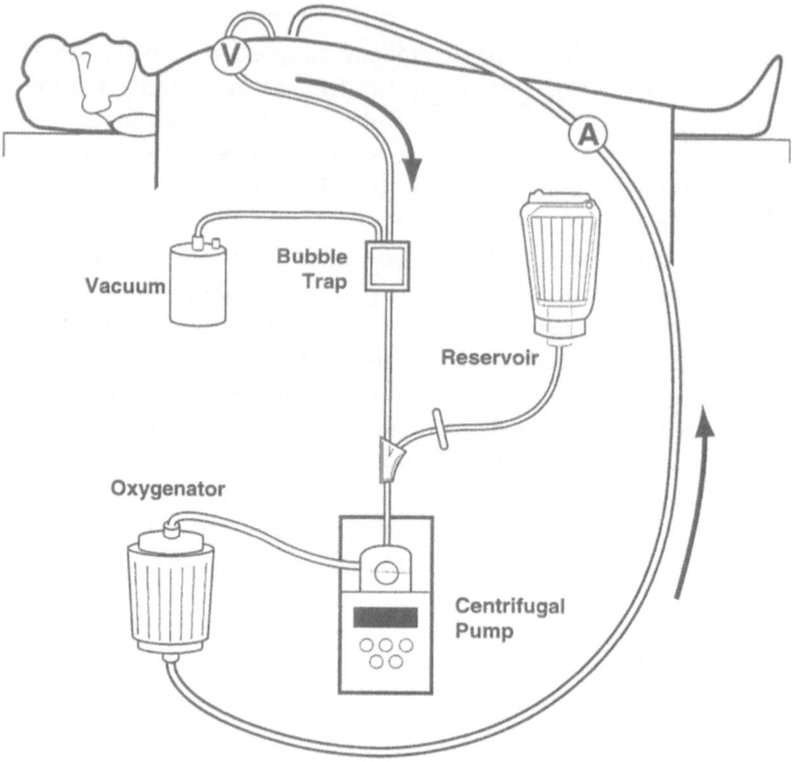

FIGURE 12.3. Circuit with venous pumping. (From Riva[45]).

volume led to significant reduction in homologous transfusions.[47] Prior to our bloodless surgery initiative our standard prime volume was 2,220 ml, regardless of adult patient size. Subsequently, we prepared a circuit using a low-prime hollow fiber oxygenator, reduced-length A-V loop, and a reduced-diameter venous line, from $\frac{1}{2}$ to $\frac{3}{8}$ inch. The changes resulted in a prime reduction of 800 ml. Eighty consecutive adult patients (70 kg or less) undergoing nonemergent cardiopulmonary bypass (CPB) were randomly divided into two groups. The low prime (LP) ($n = 40$) utilized a 1400 ml prime, and the control group ($n = 40$), our standard setup, had a 2,220-ml prime volume (Table 12.11). Data were collected during the preoperative, intraoperative, and postoperative periods. Patients were closely matched for age, gender, preoperative risk, and procedure. Table 12.12 illustrates the patient characteristics. Mean weight (kg) was less in group LP (59.2 vs 62.2, $p < .02$). Pre-CPB hematocrits (HCT) were similar in both groups. Initial on CPB HCT was higher in group LP (19.8 vs 18.4, $p < .04$) as seen in Table 12.13. Group LP had a higher frequency of initial on CPB HCTs of 20% of greater (55% vs 33%, $p < .04$). LP had a lower packed red blood cell (PRBC) transfusion rate on CPB (0.4 vs 0.9 unit, $p < .03$). LP had a

TABLE 12.11. Prime constituents of adult routine and low-prime systems (70-kg example).

Low prime		Routine prime	
Normosol 7.4	1125 ml	Normosol 7.4	1825 ml
25% normal serum albumin	100 ml (25 g)	25% normal serum albumin	200 ml (50 g)
20% osmitrol	175 ml (0.5 g per kg)	20% osmitrol	175 ml (0.5 g per kg)
Heparin (1000:1)	10 ml (10,000 U)	Heparin (1000:1)	10 ml (10,000 U)
Total	1410 ml		2210 ml

higher percentage of patients that did not require transfusion CPB (78% vs 55%, $p < .03$). Oxygen delivery and consumption were similar in both groups. Despite fewer transfusions, group LP had a higher post-CPB (20.6 vs 19.3, $p < .04$). No significant differences were noted postoperatively, although a trend was noted with a lower total PRBC transfusion rate in group LP (1.9 vs 2.4, $p = .10$). Chest drainage, 24-hour HCT, and discharge HCT were similar in both groups. Transfusion of platelets, fresh frozen plasma, and cryoprecipitate were similar in both groups. There were no deaths in either group.

We concluded that a significant reduction in prime volume appears to be safe, simple, and reduces blood transfusion (HBTs) in the smaller patient population undergoing CPB. As a result prime reduction has become part of our comprehensive multimodality blood conservation program.

Heparin-Coated Circuits

Extracorporeal circulation is a potent stimulus for clot formation, and blood will clot within minutes when exposed to an untreated, unheparinized circuit. For this reason patients are heparinized prior to the initiation of cardiopulmonary bypass, and typical doses are 3 to 5 mg/kg. Even in the

TABLE 12.12. Patient characteristics of low-prime and control groups mean (and standard deviation).

Variable	Low prime (n = 40)	Control (n = 40)	p value
Sex (m/f)	22/18	24/16	NS
Age (yrs)	65 (10.1)	69 (7.8)	NS
Bypass time (min)	79 (27.2)	74 (22.3)	NS
Ejection fraction (%)	39 (9.0)	40 (9.5)	NS
Weight (kg)	59 (6.3)	62 (4.4)	<.05
Preoperative hematocrit (%)	34.7 (4.2)	34.3 (4.3)	NS
Procedure			
CABG	34	36	NS
Valve	6	4	

TABLE 12.13. Hematologic values on cardiopulmonary bypass of low-prime and control groups: mean (and standard deviation).

Variable	Low prime ($n = 40$)	Control ($n = 40$)	p value
Precardiopulmonary bypass hematocrit (%)	34.7 (4.2)	34.2 (4.3)	.60
Initial hematocrit on cardiopulmonary bypass (%)	19.8 (3.4)	18.4 (3.3)	<.04
Hematocrit decrease on cardiopulmonary bypass (%)	43 (8.3)	45 (11.6)	.24
Number of patients with cardiopulmonary bypass hematocrits > 20%	22	13	<.05
Number of patients transfused PRBC on cardiopulmonary bypass	9/40	18/40	<.04
Units of PRBC on cardiopulmonary bypass	0.4 (0.8)	0.9 (1.2)	<.03
Immediate postcardiopulmonary bypass hematocrit (%)	20.6	19.3	.08
Number of patients transfused during hospital stay	26/40	34/40	<.04
Units PRBC during hospital stay	1.9	2.4	.10

presence of heparinization there is activation of the complement system and coagulatory mechanisms, which lead to a total body inflammatory response.[48,49]

The two most commonly available heparin-coated systems are the Carmeda (Medtronics) and Duraflow (Baxter) circuit treatments. In the Carmeda systems, heparin is covalently bonded to surfaces via end-point attachment. By depositing polyethylenimine (PEI) spacer onto the various extracorporeal surfaces, porcine mucosal heparin fragments can then be attached, resulting in an unleachable heparin-coated surface.[50] In the other process, Duraflow II, unfractionated porcine mucosal heparin is ionically bound to a carrier. Following this process the extracorporeal surfaces are then rinsed with the heparin-carrier complex.[51] As well as the processes, costs vary significantly for both treatments. Presently, Duraflow II coating can add approximately 25% to the cost of a complete bypass circuit. In contrast, Carmeda can increase the cardiopulmonary bypass circuit costs by as much as 100%.

Until recently, there has been little clinical experience with heparin-coated circuits. Manufacturers have stated that heparin-coating decreases the inflammatory response of cardiopulmonary bypass. They claim that transfusion requirements, postoperative bleeding, and complement activation are also decreased, but results in the literature are unclear.[52–55] Inconsistencies in the studies may be due to the small sample sizes, differences in systemic anticoagulation, and differences in the techniques used for cardiopulmonary bypass circuit coating.[51]

When the risk of anticoagulation is high, heparin-coated circuits appear

TABLE 12.14. Uses for heparin-coated circuits.

Clinical condition	Considerations
Heparin-induced thrombocytopenia	Use nonleaching heparin coating similar to Carmeda[58]; must avoid all other sources of heparin including coated Swan-Ganz catheters
Protamine allergy	Use of low-dose heparin to reduce or even eliminate protamine requirements[59]
Recent stroke or trauma	No or low heparin administration[60,61]
Descending thoracic and thorcoabdominal aortic aneurysm repairs	Use of left heart or partial cardiopulmonary bypass[62,63]

to offer a significant benefit. Yet, because of the increased costs and lack of large clinical trials data, we do not use this technique for routine cardiopulmonary bypass procedures. Additionally, we have found that aprotinin has a significant impact on postoperative blood loss in high-risk patients.[56,57] Table 12.14 lists our indications for heparin-coated circuits. Chapter 18 discusses heparinless bypass.

Conclusions

Using common bypass equipment and techniques, several technical options are available for the perfusionist to reduce homologous requirements during cardiopulmonary bypass. These include low-prime circuits for small adults, minimum transfusion triggers, retrograde autologous priming, and optimal matching of flow rate to metabolic demand. We have shown that an optimally designed perfusion circuit can have a significant impact on blood usage in a cardiac surgery program. Although these benefits are most significant in small adults and children, larger patients can also benefit because the use of low-prime circuitry decreases hemodilution and allows for removal of increased amounts of autologous blood.

It is of paramount importance that extensive training and support is provided for perfusion personnel involved in an aggressive blood conservation program. Complacency with the status quo must be overcome. Weekly in-service training was held in our institution to demonstrate the new perfusion setup and techniques. In a wet lab setting, the staff received training in the safe application of the new equipment. Concerns related to the low transfusion triggers and the safety of retrograde autologous priming (RAP) and the smaller circuits had to be addressed. Involvement and discussion with the attending surgeons and anesthesiologists were helpful to encourage commitment to the new program.

Although low-prime techniques will not revolutionize cardiac surgery, they play a critical role in a multimodality blood conservation program.

Our results with low-prime circuitry demonstrated significant reductions in the number of patients requiring transfusions. If bloodless cardiac surgery is to become a reality in the new millennium, perfusionists must work shoulder to shoulder with cardiovascular surgeons and anesthesiologists to redefine and revise perfusion techniques with the hope of ultimately providing the best possible patient care.

References

1. Melrose DG. A mechanical heart-lung machine for use in man. *Br Med J* 1953;2:57.
2. Zudhi N, McCollough B, Carey J, et al. Hypothermic perfusion for open-heart surgical procedures. Report of the use of a heart-lung machine primed with five percent dextrose in water inducing hemodilution. *J Int Coll Surg* 1961; 35:319–326.
3. Green AE, Carey JM, Zudhi N. Hemodilution principle of hypothermic perfusion. A concept of obviating blood priming. *J Thorac Cardiovasc Surg* 1962;43:640–648.
4. Cooley DA. Fifty years of cardiovascular surgery. *Ann Thorac Surg* 1994; 57:1059–1063.
5. Panico FG, Neptune WB. A mechanism to eliminate the donor blood prime from the pump oxygenator. *Surg Forum* 1960;10:605–609.
6. Gadboys HL, Slonim R, Litwak RS. Homologous blood syndrome. *Ann Surg* 1962;155;5:794–804.
7. Cooley DA, Beall AC, Grondin P. Open-heart operations with disposable oxygenators, 5 percent dextrose prime, and normothermia. *Surgery* 1962; 713–718.
8. Cosgrove DM, Loop FD, Lytle BW, et al. Determinants of blood utilization during myocardial revascularization. *Ann Thorac Surg* 1985;4);380–384.
9. Utley JR, Wallace DJ, Thomason ME, et al. Correlates of preoperative hematocrit value in patients undergoing coronary artery bypass. *J Thorac Cardiovasc Surg* 1989;98:451–453.
10. Buckberg GD. Oxygenated cardioplegia: blood is a many splendored thing. *Ann Thorac Surg* 1990;50:175–177.
11. Williams DR, Tyers GF, Williams EH, et al. Similarity of clinical and laboratory results obtained with microporous Teflon membrane oxygenator and bubble-film hybrid oxygenator. *Ann Thorac Surg* 1978;25:30–35.
12. Liddicoat JE, Bekassy SM, Beall AC, et al. Membrane versus bubble oxygenator: clinical comparison. *Ann Surg* 1975;181:747–753.
13. Fenchel G, Seybold-Epting W, Schmidt K, et al. Clinical comparison between membrane and bubble oxygenators in cpb. *J Cardiovasc Surg (Torino)* 1979; 20:419–422.
14. Clark RE, Beauchamp RA, Magrath RA, et al. Comparison of bubble and membrane oxygenators in short and long perfusions. *J Thorac Cardiovasc Surg* 1979;78:655–666.
15. Hicks GL, Zwart HH, DeWall RA. Membrane versus bubbler oxygenators: a prospective study of 52 patients. *Arch Surg* 1979;114:1285–1287.
16. Hessel EA, Johnson DD, Ivey TD, et al. Membrane versus bubble oxygenator for cardiac surgery. A prospective randomized study. *J Thorac Cardiovasc Surg* 1980;80:111–122.

17. Beall AC, Solis RT, Kakvan M, et al. Clinical experience with the Teflon disposable membrane oxygenator. *Ann Thorac Surg* 1976;21:144–150.
18. Karlson KE, Massimino RM, Cooper GN, et al. Initial clinical experience with a low pressure drop membrane oxygenator for cpb in adult patients. *Ann J Surg* 1984;147:447–450.
19. Blauth CI, Smith PL, Arnold JV, et al. Influence of oxygenator type on the prevalence and extent of microembolic retinal ischemia during cpb. Assessment by digital image analysis. *J Thorac Cardiovasc Surg* 1990;99:61–69.
20. Zadeh BJ, Holazo R, Conlon C, et al. A clinical evaluation of three modern blood oxygenators. *Perfusion* 1987;2:263–270.
21. Kolff J, McClurken JB, Alpern JB, et al. Beware centrifugal pumps: not a one-way street, but a dangerous siphon. *Perfusion* 1990;5:225–226.
22. DeBois WJ, Brennan R, Wein E, et al. Centrifugal pumping: the patient outcome benefits following coronary artery bypass surgery. *J Extracorp Tech* 1995;27:77–80.
23. Wheeldon DR, Bethune DW, Gill RD. Vortex pumping for routine cardiac surgery: a comparative study. *Perfusion* 1990;5:135–143.
24. Salama A, Hugo F, Heinrich D, et al. Deposition of intimal C5b-9 complement complexes on erythrocytes and leukocytes during cardiopulmonary bypass. *N Engl J Med* 1988;318:408–414.
25. Parault BG, Conrad SA. The effect of extracorporeal circulation time and patient age on platelet retention during cardiopulmonary bypass: a comparison of roller and centrifugal pumps. *J Extracorp Tech* 1992;23:34–38.
26. Kurusz M, Schneider B, Brown JP, et al. Filtration during open-heart surgery: devices, techniques, opinions and complications. *Am Acad Cardiovasc Perfusion* 1983;4:123–129.
27. Reed CC, Stafford TR. *Cardiopulmonary Bypass.* The Woodlands, TX: Surgimedics/TMP, 1989.
28. Gravlee GP. Heparin-coated cardiopulmonary bypass circuits. *J Cardiothorac Vasc Anesth* 1994;8:55–92.
29. Buckberg GD. Update on current techniques of myocardial protection. *Ann Thorac Surg* 1995;60:805–814.
30. Ihnkken K, Morita K, Buckberg GD. New approaches to blood cardioplegic delivery to reduce hemodilution and cardioplegic overdose. *J Cardiovasc Surg* 1994;9:26–36.
31. DeBois WJ, Gold JP, Rosengart TR, et al. Blood conservation for infants and children: the impact of a low prime cardioplegia set. *Perfusion* (in press).
32. Sistini JJ, Feiner CJ. Survey of blood conservation techniques during open-heart surgery. *J Extracorp Tech* 1988;119–123.
33. Kaneko Y, Miyauchi Y, Goto H, et al. Benefits and limitations of extracorporeal circulation with autologous blood using low prime membrane oxygenator. *Nippon Kyobu Gaka Gakkai Zasshi* 1989;37:2359–2266.
34. Carrel A. On the experimental surgery of the thoracic aorta and the heart. *Ann Surg* 1910;52:83–92.
35. Fanning WJ, Kakos GS, Williams TE. Reoperative coronary artery bypass grafting without cardiopulmonary bypass. *Ann Thorac Surg* 1993;55:486–489.
36. Cosgrove DM. Is coronary reoperation without the pump an advantage? *Ann Thorac Surg* 1993;55:329.
37. Benetti FJ, Naselli G, Wood M, et al. Direct myocardial revascularization

without extracorporeal circulation. Experience in 700 patients. *Chest* 1991; 100:312–316.
38. Schill DM. The optimal preservation of the patient's hematocrit when cpb is required. *J Extracorp Tech* 1990;22:73–78.
39. DeBell RH. Improved fluid management by a simple extracorporeal circuit design change. *J Extracorp Tech* 1993;25:58–60.
40. Rosengart TR, DeBois WJ, Helm RE, et al. Retrograde autologous priming (RAP) for cardiopulmonary bypass: a safe and effective means of decreasing hemodilution and transfusion requirements. *Circulation* 1995;92(8 Suppl)I763.
41. Tyndal CM, Berryessa RG, Campbell DN, et al. Micro-prime circuit facilitating minimal blood use during infant perfusion. *J Extracorp Tech* 1987;19:352–357.
42. Sistino JJ, Michler RE, Mongero LB, et al. Laboratory evaluation of a low prime closed-circuit cpb system. *J Extracorp Tech* 1993;24:116–119.
43. Gorney R, Molina J, Reynolds T. A modification of the Sarns conducter heat exchanger as a low prime pediatric cardioplegia system. *J Extracorp Tech* 1994;26:37–39.
44. Galletti PM, Brecher GA. *Heart-Lung Bypass: Principles and Techniques of Extracorporeal Circulation*. New York: Grune and Stratton, 1962.
45. Personal communiation, Randy Riva, October 17, 1994.
46. McCusker K, Hoffmann D, Maladarelli W, et al. Biopump on venous line. *Perfusion* 1994.
47. DeBois WJ, Sukhram Y, McVey J, et al. Low circuit prime reduces homologous blood transfusions. *J Extracorp Tech* 1996;28:58–62.
48. Kirlin JK, Westaby S, Blackstone EH, et al. Complement and the damaging effects of CPB. *J Thorac Cardiovasc Surg* 1983;86:845–857.
49. Gu YJ, van Oeveren, et al. Heparin-coated circuits reduce the inflammatory response to cardiopulmonary bypass. *Ann Thorac Surg* 1993;55:917–922.
50. Larm O, Larsson R, Olsson P. A new non-thrombogenic surface prepared by selective covalent binding of heparin via a modified reducing terminal residue. *Biomater Med Devices Artif Organs* 1983;11:161–173.
51. Gravlee GP. Heparin-coated cardiopulmonary bypass circuit. *J Cardiothorac Vasc Anesth* 1994;8:213–222.
52. Boroweic L, Thelin S, Bagge L, et al. Heparin-coated circuits reduce activation of granulocytes during cpb. *J Thorac Cardiovasc Surg* 1992;104:642–647.
53. Mollnes TE, Videm V, Gotze, et al. Formation of C5a during cpb: inhibition by precoating with heparin. *Ann Thorac Surg* 1991;52:92–97.
54. Boonstra PW, Gu YJ, Akkerman C, et al. Heparin coating of an extracorporeal circuit partly improves hemostasis after cpb. *J Thorac Cardiovasc Surg* 1994; 107:289–292.
55. Svennevig JL, Odd R, Karlsen H, et al. Complement activation during extracorporeal circulation. *J Thorac Cardiovasc Surg* 1993;106:466–472.
56. Rosengart TK, Helm RE, Klemperer J, et al. Combined aprotinin and erythropoietin use for blood conservation: results with Jehovah's Witnesses. *Ann Thorac Surg* 1994;58:1397–1403.
57. Westaby S. Aprotinin in perspective. *Ann Thorac Surg* 1993;55:1033–1041.
58. Couyant MA, Beemer GH, Tatoulis J, et al. A proposed protocol for the management of cpb for patients with heparin-induced thrombosis thrombocytopenia syndrome. *Aust Perfusion Soc J* 1992.
59. Jones DR, Hill RC, Hollingsed MJ, et al. Use of heparin-coated cardiopulmonary bypass. *Ann Thorac Surg* 1993;56:566–568.

60. Jones DR, Hill RC, Vasilakis A, et al. Safe use of heparin-coated bypass circuits incorporating a pump-oxygenator. *Ann Thorac Surg* 1994;57:815–819.
61. Bennett J, Hill J, Bruhn P, et al. Heparin-free cardiopulmonary support, utilizing a Carmeda coated circuit, for a patient with pulmonary hemorrhage and multiple trauma. *J Extracorp Tech* 1992;24:6–11.
62. von Segesser LK, Weiss BM, Garcia E, et al. Reduction and elimination of systemic heparinization during cardiopulmonary bypass. *J Thorac Cardiovasc Surg* 1992;103:790–799.
63. Bianchi JJ, Swartz MT, Raithel SC, et al. Initial clinical experience with centrifugal pumps coated with the Carmeda process. *ASAIO J* 1992; 38:M143–146.

13
Intraoperative Blood Salvage

JOHN D. KLEMPERER AND O. WAYNE ISOM

Intraoperative blood salvage is an essential component of blood conservation efforts in cardiac surgery. Traditionally, cardiac surgical procedures necessitated the administration of large volumes of homologous blood products.[1] The development of effective salvage techniques along with the introduction of nonblood priming solutions for the bypass circuit have played a major role in reducing and frequently eliminating the need for perioperative transfusion. Autotransfusion has been employed in a variety of noncardiac settings, such as vascular, trauma, and orthopedic surgery. However, the most extensive experience and the greatest benefits have been achieved in the field of cardiopulmonary bypass surgery. Several options exist for the processing of both intraoperative losses and residual bypass circuit blood. Each is associated with distinct advantages and disadvantages. The optimization of intraoperative blood salvage strategies may require a degree of flexibility, with specific techniques selected on an individual basis. This chapter reviews the major types of available salvage systems and discusses their benefits and limitations. In addition, we describe an approach that has worked well in our institution's comprehensive blood conservation program.

History

The concept of autologous transfusion as a response to major hemorrhage was introduced in England in 1818 by Blundell[2] and documented in the medical literature in 1874 by Highmore.[3] Reinfusion of surgical blood loss slowly became an accepted technique. By 1936 a review of the American literature documented 272 cases of autotransfusion.[4] Interest in autotransfusion waned in the 1940s and 1950s due to the boom in modern blood banking services. It was not until the 1960s that new progress and the modern era of intraoperative blood salvage emerged. During the 1960s and 1970s, the advent of the Vietnam War, the increase in cardiac surgical procedures, and concern regarding transmission of infectious diseases revived interest in improving autotransfusion techniques. Experimental work performed by Dyer[5] and Klebanoff[6] culminated in the production of the first commercial intraoperative blood salvage device, the Bentley ATS-100 autotransfusion system (Bentley Laboratories, Santa Ana, CA). The device consisted of a sterile cardiotomy reservoir equipped with an integral filter. A variable-speed roller pump was used to aspirate and reinfuse salvaged blood under pressure. The apparatus was designed to facilitate the rapid return of massive intraoperative blood losses. Initial experience obtained in Southeast Asia was encouraging,[6] and it was subsequently utilized in many trauma and vascular surgery centers. Although the Bentley system was easy to operate and effective, its usefulness was overshadowed by associated complications. The high-pressure system added to the destruction of blood elements. Blood collected from the surgical field was merely filtered, so tissue debris, free hemoglobin, red cell stroma, and activated coagulation products were directly reinfused into patients. An unacceptable incidence of coagulopathy as well as impaired renal function resulted.[7-9] The high-pressure system inadvertently led to several cases of fatal air embolism.[10] Production of the Bentley autotransfuser was discontinued. By the mid-1970s, improved devices were introduced—the centrifuge and canister-based collection devices. Along with increasing experience in the use of ultrafiltration, these methods represent the mainstays of modern intraoperative blood salvage protocols in cardiac surgery.

Techniques of Intraoperative Blood Salvage

This section discusses the technical aspects of the major blood scavenging systems. Available methods are applicable both during cardiopulmonary bypass as well as during the pre- and post-bypass phases of the operation. An appreciation of the mechanisms by which the various modalities work is essential for optimizing approaches to intraoperative blood salvage. In aggressive blood conservation protocols, salvage techniques are routinely employed from the beginning to the end of the operation.

Cardiotomy System

During cardiopulmonary bypass, the reinfusion of shed blood is simplified by the continuity of the extracorporeal circuit and full systemic heparinization. A standard cardiotomy apparatus, consisting of a suction wand, roller pump, and filter, returns blood directly to the venous/cardiotomy reservoir. The patient must be fully heparinized and the surgeon must be careful to avoid the aspiration of any potentially thrombogenic material that could produce clot formation within the bypass circuit. Cardiotomy salvage is most applicable for the clearance of fresh intracardiac blood during valve procedures. Use of cell washing devices are preferable for the aspiration of intrapericardial blood when debris or cold crystalloid/slush solution is present.

Cannister Systems

Intraoperative autotransfusion techniques have been characterized by two principal approaches. Salvaged blood has been either recovered, filtered, and reinfused as whole blood, or concentrated and washed prior to reinfusion.[11] A passive cannister collection system, developed by the Sorensen Research Corp. (Salt Lake City, Utah) typifies the former approach[11,12] (Fig. 13.1). Its construction, although conceptually similar to the Bentley device, is less damaging to blood elements and offers improved filtration and safety features. The system consists of a disposable, dual function 1900 ml capacity reservoir-transfusion bag, a rigid outer cannister, and a special suction tip that mixes blood with anticoagulant as it is aspirated (usually citrate-phosphate-dextrose solution). Whole blood is collected from the operative field by vacuum suction, and is filtered through a 170-υ screen upon entering and exiting the upper reservoir. The filtered blood passes by gravity into the lower reservoir, which serves as a standard

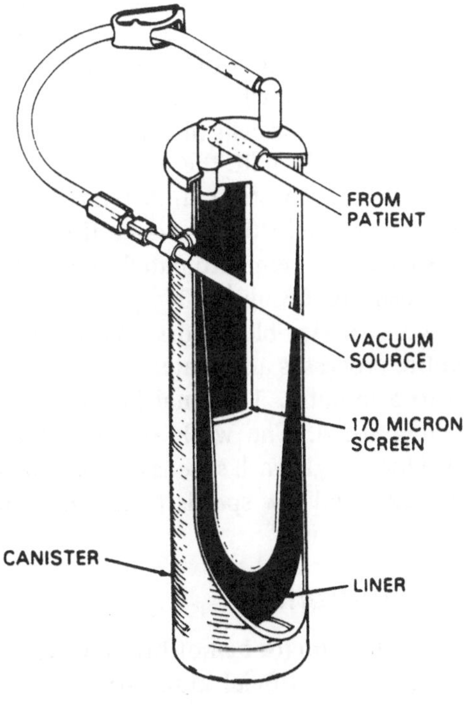

FIGURE 13.1. Sorensen autotransfusion cannister collection system. Blood enters the cannister and passes through a 170-υ filter. After collection, the liner bag is removed, and an infusion set and microaggregate filter is inserted in the bottom. (From Williamson and Taswell,[12] by permission of *Transfusion*.)

blood administration bag. Whole filtered blood can be reinfused immediately to the patient as was originally reported[13] or first be washed and concentrated at the central blood bank.[11,12] The related Solcotrans (Cabot Ltd., High Wycombe, UK) device operates in a similar fashion[14]; however, experience in cardiac surgery has not yet been reported. As will be discussed, the development of efficient red cell washing devices has largely replaced the intraoperative use of cannister-based devices in cardiac surgery. The Sorensen collection system remains in frequent use for postoperative mediastinal shed blood collection.[15–17]

Cell Saver

In 1976 the Haemonetics Corporation (Braintree, MA) introduced the first centrifuge-based cell collection/washing unit, the Cell Saver. Since that time, other companies have introduced competing products, yet for the purpose of this chapter, an outline of the operation of the Cell Saver (Fig. 13.2) will serve as a prototype for cell washing systems.[7] As with the cannister based systems, blood is aspirated through double-lumen suction tubing and mixed with anticoagulant solution (usually heparinized saline), permitting collection before systemic heparinization or after reversal with protamine. The anticoagulated blood is then filtered and pumped from the collection reservoir into a Latham centrifuge bowl in which the cellular components are separated (Fig. 13.3). The red cell mass migrates outward and is separated from the lighter plasma and "buffy coat" layers. As centrifugation progresses, the lighter components are displaced through the bowl outlet into the waste chamber. The remaining red cells are then washed with saline solution to remove residual debris, anticoagulant, and plasma. Each 225-ml bowl requires a minimum of 700 ml of saline to effectively wash the packed cells of debris and heparin.[18,19] Under standard operation, approximately half the amount of blood suctioned from the patient is ultimately reconstituted. After washing is complete, the resulting red cell product is pumped into a collection bag for reinfusion. The early Cell Saver systems were semiautomated and required almost 45 minutes to complete red cell processing.[18] This greatly restricted applicability in the setting of ongoing major blood loss. With the current generation, Cell Saver 4, the entire process is automated and can process up to 500 ml of whole blood in 3 to 5 minutes. The final hematocrit achieved is inversely related to the filling speed. The wash speed will also affect the content of the final product. High wash speeds ($>$600 ml/min) can lead to red blood cell (RBC) spillage, and low speeds ($<$200 ml/min) inadequately cleanse the packed cells of debris.[20]

Ultrafiltration

Ultrafiltration (or hemofiltration) refers to the hemoconcentration of blood utilizing an artificial kidney-type device, and was initially developed as a

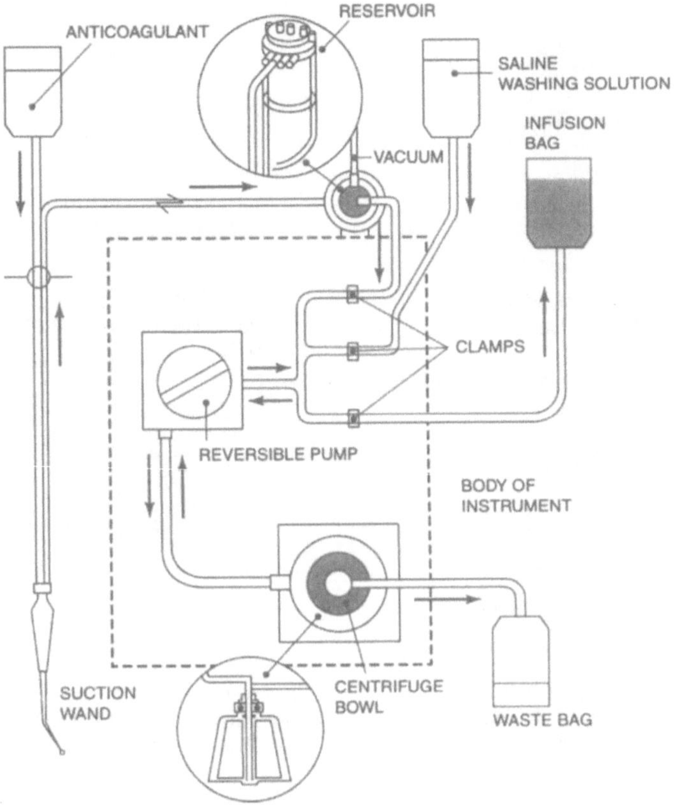

FIGURE 13.2. Design of a cell salvage/washing device such as the Haemonetics Cell Saver. The instrument includes a dual-lumen suction wand, reservoirs for aspirated blood and saline wash solution, an infusion bag for collecting the washed blood, and serial tubing clamps controlled by a microprocessor. A reversible pump head allows blood to flow either into or out of the centrifuge bowl. (From Williamson and Taswell,[12] by permission of *Transfusion*.)

component of hemodialysis in renal failure patients. The indications for ultrafiltration have broadened, however, and it is now applied in a variety of clinical settings where critical volume overload exists.[21] Although not a blood salvage technique in the pure sense, it is an effective method for limiting the dilutional anemia that may arise as a consequence of cardiopulmonary bypass (CPB). Ultrafiltration has been employed during CPB[22-24] as well as in the pre- and post-CPB phases of the operation.[25] The technique is based on the principle of convective solute transport.[22,23] Water, electrolytes, and small molecules are driven across a semipermeable membrane by hydrostatic pressure. Large molecular substances, such as blood cells and plasma proteins, remain well preserved while surplus fluid is removed.[21-23] Removal of solutes is determined by the pore size of the

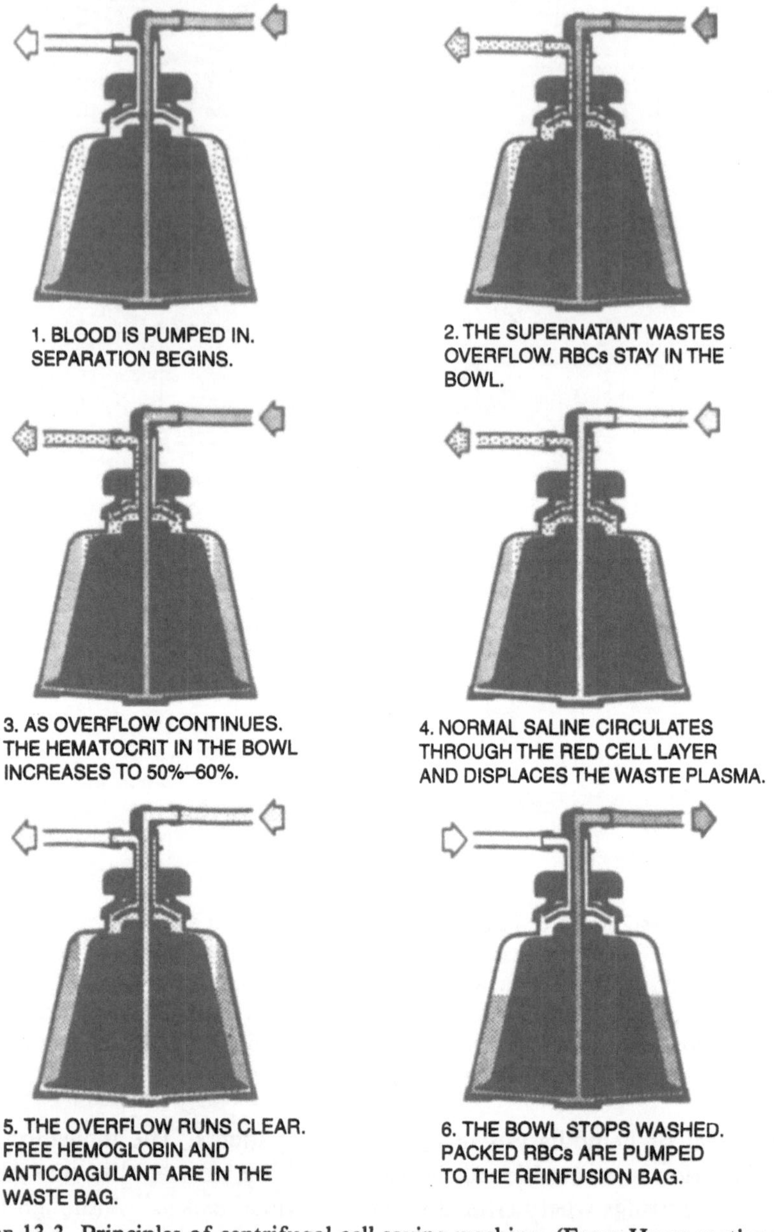
1. BLOOD IS PUMPED IN. SEPARATION BEGINS.
2. THE SUPERNATANT WASTES OVERFLOW. RBCs STAY IN THE BOWL.
3. AS OVERFLOW CONTINUES. THE HEMATOCRIT IN THE BOWL INCREASES TO 50%–60%.
4. NORMAL SALINE CIRCULATES THROUGH THE RED CELL LAYER AND DISPLACES THE WASTE PLASMA.
5. THE OVERFLOW RUNS CLEAR. FREE HEMOGLOBIN AND ANTICOAGULANT ARE IN THE WASTE BAG.
6. THE BOWL STOPS WASHED. PACKED RBCs ARE PUMPED TO THE REINFUSION BAG.

FIGURE 13.3. Principles of centrifugal cell saving-washing. (From Haemonetics Cell Saver 4 Operator's Manual.[20])

membrane. Available filters differ with respect to chemical composition, surface area, and efficiency.[26] The composition of the ultrafiltrate is similar to glomerular filtrate and the process does not alter serum electrolyte concentrations or acid-based status.[21] The amount of fluid removed depends on the flow and transmembrane pressure and can be controlled by the operator.[22,23] Placement of a filter in parallel to the CPB circuit on the

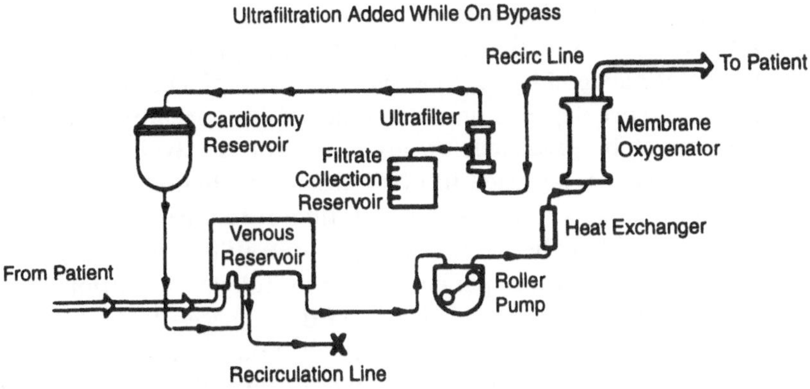

FIGURE 13.4. Schematic of a typical CPB circuit with incorporation of an ultrafilter. The ultrafilter is placed distal to the oxygenator to obviate the need for an additional pump. Filtered blood is returned to the circuit by a recirculation line. (From Magilligan,[25] by permission of *Journal of Thoracic and Cardiovascular Surgery*.)

arterial side obviates the need for an additional pump (Fig. 13.4).[27] After separation from CPB, up to 50% of the crystalloid content in the residual circuit blood can be removed with a "one-pass" ultrafiltration.[28] Processed blood can be returned directly to the cardiotomy reservoir or into a transfusion bag for post-CPB reinfusion.

Indications

Over the past two decades, the role of intraoperative salvage techniques in cardiac surgery has expanded and contributed significantly to reducing the reliance on homologous blood products. Several investigators have reported their experience with intraoperative autotransfusion. A moderate decrease in perioperative transfusion requirements was documented in an early study using a Sorensen-type cannister system.[29] Keeling and colleagues[30] reported more dramatic results with their experience using the Haemonetics Cell Saver in 539 patients undergoing cardiac surgery. Patients received a mean of 537 ml of processed blood, which contributed to a 50% decrease in the intraoperative use of homologous packed red cells compared to a historical cohort. A reduction in mean packed red cell use by 67% at the Mayo Clinic was attributed to the introduction of intraoperative salvage techniques.[31] Several prospective studies have demonstrated the effectiveness of the Cell Saver in decreasing intra- and postoperative homologous blood requirements.[17,29,32–34] Although reduction in transfusion requirement has not been the universal experience,[35] the majority of reports in the cardiac surgery literature clearly support the routine practice of intraoperative blood salvage and autotransfusion.

Exclusive use of cell saver suction from the onset of the operation, with minimal use of discard suction or laparotomy pads, has been advocated as a component of maximal blood conservation efforts.[36] The benefit derived from such a practice depends on the amount of intraoperative blood loss. Since this cannot be predicted, an argument for the availability of cell salvage capability can be made in every case, including routine, primary coronary bypass surgery.[37] Hemoconcentration of residual oxygenator and tubing volume, with either a cell saver or ultrafilter, is essential with nonblood prime CPB. Most patients can only tolerate a portion of this dilute volume during separation from CPB. If necessitated by a low hematocrit or excess reservoir volume, circuit blood can be hemoconcentrated during CPB either with the Cell Saver or ultrafilter.[26,38] Ultrafiltration has been employed preoperatively to manage volume overload or pulmonary edema in patients with coexisting renal insufficiency.[25] Ultrafiltration has been suggested to be particularly beneficial in controlling excessive hemodilution following long (>2 hour) CPB times or the administration of large volumes of cardioplegia or other crystalloid solutions.[27]

Contraindications

Few contraindications exist with respect to the practice of intraoperative blood salvage in cardiac surgery. The two most frequently cited are the presence of malignancy or infection. Recovery of viable tumor cells following passage through a Bentley-type apparatus and its filters has been reported.[39] Whether salvaged malignant cells are capable of initiating distant metastases following reinfusion is not clear. The theoretical possibility, however, has influenced recommendations regarding the use of salvage techniques during cancer surgery despite reports in which autotransfusion was employed without apparent detrimental effects.[40,41] Most cardiac surgery operations do not involve malignant disease, yet in those that do (i.e., resection of primary or metastatic cardiac or mediastinal tumors), blood salvage techniques should probably not be used. Similarly, if a diagnostic procedure for malignancy is to be performed following cardiopulmonary bypass, such as biopsy of a lung mass, use of the Cell Saver should be discontinued.

The second major contraindication to the use of intraoperative blood salvage is the presence of infection. Washing of salvaged blood decreases the number but does not completely remove contaminating bacteria.[42] Although the reinfusion of washed, contaminated blood in conjunction with appropriate systemic antibiotic coverage has been reported,[43] it seems prudent to avoid this practice except in emergency situations where alternative therapy is not available. Screening cultures have routinely documented the presence of bacterial organisms, usually staphylococcal species, within supposedly uncontaminated salvaged blood.[44-46] This finding, however, has rarely been linked to clinically significant infectious complications.[45,46] We will use Cell Saver suction during valve replacement in the setting of endocarditis, but avoid aspiration of grossly infected material.

Blood exposed to topical clotting agents such as Avitene (Alcon Inc., Humancao, Puerto Rico) or Surgicel (Johnson and Johnson, Arlington, TX) should not be salvaged. Separation of microfibrillar collagen hemostat with red cells during centrifugation and washing was documented in experimental animals, and reinfusion was associated with cerebral infarction.[47] Intraoperative salvage should be discontinued after the application of topical hemostatic substances. Similarly precaution should be taken if topical bacitracin or neomycin antibiotic solutions have been employed. These are not recommended for parenteral administration and can produce renal and neurologic toxicity.[48]

Quality of the Salvaged Blood

Blood salvaged from cannister-type systems that is not washed prior to reinfusion contains potentially injurious components. Plasma hemoglobin concentrations typically range from 66 to 245 mg/dl, with values as high as 2000 mg/dl having been reported,[12,49] suggesting the potential for nephrotoxicity. The presence of activated clotting factors and high concentrations of heparin could worsen coagulation abnormalities following reinfusion.[12] The salvaged blood can undergo further processing with standard blood bank equipment,[11,12] but this is cumbersome and time-consuming compared to the speed and ease with which the current generation centrifuge systems accomplish the task. Application is then limited to situations where the processed blood is not acutely needed.

Centrifugal cell washing has largely supplanted the use of the cannister-based systems in cardiac surgery. Advantages of cell washing include the removal of excess water, heparin, free hemoglobin, potassium, cellular debris, and thromboplastic substances. Blood salvaged with the Cell Saver has a hematocrit in the range of 45% to 65% when processed according to the manufacturer's recommendations, and is readily available in the operating room for swift reinfusion. Red blood cell survival after salvage, centrifugation, and washing does not differ significantly from normal.[50] Oxygen-carrying capacity is well preserved, and the concentration of 2,3-diphosphoglycerate is higher than that typically found in banked blood.[51] Washing removes up to 70% of the free hemoglobin,[48] and heparin concentration is reduced to levels insufficient to cause systemic anticoagulation.[18,19]

The principal recognized deficiency with centrifugal hemoconcentration is the loss of plasma proteins. A dilutional coagulopathy may arise if large volumes of Cell Saver blood are processed. This led some authors to recommend the routine administration of clotting factors and platelets under such conditions.[52] There is no clear consensus, however, as to what volume of blood can be processed with the Cell Saver before the loss of plasma proteins and platelets outweigh the benefit of red cell salvage. The impression that infusion of salvaged blood itself promotes a coagulopathy probably arose from early experience with the Bentley apparatus. Biochemical and tissue debris present in unprocessed whole blood, as discussed above, were likely the source of this disturbing problem.[8,9] Association of Cell Saver blood administration per se with bleeding is unfounded and in discordance with published clinical experience.[53]

The use of ultrafiltration to hemoconcentrate circuit blood during and after CPB has been promoted as a strategy for preserving clotting factors and perhaps attenuating postoperative coagulopathies. Several studies have documented significantly greater retention of clotting factors and platelets with ultrafiltration compared with the Cell Saver.[26,54–56] Although laboratory parameters of coagulation have been reported to be less deranged following hemofiltration,[54,56,57] clinically meaningful differences in postoperative bleeding have not been demonstrated.[27,38,54,58] Ultrafiltration removes plasma water only; it does not cleanse salvaged blood of contaminants such as tissue debris, activated coagulation factors and complement, free hemoglobin, or heparin. Applicability is therefore most suited for incorporation within the extracorporeal circuit, not for the processing of blood aspirated from the surgical site pre- or post-CPB.

New York Hospital Protocol

Our current intraoperative blood salvage protocol is centered on use of the Haemonetics Cell Saver 4. Cell salvage is begun at the onset of the operation and continued until the sternum is closed. During CPB, the Cell Saver is utilized for aspiration of pericardial contents. Cardiotomy suction is employed predominantly for clearing the surgical field during valve surgery or for return of fresh blood lost to the circuit during CPB.

We feel that it is important to minimize trauma to the salvaged red blood cells. Efforts are made to avoid squeezing out lap pads, suctioning air, or employing a high vacuum. Cell spinning and washing are conducted according to the manufacturer's instructions by our perfusion team. Salvaged blood is spun after collection of 500 to 1000 cc depending on the hematocrit and quality of the recovered blood. A 1000-cc wash is generally performed. Except for reoperative surgery and cases with inadvertent major blood loss pre-CPB, there is typically not enough salvaged blood to process before the addition of the residual pump volume. Hemoconcentration of circuit blood during CPB is performed only in the setting of a full venous reservoir and significant volume overload or a precipitously low hematocrit.

In our experience, especially with a low prime circuit, this is usually not feasible except in some cases of mitral or aortic valve replacement. When major, unexpected blood loss is encountered, in either the pre- or post-CPB phases of the operation, we have employed two Cell Saver devices simultaneously. Under such circumstances, an incomplete wash may be unavoidable in order to rapidly return the salvaged blood to maintain hemodynamic stability while avoiding homologous transfusion. After termination of CPB, circuit volume is returned to the patient as hemodynamics allow. Residual oxygenator and tubing volume is hemoconcentrated with the Cell Saver as soon as possible following decannulation. We do not routinely transfuse clotting factors when a large amount of Cell Saver blood has been salvaged, but instead assess the degree of bleeding on a per case basis and administer plasma or platelets according to the principles outlined in Chapter 20. In fact, we have processed up to 10 L of Cell Saver blood without concomitant homologous transfusion (unpublished data). Cell Saver blood is not withheld from the bleeding patient because of concerns regarding the potentiation of post-CPB coagulopathy. A summary of our protocol is outlined in Table 13.1.

Optimizing Intraoperative Blood Salvage

Recently, interest has focused on ways to maximize blood conservation during and after CPB. As discussed above, when addressing intraoperative loss into the surgical wound, the presence of potentially toxic and coagulopathic contaminants must be recognized. The cannister-based systems have been used successfully in cardiac surgery,[11,29] and although significantly less expensive, they cannot be recommended over the Cell Saver. The use of washed blood has been clearly demonstrated to be safe and efficacious, and should be considered superior to an unwashed product. Some centers have chosen to use the simple and inexpensive cannister devices and subsequently wash the salvaged blood in the central blood bank. The limitations of this practice, however, are significant. In our

TABLE 13.1. The New York Hospital intraoperative blood salvage protocol.

Cell Saver used in every case
Blood salvage employed from initial skin incision to sternal closure
Minimal use of lap pads and discard suction
Return of as much residual circuit blood to the patient as possible before hemoconcentrating
Attempt to process and reinfuse residual circuit volume as quickly as possible after decannulation
Cell Saver blood is not withheld from the bleeding patient
Clotting factors are not routinely administered when a large volume of Cell Saver blood is processed

experience, Cell Saver blood is typically needed early after the termination of CPB in order to raise the hematocrit to an acceptable level and provide needed colloid volume and oxygen carrying capacity.

The Cell Saver and ultrafilter both achieve hemoconcentration, but via fundamentally different mechanisms. Since ultrafiltration preserves clotting factors, investigators have sought to demonstrate a decrease in postoperative blood loss with its use. Several randomized studies have addressed this issue, but did not find significant differences in the degree of bleeding or blood utilization between the two methods. The ultrafilter is less expensive, more compact, and does not involve the major capital investment of the Cell Saver. It is, however, a more operator-intensive methodology, and is less appropriate for processing blood from the surgical site where free hemoglobin, heparin, activated coagulation factors, and other contaminants are present. The relative advantages and disadvantages of ultrafiltration and centrifugal cell washing are summarized in Table 13.2.

Further advancement of intraoperative blood conservation may require flexibility and the ability to employ several techniques of blood salvage. A Cell Saver system could be set up and used to collect blood from the chest throughout the operation. A hemofilter placed in line within the extracorporeal circuit would allow this option to be exercised if an appropriate indication was encountered. The residual circuit blood could be processed by either system, basing the decision on the volume involved, the immediacy of the need for the processed blood, and an assessment of clotting function.

The costs associated with routinely incorporating two salvage systems

TABLE 13.2. Ultrafiltration versus cell washing.

Centrifugal cell washing (i.e., Cell Saver)
Advantages
Salvaged blood is cleansed of debris and activated coagulation factors
Heparin is removed
Useful for blood salvage before and after CPB
Disadvantages
Loss of plasma proteins including clotting factors
Loss of platelets
Major capital investment required
Ultrafiltration
Advantages
Only removes excess plasma water
Retention of clotting factors, plasma proteins, and platelets
Relatively inexpensive
Can be used for pre- or perioperative volume overload, especially with coexistent renal failure
Disadvantages
Salvaged blood is not cleansed of debris, activated coagulation factor, or heparin
Applicability is restricted to blood obtained from the CPB circuit
More operator intense
Possible increased risk of contamination due to additional circuit connections

may be prohibitive, and a more efficient practice may be to identify those patients in whom a combination of methods would most likely be beneficial and implement them in a selective manner. In our opinion, the speed, safety, and applicability during all phases of the cardiac operation make the Cell Saver the most versatile and easiest system to adapt to a wide variety of clinical scenarios. Although it is the most expensive of the three major available techniques because of the initial capital investment of approximately $50,000, several studies have demonstrated overall cost benefits associated with the Cell Saver's ability to decrease homologous transfusion.[17,59,60] Additional cost-benefits, both medical and legal, derived from the prevention of the small but real occurrence of homologous transfusion-related illness and mortality have not been directly addressed.

An example of an imaginative approach to a difficult clinical problem was recently reported by Dekkers and colleagues.[61] They described a system (Fig. 13.5) designed for blood salvage during thoracic aortic aneurysm repair, which incorporates a standard Cell Saver apparatus, an ultrafilter,

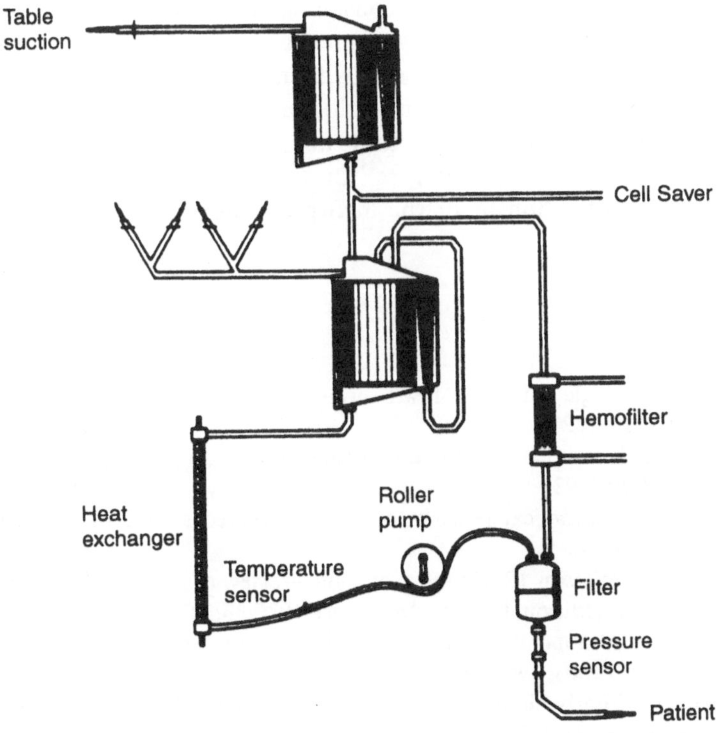

FIGURE 13.5. A novel blood salvage and autotransfusion system that incorporates several techniques for the processing of shed blood: use of the Cell Saver, an ultrafilter, and a rapid infusion system for unprocessed whole blood. (From Dekkers et al,[61] by permission of *Annals of Thoracic Surgery*.)

and a rapid infusion system (RIS, Haemonetics Corp.) capable of returning up to 1500 ml of whole, salvaged blood per minute if required by sudden, massive hemorrhage. The operator has the option to use the Cell Saver to wash salvaged blood, the ultrafilter to hemoconcentrate blood if it is too dilute, and the RIS to rapidly infuse warm, whole blood if needed. This versatile system would rarely be necessary for routine coronary or valve cases, but demonstrates how the cardiac surgeon can manipulate salvage techniques to maximize blood conservation in even the most challenging settings.

Conclusion

Intraoperative blood salvage is an established and important blood conservation measure in cardiac surgery. Along with nonblood prime hemodilution, it has had a major impact on perioperative homologous blood product requirements. Several effective techniques are available, including the Cell Saver, which in our practice is considered the standard of care. Cost considerations are expected to play an increasingly important role in cardiac surgery, yet an equally strong impetus will undoubtedly remain to minimize exposing patients to the risks of homologous transfusion. Future progress in intraoperative blood salvage may depend on implementing flexible protocols capable of responding to various clinical scenarios. This may involve the modification of or the incorporation of several existing techniques.

References

1. Roche JK, Stengle JM. Open-heart surgery and the demand for blood. *JAMA* 1973;225:1516–1521.
2. Blundell J. Experiments on the transfusion of blood by the syringe. *Med Chir Trans* 1818;9:56–92.
3. Highmore W. Practical remarks on an overlooked source of blood supply. *Lancet* 1874;1:89.
4. Watson CM, Watson JR. Autotransfusion—review of American literature with report of two additional cases. *Am J Surg* 1936;33:232–237.
5. Dyer RH. Intraoperative autotransfusion: a preliminary report and new method. *Am J Surg* 1966;112:874–878.
6. Klebanoff G. Early clinical experience with a disposable unit for the intraoperative salvage and reinfusion of blood loss (intraoperative autotransfusion). *Am J Surg* 1970;120:718–722.
7. Housman LB. Hemofiltration, dialysis, and salvage techniques. In: Utley J, ed. *Pathophysiology of Cardiopulmonary Bypass.* Baltimore: Williams & Wilkins: 1993;113–123.
8. Duncan SE, Klebanoff G, Rogers W. A clinical experience with intraoperative autotransfusion. *Ann Surg* 1974;180:296–304.

9. Duncan SE, Edwards WH, Dale WA. Caution regarding autotransfusion. *Surgery* 1974;76:1024–1029.
10. Bretton P, Reines HD, Sade RM. Air embolization during autotransfusion for abdominal trauma. *J Trauma* 1985;25:165–166.
11. Thurer RL, Hauer J. Autotransfusion and blood conservation. *Curr Probl Surg* 1982;19:98–156.
12. Williamson KR, Taswell HF. Intraoperative blood salvage: a review. *Transfusion* 1991;31:662–675.
13. Noon GP, Solis RT, Natelson EA, et al. A simple method of intraoperative autotransfusion. *Surg Gynecol Obstet* 1976;143:65–70.
14. Clifford PC, Kruger AR, Smith A, et al. Salvage autotransfusion in aortic surgery: initial studies using a disposable reservoir. *Br J Surg* 1987;74:755–757.
15. Schaff HV, Hauer JM, Bell WR, et al. Retransfusion of shed mediastinal blood following cardiac surgery: a prospective study. *J Thorac Cardiovasc Surv* 1978;75:4–12.
16. Cosgrove DM, Thurer RL, Lytle BW, et al. Blood conservation during myocardial revascularization. *Ann Thorac Surg* 1979;28:184–188.
17. Breyer RH, Engelman RM, Rousou JA, et al. Blood conservation for myocardial revascularization. Is it cost effective? *J Thorac Cardiovasc Surg* 1987;93:512–522.
18. Umlas J, O'Neill TP. Heparin removal in an autotransfuser device. *Transfusion* 1981;21:70–73.
19. Gravlee GP, Hopkins MB, Yetter CR, et al. Heparin content of washed red blood cells from the cardiopulmonary bypass circuit. *J Cardiovasc Anesth* 1992;6:140–142.
20. Haemonetics Cell Saver 4 Owner's Operating Maintenance Manual. Massachussetts: Haemonetics Corporation, 1987.
21. Silverstein ME, Ford CA, Lysaght MJ, et al. Treatment of severe fluid overload by ultrafiltration. *N Engl J Med* 1974;291:747–751.
22. Klineberg PL, Kam CA, Johnson DC, et al. Hematocrit and blood volume control during cardiopulmonary bypass with use of hemofiltration. *Anesthesiology* 1984;60:478–480.
23. Magilligan DJ, Oyama C. Ultrafiltration during cardiopulmonary bypass: laboratory evaluation and initial clinical experience. *Ann Thorac Surg* 1984;37:33–39.
24. Hakim M, Wheeldon WD, Bethune DW, et al. Haemodialysis and haemofiltration on cardiopulmonary bypass. *Thorax* 1985;40:101–106.
25. Magilligan DJ. Indications for ultrafiltration in the cardiac surgical patient. *J Thorac Cardiovasc Surg* 1985;89:183–189.
26. Boldt J, Zickmann B, Fedderson B, et al. Six different devices for blood conservation in cardiac surgery. *Ann Thorac Surg* 1991;51:747–753.
27. Page PA. Ultrafiltration versus cell washing for blood concentration. *J Extracorp Tech* 1990;22:142–150.
28. Tamari Y, Nelson R, Hall M, et al. Conversion of dilute whole blood by single pass ultrafiltration. *J Extracorp Tech* 1983;15:126–131.
29. Cordell AR, Lavender SW. An appraisal of blood salvage techniques in vascular and cardiac operations. *Ann Thorac Surg* 1981;31:421–425.
30. Keeling MM, Gray LA, Brink MA, et al. Intraoperative autotransfusion. Experience in 725 consecutive cases. *Ann Surg* 1983;197:536–540.
31. McCarthy PM, Popovsky MA, Schaff HV, et al. Effect of blood conservation

efforts in cardiac operations at the Mayo Clinic. *Mayo Clin Proc* 1988; 63:225–229.

32. Mayer ED, Welsch M, Tanzeem A, et al. Reduction of postoperative donor blood requirement by use of the cell separator. *Scand J Thorac Cardiovasc Surg* 1985;19:165–171.
33. Parrot D, Lancon JP, Merle JP, et al. Blood salvage in cardiac surgery. *J Cardiothorac Vasc Anesth* 1991;5:454–456.
34. Moran JM, Babka R, Silberman S, et al. Immediate centrifugation of oxygenator contents after cardiopulmonary bypass. *J Thorac Cardiovasc Surg* 1978; 76:510–517.
35. Winton TL, Charrette EJP, Salerno TA. The cell saver during cardiac surgery: Does it save? *Ann Thorac Surg* 1982;33:379–381.
36. Rosengart TK, Helm RE, Klemperer J, et al. Combined aprotinin and erythropoietin use for blood conservation: results with Jehovah's Witnesses. *Ann Thorac Surg* 1994;58:1397–1403.
37. Giordano GF, Goldman DS, Mammana RB, et al. Intraoperative autotransfusion in cardiac operations. Effect on intraoperative and postoperative transfusion requirements. *J Thorac Cardiovasc Surg* 1988;96:382–386.
38. Sutton RG, Kratz JM, Spinale FG, et al. Comparison of three blood-processing techniques during and after cardiopulmonary bypass. *Ann Thorac Surg* 1993; 56:938–943.
39. Yaw PB, Sentany M, Link WJ, et al. Tumor cells carried through autotransfusion: contraindication to intraoperative blood recovery? *JAMA* 1975; 231:490–491.
40. Homann B, Zenner HP, Schauber J, et al. Tumor cells carried through autotransfusion: are these cells still malignant? *Acta Anaesthesiol Belg* 1984; 35(suppl):51–59.
41. Hart OJ, Klimberg IW, Wasjman Z, et al. Intraoperative auto transfusion in radical cystectomy for carcinoma of the bladder. *Surg Gynecol Obstet* 1989;165:302–306.
42. Boudreaux JP, Bornside GH, Cohn I. Emergency autotransfusion: partial cleansing of bacterial-laden blood by cell washing. *J Trauma* 1983;23:31–35.
43. Timberlake GA, McSwain NE. Autotransfusion of blood contaminated by enteric contents: a potentially life-saving measure in the massively hemorrhaging trauma patient? *J Trauma* 1988;28:855–857.
44. Kluge RM, Calia RM, McLaughlin JS, et al. Sources of contamination in open heart surgery. *JAMA* 1974;230:1415–1418.
45. Schweiger IM, Gallagher CJ, Finlayson DC, et al. Incidence of cell-saver contamination during cardiopulmonary bypass. *Ann Thorac Surg* 1989; 48:51–53.
46. Bland LA, Villarino ME, Arduino MJ, et al. Bacteriologic and endotoxin analysis of salvaged blood used in autologous transfusions during cardiac operations. *J Thorac Cardiovasc Surg* 1992;103:582–588.
47. Robicseck F, Duncan GD, Dorn GVR, et al. Inherent dangers of simultaneous application of microfibrillar collagen hemostat and blood-saving devices. *J Thorac Cardiovasc Surg* 1986;92:766–770.
48. Guidelines for blood salvage and reinfusion in surgery and trauma. American Association of Blood Banks, 1993.
49. Clifford PC, Kruger AR, Smith A, et al. Salvage autotransfusion in aortic surgery: initial studies using a disposable reservoir. *Br J Surg* 1987;74:755–757.

50. Ansell J, Parilla N, King M, et al. Survival of autotransfused red blood cells recovered from the surgical field during cardiovascular operations. *J Thorac Cardiovasc Surg* 1982;84:387–391.
51. McShane AJ, Power C, Jackson JF, et al. Autotransfusion: quality of blood prepared with a red cell processing device. *Br J Anaesth* 1987;59:1035–1039.
52. Sharp WV, Stark M, Donovan DL. Modern autotransfusion. Experience with a washed red cell processing technique. *Am J Surg* 1981;142:522–524.
53. Ottesen S, Froysaker T. Use of Haemonetics Cell Saver for autotransfusion in cardiovascular surgery. *Scand J Thor Cardiovasc Surg* 1982;16:263–268.
54. Nakamura Y, Masada M, Toshima Y, et al. Comparative study of Cell Saver and ultrafiltration nontransfusion in cardiac surgery. *Ann Thorac Surg* 1990;49:973–978.
55. Tamari Y, Nelson R, Levy R, et al. Concentration of blood in the extracorporeal circuit using ultrafiltration. *J Extracorp Tech* 1983;15:133–142.
56. Boldt J, Kling D, von Bormann B, et al. Blood conservation in cardiac operations. Cell separation versus hemofiltration. *J Thorac Cardiovasc Surg* 1989;97:832–840.
57. Breyer RH, Engelman RM, Rousou JA, et al. A comparison of Cell Saver versus ultrafilter during coronary artery bypass operations. *J Thorac Cardiovasc Surg* 1985;90:736–740.
58. Johnson HD, Morgan MS, Utley JR, et al. Comparative analysis of recovery of cardiopulmonary bypass residual blood: Cell Saver versus hemoconcentrator. *J Extracorp Tech* 1994;26:194–199.
59. Solomon MD, Rutledge ML, Kane LE, et al. Cost comparison of intraoperative autologous versus homologous transfusion. *Transfusion* 1988;28:379–382.
60. Popovsky M, Devine PA, Taswell HF. Intraoperative autologous transfusion. *Mayo Clin Proc* 1985;60:125–134.
61. Dekkers RJ, Rizzo RJ, Body SC, et al. Shed whole blood autotransfusion during aortic aneurysm operation with a modified collection infusion system. *Ann Thorac Surg* 1995;59:184–186.

14
Operative Techniques in Blood Conservation

KARL H. KRIEGER

Very little has been written about the intraoperative technical aspects of blood conservation. This subject does not lend itself to rigorous experimental study. Nonetheless, it is a critical aspect of every successful open-heart operation and becomes a key determinant of the success or failure of cardiac surgery. Most of what each surgeon knows and practices regarding intraoperative hemostasis was learned during his residency and was passed down from teaching faculty and other surgical colleagues. There are as many different ways of opening the chest and controlling intraoperative bleeding as there are surgeons, and there are no ideal techniques for achieving hemostasis. Each surgeon has his own understanding of what is meant when he writes "meticulous hemostasis was achieved throughout the operation" in his operative notes. Nonetheless, a book directed toward minimizing blood utilization during cardiac surgery should describe at least one technique of achieving meticulous hemostasis. I hope residents and junior surgeons will find this chapter useful. Cardiovascular surgeons with several thousand cases behind them may want to investigate subsequent chapters.

Begin at the Beginning

Attempts at hemostasis begin with the skin incision. We open the skin with a knife and use the electrocautery (Pfizer – Valley Lab Model E-8-003) at a low setting to coagulate point arterial bleeders. *We do not open the skin and subcutaneous tissue with the electrocautery at a high setting*. This will stop bleeding, but we believe the associated thermal injury to the subcutaneous tissues increases the incidence of subcutaneous and sternal infections. When the sternum is encountered, the midline is marked with the electrocautery, but again, a line is not drawn along the anterior periosteum. This does limit bleeding but we feel this technique also devascularizes the anterior edges of the sternal bone. The upper portion of the skin incision is extended to the sternal notch and the lower margin is the xiphoid. Obvious transverse veins superior to the sternal notch are cauterized. The sternum is then opened with a saw and again the electrocautery is used to control arterial bleeders on the underside of the sternum. It is critical that the sternal incision is midline. We deplore devascularizing the lower sternal periosteum by cauterizing continuously along this edge. Nonetheless, careful observation throughout the operation of the posterior sternal table is critical as this is a common site of postoperative bleeding. Care is taken to point cauterize bleeding sites just above the sternal notch.

Bone bleeding is treated with a light coating of bone wax (Ethicon). Excess bone wax is contraindicated. The elderly patient with a friable, "saltine cracker"-type sternum may require the packing of oxidized cellulose (Oxycel, Parke-Davis) into the void between the sternal tables. This material (oxidize cellulose) and the bone wax may or may not be removed before sternal rewiring. Placing towels or drapes along the sternal edges underneath the retractor blades may decrease "pesky" bleeding from the bone during the procedure.

Anterior Mediastinum

Attention is directed to the soft tissues beneath the sternum. Thymic arteries and veins crossing the midline may need to be cauterized or clipped. Any thymic tissue that can be retracted out of the operative space and not divided will decrease bleeding. Anterior mediastinal soft tissue is a common site of postoperative bleeding and care should be taken during its division. Watch for the innominate vein, which is crossing transversely. The soft tissue in the plural spaces seldom bleeds except in reoperative cases. *Collateral arteries and veins may grow into any tissue area in a reoperative case and potential bleeding sites should be suspected everywhere.* The pericardium is usually opened with the cautery or scissors. This is a vascularized tissue and will bleed profusely if not appropriately cauterized. Do not cauterize the heart.

Internal Mammary Arteries

In bypass operations where internal mammary arteries (IMAs) are utilized, *the dissection should be performed in a non-"hurry up" environment.* The IMA bed should be carefully visualized with appropriate retraction and lighting and side branches of the mammary pedicle can be clipped, tied, or cauterized. When the distal IMA is divided, it is helpful to double clip or double tie the pedicle. This is another common bleeding site after coronary bypass surgery. During the proximal dissection of the internal mammary pedicle, care should be taken not to injure the left subclavian artery or vein. Again, adequate lighting and visualization is vital at this stage of the operation.

Cannulation

Choosing appropriate sites for cannulation is a critical decision in every cardiac operation. The arterial cannulation site should be chosen so that it is accessible for repair and control. In a reoperation or in a patient with a short aorta, cannulation of the transverse arch may be required. Again, it is important to choose a site that, after decannulation, can be exposed. We place a double purse-string suture with a 4-0 prolene. It is important that these sutures are not placed full thickness into the aortic wall. Pass the needles into the media but not through the intima. We put in the aortic purse strings before heparinizing the patient so that if bleeding is encountered, it can be controlled with local pressure. Many centers like to use Teflon felt pledges (PTFE Felt, Bard) on their purse-string sutures. We do not dissect away the adventitial tissue surrounding the aorta in the area of the cannulation site. We use this tissue as "pledget material" when oversewing at the conclusion of the case.

Right atrial cannulation sites are also carefully chosen for easy repair at the conclusion of the case. Sites at least a centimeter away from the atrial ventricular groove will prevent injury to the right coronary artery during closure. Routinely, 4-0 prolene is utilized in our center but very thin right atrial walls may require 5-0 sutures. With bicaval cannulation care is taken to keep the inferior vena cava (IVC) cannula site at least a centimeter above the pericardial reflection. A tear into the IVC may be lethal. When snares are placed around the caval cannulas great care is taken and this procedure may be completed more easily once cardiopulmonary bypass has been initiated. Again, a tear on the posterior aspect of the IVC is difficult to repair. Blood lost during the cannulation is returned to the circuit via the cardiotomy sucker or via the Cell Saver suction device.

Saphenous Vein Harvest

In coronary bypass procedures where the saphenous vein is harvested, skin incisions are usually made simultaneously with the sternal incision. Again, hemostasis begins with the skin incision and the electrocautery is used for point hemostasis. Saphenous veins are removed with double ligatures proximally and clips distally. Care is taken with aseptic technique and with hemostasis. Pooling of blood in large leg incisions is inappropriate and should bc avoided. With adequate exposure and lighting the dissection of the saphenous vein can be completed expeditiously with minimal blood loss.

The resected ends of the saphenous vein are doubly ligated with a suture ligature at the most proximal division site. The subcutaneous tissues of the leg incision are then closed in two or more layers. The patient may be heparinized and we do not delay the leg closure until heparin has been reversed.

When an unusual coagulopathy is diagnosed, drainage catheters may be placed or the leg closure may be delayed. This is seldom necessary. At the completion of the surgery, the legs are wrapped with a pressure dressing.

Coronary Artery Bypass Surgery

Coronary artery bypass operations are the most commonly performed cardiac operations in the country. We place the cardioplegic profusion catheter at a site that can be converted to a proximal anastomosis. This eliminates a potential bleeding site on the ascending aorta. Retrograde catheters passed into the coronary sinus should be carefully placed and the balloon not expanded until the location is confirmed. Coronary sinus rupture is difficult to repair. All distal anastomotic sites are tested for leakage with saline infusion after completion of the suture line. This technique helps evaluate anastomotic patency and is a time proven test to eliminate anastomotic bleeding. Distal anastomosis are reexamined after the completion of proximal anastomosis with a mean blood pressure between 60 and 80 mm Hg. Bleeding can usually be controlled with interrupted tacking 7-0 prolene sutures. Careful placement of repair sutures is mandatory to prevent anastomotic obstruction. Decreasing pump flow will aid in suture placement on the back of the heart. Again, dry anastomotic sites should be visualized.

Once we are confident that patients are not bleeding from their anastomoses, patients are weaned from bypass. If the patient stabilizes with an adequate cardiac output and no evidence of dramatic bleeding, protamine is given. Distal anastomoses are examined a third time after protamine is administered. Seldom are repair stitches necessary after the first examination.

Valvular Surgery

The most common valvular operations require incisions in the aorta, the left atrium, and at times the right atrium. When opening these structures, the surgeon should be thinking that all incisions require closure. *Exposure is key to successful valvular surgery, but the surgeon should always be aware that a perfect operation in a patient who bleeds to death is a catastrophe.*

Generally, the aortic incision should not extend down to the aortic annulus, yet it should be long enough so that tearing does not complicate the valve replacement. Aortotomy closure is initiated with sutures placed inside out on the aorta distal to the V point of the incision (Fig. 14.1). This seems a simple concept but adequate visualization of the V point in the left atrium (LA), for example, may be difficult and critical for hemostasis. Again, two separate suture lines starting at each end of the incision run to the middle aorta. We tie these suture lines against zero pressure and vent the aorta through a separate stab incision. The vent hole, placed on the most elevated aspect of the ascending aorta is 3 mm in length, and is oversewn with 5-0 prolene. Alternatively, it may be utilized as a proximal anastomotic site.

During mitral valve surgery, adequate exposure is again mandatory. The most commonly used lateral incision should be extended upward underneath the superior vena cava and inferiorly behind the inferior vena cava. In mitral valve replacement, sutures should be carefully placed in the posterior annulus to prevent bleeding from the posterior ventricle. Tissue in this area may be very thin, so only gentle traction should be exerted when tying the mitral valve into place.

Closure of the left atrium necessitates clear visualization at each end of the incision. We use 3-0 prolene with the first sutures placed inside out

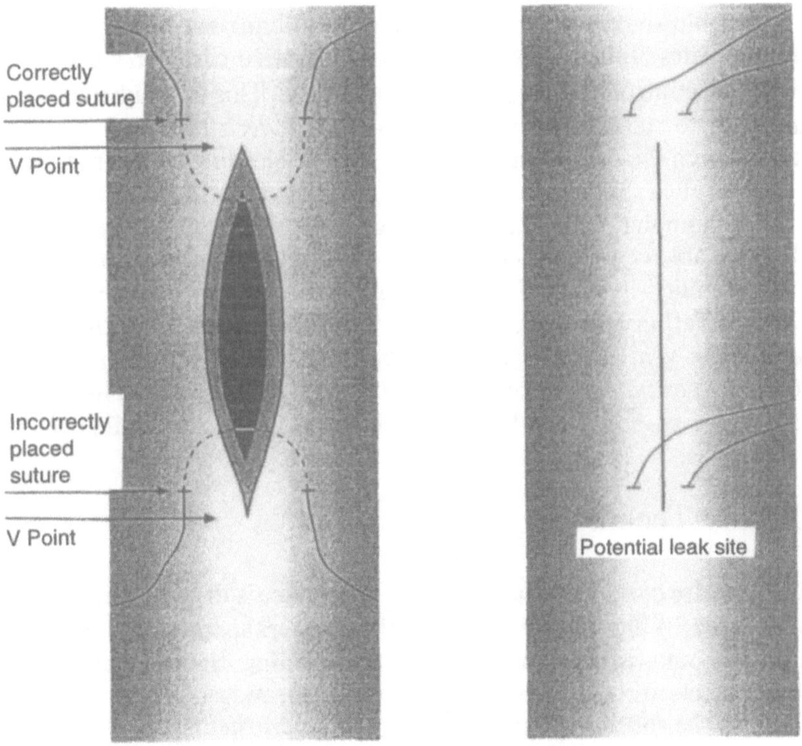

FIGURE 14.1. Schematic of vascular closure technique.

beyond the V point of the incision. We use a double layer running suture line. At the completion of the procedure, before weaning the patient from bypass, all suture lines are carefully examined. It may be necessary to increase the systemic blood pressure to carefully evaluate the aortic suture line. Likewise, repair of the left atrial suture line may be impossible once the patient is "off bypass." If left atrial catheters are placed, a small purse-string suture is tied around the insertion site. Multiple studies have noted that platelet function decreases with temperature so we routinely warm to 36°C before weaning bypass. If no obvious bleed sites are seen off bypass, time is not wasted trying to prevent needle hole bleeding, and protamine is administered.

Off Bypass

A surprising number of bleeding sites will stop with heparin reversal. Superficial venous bleeding on the posterior surface of the heart secondary to heart retraction will routinely stop with anticoagulation reversal. *Too often operating time is wasted trying to control all venous bleeding*. Benign observation will usually suffice. Topical agents like oxidized cellulose are routinely used on oozing suture lines.

Thrombin-soaked gel pads (Gelfoam, Upjohn) may also be helpful at bleeding sites. Fibrin glue is used in reoperative cases or where bleeding cannot be controlled with standard techniques. This is sprayed on the heart just prior to sternal closure. Using the Cell Saver sucker and 4 × 4 gauze pads to keep the pericardial space dry, occult bleeding sites can be localized and controlled. Saline irrigation may also help identify persistent bleeding. Venous cannulae are removed before protamine is administered. Arterial cannulae are removed after protamine administration and after cardiovascular stability is assured. All cannulation sites are oversewn with 4-0 prolene. Teflon felt pledgets may be helpful with the difficult aorta. *Left ventricular vent sites, which are routinely closed with Teflon felt, are difficult to examine after weaning the patient from bypass*. This site should be a major suspect when blood is welling up in the pericardium.

Closure Technique

When we are confident that the pericardial space is dry, the sternal retractor is removed. A lap pad is placed in the substernal space and the skin and subcutaneous tissues are reexamined for bleeding. Spot cautery is utilized. Using the electrocautery in a continuous or spray fashion increases thermal injury to the subcutaneous tissue, skin, and periosteum and is unnecessary. Only significant bleeding from the sternal bone is investigated. Oxidized cellulose laid between the sternal tables may be helpful. Large chunks of bone wax interfere with sternal healing and should be removed. The anterior and the posterior tables of the sternum and the IMA resection sites are carefully examined. The IMA ligation site is inspected and the mammary pedicle is examined. If a tunnel through the left pericardium for the IMA pedicle is needed, the left mediastinal tissues are divided with the electrocautery. This tissue is well vascularized and must be carefully perused. Avoid the phrenic nerve.

When we are confident that the skin, subcutaneous tissues, and bone are not bleeding, the sternum is reopened with the sternal retractor. The lap pad is removed and blood on the lap pad will help localize bleeding within the pericardial space. If hemostasis is adequate, the anterior mediastinal fat may be closed over the aorta. Chest tube insertion sites are carefully examined for bleeding. Pacing needles are placed to avoid the intercostal and IMAs. Sternal wires are carefully placed to avoid the same arteries. Depending on the size of the sternum, these wires may be placed through the sternum or through the intercostal spaces.

Each wire should be examined individually and bleeding can usually be controlled with a figure-8 stitch of 2-0 Vicryl. Rarely, persistent bleeding may require wire removal. As the sternal wires are examined for potential bleeding, the posterior periosteum is once again visualized.

This completes the third and final examination of the periosteum. Likewise, the mammary bed is examined for a third time. The sternum is then closed. We routinely irrigate the subcutaneous tissue with a liter of warm saline. The subcutaneous tissues are closed in several layers and the skin is closed with a subcuticular closure technique or with staples. During this external closure, bleeding from the substernal tube and the pleural tubes is carefully observed. A separate suction catheter is placed into these tubes and the total amount of bleeding is grossly evaluated. If it is felt to be unacceptable, the sternal incision can be reopened for reexamination of the mediastinum or the pleural spaces. *Bleeding over 100 cc in 15 minutes is of significant concern.* It is important to keep the drainage tubes unclotted with periodic suctioning.

Postoperative Bleeding

If significant bleeding is anticipated, because of a long or difficult operation or because of a preexisting coagulopathy, fresh frozen plasma (FFP), platelets, and cryoprecipitate may be ordered before weaning the patient from bypass. When confident that bleeding will be encountered in the postoperative setting, these factors should be given after protamine administration (Table 14.1).

TABLE 14.1. Common bleeding sites in cardiac surgery.

Lower table sternal bone	Costophrenic arteries above diaphragm
Veins of suprasternal notch	Cannulation sites
Thymic remnant tissue	LV vent site
IMA pedicle and ligation site	Distal anastomotic sites
IMA bed	Posterior angle of aortotomy incisions
Pericardial edge	Saphenous vein vasovasorum

Conclusion

Hasty closure techniques are often rewarded with significant bleeding in the intensive care unit. A complex operation and a fatigued surgeon should not add up to a hasty closure. Instead, the opposite is demanded and a careful point-by-point reexamination of bleeding sites is mandatory to guarantee hemostasis. In particularly complex or prolonged operations, a separate closure team may be indicated. At times a surgeon should "scrub out" for a cup of coffee before resuming the battle. Semirefreshed, he can complete the search for bleeding sites that might then allow him to honestly dictate "meticulous hemostasis was achieved at the completion of the procedure."

15
Pharmacologic Approaches to Coagulation (Aprotinin, Epsilon Amino Caproic Acid, DDAVP, Tranexamic Acid Therapy)

TODD K. ROSENGART

Bleeding and blood transfusion have long been associated risks of open-heart surgery. The source of this risk is twofold, being related both to the hemodilution and the coagulopathy that have to the present time been inherent components of cardiopulmonary bypass (CPB). The prevention and treatment of coagulopathy is the focus of this chapter.

The nonphysiologic mechanics of CPB and the artificial surfaces of the bypass circuit are the two most important contributors to the development of a coagulopathic state in open-heart surgery. These elements lead to massive platelet aggregation and depletion, activation of the coagulation cascades and coagulation factor depletion, and activation of the fibrinolytic and inflammation pathways. Although both pro- and anticoagulant pathways are stimulated by CPB, the net outcome is anticoagulation, as manifested in prolonged indices of coagulation function—bleeding time, prothrombin time (PT), partial thromboplastin time (PTT), etc.—and increased postoperative bleeding.

Until recently, the capability to prevent or treat these derangements was limited. Treatment ultimately was limited to the transfusion of platelets or coagulation factors. In the last few years, however, there has developed a rapidly increasing interest in the pharmacologic manipulation and reversal of coagulation defects associated with CPB. Isolated reports of pharmacologic interventions to restore normal coagulation were scattered through the cardiac surgical literature during the 1960s and 1970s. The modern era of management of coagulation function in CPB, however, probably dates to the article of Salzman et al[1] in 1986 regarding desmopressin pretreatment of patients undergoing open-heart surgery.

The publication in 1987 by Royston et al[2] and van Oeveren et al[3] of studies regarding the efficacy of aprotinin in inhibiting bleeding and blood transfusions in open-heart surgery accelerated the current expansion of interest in this drug and the other antifibrinolytics, epsilon amino caproic acid (EACA; Amicar), and tranexamic acid (TA). Each of these agents may play an important role in preventing bleeding and blood transfusion in open-heart surgery. The specific structure and function of these agents, and their relative efficacy, safety, and cost are discussed in this chapter.

Aprotinin

Aprotinin is a low molecular weight serine-protease inhibitor that was first introduced into clinical use in 1953 for the treatment of acute pancreatitis. Use of aprotinin in cardiac surgery dates back to the observations reported by Tice et al[4] in 1963. In his report, the administration of 10,000 to 20,000 kallikrein inhibitory units (KIU) of aprotinin in five patients presenting with increased fibrinolytic activity and increased bleeding after CPB resulted in the rapid remission of this bleeding. Similar inhibition of fibrinolysis was noted by Mammen et al[5] in 1968 with doses of 100,000 units per hour of aprotinin given during CPB. Decreased postoperative bleeding was also noted by Ambrus et al[6] in 1971 with prophylactic aprotinin administration, given prior to sternotomy, that more closely resembles the currently recommended dosing regimen.

The current era of high-dose aprotinin therapy (5–6 million unit average total dose) dates to the serendipitous discovery by the Hammersmith group[2] that this high-dose regimen significantly reduces bleeding in cardiac surgical patients. It is interesting that this discovery was made while the drug was being used to assess its ability to reduce kallikrein-mediated lung inflammation that occurs during CPB. The Hammersmith regimen, based upon these studies, represents the current standard of reference for all aprotinin treatment strategies.

Structure, Function, and Pharmacology

Aprotinin is a naturally occurring, highly basic polypeptide isolated from bovine lung. Its molecular weight is 6512. A lysine residue occupies its active center. The specificity of aprotinin is restricted mainly to enzymes with trypsin-like substrate specificity. Aprotinin has been shown to be effective in humans against trypsin, plasmin, streptokinase-plasma complex, tissue kallikrein, and plasma kallikrein. Aprotinin forms reversible enzyme-inhibitor complexes with various proteases, each of which has a specific dissociation constant that influences the aprotinin concentration necessary to produce enzymatic inhibition. Effective inhibition of plasmin and plasma kallikrein consequently requires 125 KIU/ml and 250 to 500 KIU/ml of aprotinin, respectively.[7]

Aprotinin demonstrates a two-phased elimination half-life with an initial half-life of 0.7 hour and a terminal half-life of 7 hours. The initial half-life represents the distribution of aprotinin in the extracellular compartment, and the terminal half-life corresponds to aprotinin accumulation in the kidneys and cartilage. The renal proximal tubules demonstrate significant aprotinin uptake and this in part translates into aprotinin-mediated renal effects.

The standard aprotinin dosage regimen, designated the "Hammersmith regimen," was based on calculations conceived at Hammersmith designed to yield a 4μM plasma concentration of aprotinin in order to block plasma kallikrein activity.[8] The high-dose aprotinin regimen is as follows: a small (10,000 KIU) intravenous test dose is given at the initiation of the surgery to assess for anaphylaxis. This is followed approximately 10 minutes later by an intravenous loading dose of 2 million KIU (280 mg) of aprotinin, and a CPB pump prime load of 2 million units. An intravenous maintenance infusion of 0.5 million units (70 mg) per hour is then continued until the end of the operation. This dosage regimen yields aprotinin plasma concentrations of 185 to 335 KIU/ml at the start of cardiopulmonary bypass and 80 to 190 KIU/mL at the end of bypass.[2,9–11] Since this aprotinin dosage is based on the plasma kallikrein inhibitory concentrations, the inhibition of plasmin should also be demonstrated at these dosage levels.

Recent data also suggest that a "half-Hammersmith" regimen may be effective in decreasing bleeding in all but the highest-risk cases, such as those patients undergoing reoperation who are also taking aspirin (J. Levy, personal communication). This regimen consists of a 1 million unit pump prime and intravenous load, followed by a maintenance infusion of 250,000 units/hour. These data are consistent with the theory that, because of the complex interrelationships between the coagulation cascades in vivo, aprotinin concentrations necessary to yield in vitro inhibition of kallikrein may not necessarily correlate with dosages that are effectively hemostatic clinically. In fact, these higher dosages may be excessively thrombogenic. Additional data supporting the efficacy of very low dose pump prime[9,12] or topical aprotinin[13] regimens have been initially promising, but must be viewed as incomplete.

Mechanism of Action

Because aprotinin is a nonspecific serine antiprotease, it intervenes in the coagulation cascade in multiple loci (Fig. 15.1). Aprotinin probably works to decrease bleeding in open-heart surgery predominantly by way of its antiplasmin and antikallikrein effects during CPB. Blood exposure to the surface of the CPB circuit activates the contact phase of coagulation, resulting in an increase in activation of factor XII and kallikrein, which in turn transform plasminogen into plasmin. Plasminogen activation by extrinsic (tissue type) plasminogen activator is also enhanced during CPB. Increased fibrinolytic activity increases the concentration of fibrin degradation products, which further accelerate the tendency toward anticoagulation. Plasmin is also thought to cleave the platelet adhesion receptor

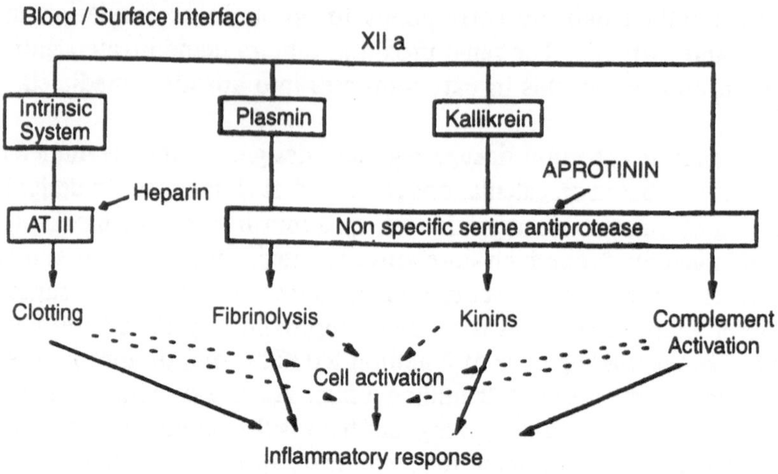

FIGURE 15.1. Effects of nonspecific protease inhibition (such as aprotinin therapy) on contact activation pathways. (Reprinted with permission from Pifarre[42])

glycoprotein (Gp) Ib, reducing platelet adhesion during and after CPB.[14] Aprotinin works to block the activation of kallikrein at the top of the cascade, plasmin at the bottom, and all the intermediary outcomes normally ensuing from these events.

In support of the importance of prophylactic aprotinin therapy, as opposed to its use after the development of a coagulopathic state, it is interesting to note that a mean decrease in the number of Gp Ib platelet receptors of 50% has been noted in control versus aprotinin-treated patients as soon as 5 minutes after the initiation of CPB.[9,12] Furthermore, aprotinin administration was shown to eliminate the increase in fibrin degradation products normally seen in nontreated patients.[12] The mechanism of action of aprotinin therefore would appear to be related to preservation of platelet function, reflected in a decrease in bleeding times in aprotinin-treated versus control patients, and an inhibition of fibrinolysis, thereby preserving clot formation.

Dietrich et al[10] have further postulated that through its antikallikrein effects, aprotinin inhibits the contact phase of coagulation, leading to diminished generation of thrombin. This would initially be perceived as an anticoagulant property of aprotinin and, in fact, may be so to some degree. Thrombin, however, is also a powerful platelet aggregator. Since excessive, consumptive platelet aggregation during CPB is thought to lead to postoperative platelet dysfunction,[15] aprotinin may work to preserve platelet function and availability following CPB by inhibiting platelet aggregation during bypass.

Perhaps an incidental effect of aprotinin in terms of coagulation testing is its ability to prolong activated clotting times (ACT) in patients on heparin (Fig. 15.2), compared with patients receiving a dose of heparin without aprotinin.[9,10,16] This finding was originally attributed to the potential

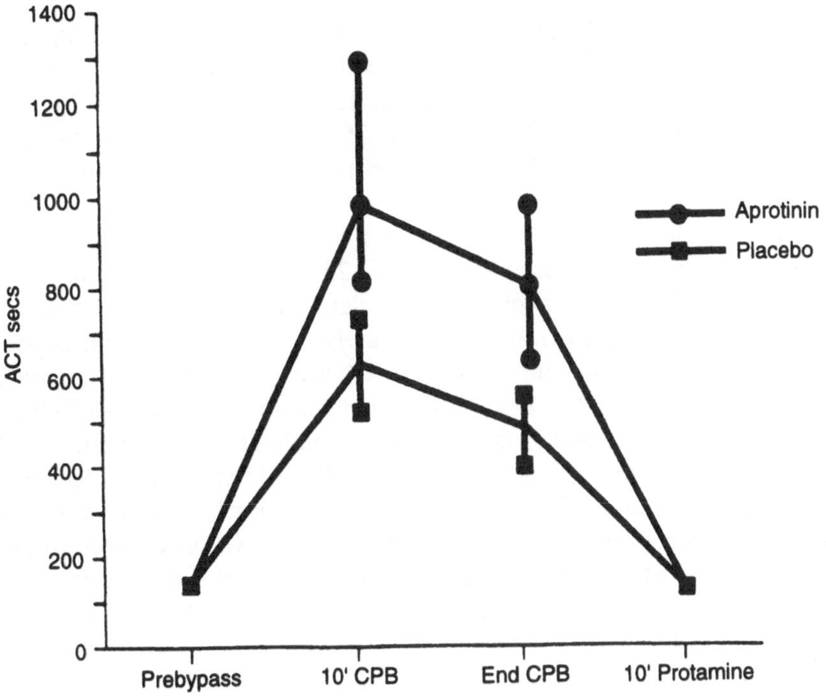

FIGURE 15.2. Effect of heparin (■) and heparin plus aprotinin (•) on automated clotting time (ACT) during cardiopulmonary bypass (CPB). (Reprinted with permission from Taylor[41])

anticoagulant properties of aprotinin, and it was initially suggested that decreased heparin dosing might be possible with aprotinin use.[16] Subsequent data suggested that the prolonged ACT phenomenon was a result of an artifactual aprotinin interaction with the diatomaceous earth (Celite) used as the activator in the Hemochron ACT testing device (International Technodyne, Edison, NJ). This consensus was the result of an observation that the substitution of kaolin for the Celite as the activator for the ACT assay reversed the ACT prolongation effect with aprotinin concentrations up to 180 KIU/ml.[17] More recently, however, Dietrich and Jochum[18] have presented evidence that kaolin, not Celite, is actually the substrate interacting with aprotinin, in fact absorbing aprotinin and thereby blocking a net anticoagulant in vitro effect. Again, these data highlight the difficulty of interpreting in vitro assays, apparent anticoagulant in effect, in light of chemical evidence of the procoagulant effects of aprotinin interactions with hemostatic pathways in vivo.

Efficacy Studies

Three studies represent the initial database demonstrating the efficacy of high-dose aprotinin. The first was a placebo-controlled, randomized, double-blinded study involving 80 patients undergoing primary coronary bypass.[11] Total blood loss was decreased from almost 600 ml to approximately 300 ml ($p < .01$) for patients in the placebo and aprotinin treatment groups, respectively. Hemoglobin loss was decreased from 37 g to 12 g, and transfusion requirement decreased from 75 units to 13 units in the two respective groups. The number of patients transfused was decreased from 95% to 20%.

More dramatic results were obtained in a prospective, randomized study of reoperative cardiac surgery patients ($n = 22$), presumably because of the increased risk of nonsurgical bleeding associated with reoperations.[2] In this study, bleeding decreased from approximately 1500 ml to less than 300 ml ($p < .001$) and there was reported almost a tenfold decrease in hemoglobin loss (78 ± 23 g vs 8 ± 2 g, $p < .001$). The total number of units of blood transfusion were decreased from 41 units to 5 units, and the percentage of patients transfused decreased from 100% to 36%, in spite of the fact that each group was discharged with similar hemoglobin levels. Interestingly, the mean chest closure time was halved in the aprotinin versus control group, from 60 minutes to 30 minutes, reflecting the dryness of the operative field and indicating that decreased blood loss was not related to increased attention to hemostasis.

These results were confirmed in a trial at the Cleveland Clinic by Cosgrove et al[19] involving 169 reoperative coronary bypass surgery patients. In this study, a low-dose protocol was introduced in which the loading and infusion rates were decreased by half. Blood loss was significantly reduced in both of the high- and low-dose treatment arms, 720 ml and 866 ml, respectively compared with 1121 ml in the clinical group (Table 15.1). A statistically significant decrease in transfusion requirement was noted both in the high- and the low-dose treatment groups. However, this report included anecdotal evidence of increased myocardial infarction rate and evidence of an increased rate of graft thrombosis in aprotinin-treated patients (Table 15.2).

Safety Data

Partly in answer to this problem, another large multicenter study was conducted in the United States. This study demonstrated similar efficacy to that found in the previous studies and in fact demonstrated efficacy for the

TABLE 15.1. Effect of aprotinin dose on postoperative bleeding and blood and blood product usage.

Dosage	Chest drainage (ml)	RBC (units)	Platelets (units)
Full dosage	720 ± 753	2.1	1.6
Half dosage	866 ± 1,636	4.8	3.3
Placebo	1,121 ± 683	4.1	5.4

RBC, red blood cells.
Data from Taylor.[41]

TABLE 15.2. Morbidity and mortality results for each aprotinin study group.

Variable	High dose	Low dose	Placebo	*p* value*
Mortality	4 (7.0%)	5 (8.9%)	4 (7.1%)	NS
MI	9 (15.8%)	5 (8.9%)	4 (7.1%)	NS
Reoperation for bleeding	1 (1.8%)	3 (5.4%)	0 (0%)	NS
Creatinine increase > 0.5 mg/dl	14 (2.6%)	11 (19.6%)	10 (17.9%)	NS
Creatinine clearance (mL/min)	132.9 ± 77.8	122.0 ± 61.5	110.7 ± 46.5	NS
Median SGOT (IU/L)	93.0	92.0	79.5	NS

*Tests for statistical significance compare aprotinin versus placebo.
MI, myocardial infarction; NS, not significant; SGOT, serum glutamic-oxaloacetic transaminase.
Data from Cosgrove et al.[19]

half-dose regimen, both in terms of bleeding and transfusion requirements, except in reoperated patients who were on preoperative aspirin, in which only the high-dose regimen was significantly effective (J. Levy, personal communication). A critical component of this study was a blinded prospective analysis examining the rate of myocardial infarction. Serial creatinine kinase and electrocardiographic determinations yielded no evidence of a significant increase in the myocardial infarction rate for either low- or high-dose aprotinin treatment compared with placebo controls.

In separate studies, both ultrafast computed tomography (CT) and magnetic resonance imaging (MRI) examinations of bypass vein grafts provided further confirmatory evidence for the lack of a significant increase in graft thrombosis with aprotinin therapy.[20,21] Small but nonstatistical increases in graft thrombosis were, however, noted with aprotinin therapy in each of these studies.

Much emphasis has been placed in the past decade on perioperative antiplatelet therapy to induce a degree of anticoagulation adequate to preserve graft patency. It therefore seems intuitive that complete restitution of the procoagulant processes following coronary bypass surgery may be undesirable in terms of graft patency. It is the author's opinion that the utilization of aprotinin probably does carry some risk of increased thrombosis compared with untreated patients, whether involving the bypass grafts or the native circulation. It is likely that the clinical significance of this risk is incremental, and must be viewed in context of the potential benefit from decreased postoperative bleeding and blood transfusion (Fig. 15.3). In most cases except in the extreme circumstances such as Jehovah's Witnesses where any bleeding carries great risk, it is the author's practice to use a half-dose aprotinin regimen. In this manner, a perhaps somewhat increased risk of bleeding is traded for a proportionately decreased potential for thrombogenicity.

Aprotinin therapy is also associated with some risk of renal dysfunction, which in general is reversible and appears to be dose related and associated with aprotinin uptake by the kidney.[20,22] A recent review of 216 patients

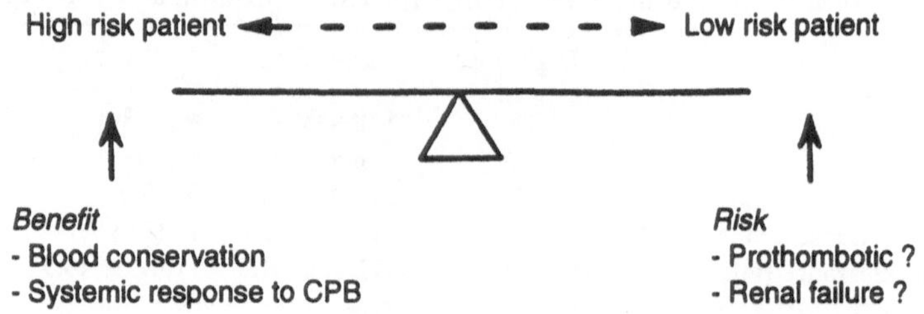

FIGURE 15.3. Schematic of risk-benefit ratio for aprotinin therapy. (Reprinted with permission from Taylor[41])

undergoing coronary bypass procedures randomized to receive high-dose aprotinin or placebo in fact found no significant differences in postoperative creatinine increases between the two groups.[23] Finally, because aprotinin is a foreign protein, treatment also carries a small (<1%) risk of anaphylaxis, which increases with reexposure. It should be noted that the recommended test dose given prior to aprotinin loading does not completely eliminate the risk of subsequent anaphylaxis.

Amicar and Tranexamic Acids

Structure and Function

The clinical use of epsilon amino caproic acid (EACA), Amicar, was first described in 1959, and the antifibrinolytic activity of tranexamic acid (TA) was elucidated in 1964. EACA and TA are both synthetic antifibrinolytics, and both have similar pharmacologic properties. They are small molecules, with weights of 131 and 157 daltons, respectively. These agents form a reversible complex with either plasminogen or plasmin. Saturation of the lysine binding site of plasminogen by EACA or TA displaces plasminogen, and therefore its active moiety plasmin, from the surface of fibrin. The in vivo activation of plasminogen is slow unless it is bound to fibrin, which in turn also binds tissue plasminogen activator to accelerate the process. The blockage of plasminogen binding to fibrin therefore effectively blocks plasminogen activation, and, consequently, fibrinolysis.[24–26] In contrast, aprotinin works directly to irreversibly bind to and inhibit the active plasmin enzyme. Both EACA and TA thereby block the premature dissolution of the normal fibrin clot, but both of these drugs are also ineffective until clotting has occurred.

EACA and TA are both different from aprotinin in their inability to inhibit kallikrein activity and in that they are without the general antiproteolytic activity of aprotinin. The only significant difference between TA and EACA is that TA is approximately 10 times as potent as EACA.[15] Dosing regimens are therefore approximately 100 to 250 mg/kg followed by a loading dose of 10 to 15 mg/kg per hour for EACA, and approximately one tenth of this dosing regimen for TA. Both drugs have an elimination half-life between 1 and 2 hours, and both are rapidly excreted in urine in the active form.

Efficacy

The first reports regarding the efficacy of EACA in reducing bleeding following open-heart surgery dates to the 1960s.[26] The use of tranexamic acid in cardiopulmonary bypass was first advocated by Horrow et al[27] in 1990. Advocacy of the use of these agents in open-heart surgery was in part related to the correlation by Marin[26] of increased fibrinolysis with prolonged CPB times, and the finding of subsequent investigators that increased fibrinolysis could be demonstrated with such minimal interventions as skin incision.

EACA was initially employed as a therapeutic modality for excessive bleeding noted after the cessation of CPB. In this fashion, Lambert et al[28] in 1979 identified patients with coagulation disorders (20% of total primary coronary bypass patients) and successfully treated these patients with EACA. Similar results were obtained by VanderSalm et al[29] in a double-blind, placebo-controlled trial involving randomized administration of EACA after weaning from CPB.

In contrast, Del Rossi et al[30] demonstrated the efficacy of *prophylactic* EACA administration in 350 patients undergoing CPB. In their study, 5 g of EACA was given prior to skin incision, followed by 1 g per hour for 6 to 8 hours. Average blood loss for 24 hours decreased from almost 900 ml to approximately 600 ml ($p < .05$), and blood transfusions in the first 72 hours postoperatively decreased from 4.2 ± 2.3 to 2.8 ± 2.0 units ($p < .05$). In light of the above discussion about prevention of Gp Ib platelet receptor cleavage as a mechanism of action of the antifibrinolytics, it is not surprising that the prophylactic use of EACA or TA would be of importance. Similar decreases in postoperative bleeding were noted with prophylactic TA therapy by Horrow et al[27] in 1990 in 38 patients undergoing CPB.

As with aprotinin, some concern has been raised regarding the potential risk of these agents in causing increased, possibly pathologic, thrombosis. Based on adverse event reporting in the literature, this risk seems less pronounced than that addressed with aprotinin, perhaps because of the more limited focus of action of the synthetic antifibrinolytics and the relatively lesser degree of prothrombotic activity of these agents. As with aprotinin, the risk of inappropriate thrombosis is perhaps most properly viewed as being in indirect proportion to these agents' procoagulant efficacy.

Desmopressin

Desmopressin acetate (DDAVP) is a synthetic analogue of the hormone vasopressin that is devoid of the vasoconstrictor effects of the native hormone. In terms of its hematologic effects, desmopressin appears to function by augmenting the release from endogenous stores in endothelial cells and increasing the circulating levels of von Willebrand factor (VWF) and factor VIII coagulant protein (FVIII:c). These substances act to increase platelet adhesion. Sloand et al[31] have further demonstrated that DDAVP increases the in vitro expression of platelet membrane GpIb, which is the VWF platelet receptor. Secretion of tissue plasminogen activator (TPA), responsible for activation of the fibrinolytic system, is also stimulated by DDAVP, and this may represent a potentially deleterious effect of DDAVP in regard to increasing hemostasis.[32]

Czer et al[33] initially reported on the effects of DDAVP in CPB surgery, demonstrating that in selected patients with excessive bleeding after cardiopulmonary bypass, less blood component transfusion (15 ± 13 vs. 29 ± 19 units, $p = .02$) and fewer reoperations for bleeding (9% vs. 75%) were required if patients were treated with DDAVP. Salzman et al[1] performed the first prospective randomized, double-blind trial in unselected patients undergoing cardiopulmonary bypass, and demonstrated a 40% reduction in 24-hour blood loss (2210 ± 1415 ml vs. 1317 ± 487 ml, $p < .001$) and a 34% decrease in transfusion requirement (3.7 ± 3.3 vs. 2.6 ± 2.1 units, $p = .079$). Desmopressin in this study was administered as a dose of 0.3 μg/kg given at the conclusion of cardiopulmonary bypass. These results appeared to correlate with an elevation of circulating levels of VWF. The increased blood transfusion and bleeding rates in the control population of both these studies, however, raises some concern regarding their general applicability. In fact, multiple subsequent studies generally fail to demonstrate similar efficacy, and have placed the role of DDAVP in cardiac surgery in serious doubt.[34]

Although most recent studies have failed to demonstrate the efficacy of desmopressin, it is conceivable that DDAVP may nevertheless prove to be effective in subsets of patients at risk for increased bleeding, especially those patients with a functional platelet defect because of aspirin therapy or from other causes. A reexamination of DDAVP in these patients is the subject of current investigations. In fact, Monogan and Hosking,[35] by selecting for such patients with the aid of thromboelastography, did demonstrate a decrease in chest tube drainage in patients treated with DDAVP as compared with a control population. Salzman et al[36] have most recently advocated such a selective approach, suggesting as well the utilization of a prophylactic regimen.

Cost and Efficacy: Comparative Considerations

Aprotinin and the antifibrinolytics, and possibly DDAVP as well, will most likely provide significant clinical efficacy at decreasing bleeding and blood transfusions in patients undergoing open-heart surgery, especially in patients at increased risk for bleeding. In fact, this observation was recently confirmed in a study performed by Fremes et al,[37] in which the results of essentially all clinical trials involving these agents completed since 1980 were pooled and subjected to metanalysis. They concluded that each of these drugs significantly reduced chest tube drainage compared with a placebo. This reduction, however, was only 86 ml in DDAVP studies ($p = .0021$, 11% reduction), compared with a reduction of 225 ml in the antifibrinolytic trials ($p < .0001$, 30% reduction, and a 252-ml reduction in the aprotinin studies ($p < .0001$, 36% reduction). The difference in decrease in chest tube drainage between the aprotinin and the antifibrinolytic trials was not significant ($p = .5003$), although all three drugs were significantly more effective than DDAVP in decreasing chest tube drainage (Fig. 15.4).

In the metanalyses by Fremes et al,[37] DDAVP use failed to demonstrate a decrease in blood transfusion requirements (Table 15.3). The antifibrinolytics and aprotinin decreased transfusion requirements by 32% and 53%, respectively ($p < .0001$). Differences between aprotinin and antifibrinolytics were not statistically different. However, only aprotinin decreased the absolute frequency of postoperative transfusion requirements in terms of the percentage of patients transfused compared with a placebo ($p < .0001$, 23% reduction). Nonoverlapping 95% competence intervals also suggested that aprotinin was significantly better in this regard than the other drugs studied. Although thrombosis and myocardial infarction rates could not adequately be compared in this analysis, each drug treatment actually *decreased* overall mortality (odds ratio .78 to .85) compared with a placebo, although these differences were not statistically significant.

One recent study directly comparing the efficacy of aprotinin and TA demonstrated that both exhibited similar antifibrinolytic activity, but aprotinin was nevertheless significantly more effective than TA in decreasing blood loss and required transfusions.[38] A second recent study comparing the two agents demonstrated results similar to the metanalysis of Fremes et al.[37] Both were more effective than placebo in decreasing postoperative blood loss and perioperative blood component therapy.[39] Aprotinin demonstrated better efficacy in both outcomes than did TA, although the differences could not be resolved statistically because of the small study population ($n = 15$). A third study, comparing the efficacy of TA and EACA, further demonstrated a small relative advantage in terms of blood loss and transfusion requirement in TA- versus EACA-treated patients.[40] Aprotinin may most appropriately be viewed as a general procoagulant, possessing synergistic mechanisms of action, while EACA and TA, and finally DDAVP would seem to have relatively more specific effects, and therefore correspondingly less dramatic efficacy. Both EACA and TA nevertheless appear to be effective hemostatic agents for open-heart surgery, as well. In selected cases, DDAVP may also have some efficacy, although the role of this agent may be limited compared with the others.

Thrombotic complications may be proven to occur in a reciprocal relationship to the hemostatic efficacy of these agents. To date, statistical

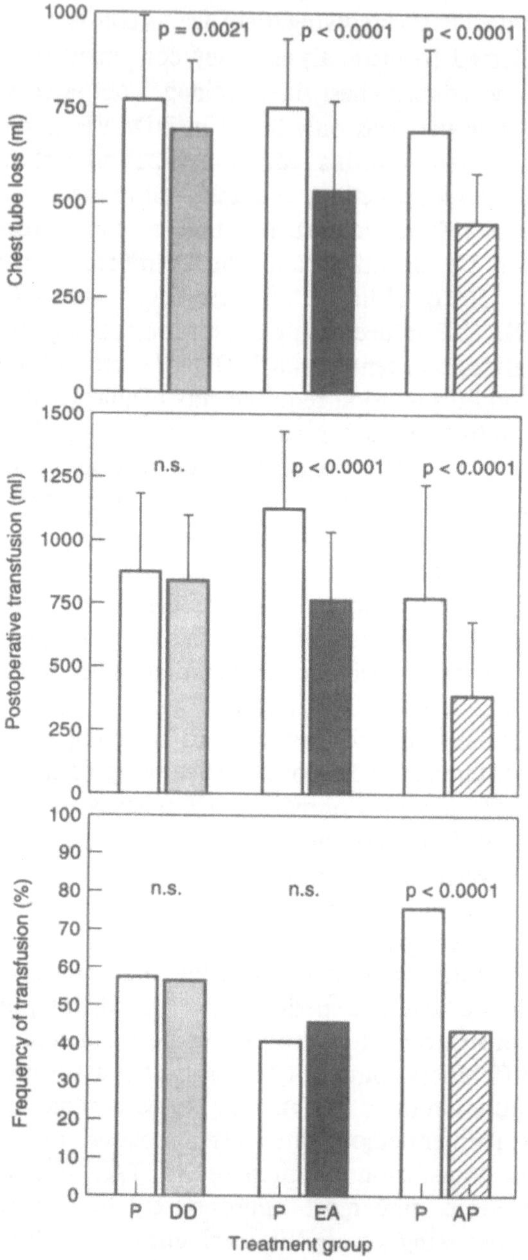

FIGURE 15.4. Comparative analysis of placebo (P), desmopressin (DD), ϵ-aminocaproic acid or tranexamic acid (EA), or aprotinin (AP). (Reprinted with permission from Fremes et al[37])

TABLE 15.3. Volume of postoperative transfusion.*

Comparison	Trials	Patients	Mean difference between groups (ml)	Percent reduction	p value
DD versus P	8	460	45.4	0.05	.7992
EA versus P	2	388	358.3	0.32	<.0001
AP versus P	11	631	417.9	0.53	<.0001
ΔEA versus ΔDD	10	848	312.9	6.89	<.0001
ΔAP versus ΔDD	19	1091	372.5	8.20	<.0001
ΔAP versus ΔEA	13	1019	59.6	0.17	.5037

AP, aprotinin; DD, desmopressin; EA, ϵ-aminocaproic acid or tranexamic acid; P, placebo.
*Results of the metanalysis for postoperative red cell transfusions are reported as the mean difference between groups. There was a significant reduction identified for the antifibrinolytic drugs and aprotinin compared with placebo or desmopressin.
Data from Fremes et al.[37]

verification of an increased thrombotic potential with any of these agents has not been demonstrated. Finally, the cost of TA and EACA are about tenfold less than that of aprotinin. On the other hand, some of these costs may be recouped in decreased transfusion costs. Except in extreme risk cases where hemostasis is critical, such as for Jehovah's Witnesses or patients with significant coagulation defects undergoing reoperation, the cost-benefit ratio may therefore not favor aprotinin use. Similarly, in most cases, the author would advocate aprotinin therapy in the half-dose range, rather than utilizing the full Hammersmith regimen.

References

1. Salzman EW, Weinstein MJ, Weintraub RM, et al. Treatment with desmopressin acetate to reduce blood loss after cardiac surgery: a double-blind randomized trial. *N Engl J Med* 1986;314:140.
2. Royston D, Bidstrup BP, Taylor KM, Sapsford RN. Effect of aprotinin on need for blood transfusions after repeat open heart surgery. *Lancet* 1987; 2:1289–1291.
3. Van Oeveren W, Jansen NJG, Bidstrup BP, et al. Effect of aprotinin on hemostatic mechanisms during cardiopulmonary bypass. *Ann Thorac Surg* 1987;44:640–645.
4. Tice DA, Reed GE, Clauss RH, Worth MH. Hemorrhage due to fibrinolysis occurring with open heart operations. *J Thorac Cardiovasc Surg* 1963; 46:673–676.
5. Mammen EF. Natural protease inhibitors in extracorporeal circulation. *Ann NY Acad Sci* 1968;146:754–762.
6. Ambrus JL, Schimert G, Lajos TZ, et al. Effects of antifibrinolytic agents and estrogens on blood loss and blood coagulation factors during open heart surgery. *J Med* 1971;2:65–81.
7. Fritz H, Wunderer G. Biochemistry and application of aprotinin, the kallikrein inhibitor from bovine lungs. *Arzneimittelforschung* 1983;33:479–494.

8. Taylor KM. Effects of aprotinin on blood loss and blood use after cardiopulmonary bypass. In: Roque Pifarre, ed. *Anticoagulation, Hemostasis, and Blood Preservation in Cardiovascular Surgery*. Philadelphia: Hanley and Belfus, 1993.
9. Van Oeveren W, Harder HP, Roozendaal KJ, Eijsman L, Wildevuur CRH. Aprotinin protects platelets against the initial effects of cardiopulmonary bypass. *J Thorac Cardiovasc Surg* 1990;99:788–797.
10. Dietrich W, Spannagl M, Jochum M, et al. Incidence of high dose aprotinin treatment on blood loss and coagulation patterns in patients undergoing myocardial revascularization. *Anesthesiology* 1990;73:1119–1126.
11. Bidstrup BP, Royston D, Sapsford RN, Taylor KM. Reduction in blood loss and blood use after cardiopulmonary bypass with high dose aprotinin (Trasylol). *J Thorac Cardiovasc Surg* 1989;97:364–372.
12. Wildevuur CRH, Eijsman L, Roozendaal KJ, Harder MP, Chang M, van Oeveren W. Platelet preservation during cardiopulmonary bypass with aprotinin. *Eur J Cardiothorac Surg* 1989;3:533–538.
13. O'Regan DJ, Giannopolous MD, Mediratta N, et al. Topical aprotinin in cardiac operations. *Ann Thorac Surg* 1994;58:778–782.
14. Adelman B, Michelson AD, Loscalzo J, Greenberg J, Handin RI. Plasmin effect on platelet glycoprotein Ib-von Willebrand factor interaction. *Blood* 1985;65:32–40.
15. Hardy JF, Desroches J. Natural and synthetic antifibrinolytics in cardiac surgery. *Can J Anaesth* 1992;39:353–365.
16. deSmet A, Joen M, van Oeveren W, et al. Increased anticoagulation during cardiopulmonary bypass by aprotinin. *J Thorac Cardiovasc Surg* 1990; 100:520–527.
17. Wang JS, Lin CY, Hung WT, Thisted RA, Karp RB. In vitro effects of aprotinin on activated clotting time measured with different activators. *J Thorac Cardiovasc Surg* 1992;104:1135–1140.
18. Dietrich W, Jochum M. Effect of celite and kaolin on activated clotting time in the presence of aprotinin: activated clotting time is reduced by binding of aprotinin to kaolin. *J Thorac Cardiovasc Surg* 1995;109:177.
19. Cosgrove DM III, Heric B, Lytle BW, et al. Aprotinin therapy for reoperative myocardial revascularization: a placebo controlled trial. *Ann Thorac Surg* 1992;54:1031–1038.
20. Lemmer JH Jr, Stanford W, Bonney SL, et al. Aprotinin for coronary bypass operations: efficacy, safety, and influence on early saphenous vein graft patency. *J Thorac Cardiovasc Surg* 1994;107:543–553.
21. Bidstrup BP, Underwood SR, Saprsford RN. Effect of aprotinin (trasylol) on aorto-coronary bypass graft patency. *J Thorac Cardiovasc Surg* 1993; 105:147–153.
22. Blauhut B, Gross C, Necek S, et al. Effect of high dose aprotinin on blood loss, platelet function, fibrinolysis, complement and renal function after cardiopulmonary bypass. *J Thorac Cardiovasc Surg* 1991;101:958–967.
23. Lemmer JH, Stanford W, Bonney SL, et al. Aprotinin for coronary artery bypass grafting: effect on postoperative renal function. *Ann Thorac Surg* 1995;59:132–136.
24. Verstraete M. Clinical application of inhibitors of fibrinolysis. *Drugs* 1985; 29:236–261.
25. Ogston D. Current status of antifibrinolytic drugs. *Blood Rev* 1989;3:1–4.

26. Marin HM. Hemostatic mechanism in extracorporeal circulation. *Arch Surg* 1964;88:988–998.
27. Horrow JC, Hlavacek J, Strong MD, et al. Prophylactic tranexamic acid decreases bleeding after cardiac operations. *J Thorac Cardiovasc Surg* 1990; 99:70–74.
28. Lambert CJ, Marengo-Rowe AJ, Levenson JE, et al. The treatment of postperfusion bleeding using ε-aminocaproic acid, cryoprecipitate, fresh frozen plasma, and protamine sulfate. *Ann Thorac Surg* 1979;28:440–444.
29. VanderSalm TJ, Ansell JE, Okike ON, et al. The role of epsilon-aminocaproic acid in reducing bleeding after cardiac operations: a double blind, randomized study. *J Thorac Cardiovasc Surg* 1988;95:538–540.
30. Del Rossi AJ, Cernaianu AC, Botros S, Lemole GM, Moore R. Prophylactic treatment of postperfusion bleeding using EACA. *Chest* 1989;96:27–30.
31. Sloand EM, Sloand J, Kessler C, et al. Loss of glycoprotein Ib from platelets on hemodialysis (HD) or cardiopulmonary bypass (CABG) is followed by its re-expression on the platelet membrane. *Blood* 1991;78:388a.
32. Sloand EM, Kessler CM, Sloand J, et al. DDAVP corrects the platelet dysfunction produced by cardiopulmonary bypass, hemodialysis, and prolonged storage: reexpression of glycoprotein Ib on the platelet membrane. In Mariani G, Mannucci PM, Cattaneo M, eds. *Desmopressin in Bleeding Disorders*. London: Plenum, 1993.
33. Czer L, Bateman T, Gray RJ, et al. Prospective trial of DDAVP in treatment of severe platelet dysfunction and hemorrhage after cardiopulmonary bypass. *Circulation* 1995;72(Suppl 3):111.
34. Mariani G, Arcieri P, Pizzo F. The use of desmopressin in cardiopulmonary bypass surgery. In: Roque Pifarre, ed. *Anticoagulation, Hemostasis, and Blood Preservation in Cardiovascular Surgery*. Philadelphia: Hanley and Belfus, 1993.
35. Monogan PD, Hosking MP. The role of desmopressin acetate in patients undergoing coronary artery bypass surgery. *Anesthesiology* 1992;77:38–46.
36. Salzman EW, Weinstein MJ, Reilly D, Ware A. Adventures in hemostasis: desmopressin in cardiac surgery. *Arch Surg* 1993;128:212–217.
37. Fremes SE, Wong BI, Lee E, et al. Metaanalysis of prophylactic drug treatment in the prevention of postoperative bleeding. *Ann Thorac Surg* 1994; 58:1580–1588.
38. Blauhut B, Harringer W, Bettelheim P, et al. Comparison of the effects of aprotinin and tranexamic acid on blood loss and related variables after cardiopulmonary bypass. *J Thorac Cardiovasc Surg* 1994;108:1083–1091.
39. Speekenbrink RGH, Vonk ABA, Wildevuur CRH, Eijsman L. Hemostatic efficacy of dipyrimidole, tranexamic acid, and aprotinin in coronary bypass grafting. *Ann Thorac Surg* 1995;59:438–442.
40. Karski JM, Teasdale SJ, Norman MD, et al. Prevention of postbypass bleeding with tranexamic acid and ε-aminocaproic acid. *J Cardiothorac Vasc Anesth* 1993;7:431–435.
41. Taylor KM. Perioperative approaches to coagulation defects. *Ann Thorac Surg* 1993;56:S81.
42. Pifarre R. *Anticoagulation, Hemostasis, and Blood Preservation in Cardiovascular Surgery*. Philadelphia: Hanley and Belfus, 1993.

16
Indications for Red Cell Transfusion

Robert E. Helm and O. Wayne Isom

This book describes the many methods and strategies available for decreasing the need for homologous transfusion in cardiac surgery. With respect to red cell transfusion, such techniques as preoperative autologous donation, intraoperative autologous blood donation, intraoperative salvage, and postoperative shed blood infusion clearly help to reduce homologous requirements, and are important components of a comprehensive blood conservation program. There exists, however, another fundamental and yet often overlooked technique that is simple, effective, inexpensive, and complementary to all other blood conservation measures: the technique of *minimum safe transfusion*.[1] Minimum safe transfusion is the minimization of homologous red cell transfusion through correct application of a clear set of transfusion guidelines based on physiologic principles, experimental data, and clinical experience.[2] By understanding the physiology of anemia, and then using this knowledge to transfuse the individual patient only when it is necessary to maintain adequate homeostatic function, homologous red cell transfusion can be markedly reduced. Because this reduction is achieved through elimination only of unnecessary transfusions, patient safety is in no way compromised; optimal patient care and minimal homologous blood use are simultaneously achieved.

The essential first step in applying the concept of minimal safe transfusion is to identify the point—the "transfusion trigger"—at which transfusion becomes necessary. This involves a careful analysis of the existing experimental and clinical data, a relatively large body of which has been reported. Digestion and resynthesis of this information reveals that there are three important levels of anemia: the *optimal* level of anemia, the lowest *acceptable* level of anemia, and the *lowest* level of anemia that is compatible with life. While the latter becomes of clinical interest only occasionally, it has been a general lack of distinction between the former two that has led to a sense of confusion and discordance in the clinical arena with respect to the level of perioperative anemia that should trigger red cell transfusion.[3] The traditional "10/30" (hemoglobin/hematocrit) rule was based primarily on clinical experience in World War II and Korea,[2,4-8] and subsequent rheologic studies indicating that *optimal* oxygen delivery was maintained at a hematocrit of 30%.[9] It was at this hematocrit level that decreases in oxygen carrying capacity were best balanced by increases in viscosity-related flow. Other data, however, clearly established that *optimal* oxygen delivery did not equal necessary or *acceptable* oxygen delivery. There still exists a significant reserve of oxygen at a hematocrit of 30%, and under various clinical conditions much lower hematocrit levels are able to carry the amount of oxygen necessary to meet tissue metabolic needs. The level of anemia just above that at which tissue needs begin to be compromised can be defined as the lowest acceptable level of anemia. Clearly, maintenance of hematocrit at or just above this lowest acceptable level will lead to adequate support of homeostasis and minimization of homologous blood use. Conversely, rigid application of the 10/30 rule will, under most circumstances, lead only to the same support of homeostasis, but also to a significant increase in unnecessary homologous blood use.

Obviously there is not one universal lowest acceptable level of anemia, or corresponding "magic" transfusion trigger. The lowest acceptable level of anemia varies among patients in relation to two general groups of intrinsic factors that affect oxygen supply and demand: (1) those related to the physical status of the individual patient, and (2) those related to the set of extrinsic environmental circumstances in which the patient is found at any given time. With respect to the former, a variety of factors *intrinsic* to the patient will affect the degree of anemia that can be tolerated. Age, type, and extent of cardiac disease, and the presence of concurrent illnesses are important examples. The preoperative patient with severe triple-vessel disease and poor ventricular function attributable to ongoing ischemia may not be able to tolerate the same degree of anemia as this same patient, 48 hours later, after successful coronary artery bypass grafting (CABG) has been performed. Just as important as disease status of the patient in determining the level of anemia that can be tolerated is the set of external circumstances in which the patient exists at any given time. Such *extrinsic* factors as the amount of oxygen supplied to the lungs, temperature, anesthesia, stress, and the use of cardiopulmonary bypass (CPB) can markedly affect both the amount of oxygen delivered to the tissue as well as the oxygen consumption of those tissues. The patient on hypothermic bypass can tolerate a different level of anemia than the same patient at normothermia. The supine fully anesthetized patient has different tissue oxygen requirements from the ambulating patient. All of these intrinsic and extrinsic factors affecting oxygen supply and demand and the level of anemia that can be tolerated must be assessed for each individual patient. Only then can the technique of minimal safe transfusion be safely and confidently applied.

This chapter describes a safe and effective set of perioperative red cell transfusion guidelines, based on what basic science and clinical experience have shown to be the lowest acceptable level of anemia that can be tolerated by any individual patient under any given set of conditions. The first section reviews the historical development of red cell transfusion practices to help place current red cell transfusion practices in cardiac surgery in perspective. The second section provides an overview of the physiologic concepts needed to understand the basic science and clinical research that has been performed in the area of anemia and the need for transfusion. The third section reviews these data, with an organization based on the various factors that serve to affect oxygen supply and demand and the level of anemia that can be tolerated. The effects of hemodilution on the body as a whole are examined under these various sets of conditions, as well its effects on the heart and brain as sensitive end organs. The fourth section summarizes these findings and provides a set of recommendations for red cell transfusion during each of the perioperative periods.

Development of the Red Cell Transfusion Trigger

Initial human transfusions in the seventeenth century were performed not for anemia, but for insanity, manias, melancholy, and long lasting unremitting disease.[10] It was not until the late eighteenth century investigations of Priestley and Lavoisier that the importance of oxygen and the danger of acute blood loss and anemia began to be understood. The pioneering work of Blundell[11] in the early nineteenth century stemmed from this understanding. His reinfusion of salvaged blood into patients suffering from puerperal hemorrhage was the first clear treatment of red cell loss and anemia with transfusion therapy. Blood transfusion, in several different forms, slowly increased in popularity during the nineteenth and early twentieth centuries, but little work was performed in the area of determining the lowest acceptable level of anemia, or the indications for blood transfusion.[12] Notable of the few formal investigations performed during this time were Kronecker's[13] finding that replacement of two thirds of a dog's blood volume with saline was compatible with survival, and Carrel and Lindberg's[14] finding that organ survival was possible with hematocrits as low as 3%. By World War I, advances in blood typing and anticoagulation-preservation allowed for the first consistent use of homologous blood. Blood was administered for acute hemorrhage, but specific guidelines were not recorded. The 1930s marked the development of the first blood banks, and in World War II the use of homologous blood became an essential part of battlefield resuscitation and surgical therapy. It remained the case, however, that little was known regarding the level of anemia at which transfusion became necessary. Transfusion triggers were developed based mainly on a clinical "feeling" about what was best or *optimal* for the patient, and a significant margin of safety was built into these empirical triggers.[15,16] Reports on the treatment of combat casualties that appeared in the medical and surgical literature in the 1940s and 1950s listed the use of hematocrit triggers approximating 30%.[4–8] In the words of one author reporting in *The Lancet* in 1946: "We think, but cannot prove, that the former figure (hematocrit = 30%) is more desirable and should be aimed at. The difficulty is to differentiate between what is beneficial and what is essential."[4] Other authors during this period discussed a blood volume loss of 25% (the equivalent of a drop in hematocrit from 40% to 30%) as an indication for whole blood or red cell transfusion.[6] The 30% hematocrit transfusion trigger became further entrained in perioperative transfusion medicine by a series of studies appearing over the next 20 years that showed that this hematocrit level provided for optimal oxygen transport to the tissues; this was the point at which decreases in oxygen carrying capacity were optimally countered by increases in viscosity related flow.[9,17] Initial clinical findings had finally been scientifically corroborated, and the so-called 10/30 rule became firmly entrenched in transfusion medicine. If a patient had to be anemic, this was the level that would provide for optimal oxygen delivery to the tissues, and this then was the level to which they should be transfused.

While development of the understanding of the *optimal* level of anemia was taking place, another body of research was initiated that was aimed at determining the lowest *acceptable* level of anemia—the level below which the tissue homeostasis began to be negatively affected. Because application of the 30% optimal transfusion trigger had received such universal acceptance in the clinical arena by this time, these investigations were performed primarily using animal models, and on the few patients who refused transfusion on religious grounds. These studies began to reveal that adequate tissue oxygen delivery could be maintained at hematocrit levels well below 30%, the actual extent depending on disease status and environmental conditions. The first large-scale clinical breach of the 30% transfusion trigger occurred in the rapidly developing field of cardiac surgery in the early 1960s. Efforts to reduce the often massive transfusion requirements led to a reevaluation of the level of anemia that was acceptable during cardiopulmonary bypass. Such investigators as Panico and Neptune,[18] Cooley et al,[19] and others[20] clearly showed that hemodilution during cardiopulmonary bypass was not only acceptable, but that it led to an improvement in outcome through improved tissue perfusion. Routine acceptance of hematocrits as low as 15% was found to provide clinically sound results, while at the same time markedly reducing transfusion requirements.[21]

Unfortunately, flexibility with respect to rational acceptance of the lowest safe level of anemia was difficult to extend beyond the cardiopulmonary bypass setting. Postoperative cardiac and general surgical patients continued to be subjected to routine application of the 30% rule, despite evidence that was beginning to gather that clearly indicated that lower hematocrits were acceptable under most circumstances. The first step toward acceptance of more advanced degrees of anemia in the postoperative patient was again taken by the cardiac surgeon. In response to continued interdisciplinary pressure to reduce homologous transfusion, as well as to laboratory investigations predicting the safety of hematocrits below 20% in the asymptomatic subject, cardiac surgeons began to apply lower postoperative transfusion triggers.[21,22] Reports by several investigators documented the safety of allowing hematocrits as low as 21% routinely in the postoperative patient.[23,24] The examples set by these reports were followed by some, treated with skepticism by others. The general result was moderate decrease in the postoperative transfusion triggers applied.

In the mid-1980s, the onset of HIV disease and the greater awareness by patients and physicians of the risks of transfusion that accompanied this disease, provided an important impetus for reevaluation of the traditional transfusion practices that had become so firmly ingrained in perioperative patient care. Recognizing that adherence to the 30% transfusion trigger was responsible for a large number of clinically unnecessary transfusions, in 1988 the AMA called for a reevaluation of the transfusion practices that had come to exist, and issued the statement that red cell transfusion should be based primarily on clinical symptomatology, suggesting that the trigger should lie somewhere between 21% and 30%.[25] Transfusion should not be based on achieving the theoretical optimal level of anemia, but on providing an acceptable level of anemia for the individual patient. The American College of Physicians proposed a very similar set of guidelines in 1992.[26] Other authors have published similar recommendations, emphasizing the importance of evaluating the clinical status of the individual patient when determining the need for transfusion.[27,28] The shift from optimal to acceptable had finally been made—at least on paper.[2] Actual clinical acceptance and use of these guidelines has significantly trailed their publication, however. Old habits, particularly those that appear to work adequately, are not easily eliminated.

Where does cardiac surgery stand today with respect to application of minimal safe transfusion? The answer is: somewhere in the middle. Fewer and fewer surgeons adhere rigidly to the 30% rule postoperatively, or maintain hematocrits above 24% at all times during CPB. If a national survey were to be taken it would probably show that most surgeons allow hematocrits in the 24% to 28% range in the asymptomatic postoperative patient, and in the 18% to 24% range during CPB. Younger patients are probably allowed to drift somewhat lower. But if laboratory and clinical investigations have repeatedly shown that hematocrits at least as low as 21% provide for adequate support of homeostasis in the asymptomatic postoperative patient, and that hematocrits of 15% during CPB are compatible with successful clinical outcome, then why has further reduction in the red cell transfusion trigger toward these levels not occurred, particularly when such reductions can clearly lead to a simple and very significant reduction in homologous red cell use?[29,30] The lack of further progress toward minimum safe transfusion can be attributable not to lack of information, for, as will be seen, an abundance exists, but to a lack of organization and dissemination of this information in a way that is meaningful to the practicing cardiac surgeon and anesthesiologist. For example, the transfusion guidelines put forth by the AMA suggest that transfusion should not be withheld in the patient with significant cardiovascular disease. By definition, however, the cardiac surgical patient has advanced cardiovascular disease. Should all cardiac surgical patients be transfused to a hematocrit of 28% to 30%, even postoperative patients who have had their disease corrected? Obviously not, but what should the trigger be? This chapter presents the data delineating the lowest acceptable level of anemia in a fashion that will allow the cardiac surgeon or anesthesiologist to understand the minimum safe level of anemia for the variety of patients and under the variety of conditions that he or she will encounter. By clearly understanding the lowest safe hematocrit under each of these circumstances, the physician can apply the technique of minimum safe transfusion and feel confident that he is minimizing transfusion while not adversely affecting his/her patient's perioperative course. Only through such understanding can the full potential of the technique of minimal safe transfusion be realized in today's cardiac surgical arena. But first, the following section provides a brief review of the concepts involved in understanding the physiology of anemia.

Physiology of Anemia

Oxygen Transport and Anemia

The primary role of the red blood cell is to transport oxygen to the tissues. Therefore, to define the lowest acceptable hemoglobin/hematocrit level for withholding red cell transfusion under any given set of conditions, one must necessarily define the lowest acceptable level of systemic oxygen transport. To help in this endeavor, this section provides a brief review of the basic physiology of oxygen transport under normal and anemic conditions.

Oxygen is delivered to the tissues of the body by the blood in two forms. A majority is carried complexed to red cell hemoglobin. A much smaller portion is carried as the fraction dissolved in plasma. The total *arterial oxygen content* (Ca_{O_2}) can be calculated by adding these two components:

$$Ca_{O_2} = \text{Oxygen bound to hemoglobin} + \text{Dissolved oxygen}$$
$$Ca_{O_2} = (1.35 \times \text{Hg concentration} \times \%\ O_2 \text{ saturation}) + (0.0031 \times PaO_2)$$

Here 1.35 is the estimate of the mean volume of oxygen that can be bound to 1 gram of normal hemoglobin that is fully saturated, and 0.0031 is the solubility coefficient of oxygen in human plasma at 37°C. Under normal conditions (Hg 15 mg/dL, O_2 saturation 100%, PaO_2 100 mmHg, normothermia) the total oxygen content of the blood can be calculated as:

$$Ca_{O_2} = (1.35 \times 15\ g/dL \times 1.0) + (0.0031 \times 100\ mmHg)$$
$$Ca_{O_2} = (20.25\ ml/dL) + (0.3\ ml/dL)$$
$$Ca_{O_2} = 20.55\ ml/dL, \text{ or approximately } 200\ ml/L$$

The oxygen content of the blood is decreased in direct proportion to the decrease in hemoglobin and hematocrit. While the oxygen content of the blood at a normal hemoglobin of 15 mg/dl is 200 ml/L, at a hemoglobin of 10 mg/dl (hematocrit = 30%) the oxygen content at normothermia decreases to 135 ml/L, and at a hemoglobin of 5 mg/dl the oxygen content decreases to 67 ml/L. At normothermia and with normal arterial PaO_2, the proportion of oxygen carried as dissolved oxygen is relatively small (1.5%). Under conditions of moderate or extreme hypothermia, hemodilution, and elevated arterial P_{O_2}, however, the conditions commonly seen during cardiopulmonary bypass, the fraction of oxygen carried in solution can reach 15% to 30% of the total blood oxygen content, therefore becoming an important source of oxygen for the tissues. This often overlooked phenomenon carries important implications with respect to the tolerance of hemodilution during bypass, as will be seen in subsequent sections of this chapter.

Oxygen delivery (D_{O_2}) to the tissues can be calculated by multiplying the arterial oxygen content by the cardiac output:

$$D_{O_2} = CO \times Ca_{O_2}$$

Given a normal cardiac output of 5.0 L/min, the normal calculated oxygen delivery can be calculated to be 1000 ml/min. In anemic states, when oxygen content decreases, oxygen delivery is at first maintained through increases in cardiac output and index. At more advanced degrees of anemia, increases in heart rate also help to maintain oxygen delivery. The magnitude of the increase in cardiac index required to maintain normal oxygen delivery can be seen in Figure 16.1. This increase in cardiac index is achieved through increases in stroke volume, which are attributable to both an increase in venous return to the heart, as well as to a decrease in systemic afterload that result from a decrease in hematocrit dependent viscosity.[31-33] The decrease in viscosity allows for improved flow characteristics of the blood, and allows the initial increases in cardiac output that accompany hemodilution to occur in a largely passive manner, as long as euvolemia is maintained. As previously discussed, it has been determined by several investigators, both in vitro and in vivo, that the optimal hematocrit with respect to blood rheology occurs at a hematocrit of 30% (Figs. 16.2 and 16.3).[9,34-36] This is the level of anemia at which improvement in microcir-

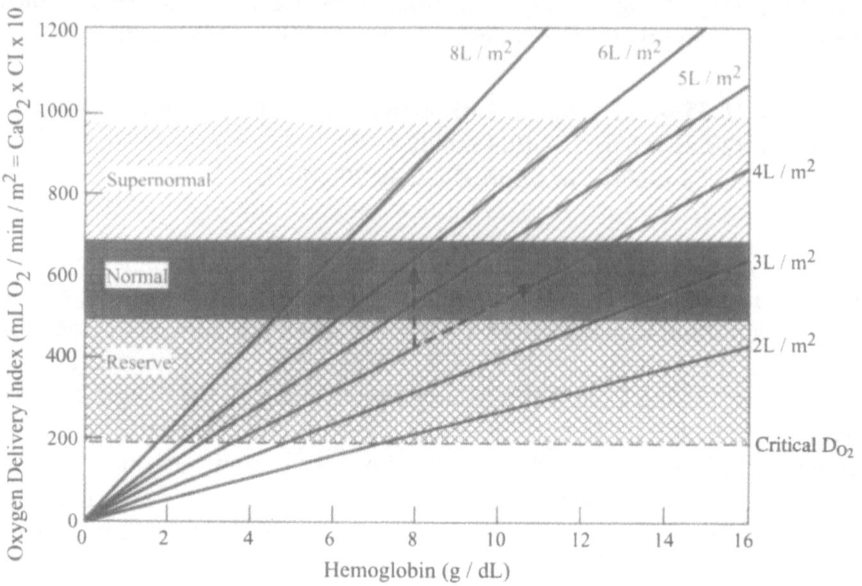

FIGURE 16.1. The interaction between hemoglobin concentration and cardiac index in determining oxygen delivery. The diagonal lines represent constant cardiac index (CI). The darkly shaded area represents the range of normal oxygen delivery at rest (indexed to body surface area). An individual with a cardiac index of 4 L/m^2 and a hemoglobin 8 g/dL would have a subnormal oxygen delivery index of approximately 430 ml $O_2/min/m^2$. Oxygen delivery could be increased to within normal range by increasing either cardiac index (vertical dashed arrow) or hemoglobin concentration (horizontal dashed arrow). The area shaded with diagonal lines above the darkly shaded normal range represents the range of increased oxygen delivery that would be required under conditions of tissue oxidative stress such as exercise, sepsis, or severe injury (marked "Supernormal"). Conversely, the horizontal dashed line well below the normal oxygen delivery ranged (marked "Critical D_{O_2}") indicates what one study found to be the critical level of oxygen delivery (determined in this particular study by measuring the level of oxygen delivery at which oxygen consumption began to decrease as an anesthesized Jehovah's Witness patient slowly bled to death).[41] The lightly shaded area between the normal range and this clinically measured critical level of oxygen delivery therefore depicts the potential oxygen delivery reserve at any given cardiac index or hematocrit under conditions of normothermic anesthesia (marked "Reserve"). (Adapted with permission from Greenberg.[120])

culatory flow optimally compensates for the decrease in oxygen content of the blood.

The *oxygen consumption* (V_{O_2}) is the amount of oxygen that the tissues being perfused by the blood extract and use for cellular metabolism. It can be calculated as the difference between the oxygen carried to the tissues by arterial blood and that carried away from the tissues by venous blood. This can be easily calculated by multiplying the cardiac output by the difference

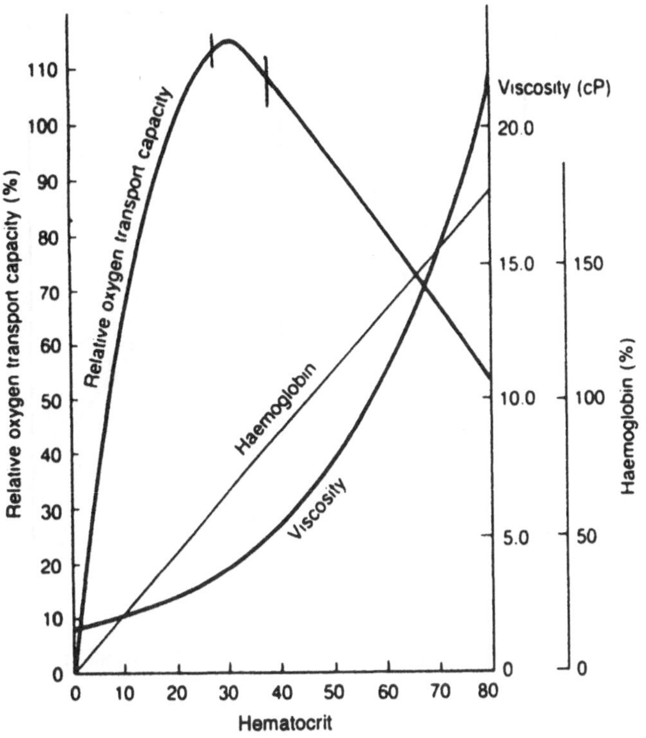

FIGURE 16.2. The relationship between hematocrit, blood viscosity, and the ability of the blood to transport oxygen. There is an exponential increase in viscosity as hematocrit increases (viscosity curve). But because oxygen content of the blood only increases linearly as hematocrit increases (hemoglobin curve), the maximum amount of oxygen is able to be transported at a hematocrit below normal (30–33%). (Adapted with permission from Hint[34] and Cooper and Elliot.[121])

in oxygen content between arterial blood (Ca_{O_2}) and the venous blood (C_{VO_2}). (The venous oxygen content is calculated in an identical fashion as the Ca_{O_2}, but the venous oxygen saturation and partial pressures are substituted for the respective arterial values):

$$V_{O_2} = CO(Ca_{O_2} - C_{VO_2})$$

Given a normal venous PO_2 of 40 mm Hg and a venous hemoglobin saturation of 73% to 75%, the normal oxygen consumption in the resting individual with a hemoglobin of 15 mg/dl can be calculated to be 250 ml/min.

The ratio of the amount of oxygen consumed to the total amount of oxygen delivered is known as the *oxygen extraction ratio* (ER):

$$ER = V_{O_2}/D_{O_2}$$

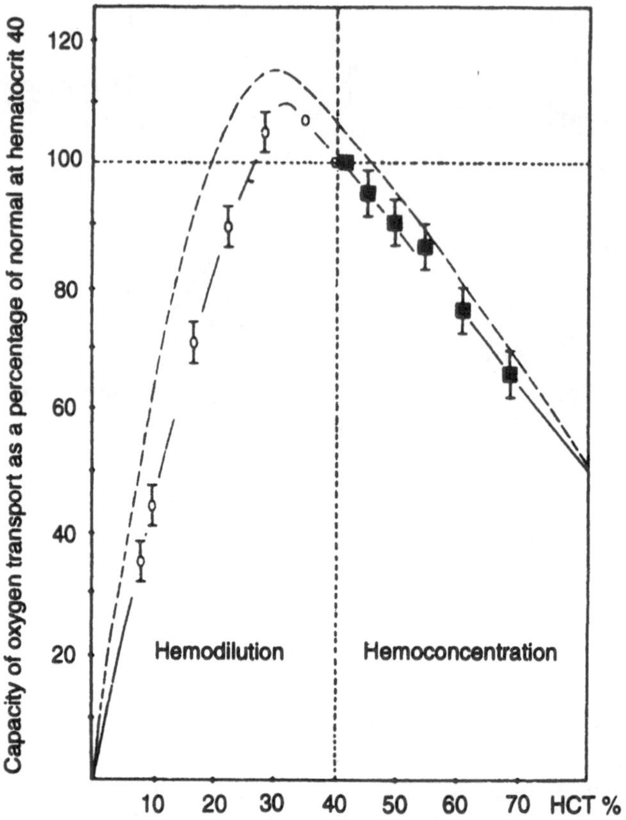

FIGURE 16.3. Experimentally derived values for oxygen transport capacity at different hematocrit levels. Note the very close correlation between these values (solid line) and the theoretical curve predicted by Hint (dashed line) and also depicted in Figure 16.2. (Adapted from Messmer et al[35] and Adhoute.[36])

The normal whole body oxygen extraction ratio is 20% to 25% under resting conditions. This whole body ratio is an average of the ERs of the various organ systems. The heart extracts the greatest amount of oxygen at baseline (55%), followed by the brain (35–40%).[31,37] The increased oxygen extraction by these organs leads to a decrease in oxygen reserves. This potentially harmful situation is countered by preferential maintenance of flow to these organs during times of increased oxygen needs.[31,38]

As anemia ensues the tissue oxygen extraction ratio is at first able to remain constant as increases in stroke volume and later heart rate maintain oxygen delivery. Increases in heart rate contribute to varying degrees, depending on the species. In adult humans the increase in cardiac output has been shown to be attributable primarily to increases in stroke volume.[39,40] Below a certain level of anemia, increases in heart rate and stroke volume can no longer maintain cardiac output, and so oxygen delivery begins to fall in direct relation to decreases in hematocrit. As oxygen delivery falls, oxygen consumption is held constant by increasing the percentage of oxygen that is extracted from the arterial blood (the oxygen extraction ratio increases). Under circumstances in which oxygen delivery is markedly reduced, tissue oxygen extraction can increase to a maximum of 50% to 75%, the extent of which varies between organ systems. At more advanced degrees of hemodilution, a rightward shift in the hemoglobin oxygen dissociation curve can contribute to oxygenation at the tissue level by improving the unloading of the oxygen that is delivered.[41,42] Beyond this point no additional increases in tissue extraction can occur, and further decreases in oxygen delivery lead to direct decreases in tissue oxygen consumption. It is this *critical level of oxygen delivery* (the *critical* D_{O_2}) that can be used to define the minimum acceptable hematocrit under any given set of physiologic conditions. This is the level of oxygen delivery below which whole body tissue oxygen needs are not adequately met, and at which anaerobic metabolism must begin to take over. The compensatory changes that occur with anemia are depicted in Figure 16.4.

The hematocrit at which the critical level of oxygen delivery is reached—the lowest acceptable level of anemia—is most appropriately assessed by measuring oxygen consumption as hematocrit is progressively decreased (measurements of the critical D_{O_2} made by decreasing cardiac output in the setting of various fixed hematocrits ignore the rheologic benefits of hemodilution, and therefore are not physiologically applicable when evaluating the critical D_{O_2} during anemia).[41,43-46] An example of determination of the critical D_{O_2} using serial hemodilution can be seen in Figure 16.5,[41] which depicts serial measurements of hematocrit D_{O_2} and V_{O_2} made as an unfortunate Jehovah's Witness patient slowly bled to death. The critical level of D_{O_2}—the level at which tissue oxygen consumption begins to progressively decrease—is clearly evident. Because such serial measurements obviously cannot be performed clinically on every patient undergo- ing cardiac surgery, other indirect measures of D_{O_2} have been sought. These include a mixed venous P_{O_2} less than 25 mmHg,[47] a mixed venous saturation of less than 45%,[47] an oxygen extraction ratio of greater than 50%,[48] and venous lactate

COMPENSATORY CHANGE	HEMATOCRIT
Increased Stroke Volume	40%
Increased Heart Rate	↓
Increased Oxygen Extraction	↓
Hemoglobin Dissociation Shift (right)	10%

FIGURE 16.4. An illustration of the adaptive changes that occur as hematocrit decreases, allowing oxygen consumption by the tissues to remain constant and sufficient until very low hematocrit levels are reached.

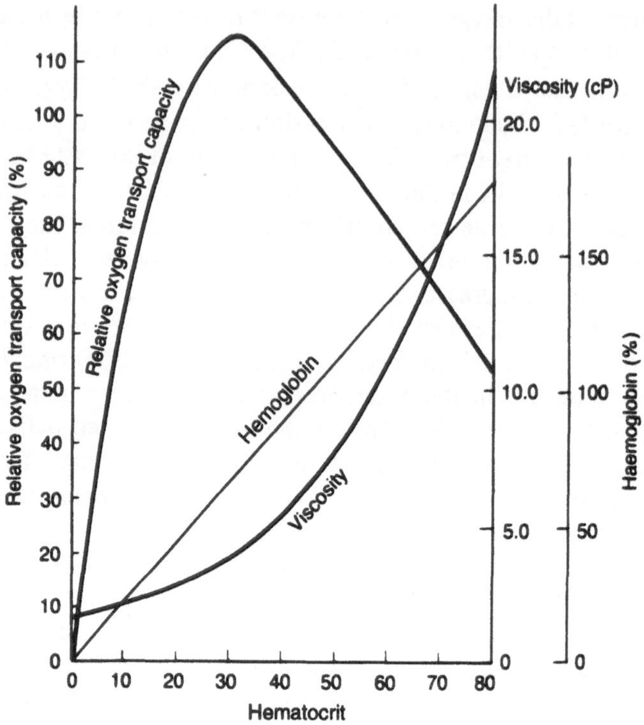

FIGURE 16.5. The critical level of oxygen delivery as delineated by the point at which oxygen consumption first begins to decrease as hemodilution proceeds. These measurements were made as an unfortunate Jehovah's Witness patient bled to death under conditions of normothermic ventilator-assisted anesthesia. Until this critical level of oxygen delivery is reached, the compensatory changes depicted in Figure 16.4 help to maintain a constant supply of oxygen to the tissues. (Reproduced with permission from van Woerkins et al.[41])

production.[49] Of these measures, only the latter has been found to be generally accurate in predicting inadequate oxygen delivery and the onset of tissue ischemia (the initiation of anaerobic metabolism).[49–52]

From this discussion it becomes apparent that the minimum safe hematocrit can be defined in theory as that which leads to oxygen delivery at or above the critical D_{O_2} – the level at which tissue oxygen needs are no longer adequately met. This critical hematocrit can be identified for any individual patient, by estimating two general categories of information: (1) the ability to deliver and unload oxygen to the tissues as hematocrit decreases – oxygen supply, and (2) the oxygen requirements of these tissues – oxygen demand. A variety of factors influence oxygen supply and demand. Those factors affecting oxygen supply in the cardiac surgical patient include the inspired oxygen content, pulmonary function and the ability to reoxygenate venous blood, cardiac function and the ability to increase cardiac output, the presence of flow-limiting atherosclerotic disease, and the ability to unload oxygen from hemoglobin at the tissue level. Factors affecting oxygen demand include temperature, stress, metabolic load, and anesthesia. It will be seen in the following section that by assessing the factors influencing oxygen supply and demand for any cardiac surgical patient at any given point in their hospital stay, and by combining this assessment with an assessment of the patient's clinical symptomatology, the technique of minimal safe transfusion can be successfully and confidently applied.

Lowest Acceptable Level of Anemia

A large body of data has been published describing the effects of anemia, and attempting to quantify the lowest safe level of anemia. Both animal models and humans have been studied. Several end points have been utilized to help determine the lowest acceptable hematocrit in these studies. These include actual measurement of the critical level of oxygen delivery (the point at which whole body or individual organ oxygen consumption begins to decrease), as well as assessment of markers of this critical level having been reached, including the onset of lactic acid production (as a marker of anaerobic metabolism resulting from insufficient oxygen supply), and whole body or individual organ functional parameters such as exercise tolerance, cardiac electrocardiographic, or wall motion changes. Studies performed assessing the tolerance of anemia can be divided into five groups based on the major factors or groups of factors influencing oxygen supply and demand under which the study was performed: (1) the normothermic healthy awake subject, (2) the healthy anesthetized subject, (3) the cardiovascular disease-*compromised* subject, (4) the hypothermic subject on cardiopulmonary bypass, and (5) the cardiovascular disease-*corrected* subject. This classification is useful when assessing the safety of anemia, as these sets of conditions – or various combinations of these conditions – are found at some point during the hospital stay of all patients undergoing cardiac surgery. By understanding what research has delineated to be the lowest acceptable anemia under each of these circumstances, the tolerance of any given patient to anemia can be predicted once the set of circumstances influencing that individual patient at that time has been determined. Combining this prediction with assessment of the patient's actual clinical status can then allow for the safe application of the technique of minimum safe red cell transfusion.

Studies assessing the tolerance to anemia have been performed by measuring whole body tolerance, as well as the tolerance of the heart as a marker end organ. During cardiopulmonary bypass when the heart is relatively protected, the brain has also been used to assess the tolerance to anemia. As discussed in the first section of this chapter, organ systems vary in the degree to which they rely on increases in blood flow and tissue extraction to maintain oxygen consumption as hematocrit decreases. The heart and brain are somewhat unique in that they extract a higher baseline percentage of their delivered oxygen (55% and 30–35%, respectively), and therefore can only minimally increase extraction as hemodilution proceeds.[37,53,54] These organs are compensated for this by receiving preferential increases in blood flow as anemia increases in severity. Coronary blood flow has been shown to increase by 420% to 650% during extreme hemodilution (hematocrit = 9–12%), this increase in flow being primarily attributable to a combination of vasodilatation and decreased viscosity.[38,54] Cerebral blood flow, through a carefully controlled system of autoregulation, can also markedly increase blood flow to help maintain oxygen delivery.[55] Organs such as the skin, muscle, and gut, which extract relatively less oxygen at baseline, have much higher oxygen extraction reserves when responding to severe anemia.[38] Because of their reliance on increases in flow to maintain oxygen delivery in the face of advancing anemia, any obstruction to flow, such as atherosclerotic stenosis, can decrease the tolerance of both the heart and brain to anemia. To apply minimum safe transfusion strategies it is imperative to have an understanding of the magnitude of this decrease in tolerance, and to be able to assess the degree of stenosis present for any given patient. The following sections present data gathered on the tolerance of the whole body, heart, and brain to anemia under conditions or groups of conditions that are commonly encountered in the perioperative setting. The rather limited data regarding the tolerance of the normal healthy awake individual to anemia are first presented in order to establish a general baseline. Data assessing the effects of anesthesia, cardiovascular compromise, hypothermic cardiopulmonary bypass, and surgical correction of cardiovascular disease are then presented.

The Normothermic Awake Healthy Subject

There are relatively few hard data delineating the lowest safe hematocrit in the healthy nonanesthetized individual, as sufficient monitoring and sampling in animals and humans typically requires the use of anesthesia. A study by Levine et al[56] assessed the effects on whole body oxygen consumption of isovolemic hemodilution to a hematocrit of 15% in baboons following sham laparotomy and placement of appropriate sampling/monitoring instrumentation. The authors found that oxygen consumption was well preserved at this hematocrit, through a combination of increased cardiac output and increased oxygen extraction. The effects of hemodilution on the heart in conscious dogs both at rest and under exercise stress conditions were evaluated by von Restorff et al.[57] In the awake nonanesthetized animal they found that at a hematocrit of 12.5% coronary flow was increased sevenfold, but that 47% of the reserve vasodilatory capacity remained, and that cardiac function was not compromised. When animals were exercised (treadmill), however, vasodilator reserve became compromised at a hematocrit between 15% and 20%. Below this level compromise in cardiac output and exercise tolerance were seen. Unfortunately, clinical correllation with respect to such advanced degrees of anemia in awake healthy humans is generally not available.

These few studies performed on awake nonanesthetized subjects indicate that, at rest, a hematocrit at least as low as 15% can be tolerated without systemic or cardiovascular compromise. Under stress conditions, however, they suggest that less severe degrees of anemia may be tolerated, and a hematocrit of 20% or greater is appropriate. These conclusions must be qualified, however, as they are based on a small amount of data. As will be seen subsequently, a much larger body of data has been published on normothermic healthy animals and humans in the anesthetized state. Because anesthesia reduces oxygen consumption by an estimated 15% to 25%,[58] the degree varying with the type of agent(s) used, estimates of the minimum safe hematocrit made in these anesthesia studies should be adjusted upward when extrapolating from the anesthetized to the awake state. Fortunately, in the awake patient clinical symptoms can be used to help guide in this adjustment.

The Healthy Anesthetized Subject

As suggested above, significantly more information exists describing the tolerance of the healthy *anesthetized* subject to anemia. Both the whole body and heart have been evaluated. Studies have been performed in a variety of mammalian systems including dogs, pigs, baboons, and humans.

Measurement of the *whole body* critical oxygen delivery—the point at which whole body oxygen consumption begins to decrease—has been used by a number of studies to identify the hematocrit at which tissue compromise begins in the healthy normothermic anesthetized subject. The results of these studies have been surprisingly consistent across mammalian species. In 1968 Michalski et al[12] acutely hemodiluted dogs to an average hematocrit of 4.7%, and then restored hematocrit to normal 1 hour later using the withdrawn autologous blood. The authors found cardiovascular function to be "well maintained," but no specific oxygen related metabolic or functional measurements were performed during the time of low hematocrit. All animals survived without obvious deficit until sacrifice 10 days following dilution. A study by Cain,[39] also using a dog model, revealed a whole body critical D_{O_2} at a hematocrit of 10%. Trouwborst et al[60] found that in pigs subjected to acute serial hemodilution to hematocrits of 15.9% ± 1.5%, oxygen consumption was found to increase, therefore indicating that the critical D_{O_2} had not yet been reached at this hematocrit. In a second study these authors continued hemodilution to a hematocrit of 9% and again found no evidence of a decrease in tissue oxygen consumption.[38] Another study of serial hemodilution in pigs revealed a critical D_{O_2} at a hemoglobin of 3.9 ± 0.7 g/dl.[61] A study by Noldge et al[62] assessed the effects of hemodilution on splanchnic and hepatic oxygenation parameters in the anesthetized pig, and found that hemodilution to a hematocrit of 15% did not adversely affect the intestine or liver. They found that compensatory reserve mechanisms were likely at their limit at this hematocrit, however, as superimposed adenosine-induced hypotension resulted in significant tissue oxygen deficits.

Similar results from measurement of the whole body tolerance to anemia under conditions of anesthesia have been obtained in humans. In a postoperative anesthetized 84-year-old Jehovah's Witness who slowly bled to death, the hemoglobin at the critical level of oxygen delivery was found to be 4.0 g/dl (hematocrit = 12%).[41] The patient expired at a hematocrit of 1.6 mg/dl (hematocrit = 4.8%). A similar study was performed on a 22-year-old Jehovah's Witness who was able to survive a nadir hemoglobin of 2.3 mg/dl without neurologic deficit or other organ injury.[63] Unfortunately, oxygen delivery and consumption were not evaluated. Measurements performed in CABG patients following separation from CPB (i.e., after revascularization) revealed that at a hematocrit of 15% no decrease in systemic oxygen consumption occurred as compared to consumption at two higher hematocrit levels.[64] It can be inferred from this that the critical D_{O_2} lay somewhere below this 15% level. Laks et al[65] hemodiluted four healthy patients undergoing elective hip replacement to an average hematocrit of 19.7%. They found that while total oxygen delivery decreased slightly following hemodilution, oxygen consumption actually increased. They found evidence of increased tissue perfusion (elevated muscle pH) during hemodilution, and no evidence of an increase in lactate production. Finally, several papers have appeared in the literature relating the safety of profound hemodilution in the anesthetized pediatric population. Fontana et al[66] evaluated oxygen consumption and lactate production during profound normothermic hemodilution in eight children undergoing scoliosis surgery. They found that at an average hemoglobin of 3.0 ± 0.8 g/dl, oxygen consumption remained constant and no increase in lactate production occurred. Similar positive results with extreme hemodilution in normothermic healthy anesthetized children have been reported.[67,68] In total, these studies of whole body oxygen consumption in healthy anesthetized subjects demonstrate a remarkable tolerance to anemia. The increase in tolerance over that seen in the awake state is attributable to a decrease in systemic oxygen demand resulting from the combination of sedation and muscular relaxation.[69,70] Under conditions of anesthesia the healthy subject likely suffers no tissue compromise until a hematocrit of less than 20% is reached, and probably not until a hematocrit of 9% to 12% is reached.

The heart, because of its relatively high oxygen requirements and decreased oxygen reserves, as well as the increased work load placed on it by anemia, is believed to be the organ at highest risk for anemia-related compromise (except during CPB).[53,71,72] A relatively large body of data has been obtained delineating the heart's tolerance to hemodilution under conditions of anesthesia. End points for these studies have included measurements of the critical level of oxygen delivery, lactate production, and vasodilator reserve, as well as assessment of functional parameters such as electrocardiographic myocardial ischemia, wall motion abnormalities, and decreases in global myocardial function. In 1974 Brazier et al[73] assessed the effects on dogs of acute hemodilution to a hematocrit of 15% on both the epicardium and endocardium, as it is the endocardium that typically is at highest risk for ischemia. Relative flow to these regions was measured using microspheres, and, in addition, electrocardiographic evidence of ischemia was evaluated using epi- and endocardial leads. The authors found no evidence of cardiac compromise with respect to global cardiac function, coronary flow, relative endocardial flow, or electrocardiographic changes at hematocrits as low as 15%. Below this level (average hematocrit 10.2%) cardiac function became compromised, and evidence of decreased endocardial flow and endocardial ischemia appeared. Geha[74] again used the dog model to examine the cardiovascular effects of hemodilution to a hematocrit of 20%. He found that while oxygen delivery was mildly decreased at this degree of anemia despite increases in coronary flow, this was compensated for by an increase in the already high oxygen extraction ratio. Oxygen consumption therefore remained constant, as did myocardial function. Crystal and Salem[75] found that myocardial oxygen consumption and segmental shortening measured by sonomicrometry remained normal at a hematocrit of 10%. Another study examined hemodilution to an average hematocrit of 21.7% and found that oxygen delivery and oxygen consumption were maintained at normal levels.[76] This study found that adenosine-induced hypotension improved rather than harmed oxygen delivery and consumption at this level of anemia, although no control group was available for comparison. A study by Bowens et al[77] examined the effects of prolonged 4-hour hemodilution to a hematocrit of 22.5%. No deterioration in cardiac function was seen.

The cardiac effects of normovolemic hemodilution to a hematocrit of 9% were evaluated in the pig model by van Woerkens et al.[38] They found that blood flow to the heart was selectively increased over baseline by 420%, this allowing for the increase in oxygen consumption required by the increase in cardiac work. Cardiac functional analysis was not performed, although regional flow analysis revealed a relative decrease in endocardial flow at this extreme level of anemia. A study in baboons by Wilkerson et al[48,53] attempted to determine the lowest safe level of anemia by measuring cardiac lactate production during serial dilution to an average hematocrit of 4%. The authors found no decrease in oxygen consumption until a hematocrit of 10% was reached, and this was also the level at which significant lactate production and a shift in the lactate-pyruvate ratio began to occur, as measured by arterial-coronary sinus differences. The authors also found that the whole body oxygen extraction ratio (ER) increased from 25% at baseline, to 50% at a hematocrit of 10% (where the deficits began to occur), and therefore suggest that a calculated whole body ER of 50% or greater might serve as a useful indicator of the tolerance to anemia. Finally, in one of the few human studies assessing cardiac parameters of adequate oxygenation during hemodilution, Mathru et al[78] found that myocardial lactate extraction was unaltered at a hematocrit of 15% immediately following separation from CPB, suggesting that anaerobic metabolism had not yet begun to occur at this level of hemodilution. Taken as a whole this group of studies evaluating the effects of hemodilution on the hearts of healthy non-disease-compromised anesthetized subjects under normothermic conditions establishes that hematocrits of at least as low as 20% are well tolerated. The first negative effects do not begin to appear until hematocrit decreases to less than 15% (endocardial ischemia), and global myocardial dysfunction and the onset of significant anaerobic metabolism likely do not begin to occur until hematocrit falls below 10% to 12%. Tolerance of these hematocrits is demonstrable acutely, as well as over sustained periods of time. These numbers generally correlate well with those obtained for whole body oxygen consumption in the anesthetized patient.

The Cardiovascular Disease-Compromised Subject

Relatively profound degrees of anemia may be well tolerated in healthy awake and anesthetized animals and humans, but such tolerance may be markedly limited in the subject who (1) cannot appropriately increase cardiac output to maintain oxygen delivery, or (2) has vascular stenoses that limit blood flow to vital organs even when output is appropriately increased. Patients with output limiting valvular disease, such as aortic stenosis, or with past myocardial infarction with resulting low ejection fraction are examples of the former. Patients with coronary arterial or cerebrovascular disease are examples of the latter. A large body of investigation has addressed the issue of the tolerance to anemia of the awake or anesthetized individual with such compromised cardiovascular function.

Decreases in cardiac pump function (e.g., myocardial infarction, cardiomyopathy) can limit the ability of the heart to increase cardiac output in response to the decreased oxygen carrying capacity of anemia. A rat myocardial infarction model has been used to provide laboratory documentation of the need for such an increase in cardiac output. Kobayashi et al[79] showed that rats with large healed myocardial infarctions had a decreased ability to increase cardiac output relative to control animals when hemodiluted to a hematocrit of 20%. Similar results were found using pharmacologic myocardial depression.[80] Studies in elderly patients treated with neuroleptic anesthesia also revealed a decreased capacity to increase cardiac output in response to anemia, and patients with low ejection fractions showed a similar blunted response.[81,82] Another study, however, revealed that older patients responded in a similar fashion to younger patients exposed to moderate hemodilution.[83] In a study of 140 patients undergoing elective hip and knee replacement, Singbartl et al[84] found that more patients in American Society of Anesthesiologists (ASA) class III had ischemic changes on continuous EKG monitoring than patients in ASA classes I and II, even though their lowest intraoperative hematocrit was higher (19% vs 14%).[84] Nevertheless, despite these low hematocrits and this measurable level of intraoperative ischemia, all 140 patients in classes I, II, and III were successfully operated on without EKG or enzyme evidence of myocardial injury. Finally, in several studies in critically ill patients a compromised ability to increase cardiac output was found to directly compromise whole body oxygen consumption.[43,44,49] These studies serve to underscore the primary importance of the normal cardiac response to anemia in allowing for successful adaptation to anemia. When this ability to increase cardiac output to maintain oxygen delivery is compromised, the organism must begin to rely on oxygen extraction at a less advanced degree of anemia, and the critical level of oxygen delivery required to maintain oxygen consumption is shifted upward.

A significant amount of research has been performed addressing the second general cardiovascular condition that can compromise the tolerance to anemia—compromised coronary blood flow. As discussed, the normal nondiseased heart functions on near maximum extraction of oxygen at baseline. It is therefore dependent primarily on increases in coronary flow to maintain oxygen delivery as hematocrit decreases. It can do so to a rather remarkable degree, increasing flow by up to sevenfold in severe anemia in the absence of coronary stenosis. This dependence on coronary flow reserve puts the heart at a significant disadvantage when flow-limiting coronary stenoses are present. Because such stenoses limit the degree to which coronary blood flow can increase in response to anemia, they also significantly decrease the cardiac tolerance to anemia. The resultant ischemia can lead to contractile dysfunction, further decreases in cardiac output, further decreases in coronary flow, and the initiation of a downward spiral. What is the level of anemia that can be tolerated by the subject with significant flow-limiting coronary vascular stenosis? Yoshikawa et al[85] used anesthetized dogs to evaluated the effects of hemodilution to a hematocrit of 6% in the presence of intermittent left anterior descending (LAD) artery occlusion. They found no evidence of electrocardiographically measured epicardial ischemia, and found that collateral flow to the occluded myocardial area was increased as compared to control animals with normal hematocrits. Crystal and Salem[75] evaluated a dog model in which a 90% LAD occlusion was simulated by selectively decreasing LAD perfusion pressure. The authors found that myocardial oxygen consumption and systolic shortening were significantly decreased when hematocrit was decreased to 17% in the presence of such a lesion. The authors commented, however, that this model differed from the real-life human situation in which collateral flow to such occluded areas is likely much more developed.

Most et al[86] evaluated the effects of a 64% LAD stenosis on myocardial blood flow, oxygen delivery, oxygen consumption, and lactate production. They found that at a hematocrit of 17% oxygen consumption was significantly decreased in the area of myocardium perfused by the stenotic vessel, but that lactate production was not significantly decreased. Spahn et al[87] found that hemodilution to a hemoglobin of 7.4 mg/dl led to mild contractile dysfunction in the myocardial region supplied by a critically stenosed (90–95%) LAD artery. Rapid pacing did not worsen this dysfunction. In another study in dogs these authors found that with serial hemodilution in the setting of a critical LAD stenosis, myocardial function (measured by systolic shortening) began to show a very mild decrease at an average hematocrit of 24%.[88] Severe dysfunction became evident at a mean hematocrit of 15%. The authors found that noncompromised myocardium was able to compensate for the dysfunctional LAD-supplied area during extreme hemodilution, thus partially preserving global myocardial function. A related study evaluating the tolerance to hemodilution with multiple vessel disease determined that this compensatory mechanism is lost when blood flow to these areas providing compensatory support is also compromised.[89] In another study the same authors found that critical LAD stenosis did not result in a fall in myocardial function until the hemoglobin was decreased to less than 7.5 mg/dl.[90] Significant contractile dysfunction and a decrease in myocardial oxygen consumption became evident at a mean hemoglobin of 6.0 mg/dl. Two important findings were demonstrated by this study: (1) contractile dysfunction was able to be *completely* reversed by the equivalent of a two-unit blood transfusion, and (2) the critical hematocrit (the point at which dysfunction was first measured) occurred over a wide range extending from 6 to 9 mg/dl of hemoglobin, pointing to the variability of the tolerance to anemia even under constant laboratory conditions. This serves to underscore the importance of attention to the clinical symtomatology of the individual patient, rather than to any given numeric trigger.

Taken as a whole, these studies of the normothermic awake and anesthetized subject with cardiovascular disease indicate that the presence of such disease clearly decreases the tolerance to anemia. It does so by partially removing the heart's primary compensatory mechanism for maintaining oxygen delivery. In the presence of severe stenosis, mild compromise can begin to be seen at hematocrits of 24% to 27%, although typically levels of 22% are well tolerated overall, partially through compensatory increases in function in nonischemic areas. Care must be taken, however, when transferring these results from the lab to the clinical arena. First, animal models of coronary stenosis are models of acute stenosis. Under these conditions little collateralization is allowed to occur. This lies in contrast to the human with coronary artery disease who is often surviving from collateral flow. Under these conditions mild improvement in collateral flow may occur with hemodilution, offsetting some of the decrease in tolerance seen in acute animal models. The same would be expected for cerebrovascular disease. Second, the patient with coronary disease proceeding to surgery typically has multiple vessel disease, as opposed to the single-vessel disease studied by many of the above models. The compromise of more than one vessel would be expected to decrease the tolerance to anemia by enlarging the amount of myocardium jeopardized by decreased flow, and decreasing the amount of myocardium that can provide compensatory increases in function.[89,90] Other considerations include the presence of valvular disease. Cardiac hypertrophy may decrease the tolerance to hemodilution by increasing oxygen requirements. On the other hand alterations in viscosity-related flow may provide for hemodynamic improvement, as demonstrated by an improved tolerance to surgically produce acute aortic insufficiency.[91] Because of the multitude of factors that can affect the tolerance of the individual with cardiovascular disease to anemia, it is likely wise to err on the side of safety. Reviewing these studies it can be seen that a safe hematocrit likely lies in the range of 22% to 25%, with adjustment upward in the setting of clinical decompensation.

Fortunately for the cardiac surgeon, the decision to transfuse such a patient does not often occur. This statement can be understood by realizing that in most patients undergoing cardiac surgery hematocrits typically do not reach this range during the patient's hospitalization until *after* corrective measures have been taken. It is the *pre*operative patient that is most at risk for decreased tolerance to anemia, and fortunately it is relatively uncommon to see hematocrits of less than 25% during the preoperative period. Should the preoperative critically ill patient with severe cardiac disease or the postoperative patient with poor surgical outcome present with a hematocrit less than 25%, then this patient *should* be transfused toward the "optimum" hematocrit of 30%, particularly if hemodynamic instability or other signs of anemia-related compromise become apparent. This is particularly true during the preoperative period as transfusion will be necessary during or following cardiopulmonary bypass anyway, given this low preoperative hematocrit. A patient with a hematocrit less than 25% will very likely need blood at some time during or following surgery, and so it is logical to administer this blood at a time when it could also provide for improved tissue oxygenation in the setting of an as yet uncorrected lesion.

The Hypothermic Subject on Cardiopulmonary Bypass

The primary concern of the cardiac surgeon is the heart. When the fully anesthetized patient is placed on bypass, cardiac decompression and progressive hypothermia markedly decrease the work requirements of the heart, and so oxygen supply to the heart is usually adequate even at relatively low hematocrits. During the time of aortic cross-clamping and hypokalemic arrest, the oxygen content of the blood becomes virtually irrelevant in respect to the heart. It follows from this, then, that during a majority of the time on cardiopulmonary bypass it is not adequate oxygenation of the heart that is of concern with respect to the minimum acceptable hematocrit, but adequate oxygenation of the entire remaining body. To determine the lowest safe hematocrit during bypass, it is necessary, therefore, to determine the necessary level of oxygen delivery required for support of the body as a whole and for such organs as the brain, liver, kidneys, and gut. A relatively large amount of information is available concerning adequate flow and pressure for such preservation during cardiopulmonary bypass, but unfortunately little is available concerning the minimum safe hematocrit. Clear guidelines for red cell transfusion during bypass have never been published, and surgeons have had to rely on personal experience and anecdotal accounts in order to develop their own transfusion practices during bypass. This section reviews the data that are available—laboratory and clinical—to help delineate the lowest safe hematocrit level for the anesthetized subject during nonpulsatile hypothermic cardiopulmonary bypass.

Hypothermic cardiopulmonary bypass under anesthesia imposes a unique set of influences on the patient's ability to tolerate anemia. First, as discussed above, during bypass, the heart, which is the organ most sensitive to the effects of severe anemia, is relieved of its burden as the main provider of compensation for anemia. The heart's myocardial oxygen demands and its risk for ischemic damage are therefore markedly reduced. Second, use of the cardiopulmonary bypass pump allows for complete control of cardiac output. This allows compensation for anemia to be manually implemented, in the form of increased flow, to whatever level is desired. Whereas prior to bypass the person with a limited ejection fraction cannot adequately compensate for low hematocrit, once on bypass this compensation can be manually instituted to maintain the level of oxygen delivery that is required for adequate organ preservation. This ability to control flow to the body during bypass plays an important role in determining the lowest safe level of anemia that can be tolerated. A third feature of cardiopulmonary bypass that allows for increased tolerance to anemia is hypothermia. Whole body oxygen requirements are estimated to be reduced by 50% for each 10° reduction in body temperature (e.g., 38° to 28°C).[92] Such a reduction in oxygen requirement directly decreases the amount of oxygen that must be delivered, and therefore increases the degree of anemia that can be tolerated. The fourth attribute of CPB that allows increased tolerance to hemodilution is the ability of the body to maintain preferential flow to organs with higher oxygen requirements, most notably the brain. During bypass, cerebral autoregulation remains intact even at temperatures of 20°C, pump flow rates as low as 1.2 L/min/m^2, and perfusion pressures as low as 30 mm Hg.[93] The method of pH/CO_2 management can affect this autoregulation, with the less preferred pH stat management providing for a relative increase in cerebral blood flow and even "luxury" perfusion.[94] The fifth aspect of cardiopulmonary bypass that increases the tolerance to anemia is the deep level of anesthesia that is obtained during CPB, often in conjunction with paralysis. This can result in an additional 20% to 30% reduction in oxygen requirements depending on the anesthetic regimen utilized.[95] The sixth and final attribute of CPB that allows for a safe decrease in hematocrit is the ability to markedly increase the amount of oxygen that is delivered to the tissues in the dissolved state.[96] During CPB, arterial PO_2 can be increased to as high as 500 mmHg with oxygenators currently available, although typically it is maintained in the range of 350 mmHg. This elevation directly increases the amount of oxygen in solution, and hypothermia serves to further increase the amount of oxygen in solution. At a hematocrit of 16%, a PO_2 of 360 mmHg, and a temperature of 30°C, it can be estimated that 15% of the oxygen delivered and 60% of the oxygen consumed is transported in the form of dissolved oxygen.[96] The ability to provide such supplementation of oxygen delivery is an important benefit of hypothermic CPB.

While the preceding indicates that hypothermic CPB increases the tolerance to anemia through at least six different mechanisms, there is ample evidence that the reverse is also true, i.e., hemodilution enhances the tolerance of the body to cardiopulmonary bypass. In fact, this was one of the two primary reasons (the other being blood conservation) that hemodilution was first used during bypass.[19] Hypothermia increases blood viscosity, which at higher hematocrits can lead to microvascular sludging, decreased tissue perfusion, and increased end organ damage. The decrease in viscosity that results from hemodilution serves to counteract these processes, and actually provides for increased organ perfusion.[35] Utley et al,[97] for example, found that the decrease in subendocardial blood flow that can be seen during CPB is largely reversed by hemodilution. At some point, however, as hematocrit decreases, the increase in viscosity-related perfusion is offset by the decrease in oxygen carrying capacity. The question then becomes at what hematocrit level are the benefits of CPB with respect to tolerance of hemodilution, and the benefits of hemodilution with respect to tolerance of CPB, no longer adequate to maintain adequate oxygen delivery? In other words what is the minimum safe hematocrit during CPB?

As stated above, despite the universal use of some degree of hemodilution during bypass, surprisingly few hard data delineating the lowest safe level of anemia exist. One of the few laboratory investigations on the whole body tolerance to hemodilution during cardiopulmonary bypass was performed by Kawashimi et al[98] in 1974. These authors serially hemodiluted dogs on full cardiopulmonary bypass under conditions of constant flow and normothermia. They found that whole body oxygen consumption was decreased and lactate production increased below a hematocrit of 20%. These results may be misleading, however, because to make comparisons the authors created hematocrit groupings of relatively broad range (40–30%, 30–20%, and 20–11%). The critical level of oxygen delivery likely occurred somewhere between 20% and 11%, for example 15%, and so hematocrits above this level may have been acceptable, while those below 15% may not have been. When the two subgroups (<15%, ≥15%) are averaged as one large group, however, the decrease in the less than 15% group may have been enough to cause a significant decrease in the entire 20% to 11% group, even though a hematocrit in the 20% to 15% range was perfectly acceptable. So while this study demonstrates that hematocrits of 20% or greater are acceptable, it unfortunately does not provide specific-enough data to delineate the actual lowest safe level of anemia during CPB. Clinical data supporting adequate whole body tissue oxygenation by hematocrits less than 20% was provided by Lilleaasen and Stokke,[99] who demonstrated that compared to a control group with an average hematocrit of 27%, patients hemodiluted to an average hematocrit of 18% did not show any adverse effects with respect to whole body venous oxygen saturation or acid-base status.

An equally small body of literature has addressed the tolerance to anemia during cardiopulmonary bypass of the brain as an end organ. Kawata et al[100] assessed brain oxygen metabolism in hemodiluted rabbits during CPB. They found that the critical level of oxygen delivery occurred at a hemoglobin of 3.0 gm/dl during hypothermic CPB, and at 4.0 gm/dl at normothermia. Breuer et al[101] found no relationship between stroke or poor neurologic outcome and the lowest hematocrit during CPB. The average low hematocrit in their group of 421 patients was 20% ± 4%. In a similar prospective study of 312 patients, Shaw et al[102] found that a large drop in hemoglobin level from baseline was related to increased incidence of poor neurologic outcome. The significance of this finding is difficult to interpret, however, as the relationship of low hematocrit itself was not determined, and because a large drop in hemoglobin could serve as a marker of intraoperative difficulty or mishap (it is interesting to note that in the several other studies addressing stroke and neurologic outcome that have appeared in the cardiac surgical and stroke literature, both prospective and retrospective, the level of hemodilution was not even mentioned as one of the assessed variables). In a study of the effects of age on cerebral blood flow during cardiopulmonary bypass, Brusino et al[103] demonstrated that use of an average low hematocrit on CPB of 17.4% was well tolerated in the patient group 65 years and older. In an important recent study, Newman et al[55] examined 197 patients undergoing CABG to determine the effects of hemodilution during CPB on cerebral oxygen delivery. Cerebral blood flow was measured at both hypothermia and following warming over a wide range of hematocrit values using the ^{133}Xenon clearance technique. It was found that cerebral oxygen delivery remained constant down to a hemoglobin of 5 mg/dl (the lowest level measured), presumably due to cerebral autoregulation.

Given the relative paucity of laboratory data delineating the lowest tolerable level of anemia during CPB, one is forced to turn to the body of largely anecdotal clinical data to assess this level. An early study by Roe et al[108] indicated that a hematocrit of 20% provided for adequate tissue oxygenation. The safety of lower hematocrits was not specifically investigated by these authors, but it appears as if a significant number of patients experienced hematocrits as low as 13% without obvious detriment. In 33 patients undergoing CABG Zubiate et al[23] allowed a hematocrit of 15% without clinical compromise. Cohn et al[105] allowed hematocrits as low as 13% during moderate hypothermic bypass in 400 patients undergoing a variety of procedures. Lilleaasen,[106] Lowenstein,[107] and Niinikowski et al[96] found that mean hematocrits of 18%, 18%, and 16%, respectively, were well tolerated. In 441 consecutive primary CABG patients Cosgrove et al[108] did not administer red cells on bypass until hematocrit reached 14% or less, with excellent clinical results (0.2% mortality, 2.3% stroke rate). Szecsi et al[109] reported the use of the same trigger in a group of 68 patients. In a study of 300 patients Ochsner et al[21] found that hematocrit during cardiopulmonary bypass "not infrequently was less than 15%" without adverse effect. Jones et al[24] randomized 300 patients to a hematocrit transfusion trigger on bypass of either 21% or 15%. They found an actual decrease in morbidity and mortality in the low hematocrit group, although this difference was not statistically significant. Finally, in the Jehovah's Witness population (n = 32) undergoing CPB using moderate hypothermia we found that an average low hematocrit of 16% ± 2% was well tolerated.[110] Six of 14 patients experienced hematocrits in the 13% to 15% range without obvious detriment. Similarly, in a study of large-volume intraoperative autologous donation, we found that hemodilution to an average low hematocrit on CPB of 17.8% ± resulted in no increase in adverse events (myocardial infarction, renal failure, stroke) as compared to a randomized control population in which the average low hematocrit was 20.4%.[111] Twenty percent of patients had hematocrits of 16% or less during CPB in this study. An additional body of data exists relating the successful use of profound hemodilution in the pediatric cardiac surgical population. In an early study, Buckley et al[112] found that an average hematocrit of 10% (range: 4% to 16%) was well tolerated by a group of 27 Jehovah's Witness children undergoing congenital heart surgery using the heart-lung apparatus. Several similar reports have appeared in subsequent years.[113]

The paucity of hard data delineating the safe low hematocrit during cardiopulmonary bypass, combined with our continued efforts to create an optimal blood conservation program at the New York Hospital–Cornell Medical Center, prompted us to perform an in-depth analysis of our own experience with low hematocrits during cardiopulmonary bypass. Knowledge of the safe level of hemodilution during bypass would allow for decreased homologous blood use during bypass, and would also help optimize the use of other blood conservation measures such as large-volume intraoperative autologous donation (the lower the acceptable hematocrit during CPB, the greater the volume of blood that can be removed).[111] We reviewed the perfusion records of all patients undergoing CABG from 1990 to 1993 (n = 3800), recording the hematocrits on bypass, as well as the times at these various hematocrits (Helm, Krieger, unpublished data). Cardiopulmonary bypass with moderate hypothermia (28°–32°C) and specified flow rates were used for all patients. Three groups were formed: those with hematocrits 20% or greater only during bypass, those with hematocrits of 16% to 19% on bypass, and those with hematocrits of 15% or less. It was found that 14% (n = 532) of patients experienced hematocrits of 15% or less at some point during CPB. When the incidence of stroke or other clinically apparent neurologic injury (as a marker for end organ damage) was assessed in these 4000 patients, no statistically significant relationship with low hematocrit could be identified. Neither could a relationship between low hematocrit and renal injury be identified. When a randomly selected subgroup of 100 patients with hematocrits of 15% or less on bypass was compared with a group of patients with hematocrits of 20% or greater, no significant differences in morbidity or mortality could be detected. Respirator time, length of ICU, and hospital stay did not differ between the two groups. In accordance with the general literature it was found that there was a significant relationship between the incidence of stroke/neurologic injury following CPB and history of stroke, cerebrovascular insufficiency, peripheral vascular disease, and insulin-dependent diabetes mellitus (IDDM).

In a second study, 240 primary CABG patients were prospectively randomized to undergo either high-pressure or low-pressure cardiopulmonary bypass (Dr. Jeffrey P. Gold, unpublished data). Complete neurocognitive testing was performed prior to surgery, and on postoperative day 6. Full data for hematocrits on bypass and oxygen delivery were recorded. Seventeen percent of patients had hematocrits of 15% or less on cardiopulmonary bypass. No correlation could be found between the incidence of stroke or neurocognitive deficit and hematocrit on bypass. An important exception occurred when those patients with markers for cerebrovascular disease were analyzed as a separate subgroup, and IDDM were at increased risk for suffering neurocognitive deficit if hematocrit on bypass was allowed to go below 18% on bypass. These data provide additional support for the contention that each patient must be assessed individually when attempting to determine the need for transfusion. We recently confirmed the above findings in a third study that evaluated the relationship between low hematocrit during CPB and several markers of morbidity and mortality.[114] A hematocrit of 15% was found to lead to no statistically significant increase in morbidity or mortality. When any of a group of preoperative risk factors for increased morbidity or mortality were present, this number increased to 16%.

Taken together, these data indicate that the lowest safe hematocrit during cardiopulmonary bypass, in the absence of significant cerebrovascular and peripheral vascular disease, is likely at least as low as 15% when moderate hypothermia and flow rates of at least 1.2 L/min/m^2 are utilized. In the presence of cerebrovascular disease, markers of cerebrovascular disease such as long-standing IDDM are very advanced age, a hematocrit of 18% should probably be used to delinate the need for transfusion. For operations under normothermia, adjustments upward are likely necessary as the protective effects of hypothermia are not provided.

The Subject with Surgically Corrected Cardiovascular Disease

This final grouping of factors influencing the tolerance to anemia is representative of cardiac surgical patients during the postoperative stage. Patients with corrected cardiovascular disease are a diverse group of individuals characterized by complete or partial reestablishment of coronary blood flow, improved valvular hemodynamics, or repaired congenital abnormality in blood flow. Persistent in these patients during the postoperative period, however, are the long-term cardiac and physiologic "side effects" of the corrected disease process (e.g., cardiac hypertrophy or dilatation in response to long-standing valvular disease). Incomplete surgical repair or correction—most notable in the case of incomplete coronary revascularization—may further compromise the postoperative cardiac surgical patient. With respect to their tolerance to anemia, therefore, these patients physiologically lie at an intermediate point between the awake or anesthetized healthy individual and the awake or anesthetized patient with as yet uncorrected cardiac disease. They may or may not still be intubated or anesthetized depending on their exact postoperative stage, and they are under variable levels of stress. At first this stress is primarily the stress of surgery, but this is soon followed by the stress of physical exertions such as coughing and ambulation. This unique set of intrinsic and extrinsic influences creates a unique and variable ability to tolerate anemia. At no point in the cardiac patient's hospital course is combined reliance on both an understanding of the tolerance to anemia and assessment of the individual patient's clinical symptomatology of greater importance. This is particularly true because this is also the time when hematocrits are in the range where transfusion becomes an issue. It is here, more than at any other time, that appropriate application of the concept of minimum safe transfusion can successfully decrease homologous blood use.

Because laboratory models simulating the unique set of circumstances in which the postoperative cardiac surgical patient is found are difficult to construe, data regarding the tolerance to anemia primarily appears in the form of clinical reports of successful outcomes using various triggers. In 1974 Zubiate et al[23] reported successful outcome using a postoperative transfusion trigger of "less than 22%." They did not comment on assessment of symptomatology in conjunction with this trigger. Patients were discharged home with hemoglobins as low as 7.5 mg/dl. Conversely, Cosgrove et al[22] focused on symptomatology: "normothermic anemia was accepted in hemodynamically stable patients without signs of perioperative myocardial injury or of neurological of respiratory complications. Bank blood was only given for a specific indication, never to maintain a predetermined hematocrit level." Jones et al[24] reported good clinical results using a postoperative red cell trigger of 21% in patients less than 70 years of age, 24% in those greater than 70 years of age, and 30% for those patients with pulmonary failure, cerebral injury, or perioperative myocardial infarction. Paone et al[29] utilized a postoperative transfusion trigger of less than 20% in the asymptomatic patient, and found an actual decrease in mortality.

More physiologic clinical data pertaining to the tolerance to anemia in the immediate post-CPB period has recently become available. Mathru et al[78] weaned seven CABG patients from CPB at a hematocrit of 15%, and measured myocardial oxygen consumption and coronary lactate extraction. Measures obtained were compared with those subsequently made at hematocrits of 20% and 25% (achieved by reinfusing autologous blood withdrawn during the pre-bypass period). It was found that while oxygen consumption was decreased at the initial hematocrit of 15%, lactate extraction was not decreased, therefore indicating that anaerobic metabolism had not begun to occur at this relatively advanced degree of normothermic anemia. Myocardial oxygen consumption values were within normal range in both the 20% and 25% hematocrit groups. Doak and Hall[115] recently examined the relationship between hemoglobin concentration and myocardial ischemia in 224 patients undergoing CABG procedures. They found that no relationship between hemoglobin concentrations (range 58 g/dL to 172 g/L) and the development of myocardial ischemia measured by mean lactate flux, and suggest that a hemoglobin level of 6 to 7 g/L may be safe in the postoperative period. Using data from a 24-institution study, Speiss et al[116] found that low hematocrits in the postoperative period were actually protective against myocardial infarction. They divided patients into three groups based on the hematocrit at the time of arrival in the ICU: (1) hematocrit less than 24%, (2) hematocrit 24% to 34%, and (3) hematocrit greater than 34%. The authors found that after correction for potentially confounding variables, patients in the low-hematocrit group had less than half the infarction rate of the high-hematocrit group, with the moderate group lying midway between the two. Interestingly, 18 patients with hematocrits of 18% or less at the time of arrival in the ICU had a zero incidence of myocardial infarction. The authors suggest that this direct relationship between hematocrit and infarction rate may be related to changes in viscosity, shear forces, and microvascular flow. These changes, coupled with an increase in platelet margination, leads to an increase in platelet-endothelium interaction, and an increased tendency toward thrombosis. A study by Weisel et al[117] evaluated the safety of hemodilution during the period 3 to 5 hours after arrival of the patient in the postoperative ICU. Using measurement of myocardial oxygen and lactate extraction as a measure of the adequacy of oxygen delivery, they found that myocardial metabolic recovery was delayed in patients randomized to a transfusion trigger of 7 gm/dl, versus a trigger of 12 gm/dl (average hemoglobin 8.9 g/dL vs 12.1 g/dL, respectively). Under stress conditions (rapid atrial pacing) additional metabolic compromise became apparent, although there was no difference between the two groups with respect to morbidity, myocardial infarction, or mortality. These findings indicate that while global measures of the safety of anemia during the postoperative period (morbidity and mortality) clearly indicate that hemodilution is safe, limited reserve capacity likely exists at these lower hematocrit levels. While the relevance of these more subtle changes in cardiac metabolism may be questioned (i.e., there was no difference between groups in overt morbidity and mortality), these findings nevertheless underscore the fact that acceptance of hemodilution in the postoperative patient does leave a decreased margin of safety, and therefore that close attention should always be paid to individual patient risk factors and symptomatology.

Despite the importance of determining the minimum safe hematocrit during the postoperative period, as can be seen few data directly addressing the unique set of circumstances present during this period are available. Interpolation between the data derived from studies in normal awake subjects, on the one hand, and in awake subjects with cardiovascular disease, on the other hand, can be used to supplement these limited data when making determinations as to the need for transfusion in any individual postoperative patient. A young patient with excellent revascularization can likely tolerate a similar hematocrit to that in the awake healthy patient. A transfusion trigger of 20% to 22% would be acceptable in such patients were they to be asymptomatic. Conversely, an elderly patient with poor distal vessels, an incomplete revascularization, and low cardiac output would be far better served with a hematocrit of 24% to 30%, depending on their postoperative clinical status. The clinical studies presented above support these conclusions. Perhaps the most appropriate set of recommendations would be a cross between those set forth by Cosgrove et al, who stress the importance of clinical symptomatology, and those suggested by Jones et al, which delineate a clear set of numerical guidelines that appropriately take into consideration age and disease status. It is through a combination of these two approaches that the best results will be achieved in safely and effectively minimizing homologous red cell use in the postoperative period.

Recommendations for Red Cell Transfusion

The preceding section presented the data that are available regarding the lowest safe hematocrit classified according to the general sets of intrinsic and extrinsic conditions that can influence tissue oxygen supply and demand and the tolerance to anemia. Each of these conditions, or combinations of these conditions, can be found to correlate with a specific perioperative phase, and therefore knowledge of the minimum safe hematocrit under these conditions facilitates determining the theoretical safe hematocrit during any point in the cardiac surgical patient's hospitalization. The normothermic awake patient with uncorrected cardiovascular disease is the equivalent of the preoperative cardiac surgical patient. The normothermic anesthetized subject with uncorrected cardiovascular disease is the equivalent of the cardiac surgical patient during the intraoperative pre-CPB period. The hypothermic anesthetized subject on CPB is the equivalent of the patient on hypothermic CPB. Finally, the normothermic anesthetized and awake subject with corrected cardiovascular disease is the equivalent of the postoperative cardiac surgical patient. The following discussion utilizes the data derived in the previous section to develop guidelines for minimum safe red cell transfusion in each of the perioperative periods. It is emphasized that these guidelines are meant to help place one in the correct hematocrit range when considering the need for transfusion. Once in this range, adjustment should then always be made, either upward or occasionally downward, depending on such factors as extent of disease present, patient's age, and risk for anemic insult. Table 16.1 provides a summary of the recommendations for each of the perioperative periods, with suggestions for upward and downward adjustment.

Preoperative Period

The preoperative cardiac surgical patient invariably suffers from compromised cardiac function and therefore demonstrates a decreased ability to both tolerate and compensate for anemia. The experimental and clinical data reviewed show that hematocrits in the range of 22% to 27% range would be expected to provide adequate tissue oxygen delivery for such patients, depending on the ability of the heart to increase blood flow, and the severity of the coronary stenosis present. Generally hematocrits are above this range in the preoperative patient, however, and so the issue of preoperative red cell transfusion does not arise. If a patient's hematocrit does fall into this range, two factors should influence the decision to transfuse. First and foremost, the patient's clinical status should be evaluated. In the setting of ongoing ischemia, for example, the patient should be transfused to a hematocrit of 30% – the level at which optimal oxygen delivery can be expected. Other symptoms that should prompt transfusion toward 30% include detrimental tachycardias or arrhythmias that are likely attributable to hypoxia, syncope of altered mental status not attributable to other causes, and poor pulmonary function with pulmonary hypoxia that further limits oxygen supply and delivery. The second consideration in whether to transfuse the patient with low preoperative hematocrit is patient body size. This can be understood by realizing that larger patients have larger blood volumes and a larger red cell mass. They therefore will experience relatively less hemodilution during CPB and are less likely to require transfusion for low hematocrits during CPB than patients with comparatively smaller red cell mass. We generally utilize a

TABLE 16.1. Guidelines for red blood cell transfusion.

Perioperative time point	Factors affecting tolerance	Recommended transfusion trigger	Adjustment of trigger upward	Adjustment of trigger downward
Preoperative	Awake Normothermic + Cardiovascular disease	25%	Ongoing ischemia Hemodynamic instability Small body size	Asymptomatic with very large body size
Intraoperative/ Pre-CPB	Anesthetized Normothermic + Cardiovascular disease	25%	Ongoing ischemia Hemodynamic instability Small body size (calculate hct on CPB)	Asmptomatic with very large body size
Intraoperative/CPB	Anesthetized Hypothermic Cardiopulmonary bypass	(1) 15% or less (2) 17% or less (+ stroke risk)		Profound hypothermia
Postoperative	Anesthetized/awake Normothermic ± Cardiovascular disease	(1) less than 22% (age 75 or less) (2) less than 24% (age 76 or greater)	Poor revascularization Low cardiac output Pulmonary failure/hypoxia Cardiac/cerebral ischemia	Young, healthy, and asymptomatic

transfusion trigger of 25% (i.e., transfuse for hematocrit = 24% or less) in asymptomatic patients if they are adequately hydrated and of large body size (e.g., weight >80 kg), as we have found that many of these patients can successfully undergo surgery without the need for homologous red cells if a comprehensive blood conservation program, as outlined in this text, is followed. Conversely, we have found that patients with small body size (e.g., weight less than 70 kg) generally will suffer greater amounts of hemodilution during CPB, and so will need homologous red cell mass support anyway once placed on bypass if their preoperative hematocrit is less than 27%. These patients are therefore transfused preoperatively to a hematocrit 27% or greater, depending on the body size and disease status of the patient. These patients will very likely require red cells intraoperatively anyway, and so it seems logical to supply them with these cells at a time when their cardiac disease is still uncorrected and when they are at increase risk for ischemic or other complications.

Intraoperative Period: Pre-Cardiopulmonary Bypass

During the pre-CPB period in the operating room, the patient is intubated, anesthetized, and often paralyzed. While these maneuvers decrease oxygen requirements, the continued presence of significant cardiovascular disease, and limited ability to monitor more subtle tissue hypoxia and ischemia create a situation for which it is likely appropriate to continue to follow the guidelines established for the preoperative period. Patients with ongoing ischemia or hemodynamic instability should be transfused to maintain a hematocrit of 27% to 30%. Patients with small body size who can be predicted to need additional red cell mass based on the calculated predicted level of hemodilution once on bypass should be transfused to the pre-CPB hematocrit that eliminates this need (generally 25–27%). If insufficient time is available before bypass is limited, then this blood can be placed in the CPB circuit as part of the priming volume. In this way very low hematocrits at the start of CPB when the patient is not yet fully protected by hypothermia are avoided. A 25% transfusion trigger should generally be observed for most patients during the pre-CPB period, as this will help to ensure safety, while at the same time only transfusing blood that would have to be given on bypass anyway.

Intraoperative Period: Cardiopulmonary Bypass

The literature indicates that the anesthetized patient on full cardiopulmonary bypass at moderate hypothermia can safely tolerate hematocrits as low as 15%. Patients at risk for compromised cerebral oxygen delivery (history of stroke, IDDM, documented significant cerebrovascular disease), can safely tolerate hematocrits as low as 18% during bypass when using moderate hypothermia. These are the numbers that we use in our own practice. When warm, prior to weaning from bypass, we generally shift these numbers upward two percentage points (17% and 20% respectively), as the safety margin provided by hypothermia is no longer present. When hematocrits fall below these stated numbers we follow a strict protocol in respect to the type of red cell product transfused. Such a protocol ensures consistent and timely correction of anemia, while at the same time minimizing homologous exposure. When a breach in the transfusion trigger occurs we first reinfuse all available Cell Saver blood. This includes the processing and concentration of excess circuit blood volume that might be present, for example, in mitral valvular disease. If this volume is insufficient to raise the hematocrit above the stated trigger, then any available autologous blood is returned. First any *preoperatively* procured autologous blood is returned in single unit aliquots as required to raise the hematocrit above the minimum level. Generally we have found that one unit of whole blood will raise the hematocrit approximately two percentage points, and we therefore use this as a guideline. After all preoperatively donated autologous blood (PAD) is returned, *intraoperatively* donated autologous blood (IAD) is used. Again, as with PAD, this IAD blood is returned in single-unit aliquots as required to raise the hematocrit above the minimum level. Only after all Cell Saver, PAD, and IAD autologous blood products have been reinfused are banked red cells utilized. We utilize this ordered regimen based on the logic that any blood that has been removed from the patient should be returned to the patient before homologous blood use is resorted to, as it is the absence of this autologous blood from the body or system that is at least partially responsible for the low hematocrit state. Some would argue that IAD blood should be saved for postoperative reinfusion, preferentially transfusing banked cells during CPB, but recent studies have clearly demonstrated that IAD as presently performed does not help with postoperative hemostasis.[11] We therefore disagree with this methodology, feeling that it automatically commits patients to homologous red cell use when it might be necessary, and when autologous blood is readily available.

Intraoperative Period: Post-Cardiopulmonary Bypass

Following separation from bypass, the patient is normothermic and the heart is again providing circulating support. The benefits of hypothermia and decreased cardiac work are no longer available, but the primary disease process has in most cases been corrected or alleviated. While relatively few data exist defining the lowest acceptable level of anemia during this period, logic dictates that it lies somewhere between what the literature has demonstrated to be the lowest acceptable level of anemia for the normal healthy anesthetized individual (15%), and the disease-compromised anesthetized individual (22–25%). We utilize a homologous red cell transfusion trigger of 20% (transfuse for hematocrit 19% or less) during the immediate post CPB period. If significant hemodynamic instability or ischemia becomes apparent during this time, or if incomplete revascularization is known or suspected, this number may be adjusted upward.

As was the case during the CPB period, during the immediate post-CPB period we use a consistent and ordered approach to maintaining the desired minimum hematocrit, generally reinfusing all available autologous blood before banked blood is utilized. The first blood to be reinfused following separation from bypass is any intraoperatively withdrawn autologous blood. If the last hematocrit before separation from bypass was less than 20%, then reinfusion of this blood is initiated immediately following separation without waiting for protamine reversal. We judge the restoration of oxygen carrying capacity to take precedence over the mainly theoretical concerns of exposing the fresh platelets contained in the IAD blood to unbound heparin, or to the mild additional red cell losses that might occur before hemostasis is fully achieved (cell salvage should be used to reclaim those lost cells anyway). If the last hematocrit on bypass is 20% or greater, then reinfusion of the IAD blood is withheld until after protamine has been administered. Reinfusion of IAD blood is immediately followed by processing and reinfusion of all intraoperatively salvaged blood, as well as any blood that can be removed from the CPB circuit (while still leaving the circuit ready for reinitiation of bypass should this be required). If no IAD blood is available, then this salvaged blood should be processed and reinfused as rapidly as possible following separation, as this lies as the only autologous red cell reservoir with which to raise or maintain the hematocrit above the desired level. Banked blood should be utilized only if the hematocrit is less than 20% after all rapidly available autologous blood has been reinfused. After removal of the arterial cannulae, the remainder of the residual circuit blood should be immediately processed and reinfused. This should elevate the hematocrit to 22% or greater. If the hematocrit is less than this number following the infusion of this remaining circuit volume, or at any subsequent time during the postoperative period, then single unit aliquots of homologous blood should be administered until this number is achieved. As stated above, if patient instability potentially related to tissue hypoxia becomes apparent during this post-CPB period, then no hesitation should occur in adjusting the stated transfusion triggers upward. Similarly, in young healthy patients, clinical status permitting the transfusion trigger can be adjusted downward.

Postoperative Period

The postoperative period can be considered to begin when the last of the salvaged CPB circuit blood has been reinfused. Typically this coincides with the time of transfer to the postoperative care area. The literature pertaining to this period suggests that hematocrits of 22% to 22% can be safely tolerated during this period, depending on the clinical status of the patient.

To err on the side of safety we utilize a hematocrit transfusion trigger of 22% (transfuse for hematocrit of 21% or less) in the asymptomatic patient, both while the patient remains anesthetized and intubated immediately postoperatively, as well as during later convalescence on the floor. For patients greater than age 80, a trigger of 24% is utilized during this typically 5- to 8-day period, as in our experience we have found that patients with such advanced age tolerate severe anemia less well. (There is little in the literature to substantiate this empirical belief, however.[118,119]) Symptoms used to designate a patient as symptomatic include tachycardia not explainable or appropriately treated by other means, hypovolemia in which administration of the appropriate crystalloid or colloid volume can be predicted to decrease the hematocrit to less than the stated trigger, the development of neurologic systems (syncope, mental status changes) not explainable by other causes, and significant pulmonary hypoxia that compounds the decrease in blood oxygen content.

An essential component of the application of minimum safe transfusion during this postoperative period is attention to individual patient needs. The triggers of 22% and 24% are meant as guidelines only, and while a majority of patients can be successfully and appropriately treated using these guidelines, there nevertheless exists an important group of patients who can benefit from elevation of their oxygen carrying capacity above these minimum levels. It should be remembered that optimal oxygen delivery from a rheologic standpoint does occur at a hematocrit of 30% and that the patient with poor revascularization who remains on a balloon pump will likely derive benefit if their hematocrit is maintained in this range (27–30%). Attention to the larger picture, as well as the clinical symptomatology, remains essential in the care of the postoperative cardiac surgical patient, particularly when assessing the need for red cell transfusion. The cardiac surgeon should be aware of the data pertaining to the lowest safe level of anemia, so that this level can be allowed when all pertinent factors have been assessed and judged to be favorable.

Conclusions

Minimum safe red cell transfusion is a blood conservation technique that serves to minimize the physiologically unnecessary transfusion of blood. To safely and appropriately apply minimum safe transfusion, the cardiac surgeon or anesthesiologist must have an understanding of the lowest safe level of anemia under the variety of conditions encountered by the cardiac surgical patient. This understanding can then be combined with an assessment of the patient's clinical status to determine the true need for red cell transfusion. Through appropriate application of the technique of minimum safe transfusion in the context of an overall comprehensive blood conservation program, homologous blood use can be maximally reduced. In today's health care environment this is desirable from a cost-effectiveness standpoint, but more importantly, it is essential when striving to deliver optimal patient care.

References

1. Goodnough LT. Blood conservation and blood transfusion: flip sides of the same coin. *Ann Thorac Surg* 1993;56:3–4.
2. Hasley PB, Lave JR, Kapoor WN. The necessary and unnecessary transfusion: a critical review of reported appropriateness rates and criteria for red cell transfusion. *Transfusion* 1994;34:110–115.
3. Spence RK, Cernaianu AC, Carson JL, Del Rossi AJ. Transfusion in surgery. *Curr Probl Surg* 1993;30(12):1103–1180.
4. Dacie JV, Homer GF. Blood-loss in battle casualties. Use of transfusion fluids. *Lancet* 1946;1:371–377.
5. Adams RC, Lundy JS. Anesthesia in cases of poor surgical risk. *Surg Gynecol Obstet* 1942;74:1011–1019.
6. Artz CP, Howard JM, Frawley JP. Clinical observation on the use of dextran and modified fluid gelatin in combat casualties. *Surgery* 1955;37(4):612–621.
7. Crosby WH, Howard JM. The hematologic response to wounding and to resuscitation accomplished by large transfusions of stored blood. *Blood* 1954;9(5):439–460.
8. Amspacher WH, Curreri AR. Use of dextran in control of shock resulting from war wounds. *Arch Surg* 1953;66:730–740.
9. Crowell JW, Smith EE. Determinations of the optimal hematocrit. *J Appl Physiol* 1967;22:501–504.
10. Diamond LK. A history of blood transfusion. In: Wintrobe MM, ed. *Blood, pure and eloguent*. New York: McGraw-Hill, 1990;660–661.
11. Blundell J. Successful case of transfusion. *Lancet* 1829;1:431–432.
12. Michalski AH, Lowenstein E, Austen WG, et al. Patterns of oxygenation and cardiovascular adjustment to acute transient normovolemic anemia. *Ann Surg* 1968;168(6):946–956.
13. Kronecker H. Ueber kochsalzwasser-infusion. *Dtsch Med Wochenschr* 1184; 10:507.
14. Carrel A, Lindberg CA. The culture of whole organs. *Science* 1935; 81(2112):621–623.
15. Clarke JH, Nelson W, Lyons C, Mayerson HS. Chronic shock: the problem of reduced blood volume in the chronically ill patient. *Ann Surg* 1947; 125(5):618–646.
16. Stewert JD, Warren F. Observations on severely wounded in forward hospitals: with special reference to wound shock. *Ann Surg* 1945;122:129–147.
17. Sunder-Plassman L, Klovekorn WP, Holper K, et al. The physiological significance of acutely induced hemodilution. In: Ditzel F, Lewis T, eds. *Sixth European Conference on Microcirculation*. Basel: Karger, 1971;23.
18. Panico FG, Neptune WB. A mechanism to eliminate the donor blood prime from the pump oxygenator. *Surg Forum* 1959;10:605.
19. Cooley DA, Beall AC, Grondin P. Open-heart operations with disposable oxygenators, 5 percent dextrose prime, and normothermia. *Surgery* 1962; 52(5):712–719.

20. Greer AE, Carey JM, Zuhdi N. Hemodilution principle of hypothermic perfusion. A concept of obviation of blood priming. *J Thorac Surg* 1962; 43:640.
21. Ochsner JL, Mills NL, Leonard GL, et al. Fresh autologous blood transfusions with extracorporeal circulation. *Ann Surg* 1973;177(6):811–817.
22. Cosgrove DM, Thurer RL, Lytle BW, et al. Blood conservation during myocardial revascularization. *Ann Thorac Surg* 1979;28(2):184–188.
23. Zubiate P, Kay JH, Mendez AM, et al. Coronary artery surgery. A new technique with the use of little blood, if any. *J Thorac Cardiovasc Surg* 1974;68(2):263–267.
24. Jones JW, Rawitscher RE, McLean TR, et al. Benefit from combining blood conservation measures in cardiac surgery. *Ann Thorac Surg* 1991;51:541–546.
25. Perioperative red blood cell transfusion [Consensus Conference]. *JAMA* 1988;260:2700–2703.
26. White LJ. Clinical guideline: practice strategies for elective red cell transfusion. *Ann Intern Med* 1992;116(5):403–406.
27. Stehling L, Zauder HL. How low can we go? Is there a way to know? [Editorial]. *Transfusion* 1990;30:1–3.
28. Robertie PG, Gravlee GP. Safe limits of isovolemic hemodilution and recommendations for erythrocyte transfusion. *Int Anesth Clin* 1990;28:197–204.
29. Paone G, Spencer T, Silverman NA. Blood conservation in coronary artery surgery. *Surgery* 1994;116:672–678.
30. Goodnough LT, Johnston MF, Toy PTCY, et al. The variability of transfusion practice in coronary bypass surgery. *JAMA* 1991;265:86–90.
31. Spahn DR, Leone BJ, Reves JG, et al. Cardiovascular and coronary physiology of acute isovolemic hemodilution: a review of non oxygen-carrying and oxygen carrying solutions. *Anesth Analg* 1994;78:1000–1021.
32. Guyton AC, Richardson TQ. Effect of hematocrit on venous return. *Circ Res* 1961;9:157–164.
33. Murray JF, Escobar E. Circulatory effects of blood viscosity: comparison of methemoglobinemia and anemia. *J Appl Physiol* 1968;25:594–599.
34. Hint H. The pharmacology of dextran and the physiological background for the use of rheomacrodex and macrodex. *Acta Anesth Belg* 1968;2:119–138.
35. Messmer K, Lewis DH, Sunder-Plassmann L, et al. Acute normovolemic hemodilution. *Eur Surg Res* 1972;4:55–70.
36. Adhoute BG. *Autotransfusion. Using Your Own Blood.* New York: Springer-Verlag, 1991;11.
37. Mollison PL, Engelfriet CP, Contreras M. *Blood Transfusion in Clinical Medicine.* Boston: Blackwell Scientific, 1993;55.
38. Van Woerkens EC, Trouwborst A, Duncker DJ, et al. Catecholamines and regional hemodynamics during isovolemic hemodilution in anesthesized pigs. *J Appl Physiol* 1992;72:760–769.
39. Catoire P, Saada M, Liu N, et al. Effect of preoperative normovolemic hemodilution on left ventricular segmental wall motion during abdominal aortic surgery. *Anesth Analg* 1992;75:654–659.
40. Mouren S, Baron JF, Hag B, et al. Normovolemic hemodilution and lumbar epidural anesthesia. *Anesth Analg* 1989;69:174–179.
41. Van Woerkins EC, Trouwborst A, van Lanschot JJB. Profound hemodilution: what is the critical level of hemodilution at which oxygen delivery-dependent consumption starts in an anesthesized human? *Anesth Analg* 1992;75:818–821.

42. Trouwborst A, Tenbrink R, van Woerkins ECSM. S35: a new parameter in blood gas analysis for monitoring the systemic oxygenation. *Scand J Clin Lab Invest* 1990;50(suppl 203):135–142.
43. Komatsu T, Shibutani K, Okamato K, et al. Critical level of oxygen delivery after cardiopulmonary bypass. *Crit Care Med* 1987;15(3):194–197.
44. Shibutani K, Komatsu T, Kubal K, et al. Critical level of oxygen delivery in anesthesized man. *Crit Care Med* 1983;11(8):640–643.
45. Fontana JL, Welborn L, Mongan PD, et al. Oxygen consumption and cardiovascular function in children during profound intraoperative hemodilution. *Anesth Analg* 1995;80:219–225.
46. Steltzer H, Heismayr M, Mayer N, et al. The relationship between oxygen delivery and uptake in the critically ill: is there a critical or optimal therapeutic value: a meta-analysis. *Anesthesia* 1994;49:229–236.
47. Gould SA, Moss GS. Administration of red cells: the transfusion trigger and red cell substitutes. In: Rossi EC, Simon TL, Moss GS, eds. *Principles of Transfusion Medicine*. Baltimore: Williams & Wilkins, 1991;397.
48. Wilkerson DK, Rosen AL, Gould SA, et al. Oxygen extraction ratio: a valid indicator of myocardial metabolism in anemia. *J Surg Res* 1987;42:629–634.
49. Rashkin MC, Bosken C, Baughman RP. Oxygen delivery in critically ill patients: relationship to blood lactate and survival. *Chest* 1985;87(5):580–584.
50. Shoemaker W, Ayres S, Holbrook B, Thompson W. *Textbook of Critical Care*. Philadelphia: W.B. Saunders, 1989;492–496, 1146–148.
51. Bilbert EM, Haupt MT, Mandanas RY, et al. The effect of fluid loading, blood transfusion and catecholamine infusion on oxygen delivery and consumption in patients with sepsis. *Am Rev Respir Dis* 1986;134:873–878.
52. McDaniel LB, Zwischenberger JB, Vertrees RA, et al. Mixed venous oxygen saturation during cardiopulmonary bypass poorly predicts regional venous saturation. *Anesth Analg* 1995;80:466–472.
53. Wilkerson DK, Rosen AL, Sehgal LR, et al. Limits of cardiac compensation in anemic baboons. *Surgery* 1988;103:665–670.
54. Holtz J, Bassenge B, von Restoriff W, et al. Transmural differences in myocardial blood flow and in coronary dilatory capacity in hemodiluted conscious dogs. *Basic Res Cardiol* 1976;71:36–46.
55. Newman MF, Leone BJ, White WD, et al. The effect of hemoglobin on cerebral oxygen delivery during hypothermic cardiopulmonary bypass and rewarming. *Circulation* 1993;88(4, part 2):I-246 (abstract 1327).
56. Levine E, Rosen A, Sehgal L, et al. Physiologic effects of acute anemia: implications for a reduced transfusion trigger. *Transfusion* 1990;30:11–14.
57. von Restorff W, Hofling B, Holtz J, et al. Effect of increased blood fluidity through hemodilution on coronary circulation at rest and during exercise in dogs. *Pflugers Arch* 1975;357:15–24.
58. Prough DS, Rogers AT. What are the normal levels of cerebral blood flow and oxygen consumption during cardiopulmonary bypass in humans. *Anesth Analg* 1993;76:690–693.
59. Cain SM. Oxygen delivery and uptake in dogs during anemic and hypoxic hypoxia. *J Appl Physiol* 1977;42(2):228–234.
60. Trouwborst A, Tenbrink R, Fennema M, et al. Cardiovascular responses, hemodynamics and oxygen transport to tissue during moderate isovolemic hemodilution in pigs. In: Piper J et al, eds. *Oxygen Transport to Tissue XII*. New York: Plenum Press, 1990.

61. Rasanen J. Supply-dependent oxygen consumption and mixed venous oxyhemoglobin saturation during isovolemic hemodilution in pigs. *Anesthesiology* 1991;75(3a):abstract A260.
62. Noldge GF, Priebe JH, Geiger K. Splanchnic hemodynamics and oxygen supply during acute normovolemic hemodilution alone and with isoflorane-induced hypotension in the anesthetized pig. *Anesth Analg* 1992;75: 660–674.
63. Chaney MA, Aasen MK. Severe acute normovolemic hemodilution and survival. *Anesth Analg* 1993;76:1369–1378.
64. Mathru M, Kleinman B, Blakeman B, et al. Gas exchange during extreme hemodilution in humans. *Anesthesiology* 1990;73(3a):A237(abstract).
65. Laks H, Pilon R, Klovekorn P, et al. Acute hemodilution: its effect on hemodynamics and oxygen transport in anesthesized man. *Ann Surg* 1974; 180(1):104–109.
66. Fontana JL, Welborn L, Mongan PD, et al. Oxygen consumption and cardiovascular function in children during profound intraoperative hemodilution. *Anesth Analg* 1995;80:219–225.
67. Martin E, Ott E. Extreme hemodilution in the Harrington procedure. *Bibl Haematol* 1981;47:322–327.
68. Schaller R, Schaller J, Morgan A, et al. The advantages of hemodilution anesthesia for major liver resection in children. *J Pediatr Surg* 1984; 19(6):705–710.
69. Harris EA, Seelye ER, Squire AW. Oxygen consumption during cardiopulmonary bypass with moderate hypothermia in man. *Br J Anesth* 1971; 43:1113–1120.
70. Trouwborst A, van Woerkens ECSM, Tenbrink R. Hemodilution and oxygen transport. In: Erdmann, W., Bruley DF, eds. *Oxygen Transport to Tissue XIV*. New York: Plenum Press, 1992;431–440.
71. Landow L. Perioperative hemodilution. *Can J Surg* 1987;30(5):321–325.
72. Leone BJ, Spahn DR. Anemia, hemodilution, and oxygen delivery. *Anesth Analg* 1992;75:651–653.
73. Brazier J, Cooper N, Maloney JV, Buckley G. The adequacy of myocardial oxygen delivery in acute normovolemic anemia. *Surgery* 1974;75(4):508–516.
74. Geha AS. Coronary and cardiovascular dynamics and oxygen availability during acute normovolemic anemia. *Surgery* 1976;80(1):47–53.
75. Crystal GJ, Salem MR. Myocardial oxygen consumption and segmental shortening during selective coronary hemodilution in dogs. *Anesth Analg* 1988;67:500–508.
76. Crystal GJ, Rooney MW, Salem MR. Myocardial blood flow and oxygen consumption during isovolemic hemodilution alone and in combination with adenosine-induced controlled hypotension. *Anesth Analg* 1988;67:539–547.
77. Bowens C, Spahn DR, Frasco PE, et al. Hemodilution induces stable changes in global cardiovascular and regional myocardial function. *Anesth Analg* 1993;76:1027–1032.
78. Mathru M, Kleinman B, Dries D, et al. Myocardial adaptation during extreme hemodilution in humans. *Anesthesiology* 1990;73(3a):A236(abstract).
79. Kobayashi H, Smith CE, Fouad-tarazi FM, et al. Circulatory effects of acute normovolemic hemodilution in rats with healed myocardial infarction. *Cardiovasc Res* 1989;23:842–851.
80. Estafanous FG, Smith CE, Selim WM, et al. Cardiovascular effects of acute

normovolemic hemodilution in rats with disopyramide-induced myocardial depression. *Basic Res Cardiol* 1990;85:227-236.
81. Roseberg B, Wulff K. Hemodynamics following normovolemic hemodilution in elderly patients. *Acta Anesthesiol Scand* 1981;25:402-406.
82. Rao TL, Montoya A. Cardiovascular, electrocardiographic, and respiratory changes following acute anemia with volume replacement in patients with coronary artery disease. *Anesth Rev* 1985;12:49-54.
83. Vara-Thorbeck R, Marcote JAGF. Hemodynamic response of elderly patients undergoing major elective surgery under moderate normovolemic hemodilution. *Eur Surg Res* 1985;17:372-376.
84. Singbartl G, Becker M, Frankenberg C. Intraoperative on-line ST-segment analysis with extreme hemodilution. *Anesth Analg* 1992;74:S295 (abstract).
85. Yoshikawa H, Powell WJ, Bland JHL, Lowenstein F. Effect of acute anemia on experimental myocardial ischemia. *Am J Cardiol* 1973;32:670-678.
86. Most AS, Ruocco NA, Gewirtz H. Effect of a reduction in blood viscosity on maximal myocardial oxygen delivery distal to a moderate coronary stenosis. *Circulation* 1986;74(5):1085-1092.
87. Spahn DR, Frasco PF, White WD, et al. Is esmolol cardioprotective? Tolerance of pacing tachycardia, acute afterloading, and hemodilution in dogs with coronary stenosis. *J Am Coll Cardiol* 1993;21:809-821.
88. Spahn DR, Smith LR, McRae RL, Leone BJ. Effects of isovolemic hemodilution and anesthesia on regional function in left ventricular myocardium with compromised coronary flow. *Acta Anasthesiol Scand* 1992;36:628-636.
89. Spahn DR, Smith R, Schell RM, et al. Importance of severity of coronary artery disease for the tolerance to normovolemic hemodilution. Comparison of single-vessel versus multivessel stenosis in canine model. *J Thorac Cardiovasc Surg* 1994;108:231-239.
90. Spahn DR, Smith LR, Veronee CD, et al. Acute isovolemic hemodilution and blood transfusion. Effects on regional function and metabolism with compromised coronary flow. *J Thorac Cardiovasc Surg* 1993;105:694-704.
91. Michalski AH, Lowenstein E, Austen WG, et al. Patterns of oxygenation and cardiovascular adjustment in acute, transient, normovolemic anemia. *Ann Surg* 1968;168(6):946-956.
92. Hickey RF, Hoar PF. Whole-body oxygen consumption during low-flow hypothermic cardiopulmonary bypass. *J Thorac Cardiovasc Surg* 1983; 86:903-906.
93. Fox LS, Blackstone EH, Kirklin JW, et al. Relationship of whole body oxygen consumption to perfusion flow rate during hypothermic cardiopulmonary bypass. *J Thorac Cardiovasc Surg* 1982;83:239-248.
94. Schell RM, Kern FH, Greeley WJ, et al. Cerebral blood flow and metabolism during cardiopulmonary bypass. *Anesth Analg* 1993;76:849-865.
95. Fiaccadori E, Antonella V, Coffrini E, et al. Cell metabolism in patients undergoing major valvular heart surgery: relationship with intra and postoperative hemodynamics, oxygen transport, and oxygen utilization patterns. *Crit Care Med* 1989;17:1286-1292.
96. Niinikoski J, Veikko L, Meretoja O, et al. Oxygen transport to tissue under normovolemic moderate and extreme hemodilution during coronary bypass operation. *Ann Thorac Surg* 1981;31(2):134-143.
97. Utley JR, Wachtel C, Cain RB, et al. Effects of hypothermia, hemodilution,

and pump oxygenation on organ water content, blood flow and oxygen delivery, and renal function. *Ann Thorac Surg* 1981;31(2):121–133.

98. Kawashimi Y, Yamamoto Z, Manabi H. Safe limits of hemodilution in cardiopulmonary bypass. *Surgery* 1974;76(3):391–397.
99. Lilleaasen P, Stokke O. Moderate and extreme hemodilution in open-heart surgery: fluid balance and acid-base status. *Ann Thorac Surg* 1978; 25(2):127–133.
100. Kawata H, Shimazaki Y, Miyamoto, et al. Limits of hemodilution in total bloodless hypothermic cardiopulmonary bypass. *Circulation* 1994;90(4, part 2):I-48(abstract 249).
101. Breuer AC, Furlan AJ, Hanson MR, et al. Central nervous system complications of coronary artery bypass graft surgery: prospective analysis of 421 patients. *Stroke* 1983;14(5):682–687.
102. Shaw PJ, Bates D, Cartlidge EF, et al. An analysis of factors predisposing to neurologic injury in patients undergoing cardiopulmonary bypass. *Q J Med* 1989;72(267):633–646.
103. Brusino FG, Reves JG, Smith R, et al. The effect of age on cerebral blood flow during hypothermic cardiopulmonary bypass. *J Thorac Cardiovasc Surg* 1989;97:541–547.
104. Roe BB, Hutchinson JC, Swenson EE, et al. High-flow body perfusion with calculated hemodilution. *Ann Thorac Surg* 1965;1(5):581–589.
105. Cohn LH, Fosberg AM, Anderson WP, et al. The effects of phlebotomy, hemodilution, and autologous transfusion on systemic oxygenation and whole blood utilization in open-heart surgery. *Chest* 1975;68:283–287.
106. Lilleaasen P. Moderate and extreme haemodilution in open-heart surgery. *Scand J Cardiovasc Surg* 1977;11:97–103.
107. Lowenstein E. Blood conservation in open heart surgery. *Cleve Clin Q* 1981;48:112–125.
108. Cosgrove DM, Loop FD, Lytle BW, et al. Determinants of blood utilization during myocardial revascularization. *Ann Thorac Surg* 1985;40(4):380–384.
109. Szecsi J, Batonyi, Liptay P, et al. Early clinical experience with a simple method for autotransfusion in cardiac surgery. *Scand J Thorac Cardiovasc Surg* 1989;23:51–56.
110. Rosengart TK, Helm RE, Klemperer JD, et al. Combined aprotinin and erythropoietin use for blood conservation: results with Jehovah's Witnesses. *Ann Thorac Surg* 1994;58:1397–1403.
111. Helm RE, Klemperer JD, Rosengart TK, et al. Intraoperative autologous donation: volume dependent red cell preservation. *Surg Forum* 1994; 45:249–252.
112. Buckley M, Austen G, Goldblatt A, et al. Severe hemodilution and autotransfusion for surgery of congenital heart disease. *Surg Forum* 1971; 22:160–162.
113. Henling C, Carmichael M, Keats A, et al. Cardiac operation for congenital heart disease in children of Jehovah's Witnesses. *J Thorac Cardiovasc Surg* 1985;89:914–920.
114. Fong WC, Helm RE, Krieger KH, et al. The impact of low hematocrit during cardiopulmonary bypass on outcome in patients undergoing coronary artery surgery. *Circulation*, 1996;94(8):Supplement I:I–170 (0990).
115. Doak GJ, Hall RI. Does hemoglobin concentration affect perioperative

myocardial lactate flux in patients undergoing coronary artery bypass surgery. *Anesth Analg* 1995;80:910–916.
116. Speiss BD, Kapitan BS, Body S, Maddi R, Seigel L, Stover P, et al. ICU entry hematocrit does influence the risk of myocardial infarction (MI) in coronary artery bypass graft surgery. *Anesth Analg* 1995;80:SCA47 (abstract).
117. Weisel RD, Charlesworth DC, Mickleborough LL, et al. Limitations of blood conservation. *J Thorac Cardiovasc Surg* 1984;88:26–38.
118. Rosberg B, Wulff K. Hemodynamics following normovolemic hemodilution in elderly patients. *Acta Anesth Scand* 1981;25:402–406.
119. Vara-Thorbeck R, Guerrero-Fernandez Marcote JA. Hemodynamic response to elderly patients undergoing major surgery under moderate normovolemic hemodilution. *Eur Surg Res* 1985;17:372–376.
120. Greenberg AG. Indications for transfusion. In: Wilmor DW, Brennan MF, Harken AH, eds. *Surgery, Vol. 1. Critical Care.* New York: Scientific American, 1989(I-6):1–19.
121. Cooper MM, Elliot MJ. Haemodilution. In: Jonas RA, Elliott MJ, eds. *Cardiopulmonary Bypass in Neonates, Infants, and Young Children.* Boston: Butterworth-Heinemann, 1994;85.

17
Fibrin Glue and Topical Hemostasis in Cardiac Surgery

David C. Mair, John P. Miller, and Paul D. Mintz

Technical limitations of suturing have provided the impetus behind the search for improved methods of providing surgical hemostasis, sealing anastomoses, and bonding tissues. Incompatibility of the suture material with tissues may trigger an inflammatory response, resulting in tissue damage around the suture site. Sutures placed in fragile tissue can lead to necrosis and dehiscence of wounds. Technologies employed to partially overcome these problems include the use of improved suture materials, cauterization, metallic staples or clips, and a variety of adhesive/hemostatic agents. A surgical glue should provide atraumatic and expedient tissue sealing and bonding. The search for the ideal sealant prompted the development of both natural and synthetic products such as fibrin glue, collagen pledgets, absorbable gelatin sponges, oxidized cellulose, and cyanoacrylate derivatives. Fibrin glue is an excellent hemostatic agent as it is readily resorbed and has minimal tissue toxicity.

Fibrin glue mimics the final stage of the coagulation cascade in which thrombin catalyzes the conversion of fibrinogen to fibrin to form a clot. Early attempts to use fibrin glue to anchor skin grafts were unsuccessful owing to the low concentration of fibrinogen in the preparation, as bonding strength increases directly with the amount of coagulant.[1-6] A commercial fibrin sealant system (e.g., Tisseel, Immuno AG, Vienna, Austria) available in Europe is prepared from pooled plasma, which provides a readily available and highly concentrated source of fibrinogen.[7,8] Although viral disease transmission (e.g., HIV, hepatitis) from the use of fibrin glue has never been reported, the United States Food and Drug Administration (FDA) has banned Tisseel in the United States because of this potential risk in a blood product prepared from multiple donors.

Improved methods for isolating and concentrating fibrinogen from autologous and single-donor plasma have minimized the infectious disease transmission risk while also increasing the bonding strength of the sealant so that fibrin glue is now used for a variety of surgical applications. General surgeons have used it to stop the bleeding from organ lacerations and to seal anastomoses of intestines, fallopian tubes, and blood vessels.[9-11] In neurosurgery, fibrin glue can prevent cerebrospinal fluid (CSF) leaks by sealing dural closures and has been used in the reattachment of peripheral nerves and the repair of arteriovenous malformations (AVMs).[11-13] Orthopedic surgeons have used this glue in hip replacement surgery, cartilage and bone grafting, and tendon repair.[13] The widest applications have been in the field of cardiovascular and thoracic surgery where fibrin glue has been used as an adhesive for vascular grafts, vessel anastomoses, persistent pneumothoraces, and postoperative bronchial esophageal fistulas. In open-heart surgery, this sealant provides excellent hemostasis in areas difficult to approach with sutures and can correct diffuse oozing within the surgical field. Bleeding from needle holes, small arterial tears, or from porous artificial grafts may also be arrested with fibrin glue.[14]

This chapter focuses on the applications of fibrin glue in cardiac surgery including the complications of its use. Preparation of the adhesive, the use of antifibrinolytics, and alternatives to fibrin glue as a topical hemostatic agent are also reviewed.

Preparation

Fibrin glue is prepared by applying equal volumes of cryoprecipitated plasma and thrombin, sometimes containing 10% calcium chloride, at the surgical site.[15] In addition to supplying fibrinogen as a substrate for clot formation, the cryoprecipitate also provides factor XIII and fibronectin. Factor XIII initiates cross-linking of fibrin, which increases the tensile strength of the clot.[16] Fibronectin appears to promote healing by stimulating fibroblasts and new tissue growth around the fibrin seal while also enhancing cross-linking.[7] Although cryoprecipitate is the most common source of fibrinogen, greater adhesive strength can be obtained by increasing the fibrinogen concentration of the glue.[4-6] On the other hand, greater quantities of fibrinogen may actually inhibit healing by blocking neutrophil and macrophage activity and by delaying revascu- larization.[8,17-19]

Improved fibrinogen yields may be obtained by modifying the cryoprecipitate technique to include additional freeze/thaw cycles and by altering centrifugation speed and duration. The use of single-donor plasma (autologous or allogeneic) minimizes the risk of infectious disease transmission. The technique developed by Spotnitz and colleagues[20] employs a closed system to avoid bacterial contamination where the cryosupernatant is transferred into an attached satellite bag leaving behind the fibrinogen-rich cryoprecipitate. Other investigators have used chemical additives (e.g., ethanol, ammonium sulfate or polyethylene glycol) to increase fibrinogen yield. Ethanol and ammonium sulfate precipitation are acceptable ways of preparing fibrinogen, but produce relatively low concentrations when compared with other methods.[8,21,22] Polyethylene glycol precipitation generates high concentrations of fibrinogen, but residual toxic chemicals may persist in the final product. The amount of factor XIII and fibronectin may also be increased by lengthening the duration of freezing, but it is unclear if this correlates with better hemostasis.[23]

As in the final step of the coagulation cascade, the formation of the glue requires thrombin and calcium, which are supplied commercially as bovine thrombin and calcium chloride solution. Increasing the thrombin concentration causes more rapid fibrin polymerization and hemostasis in the surgical field. On the other hand, procedures requiring manipulation of the glue, such as application into porous graft material, requires slower coagulation and therefore less thrombin.[10,14]

The addition of antifibrinolytics to fibrin glue to extend the duration of the clot remains controversial.[7] The inclusion of antifibrinolytic agents (e.g., aprotinin) in the glue prolong the existence of the resultant fibrin clot, but the clinical utility of retarding fibrinolysis has not been demonstrated.[10,24–27] Despite improvements in the preparation of noncommercial donor fibrinogen products such that they produce improved bonding strengths when used to make fibrin glue, many physicians perceive that the commercial product is more readily available and superior in function.[7,10] However, there are no definitive data to support the clinical superiority of Tisseel over the noncommercial preparations.

Surgical Application of Fibrin Glue

Cardiothoracic surgeons have developed several different techniques for applying fibrin glue during surgery. One of the earliest techniques involved placing the fibrinogen and thrombin solutions into two separate syringes with blunt-nose cannulas. Analogous to household epoxy, the two clotting factor solutions were simultaneously injected onto the surgical site where in situ fibrin generation produced the seal. This method provided relatively direct, controlled delivery of the sealant to focal areas of bleeding while limiting waste of the reagents. To provide more uniform mixing of the glue components, the fibrinogen and thrombin may be combined within a single syringe using a Y-connector, known as the Duplojet (Immuno AG, Vienna, Austria) device. Although use of the Duplojet and the individual syringes were effective in controlling small hemorrhages, spraying larger surfaces occasionally resulted in thicker coats of the coagulants. Increased glue thickness led to less efficient mixing of the components resulting in slower clot formation and lower tensile strength of the seal. In addition fibrin clots may obstruct the needle when mixing occurs within the delivery system (e.g., Duplojet).[28]

More uniform mixing of the glue components has been achieved through the use of commercially available atomizer bottles for each component, which produce small droplets of fibrinogen and thrombin, thereby forming a thinner layer of sealant.[28,29] Joyce and colleagues[30] have produced a similar spray effect by placing the thrombin and fibrinogen in individual syringes and then bending the needle tips. Spraying has the additional advantage of covering larger surface areas quickly, thereby more effectively managing mild diffuse oozing of blood within the surgical field. Diffuse bleeding is a frequent problem in repeat operations where torn adhesions can lead to widespread small hemorrhages. While the spray application of fibrin glue produces a uniform, thin layer of sealant, this technique requires larger volumes of fibrinogen, thereby, increasing the likelihood of exposure to a greater number of blood donors.

Spray bottles and syringes require constant applied pressure to obtain uniform distribution of the glue.[8] To overcome this limitation the Duplojet unit can also be fitted with a spray head. European investigators devised this elaborate dual-nozzle system analogous to a paint sprayer to apply a more uniform external pressure source to the syringes than can be obtained manually.[13,31] Both coagulant solutions are nebulized with sterile compressed air through a single spray head resulting in a well-mixed product. However, this applicator is cumbersome owing to the requirement of a sterile air source and the need for cleaning the spray head of clots after every application.[29]

Fibrin glue may also be applied with the aid of a collagen or cellulose sponge soaked in the sealant. The sponge transfers the sealant and is particularly effective in a wet field with active bleeding.[14,28] Similarly, porous vascular grafts may be pretreated with the sealant to control hemorrhaging from the graft and from needle holes. Development of additional application methods will likely expand the indications for the use of fibrin glue.

Indications for Fibrin Glue During Cardiac Surgery

Fibrin glue can provide effective hemostasis during cardiovascular surgery for slow bleeding including diffuse oozing. Generally, fibrin glue is not effective in controlling brisk arterial hemorrhage or bleeding from large raw surfaces where suturing is preferable.[10] The sealant was first employed in heart operations to arrest bleeding in areas considered inaccessible to suturing. Fibrin glue may also aid the bonding of tissues too fragile to withstand sutures. Borst et al[32] reported a 98% success rate at stopping low-pressure bleeding from atrial suture lines, coronary veins, puncture holes in arterial conduits, and right ventricular patches. Fibrin glue is also frequently used to seal coronary artery anastomoses.[33] Spraying around anastomosis sites has been effective for hemostasis, although direct application of the glue using a blunt-nosed cannula may be more efficacious in controlling pinpoint bleeding.

During cardiac reoperations, adhesions from the previous surgery may lead to areas of oozing from multiple sites along the epimyocardial and mediastinal surfaces, particularly in anticoagulated patients. In this setting, spraying fibrin glue by any of the methods previously described provides an expeditious way to produce a uniform seal. Hemostasis may also be enhanced through the use of absorbable cellulose or collagen sponges soaked in the sealant. This technique is particularly advantageous in a wet field where the sponge acts to tamponade the bleeding, and prevents the glue from being washed away. More conventional means of stopping bleeding such as electrocautery, sutures, or metal clips are relatively time-consuming and may lengthen the time of hemorrhage. Delayed hemostasis may prolong the time of operation and thereby may increase the need for blood products and the morbidity of surgery.[32] Prophylactic spraying of the anterior mediastinum just prior to closure has been shown to decrease postoperative hemorrhage.[34]

Vascular grafts employed as conduits during congenital heart surgery or aortic aneurysm repair are sealed by coating and massaging them with fibrinogen and thrombin.[28,32] In addition to providing a better seal, grafts prepared in this fashion are less brittle and easier to handle than previously achieved with blood preclotting or albumin pretreatment.[35] Furthermore, fibrin glue has promoted the use of more flexible Dacron and knitted grafts, which are more manageable and easier to suture.[7,13] Leakage from the graft may be minimized by applying a few drops of the glue directly over the needle holes.[14]

Other applications of fibrin glue include spraying the coagulant over more superficial areas including sternal incision and cannulation sites.[29] For example, the diffuse bleeding that can occur at the cannulation site for extracorporeal membrane oxygenation (ECMO) may be halted by the application of fibrin glue.[36]

In addition to acting as a hemostatic agent, fibrin glue may be employed to provide structural support in the bonding of tissues too weak to withstand sutures. Fibrin glue has been effective for fixation of coronary bypass grafts to the epicardial surface. Long bypass grafts need to be secured to the epicardium to prevent kinking and obstruction to flow. In this situation, suturing may cause direct constriction of the vessel or induce a hinge effect leading to kinking elsewhere along the vessel. Sutureless fixation with fibrin glue alleviates these problems.[32,37]

Complications from the Use of Fibrin Glue

Overall, fibrin glue has been successful in containing surgical bleeding with relatively few complications.[10,28,32] In fact, many of the potential risks associated with the use of fibrin glue have never been reported, yet it is prudent to keep these considerations in mind when using the sealant. As fibrinogen is derived from human plasma, transmission of blood-borne viruses (e.g., hepatitis B, hepatitis C, HIV) is possible. Virus particles present in the glue might be absorbed and infect the patient.[7] As noted, Tisseel, a European fibrin glue, has been banned from use in the United States by the FDA because it is made from pooled plasma of multiple donors, which increases the risk of viral disease transmission. Despite the concern of United States health agencies, Tisseel has had more than one million applications in Europe and has never been known to transmit viruses.[10,38] Noncommercial blood donor glue may diminish the risk of transfusion-associated viral infection, and the use of autologous fibrin glue virtually eliminates this chance of viral transmission (except in the case of clerical error). Strategies currently being investigated to minimize further the infectious risk of fibrin glue include the use of solvent/detergent-treated, heat-inactivated, or monoclonal antibody–purified plasma to produce the fibrinogen concentrate.[39,40] Bovine and recombinant fibrinogen are also being evaluated.[8,10]

Another theoretical concern relating to the user of fibrin glue involves application of too much sealant in the mediastinum, which might result in severe adhesions potentially leading to tamponade.[41] In addition, the use of large amounts of glue may inhibit neutrophil and macrophage activity and hence hinder healing.[17–19] Furthermore, the use of excessive glue increases the risk of viral disease transmission owing to an increasing number of donor exposures.

Fibrin sealant is a potential growth media for bacteria and should not be used where infections might occur. Matthew and colleagues[28] reported a nominal infection rate of 2% in patients undergoing cardiothoracic surgery.[28] Bacterial growth may be diminished by adding antibiotics to the mixture.[42]

Several adverse immunologic effects of the use of fibrin glue have been described. For example, fibrin glue has induced development of antibiotics to factor V and thrombin, which may elevate coagulation tests in the laboratory, although the clinical significance of these increases is not clear.[43,44] Fibrin glue has been associated with three cases of possible anaphylaxis, one of which was fatal.[45,46] In two cases reported by Berguer et al,[46] intravascular exposure was suspected. Such an event could also theoretically induce intravascular coagulation. The anaphylactic reaction to fibrin glue reported by Milde[45] occurred in an immunoglobulin A (IgA)-deficient patient and may have involved only surface exposure. These risks make it prudent to avoid the introduction of fibrinogen or thrombin into the intravascular space or cardiopulmonary bypass circuit.[41]

Alternative and Adjunct Therapies to Fibrin Glue

The search for the ideal surgical glue has prompted research into synthetic adhesives and alternate surgical techniques to replace or augment the function of fibrin glue. Direct application of cellulose or collagen material alone (e.g., Avitene, Avicon Inc., Humacao, PR; Gelfoam, Johnson & Johnson Products, Inc., New Brunswick, NJ; and Surgicel, Upjohn Company, Needham Heights, MA) to a surgical surface has proven ineffective in providing hemostasis in many instances.[27] Barton et al[47] demonstrated that fibrin sealant forms a superior vascular patch compared with microcrystalline collagen, thrombin-treated collagen, and oxidized cellulose. Despite its relatively poor performance in stopping hemorrhage, oxidized cellulose may be a superior choice for sutureless fixation of bypass grafts to the epicardium compared with fibrin glue owing to its lower cost, lack of disease transmission, and bacteriocidal activity.[37] Active hemorrhage may also be arrested through the use of thrombin-treated Gelfoam or Avitene in combination with fibrin glue and digital pressure.[14,28] Stark and de Leval[48] obtained excellent bleeding control by delivering the glue via a collagen substrate. In a preliminary report, Ennker et al[49] described the use of a collagen adhesive, gelatin resorcinol dialdehyde glue (GR-Dial). This product eliminates the formaldehyde present in earlier preparations. This sealant is second in strength only to the cyanoacrylates while showing bioresorption comparable to fibrin glue. However, further clinical studies are required before GR-Dial is added to the surgical adhesive armamentarium.

Another material used to bond fragile tissues or to control bleeding is Teflon felt pledgets. Teflon felt has been used routinely to control bleeding and to redistribute suture tension to prevent the tearing of vulnerable tissues. Repair of ventricular aneurysms can require a great deal of this material as the risk of a rupture is high in accordance with Laplace's hydrostatic law of wall tension.[50] Pledgets are also used in mitral valve repair to support thin leaflets.[51,52] Smaller-sized pledgets are frequently needed at vessel anastomoses and over focally hemorrhagic friable tissue to arrest bleeding.[53]

Several postoperative complications have been associated with the use of Teflon pledgets. Fibrosis induced by the use of Teflon can be extensive and may produce immobile areas around ventricular aneurysm repairs possibly impeding cardiac function.[50] Another complication of pledget use is infection of the Teflon strips, which may be surgically removed, but the degree of scarring in these sensitive surgical areas often makes their removal difficult.[50,54,55] Surrounding tissues may also become seeded with bacteria and, despite successful surgical extraction of the pledgets, there may be ongoing sepsis and ultimately death.[54,55] Vincent et al[50] suggested the use of strips and small pledgets made from resorbable polydioxane rather than Teflon might alleviate some of these problems. While polydioxane might also foster bacterial growth, the removal would be easier as resorbable substances may cause less scarring.[50,54] Additional complications associated with pledget use include hemolysis around the site of mitral valve repair and small pledgets used for pinpoint hemostasis may fall apart.[52,53]

Some surgeons have complained that fibrin glue lacks sufficient bonding strength to be an effective surgical adhesive. Concerns regarding the strength of fibrin glue bonds were based on earlier studies using low concentrations of fibrinogen. This resulted in lower tensile strength bonds. Synthetic adhesives such as the cyanoacrylates produce bonds of greater strength at low cost and will not transmit diseases.[8,56] However, as cyanoacrylate derivatives decay, they produce toxic substances such as formaldehyde that are damaging to tissues. Longer-chain derivatives (e.g., butyl and isobutyl cyanoacrylates) have lower tissue toxicity than their shorter-chain counterparts, methyl and ethyl cyanoacrylate, but tissue necrosis can still occur.[8] Furthermore, isobutyl cyanoacrylate has been shown to be carcinogenic in animals and may produce seals at anastomotic sites that are too rigid.[56] Despite the superior strength of the cyanoacrylates, fibrin glue is generally preferred because it lacks toxic side effects and promotes healing.

Conclusion

Despite improvements in intraoperative hemostasis and cardiothoracic surgical techniques, the search for an ideal glue to decrease bleeding, seal anastomoses, and bond fragile tissue continues. This sealant should be strong, biodegradable, easy to apply, and induce minimal or no tissue toxicity. Fibrin glue is the only natural sealant that combines all of these features. While fibrin glue carries the theoretical risk of viral disease transmission, this has never been demonstrated. The use of single-donor or autologous fibrin glue reduces this risk and future plasma modifications including solvent detergent treatment, heat inactivation, or monoclonal antibody purification may further decrease the chance of viral disease transmission. In summary, fibrin glue is a safe, effective alternative to suturing to provide hemostasis in areas of slow bleeding during cardiovascular surgery and may be used to provide structural support to tissues too weak to support, or inaccessible to, sutures.

Acknowledgments. We wish to acknowledge the word processing expertise of Ms. Susan Bywaters and the technical input of Dr. William Spotnitz.

References

1. Tidrick R, Warner E. Fibrin fixation of skin transplants. *Surgery* 1944; 15:90–95.
2. Cronkite E, Lozner E, Deaver J. Use of thrombin and fibrinogen in skin grafting. *JAMA* 1944;124:976–978.
3. Matras H. Fibrin seal: the state of the art. *J Oral Maxillofac Surg* 1985; 43:605–611.

4. Siedentop K, Harris D, Sanchez B. Autologous fibrin tissue adhesive: factors influencing bonding power. *Laryngoscope* 1988;98:731–733.
5. Saltz R, Sierra D, Feldman D, et al. Experimental and clinical applications of fibrin glue. *Plast Reconstr Surg* 1991;88:1005–1015.
6. Wan H, Huang S, Floyd D, et al. Is the amount of fibrinogen in cryoprecipitate adequate for fibrin glue? Introducing an improved recycled cryoprecipitate method. *Transfusion* 1989;29(Suppl):41S.
7. Gibble J, Ness P. Fibrin glue: the perfect operative sealant? *Transfusion* 1990;30:741–747.
8. Toriumi D, O'Grady K. Surgical tissue adhesives in otolaryngology–head and neck surgery. *Otolaryngol Clin North Am* 1994;27:203–209.
9. Ishitani M, McGahren E, Sibley D, et al. Laparoscopically applied fibrin glue in experimental liver trauma. *J Pediatr Surg* 1989;24:867–871.
10. McCarthy P. Fibrin glue in cardiothoracic surgery. *Transf Med Rev* 1993; 8:173–179.
11. Papatheofanis F, Barmada R. The principles and applications of surgical adhesives. *Surg Ann* 1993;25:49–81.
12. Shaffrey C, Spotnitz W, Shaffrey M, et al. Neurosurgical applications of fibrin glue: augmentation of dural closure in 134 patients. *Neurosurgery* 1990; 26:207–210.
13. Errett L, Walsh G. Life salvage with fibrin glue in three cases of exsanguinating hemorrhage. *Can J Surg* 1986;29:214–216.
14. Dresdale A, Rose E, Jeevanandam V, et al. Preparation of fibrin glue from single-donor fresh-frozen plasma. *Surgery* 1985;97:750–755.
15. Blood collection storage and component preparation. In: Walker R, ed. *Technical Manual.* 11th ed. Bethesda: American Association of Blood Banks, 1993;717–747.
16. Stemberger A, Blümel. Fibrinogen-fibrin conversion and inhibition of fibrinolysis. *Thorac Cardiovasc Surg* 1982;30:209–214.
17. Ciano P, Colvin R, Dvorak A, et al. Macrophage migration in fibrin gel matrices. *Lab Invest* 1986;54:62–70.
18. Houston K, Rotstein O. Fibrin sealant in high-risk colonic anastomoses. *Arch Surg* 1988;123:230–234.
19. Byrne D, Hardy J, Wood R, et al. Effect of fibrin glues on the mechanical properties of healing wounds. *Br J Surg* 1991;78:841–843.
20. Spotnitz W, Mintz P, Avery N, et al. Fibrin glue from stored human plasma. *Am Surg* 1987;53:460–462.
21. Weis-Fogh U. Fibrinogen prepared from small blood samples for autologous use in a tissue adhesive system. *Eur Surg Res* 1988;20:381–389.
22. Kjaergard H, Weis-Fogh U, S;ohrensen H, et al. A simple method of preparation of autologous fibrin glue by means of ethanol. *Surg Gynecol Obstet* 1992;175:72–73.
23. DePalma L, Criss V, Luban N. The preparation of fibrinogen concentrate for use as fibrin glue by four different methods. *Transfusion* 1993;33:717–720.
24. Harris D, Siedentop K, Ham K, et al. Autologous fibrin tissue adhesive biodegradation and systemic effects. *Larynogoscope* 1987;97:1141–1144.
25. Pipan C, Glasheen W, Matthew T, et al. Effects of antifibrinolytic agents on the life span of fibrin sealant. *J Surg Res* 1992;53:402–407.
26. Ismal S, Glasheen W, Gonias S, et al. Bovine fibrin sealant: the intraperitoneal life span of a new hemostatic agent. *Am Coll Surg* 1993;44:572–574.

27. Rousou J, Engelman R, Breyer R. Fibrin glue: an effective hemostatic agent for nonsuturable intraoperative bleeding. *Ann Thorac Surg* 1984;38:409–410.
28. Matthew T, Spotnitz W, Korn I, et al. Four years' experience with fibrin sealant in thoracic and cardiovascular surgery. *Ann Thorac Surg* 1990;50:40–44.
29. Baker J, Spotnitz W, Nolan S. A technique for spray application of fibrin glue during cardiac operations. *Ann Thorac Surg* 1987;43:564–565.
30. Joyce D, McGrath L, Gonzalez-Lavin L. A method of applying fibrin sealant using an atomizing agent. *Ann Thorac Surg* 1989;47:320.
31. Redl H, Schlag G, Dinges H. Methods of fibrin seal application. *Thorac Cardiovasc Surg* 1982;30:223–227.
32. Borst H, Haverich A, Walterbusch G, et al. Fibrin adhesive: an important hemostatic adjunct in cardiovascular operations. *Thorac Cardiovasc Surg* 1982;84:548–553.
33. Lerner R, Binur N. Current research review. Current status of surgical adhesives. *J Surg Res* 1990;48:165–181.
34. Spotnitz W, Dalton S, Baker J, et al. Reduction of perioperative hemorrhage by anterior mediastinal spray application of fibrin glue during cardiac operations. *Ann Thorac Surg* 1987;44:529–531.
35. Gundry S, Behrendt D. A quantitative and qualitative comparison of fibrin glue, albumin, and blood as agents to pretreat porous vascular grafts. *J Surg Res* 1987;43:75–77.
36. Moront M, Katz N, O'Connell J, et al. The use of topical fibrin glue at cannulation sites in neonates. *Surg Gynecol Obstet* 358–359.
37. Di Lello F, Mullen D, Flemma R. Sutureless fixation of long aortocoronary saphenous vein grafts with oxidized regenerated cellulose. *Ann Thorac Surg* 1989;47:473–474.
38. Rousou J, Gonzalez-Lavin L, Cosgrove D, et al. Randomized clinical trial of fibrin sealant in patients undergoing resternotomy or reoperation after cardiac operations. *J Thorac Cardiovasc Surg* 1989;97:194–203.
39. Clark D, Drohan W, Miekka S, et al. Strategy for purification of coagulation factor concentrates. *Ann Clin Lab Sci* 1989;19:196–207.
40. Burnouf-Radosevich M, Burnouf T, Huart J. Biochemical and physical properties of a solvent-detergent-treated fibrin glue. *Vox Sang* 1990;58:77–84.
41. Lupinetti F, Stoney W, Alford W, et al. Cryoprecipitate-topical thrombin glue. *J Thorac Cardiovasc Surg* 1985;90:502–505.
42. Kram H, Bansal M, Timberlake O, et al. Antibacterial effects of fibrin glue-antibiotic mixtures. *J Surg Res* 1991;50:175–178.
43. Bänninger H, Hardegger T, Tobler A, et al. Fibrin glue in surgery: frequent development of inhibitors of bovine thrombin and human factor V. *Br J Haemost* 1993;85:528–532.
44. Berruyer M, Amiral J, Ffrench P, et al. Immunization by bovine thrombin used with fibrin glue during cardiovascular operations. *J Thorac Cardiovasc Surg* 1993;105:892–897.
45. Milde L. An anaphylactic reaction to fibrin glue. *Anesth Analg* 1989; 69:684–686.
46. Berguer R, Staerkel R, Moore E, et al. Warning: fatal reaction to the use of fibrin glue in deep hepatic wounds. Case reports. *J Trauma* 1991;31:408–411.
47. Barton B, Moore E, Pearce W. Fibrin glue as a biologic vascular patch—a comparative study. *J Surg Res* 1986;40:510–513.

48. Stark J, de Leval M. Experience with fibrin seal (Tisseel) in operations for congenital heart defects. *Ann Thorac Surg* 1984;38:411-413.
49. Ennker I, Ennker J, Schoon D, et al. Formaldehyde-free collagen glue in experimental lung gluing. *Ann Thorac Surg* 1994;57:1622-1627.
50. Vincent J, Skotnicki S, van der Meer J, et al. Resorbable suture support for ventricular aneurysmectomy. *J Thorac Cardiovasc Surg* 1987;94:430–433.
51. Feikes H, Daugharthy J, Perry J, et al. Preservation of all chordae tendineae and papillary muscle during mitral valve replacement with a tilting disc valve. *J Cardiac Surg* 1990;5:81–85.
52. Dilip K, Vachaspathy P, Clarke B, et al. Haemolysis following mitral valve repair. *J Cardiovasc Surg* 1992;33:568–569.
53. Shapira N. An alternative to felt pledgets in cardiac surgery. *Ann Thorac Surg* 1986;41:219–221.
54. Borst H. Dire consequences of the indiscriminate use of Teflon felt pledgets. *J Thorac Cardiovasc Surg* 1987;94:442–443.
55. Bojar R, Payne D, Sheffield A, et al. Successful repair of postoperative ascending aortic mycotic false aneurysms using circulatory arrest. *Ann Thorac Surg* 1988;46:182–186.
56. Barbalinardo R, Citrin P, Franco C, et al. A comparison of isobutyl 2-cyanoacrylate glue, fibrin adhesive, and oxidized regenerated cellulose for control of needle hole bleeding from polytetrafluoroethylene vascular prostheses. *J Vasc Surg* 1986;4:220–223.

18
Routine Use of Heparin-Bonded Circuits with Minimal Anticoagulation for Coronary Artery Bypass Surgery

GABRIEL S. ALDEA, PATRICK R. TREANOR, AND
RICHARD J. SHEMIN

Many advances in blood conservation techniques are currently being applied during coronary artery bypass grafting (CABG). These include the use of cell saving to enhance intraoperative blood salvage,[1-3] the use of large-bore directional cannulae to minimize shear forces and platelet activation and loss,[4] the routine use of antifibrinolytic agents,[5-7] normothermic bypass to diminish coagulopathy,[8] low-prime cardiopulmonary bypass to diminish dilution of coagulation factors, the use of "tip-to-tip" heparin-bonded cardiopulmonary bypass circuits,[9] and postoperative reinfusion of shed blood.[10] Despite the proven efficacy of these blood conservation techniques, they have been uniformly applied to all patients undergoing CABG because of their complexity and cost. Consequently, as many as 30% to 70% of patients undergoing CABG still require transfusions.[1-3]

Background

During cardiac surgery, blood comes into contact with the very large nonendothelialized surface area of the cardiopulmonary bypass extracorporeal circuit. The artificial materials that line the circuit are recognized by the blood as being "foreign." Consequently, a surface interaction is initiated by formed and unformed blood elements, which is further amplified by stimulating many biologic reactions. These biologic reactions involve activation of the entire autoimmune defensive system of the body including the coagulation, fibrinolytic, complement, kallikrein, and kinin systems[11,12] (Fig. 18.1). This cross-stimulation and amplification results in activation and consumption of platelets, activation and degranulation of leukocytes, destruction of red blood cells, as well as the release of anaphylaxins, oxygen free radicals, endotoxins, etc.[13] The biologic effects of these reactions to the extracorporeal circuit have complex effects on many organs that are clinically described as "postperfusion syndrome." These responses can be characterized as changes in homeostasis in two principal categories: (1)

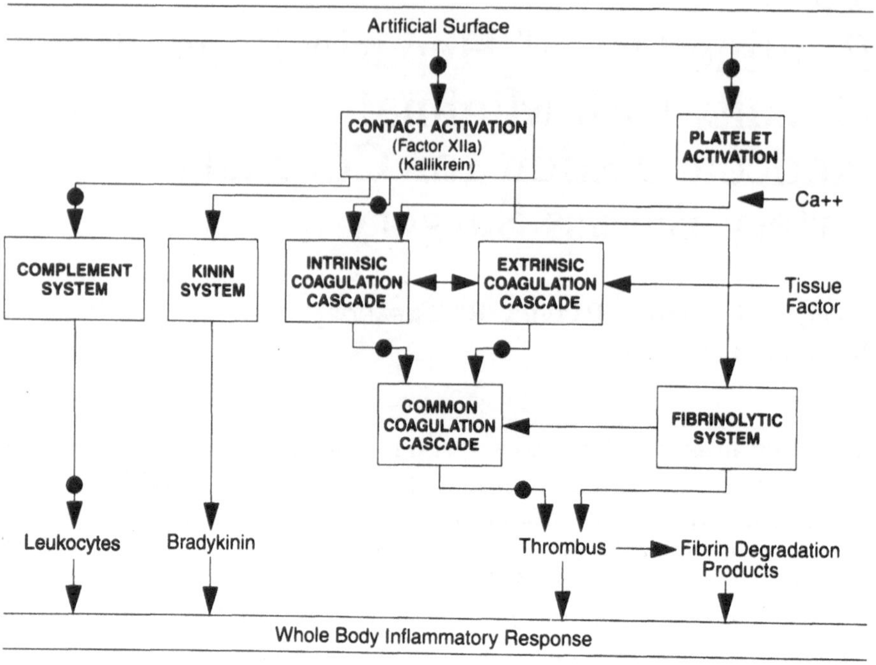

FIGURE 18.1. Interaction between formed and unformed blood elements to the "foreign" surface of the extracorporeal system. •, Research indicates mitigating effects by HBC. (From Compendium II of Clinical and Scientific Information,[12] with permission.)

coagulation and thrombosis, and (2) generalized inflammation. The role of novel extracorporeal surfaces is therefore to attenuate coagulation and thrombosis by being more thromboresistant and to diminish the inflammatory response by enhanced biocompatibility.

Thromboresistance

Thrombogenesis occurs at a site of injury (endothelial disruption) or foreign material (nonendothelial surface) and involves a complex interaction involving platelet adherence, aggregation, and granule release; thrombin generation; and fibrin formation. Thrombin cleaves fibrinogen to fibrin, which is the substructure for thrombus. The thrombus-forming effects of thrombin are naturally and normally limited by (1) inactivation of circulating thrombin by plasma proteases; (2) inhibition of thrombin by the thrombin–antithrombin III complex, and (3) neutralizing thrombomodulin. Thrombin modulation represents a normal hemostatic mechanism for balancing the coagulation system at the site of an injury. Nonthrombogenic surfaces attempt to mimic these properties to limit activation of the coagulation system.

Antithrombin III (AT) is naturally produced in the microvasculature and its effects are enhanced in the presence of heparin sulfate (natural) or heparin (circulating or surface bound). AT affects both the intrinsic and extrinsic systems at multiple points (Fig. 18.2). Heparin is a naturally occurring, heavily sulfated polysaccharide, whose main biologic effect occurs primarily through its interaction with antithrombin III. A small portion of this large molecule (referred to as the AT binding site) is responsible for a high-affinity binding to antithrombin III (Fig. 18.3), thereby accelerating the binding to circulating thrombin and its inactivation of coagulation factors by enzyme-protease inhibitor interaction (Fig. 18.2).

Full systemic anticoagulation to prevent the activation of the coagulation system has been the standard of practice during cardiopulmonary bypass (CPB). The work of Young et al[14] has shown suppression of fibrin monomer production in a primate model when the activated clotting time (ACT) exceeds 400 seconds, establishing an industry "gold standard" and the current recommendation of ACT greater than 480 seconds. Many recent investigators have questioned this standard, and have suggested that ACT of around 300 seconds is equally safe.[9,15,16] The binding of heparin to

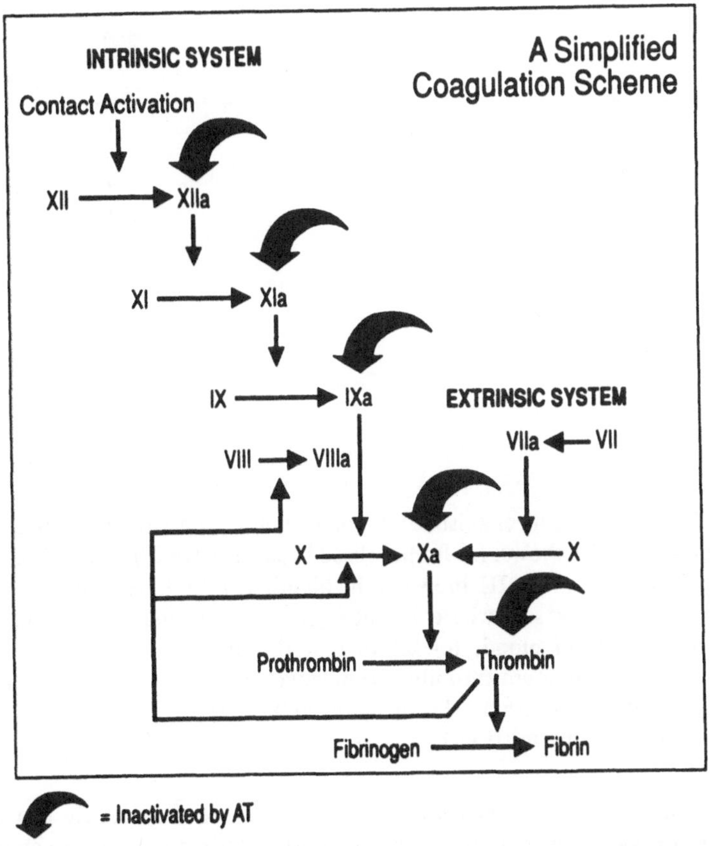

FIGURE 18.2. Antithrombin III (AT) inhibition points on the coagulation cascade. (From Compendium of Scientific Information,[11] with permission.)

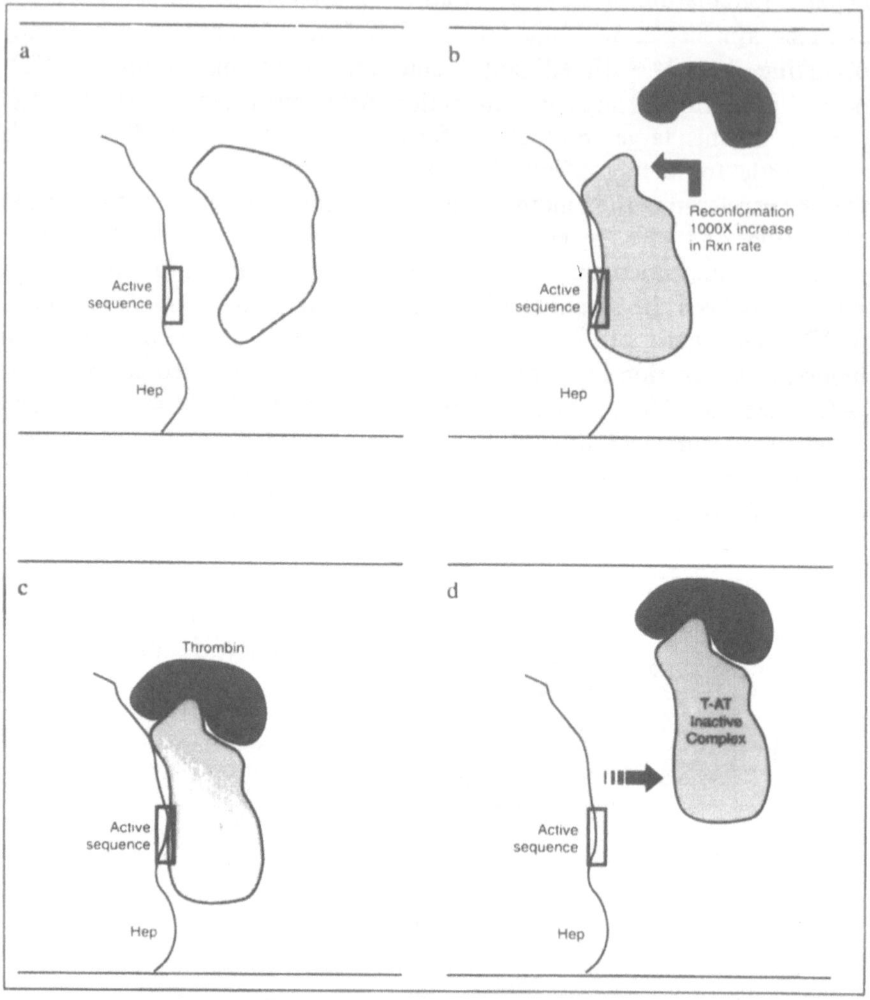

FIGURE 18.3. Proposed mechanism of action of bound heparin on antithrombin III. This simplified series shows: (a) Immobilized heparin (CBAS®) containing an active site and an antithrombin III molecule in blood. (b) Antithrombin III bound to heparin at the active site where it undergoes a conformational change and a thrombin molecule in blood. (c) Binding of thrombin to antithrombin III. (d) Release of the thrombin-antithrombin III inactive complex leaving heparin available to catalyze another reaction. (From Compendium II of Clinical and Scientific Information,[12] with permission.)

artificial surfaces was first reported by Gott et al.[17] Recently the heparin binding process was extended to the entire ("tip-to-tip") extracorporeal circuit. The thromboresistant properties of the heparin-bonded circuits (HBC) led to a resurgence of interest in reassessing the lower safe limits of anticoagulation.[9] Heparin is bound to artificial surfaces by one of several

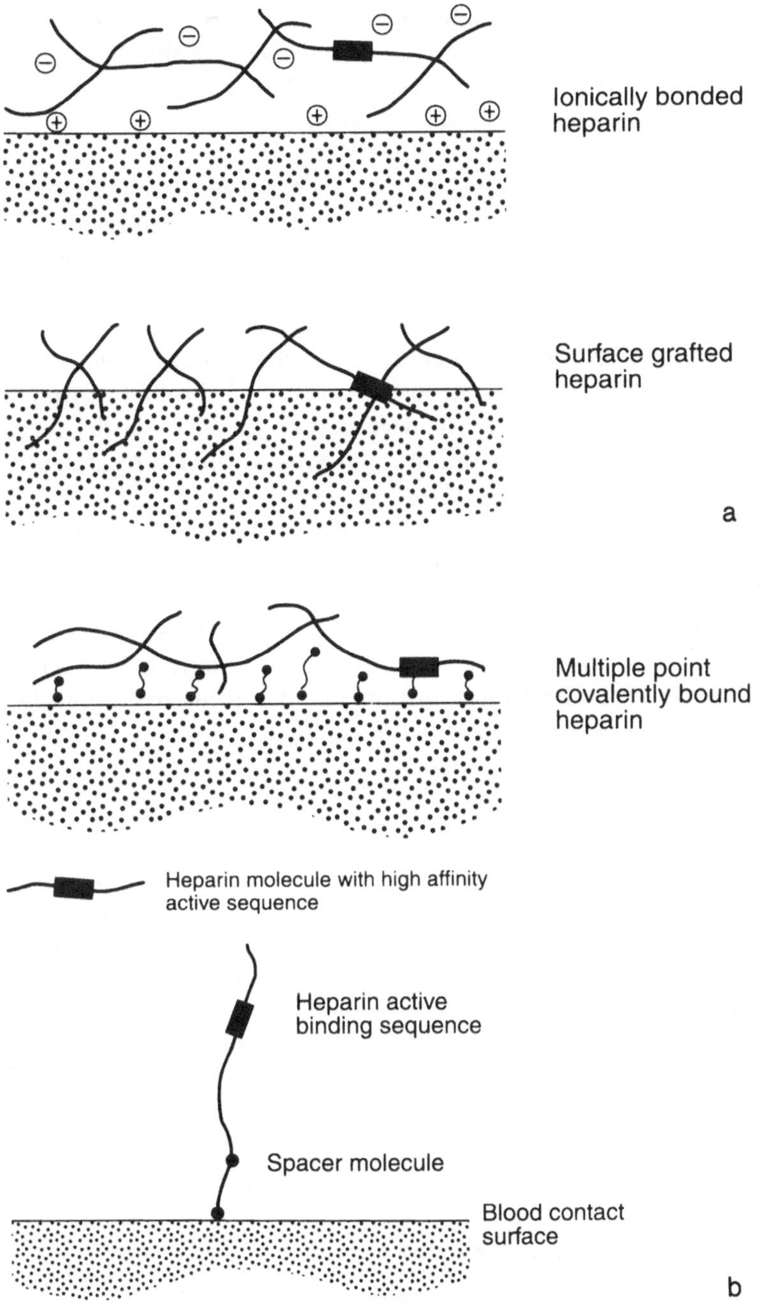

FIGURE 18.4. Different modalities of heparin binding to extracorporeal circuits. (a) Ionically bound, surface grafting and multiple point covalently bound. (b) End-point covalent attachment. (From Compendium II of Clinical and Scientific Information,[12] with permission.)

mechanisms: ionic binding, grafting, multiple point covalent binding, and end-point covalent attachment (Fig. 18.4). The specific method of attachment may have important implications for the function and durability, as well as for the cost of these extracorporeal surfaces. Published results have to be carefully interpreted since laboratory findings may be related to the specific method of heparin binding and to the particulars of the experimental design. Finally, these laboratory findings have to be translated to clinically relevant end points. Despite all these limitations, there is an overwhelming body of literature that suggests that heparin-bonded circuits (HBC) with lower levels of anticoagulation are more thromboresistant than conventional circuits with full anticoagulation nonheparin-bonded circuits (NHBC).[9,18–20] In comparison to conventional circuits with full anticoagulation, HBCs with lower anticoagulation have been demonstrated to diminish platelet activation and loss, hemolysis,[21] thrombin formation,[19] fibrinopeptide A formation[22] (a degradation product of fibrinogen, an indicator of coagulation activation), and arterial filter thrombi visualized with scanning electron microscopy.[20]

At the Boston University Medical Center Hospital there is an extensive experience (over 500 patients) equally distributed among the two commercially available HBCs using either Carmeda (Medtronic, Minneapolis, MN) or Duraflo II (Baxter, Irvine, CA) circuits. In our experience, the lower anticoagulation in conjunction with enhanced thromboresistance is not only an interesting laboratory phenomenon but has translated clinically into concrete clinical end points such as a significant decrease in transfusion requirements (see Results, below).

Biocompatibility

When compared to NHBC with full anticoagulation, HBC with diminished anticoagulation was demonstrated to result in less platelet activation, complement activation (C3a, C5a), and leukocyte degranulation. In a pig model, these laboratory end points resulted in a decrease in lung permeability and free-water content, and an increase in pulmonary compliance and post-pump function.[23] The clinical experience at our hospital revealed a significant decrease in perioperative weight gain (see Results), which may translate into a further decrease in hospital morbidity, length of stay, and hospital cost.

Methods

CPB Circuit and Technique

The entire ("tip-to-tip") cardiopulmonary bypass circuit was heparin bonded. The heparin-bonded circuit consisted of a two-stage atrial cannula (34/48 Fr), a directional arterial cannula (20 Fr), a cardioplegia multiple perfusion set, cardioplegia antegrade and retrograde administration catheters (DLP, Grand Rapids, MI), all the cardiopulmonary bypass tubing and connectors, a low-prime (1200–1500 ml) membrane oxygenator with closed venous reservoirs, a heater-cooler, a cardiotomy reservoir, and suckers. Patients were treated with either an ionically bonded heparin circuit (Duraflo II, Baxter, Irvine, CA) or a covalently bound heparin circuit with end-point attachment (Carmeda, Medtronic, Minneapolis, MN). Centrifugal pumps were used exclusively.

Anticoagulation Protocol

In patients treated with HBC, anticoagulation was achieved with 1 mg/kg (100 IU) of heparin (dose ranged from 0.8 to 1.5 mg/kg), achieving and maintaining an ACT of greater than 280 seconds as measured by a dose-response assay using the Hepcon Heparin Management System (Medtronic, Minneapolis, MN). ACT was checked every 20 minutes for the duration of the bypass run. CPB was initiated slowly with an empty (closed) venous reservoir and low Plasmalyte prime (1200–1500 ml, Travenol, Baxter, Irvine, CA). Once the venous reservoir was filled, flow was increased to maintain venous saturation of 60% to 75%. Core temperature was not allowed to drift below 34°C and active cooling was avoided. During the entire procedure all field drainage was directed to the Cell Saver (Haemonetics, Braintree, MA). No discard suckers were utilized. All sponges were soaked in saline, wrung into a sterile reservoir by the scrub nurse, and directed to the Cell Saver. A half to a full unit of autologous blood was thus harvested; the amount varied with duration of the bypass run. Pump suckers were used sparingly.

Myocardial Protection

Priming of the blood cardioplegia line was performed on cardiopulmonary bypass with blood, avoiding crystalloid priming. Cold (4°C) blood cardioplegia was administered in an antegrade fashion and supplemented in all patients with retrograde cardioplegia. In all patients cardioplegia was also administered down the saphenous grafts. Cardioplegia was readministered every 20 minutes while the cross clamp was applied. Cardioplegia stagnant in the tubing between doses was discarded onto the field prior to each repeated cardioplegia administration. A "hot shot" of blood cardioplegia was administered in an antegrade and retrograde fashion, prior to the release of the cross clamp. Topical cooling with cold saline was used to supplement myocardial protection.

Weaning from CPB and Reversal of Anticoagulation

Patients were actively warmed to a core temperature of 37°C before weaning from CPB. Once weaned from bypass, a test dose of protamine was administered (Elkins-Sunn, Cherry Hill, NJ) and after hemodynamic stability was ensured the cannulae were promptly removed. To avoid blood stagnation, the arterial, venous, pump sucker, and cardioplegia lines were quickly drained of blood by retrograde siphoning and directed to the Cell Saver. The arterial and venous cannulae were refilled (and de-aired) with crystalloid solution and a crystalloid primed circuit was made available for possible intervention in the event of hemodynamic deterioration. The appropriate protamine reversal dose was verified and titrated by the Hepcon Heparin Management System. Protamine dose ranged from 40 to 90 mg. After protamine administration, Amicar (American Reagent, Shirley, NY) was administered. A 10-g IV infusion dose was infused over 30 minutes followed by 10 g IV administered as a continuous infusion over 5 hours.

Transfusion Practice

Patients were transfused red blood cells if intraoperative hematocrits fell below 20% or postoperative hematocrits fell below 23%. Following protamine administration, ACT were checked, and circulating heparin was identified and reversed with doses titrated by the Hepcon Heparin Management System. All surgically correctable bleeding was carefully addressed. Persistent postoperative bleeding in excess of 300 ml in the first hour or 500 ml in the first 2 hours was considered an indication for transfusion of platelets (10 units) and fresh frozen plasma (2 units). Persistent bleeding despite therapy with platelets and fresh frozen plasma in the presence of fibrinogen levels of less than 20 g/dl was considered an indication for cryoprecipitate therapy (10 units). Aprotinin was not used.

Statistics

All data and figures are presented as mean ± SD. Continuous variables were evaluated by Student's *t*-test and categorical variables were tested by chi-square analysis, where appropriate. Absolute *p* values were reported.

Results

The records of all patients undergoing primary, first-time CABG at our institution operated on within a 14-month period were retrospectively reviewed. Patients were treated with either a conventional circuit and full anticoagulation (NHBC, ACT >480 seconds) or heparin-bonded circuits with low anticoagulation (HBC, ACT >280 seconds). HBCs were equally divided between Carmeda and Duraflo II. The patients' preoperative risk and hematologic profiles were comparable in NHBC and HBC patients (Tables 18.1 and 18.2).

No significant differences in preoperative hematologic parameters between the groups were noted (Table 18.2). The total amount of shed pleural and mediastinal blood differed significantly between NHBC and HBC

TABLE 18.1. Comparisons of patient profile and risk characteristics of NHBC and HBC groups.

Variable	NHBC	HBC	*p* value
Number	455	102	
Age (years)	68.00 ± 13.0	65.0 ± 5.4	NS
% Female	29.4	33.3	NS
% Urgent	65.9	65.0	NS
% Low ejection fraction (EF) (<45)	31.9	34.2	NS
% Diabetic	31.9	29.0	NS
% Preoperative IV heparin ± aspirin (ASA)	41.3	39.2	NS

TABLE 18.2. Comparisons of preoperative hematologic profiles of NHBC and HBC groups.

Variable	NHBC	HBC	*p* value
Hgb (g/dl)	13.61 ± 1.48	13.7 ± 6.50	NS
HCT (%)	38.9 ± 4.67	39.7 ± 2.66	NS
Platelets (10^3)	244 ± 74	248 ± 96	NS
Prothrombin time (PT) (seconds)	12.7 ± 0.42	12.7 ± 0.33	NS
Partial thrombin time (PTT) (seconds)	35.0 ± 2.77	34.2 ± 3.33	NS

groups at 12 hours (721 ± 486 vs. 520 ± 467, $p < .0001$) and 24 hours (984 ± 616 vs. 683 ± 561, $p < .00001$) (Fig. 18.5). The percent of patients not transfused was substantially higher in the HBC-treated group (48.0% vs. 31.9%, $p < .002$) (Fig. 18.6). The transfusion requirements for packed red blood cells (PRBC), platelets (PLT), fresh frozen plasma (FFP), as well as the total donor transfusion exposure and the total donor unit transfusion

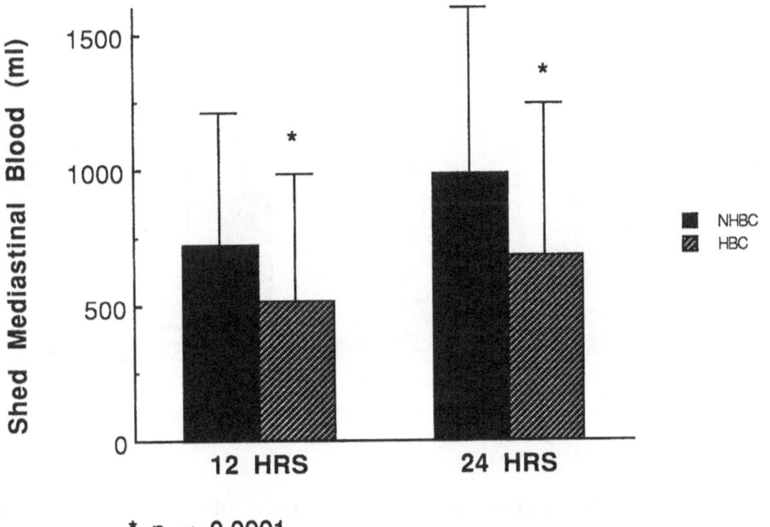

FIGURE 18.5. Analysis of shed mediastinal blood.

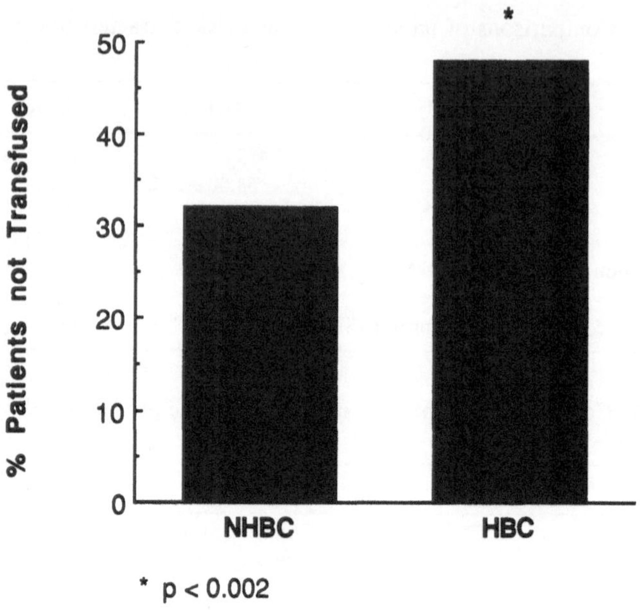

FIGURE 18.6. Percent of patients undergoing CABG not requiring transfusions. Comparison between NHBC and HBC groups.

exposure per patient undergoing CABG was reduced by 56% with routine use of HBC (Figs. 18.7 and 18.8). The donor unit exposure per patient undergoing CABG was reduced by 56% with routine use of HBC (41.0 ± 8.42 vs. 9.33 ± 10.81, $p < .00003$). The differences between HBC and

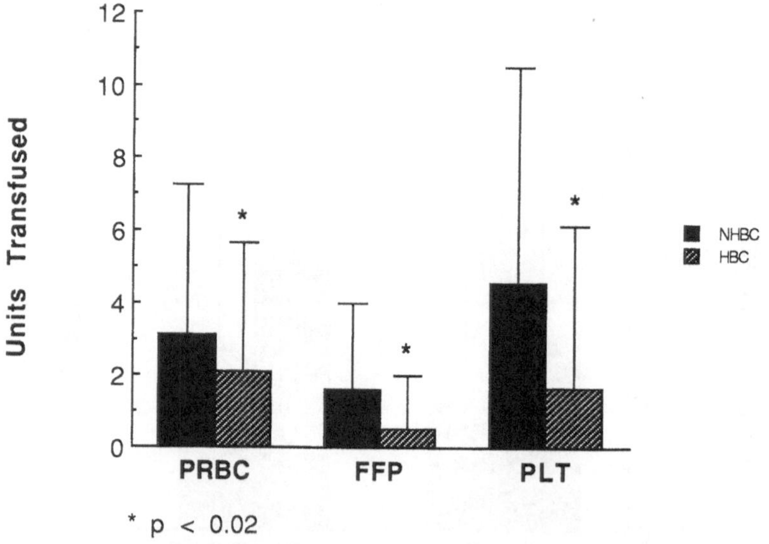

FIGURE 18.7. Transfusion requirements of packed red blood cells (PRBS), fresh frozen plasma (FFP), and platelets (PLT) measured in units. Comparison of NHBC and HBC groups.

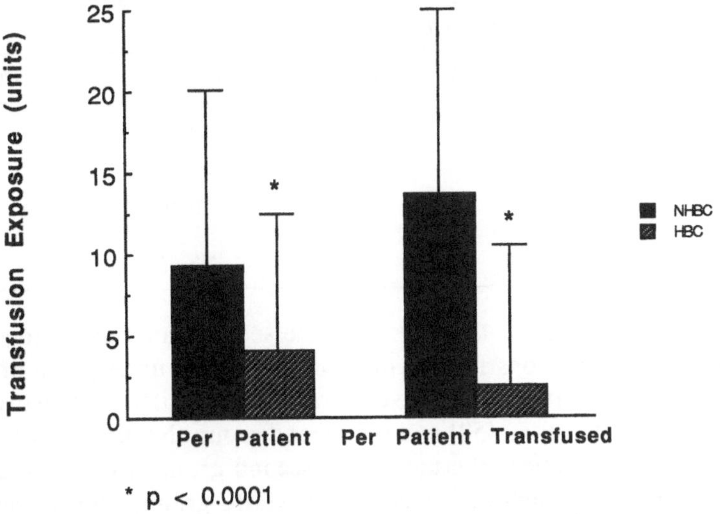

FIGURE 18.8. Transfusion exposure (units) per patient and per patient transfused. Comparison between NHBC and HBC groups.

NHBC groups persisted in patients not on aspirin and IV heparin preoperatively (nonanticoagulated patients) and were further accentuated in patients receiving preoperative anticoagulants (IV heparin and aspirin [ASA]) (Table 18.3).

A limited cost and charge analysis was performed to determine the savings resulting only from the added transfusion requirement in the NHBC group compared to the HBC group (Table 18.4). This figure does not take into consideration the cost of additional laboratory tests triggered by excessive mediastinal drainage, the labor and disposable equipment costs, the cost of the short- or long-term side effects of transfusions, or the cost of reoperations for postoperative bleeding.

TABLE 18.3. Comparison of transfusion requirements in the presence and absence of preoperative anticoagulation (IV heparin ± ASA) between NHBC and HBC groups.

Variable	NHBC	HBC	*p* value
Anticoagulated patients			
% not transfused	23.4	40.5*	.01
Donor units per patient	9.48 ± 11.57	3.80 ± 6.64*	.0001
Donor units per patient transfused	13.66 ± 11.65	7.44 ± 7.33*	.000001
Nonanticoagulated patients			
% not transfused	31.9	48.0*	.01
Donor units per patient	9.32 ± 839	4.02 ± 3.27*	.0029
Donor units per patient transfused	13.67 ± 8.82	7.88 ± 6.52*	.000008

*Donor units include banked packed red blood cells, platelets, fresh frozen plasma, and cryoprecipitate.

TABLE 18.4. Cost analysis of the effect of reduction in the transfusion requirement in patients treated with HBC.

	Units saved	Cost ($)	Charge ($)
PRBC	1.02	68.54	98.40
FFP	1.13	28.25	82.45
PLT	2.88	144.00	199.20
Type and cross match		36.00	36.00
Total		276.79	416.05

The effect of Amicar therapy was assessed by comparing the yearly incidence of reoperations for bleeding in all patients undergoing primary, first-time CABG in two consecutive years. The only difference between the first group (NHBC, $n = 450$) and the second group (NHBC, $n = 455$) was the institution of Amicar therapy in the second group. In the NHBC-Am group no Amicar therapy was given. In the NHBC group, Amicar was given after heparinization (prior to institution of cardiopulmonary bypass) as a 10-g IV loading dose infused over 30 minutes, followed by a 10-g IV infusion administered over 5 hours. The routine administration of pre-bypass Amicar therapy resulted in a decreased rate of return to the operating room for postoperative bleeding in NHBC patients (3.6% to 2.5%, $p < .05$). When compared with the NHBC group, Amicar therapy in the HBC group was limited to the post-bypass period after decannulation and reversal of heparin with protamine. Despite less aggressive pre-bypass Amicar therapy in the HBC group, return to the operating room for postoperative bleeding was significantly lower in the HBC group compared with the NHBC group (0.9% vs. 2.5%, $p < .001$) (Fig. 18.9).

We propose that postoperative weight gain may reflect the inflammatory response to extracorporeal bypass. An analysis of our current experience with 557 patients (NHBC + HBC groups) noted a significant correlation between excessive postoperative weight gain (>10% of preoperative weight) and prolonged hospital length of stay (Fig. 18.10). A comparison of weight gained measured on postoperative day 1 (represented as a percent of preoperative weight) between NHBC and HBC patients demonstrated less postoperative weight gain in HBC patients (4.98% vs. 6.84%, $p < .002$) (Fig. 18.11). In addition a larger proportion of patients in the HBC group gained less than 5% of their preoperative weight (60.7% vs. 42.2%, $p < .0003$) (Fig. 18.12).

Hospital mortality, morbidity, and length of stay were not significantly different between NHBC and HBC groups. The overall 30-day perioperative mortality was 1.6%, with 1.7% incidence of perioperative myocardial infarction (MI), 0.6% incidence of cerebrovascular accident (CVA), and a 0.9% incidence of sternal infection. In both groups 41% of patients were discharged before the fifth postoperative day and 83% of patients were discharged before or on the seventh postoperative day.

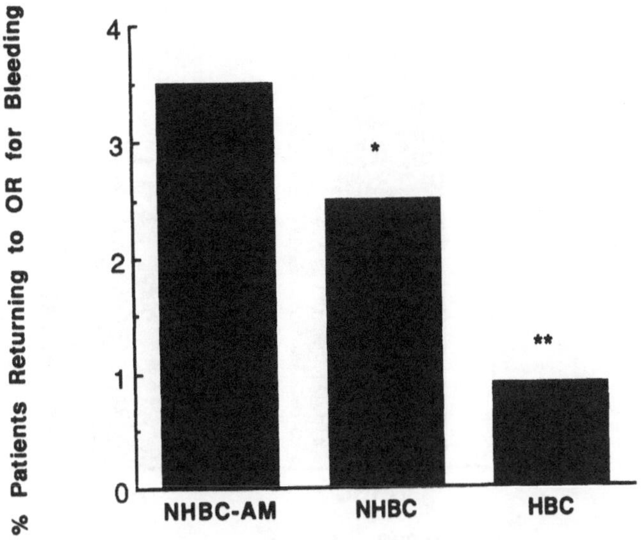

* $p < 0.05$, ** $p < 0.02$

FIGURE 18.9. Percent of patients returning to the operating room for postoperative bleeding following CABG. Comparison of NHBC treated without Amicar (NHBC-Am), NHBC treated with aggressive Amicar therapy (NHBC), and HBC groups.

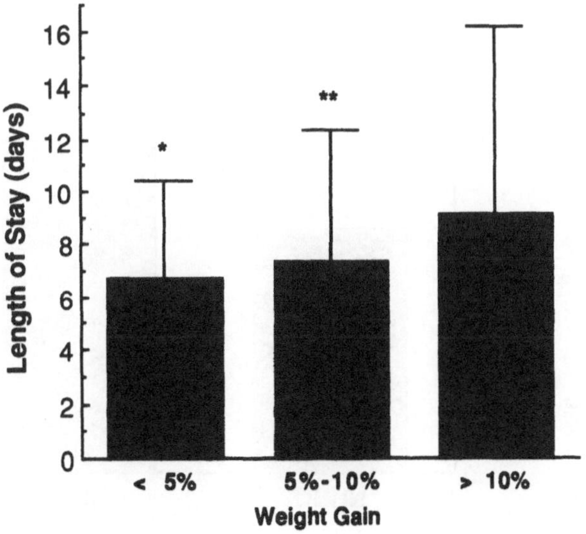

* $p < 0.000046$ vs. > 10%, ** $p < 0.01$ vs. > 10%

FIGURE 18.10. Analysis of length of hospital stay in patients with less than 5% postoperative weight gain, 5% to 10% postoperative weight gain, and greater than 10% postoperative weight gain.

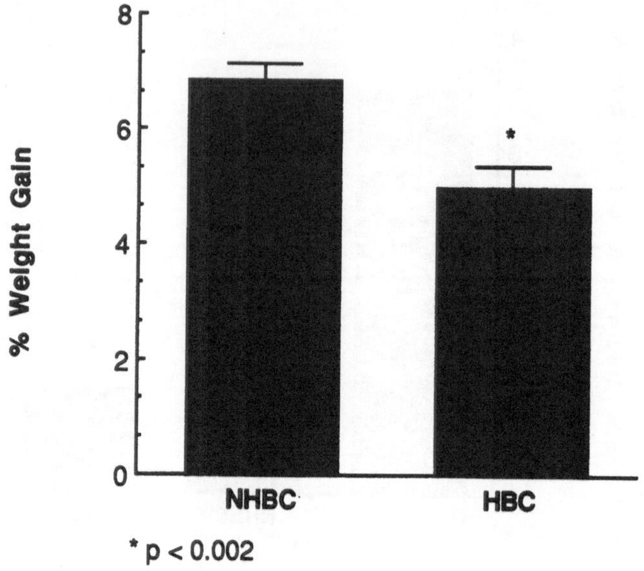

FIGURE 18.11. Weight gain on postoperative day 1 following CABG expressed as a percent of preoperative weight. Comparison of NHBC and HBC groups.

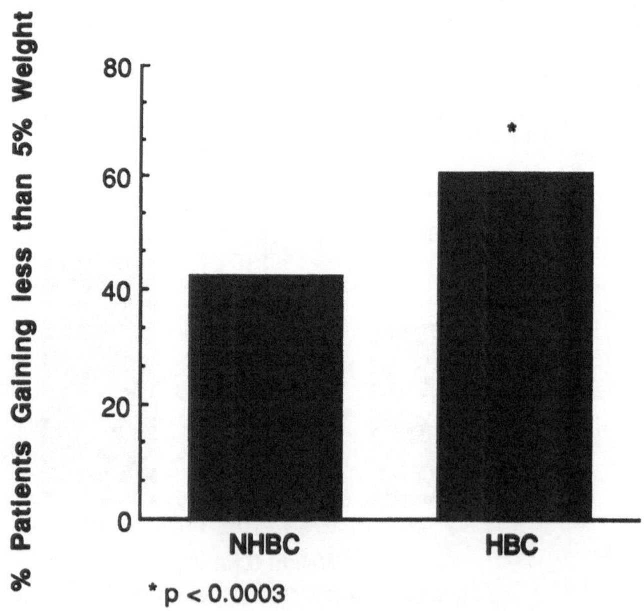

FIGURE 18.12 Percent of patients undergoing CABG gaining less than 5% of their preoperative weight by postoperative day 1. Comparison of NHBC and HBC groups.

Discussion

Despite the development of many techniques and strategies to enhance blood conservation during cardiac surgery, as many as 30% to 70% of patients still require blood transfusions.[1-3] Many of these strategies have not been routinely implemented because of their perceived complexity or added costs. Recently, these modalities have been shown to be relatively simple to implement and highly effective in diminishing perioperative blood loss.

Two alternative approaches and strategies to blood conservation during CABG can be undertaken. The first strategy is to alter the postoperative coagulation profile in patients undergoing CABG.[7,24] Recently the efficacy of potent protease inhibitors, which enhance post-bypass coagulation by affecting fibrinolysis, have been documented.[5] Aprotinin (Trasylol, Miles, West Haven, CT), the most potent and commonly used agent, inhibits plasmin and kallikrein and preserves platelet membrane adhesion glycoprotein. The use of prophylactic aprotinin is associated with concerns of potentially significant side effects such as alteration in the efficacy of monitoring of anticoagulation during CPB (Celite ACT).[25] Early experience noted a trend toward a higher incidence of perioperative Q-wave MI and graft occlusion on postmodern examination, which was thought to be related to the potential for a hypercoagulable state.[7] More recently a very low incidence of adverse events and a low incidence of graft thrombosis and renal failure has been reported.[26] These discrepancies have raised the issue of inadequate anticoagulation in earlier series perhaps related to the direct effect of aprotinin on Celite ACT. Finally, aprotinin is expensive, imposing an additional cost of nearly $1000 per patient when used as recommended, with a full (Hammersmith) loading dose.[5,26] Amicar, a substantially weaker antifibrinolytic, has also been demonstrated to decrease perioperative blood loss and transfusion requirements.[5,6] We routinely use it in all patients undergoing CPB, although the protocol is modified when a heparin-bonded extracorporeal circuit is used with low-dose heparin administration.

Our approach is to offer an alternative strategy to enhance blood conservation during cardiac surgery. Instead of altering the perioperative coagulation balance with hemostasis-promoting drugs,[5,26] we use more thromboresistant circuits (heparin-bonded) in conjunction with lower systemic anticoagulation. Thromboresistance of heparin-bonded cardiopulmonary bypass circuits has been documented at low flow rates even in the absence of heparin, as long as flow is continuous.[9,22] We agree with Edmunds[27] that flow in nonendothelialized surfaces may lead to thrombin formation, particularly when flow is intermittent (rather than continuous) and in areas of blood turbulence and stagnation. Currently we strongly condemn "heparin-free" bypass for routine cardiopulmonary bypass procedures and instead advocate lower levels of anticoagulation with frequent and careful monitoring. In addition, we are very concerned with promoting coagulation during cardiopulmonary bypass when using low-dose heparinization with HBC despite reports in the literature describing the safety of pre-bypass administration of aprotinin and Amicar in patients treated with HBC.[28] Instead we specifically and deliberately choose to implement Amicar therapy only *after* decannulation and heparin reversal. Based on our experience combined with current experimental and clinical data, *we strongly believe that a heparin-bonded circuit with lower levels of anticoagulation are more thromboresistant than equivalent, conventional (nonparin bonded) circuits with full anticoagulation.*[18-20]

In our experience, postoperative weight gain is an accurate predictor of length of hospital stay and cost. Patients who gain less than 5% of their preoperative weight post-bypass are more likely to be discharged prior to the fifth postoperative day, and patients gaining more than 10% of their preoperative weight post-bypass are more likely to have complications and a longer hospitalization. We believe postoperative weight gain reflects the intensity of the inflammatory response of the body to the extracorporeal system. We conclusively demonstrated that the routine use of HBC diminished postoperative weight gain. The mechanism for this remains to be determined. Previous work with HBC demonstrated enhanced biocompatibility and a significant attenuation of platelet activation, complement activation, and leukocyte degranulation.[9-11,23] In our experience the postoperative transfusion requirement highly correlates with postoperative weight gain. Thus, the diminished postoperative weight gain seen in the HBC group can either reflect a diminished transfusion requirement in this group or a direct effect of enhanced biocompatibility of the circuit.

As with all modifications, the techniques of CPB have to be adjusted to ensure patient safety, and the limitations of these techniques have to be clearly understood.[9] These concerns are shared by all extracorporeal circulation modalities, but are accentuated in the presence of lower anticoagulation. These concerns include identification of patients with antithrombin III deficiencies or other hypercoagulable states, avoidance of intraoperative administration of drugs that shift the balance of hemostasis and promote thrombosis, and avoidance of blood stagnation.

We reported the largest clinical experience with HBC and lower anticoagulation for routine CABG to date and conclusively demonstrated that the integrated multicomponent strategy outlined above is safe and extremely effective. Minimizing perioperative blood loss not only diminishes the potential risk of transfusion reactions,[1-3,24] but also is cost-effective and outweighs the additional cost of heparin-bonded circuits. Because of an overwhelming positive clinical experience, we are in the process of conducting a large, randomized, clinical trial to study the effect of the use of heparin-bonded circuits in all patients undergoing routine CABG.

We anticipate that the routine use of HBC will potentially be expanded to all patients requiring cardiopulmonary bypass, regardless of the surgical procedure, with gratifying results.

References

1. LoCicero J III, Massad M, Gandy K, et al. Aggressive blood conservation in coronary artery surgery: impact on patient care. *J Cardiovasc Surg (Torino)* 1990;31:559–563.
2. Jones JW, Rawitscher RE, McLean TR, et al. Benefits from combining blood conservation measures in cardiac operations. *Ann Thorac Surg* 1991; 51:541–546.
3. Scott WJ, Rode R, Castelmain B, et al. Efficacy, complication and cost of a comprehensive blood conservation program for cardiac operations. *J Thorac Cardiovasc Surg* 1992;103:1001–1007.
4. Pfaender LM. Hemodynamics in extracorporeal aortic cannula: review of factors affecting choice of appropriate size. *J Extracorp Tech* 1981;13:224–232.
5. Fremes SE, Wong BI, Lee L, et al. Metaanalysis of prophylactic drug treatment in the prevention of postoperative bleeding. *Ann Thorac Surg* 1994; 58:1580–1588.
6. Daily PO, Lamphere JA, Dembitsky WP, et al. Effect of prophylactic epsilon-aminocaproic acid on blood loss and transfusion requirements in patients undergoing first-time coronary artery bypass grafting. A randomized, prospective, double-blinded trial. *J Thorac Cardiovasc Surg* 1994;108:99–108.
7. Cosgrove DM III, Heric B, Lytle BW, et al. Aprotinin therapy for re-operative myocardial revascularization: a placebo controlled study. *Ann Thorac Surg* 1992;54:1031–1038.
8. Yau TM, Carson S, Weisel RD, et al. The effect of warm heart surgery on post-operative bleeding. *J Thorac Cardiovasc Surg* 1992;103:1155–1163.
9. von Segesser LK, Weiss BK, Pasic M, et al. Risk and benefits of low systemic heparinization during open heart operations. *Ann Thorac Surg* 1994; 58:391–398.
10. Morris JJ, Tan YS. Autotransfusion: Is there a benefit in a current practice of aggressive blood conservation? *Ann Thorac Surg* 1994;58:502–508.
11. Compendium of Scientific Information. Medtronic/Carmeda Bioactive Surface. Medtronic Inc., Minneapolis, MN, 1991.
12. Compendium II of Clinical and Scientific Information. Carmeda Bioactive Surface. Medtronic Inc., Minneapolis, MN, 1994.
13. Kirklin JK, George JP, Holman W. The inflammatory response to cardiopulmonary bypass. In: Gravlee GP, Davis RF, Utley JR, eds. *Cardiopulmonary Bypass, Principles and Practice.* Baltimore: Williams & Wilkins, 1993; 223–248.
14. Young JA, Kisher CT, Doty DB. Adequate anticoagulation during cardiopulmonary bypass determined by activated clotting time and appearance of fibrin monomer. *Ann Thorac Surg* 1978;26:231–240.
15. Gravlee GP, Haddon WS, Rothberger HK, et al. Heparin dosing and monitoring during cardiopulmonary bypass. *J Thorac Cardiovasc Surg* 1990; 99:518–527.
16. Cardoso PFG, Yamazaki F, Keshavjee S, et al. A reevaluation of heparin requirement during cardiopulmonary bypass. *J Thorac Cardiovasc Surg* 1991; 101:153–160.
17. Gott VL, Whiffen JD, Datton RC. Heparin bonding on colloidal graphite surfaces. *Science* 1963;142:1297–1298.
18. von Segesser LK. Experimental and clinical experience with Duraflo II heparin

surface coated perfusion equipment. *Pathophysiol Tech Cardiopulmonary Bypass Proc* 1992;15 (abstr).
19. Gu YJ, van Oeveren W, van der Kamp KWHJ, et al. Heparin-coating of extracorporeal circuits reduce thrombin formation in patients undergoing cardiopulmonary bypass. *Perfusion* 1991;6:221–225.
20. Borowiec JW, Bylock A, van der Linden J, et al. Heparin reduces blood cell adhesion to arterial filters during coronary bypass: a clinical study. *Ann Thorac Surg* 1993;55:1540–1545.
21. Belboud A, Al-Kaja N, Gudmundsson M, et al. The influence of heparin-coated and uncoated circuits on blood rheology during cardiac surgery. *J Extracorp Tech* 1993;25(2):40–46.
22. Arnander C, Olsson P. Influence of blood flow and the effect of protamine on thromboresistant properties of covalently bonded heparin surface. *Biomed Mater Res* 1988;22:859–868.
23. Redmond JM, Gillinov AV, Stuart RS, et al. Heparin-coated bypass reduce pulmonary injury. *Ann Thorac Surg* 1993;56(3):474–478.
24. Rosengart TK, Helm RE, Klempere J, et al. Combined aprotinin and erythropoietin use for blood conservation: result with Jehovah's Witnesses. *Ann Thorac Surg* 1994;58:1397–1403.
25. Tabuchi N, Njo TL, Tigchelaar I, et al. Monitoring of anticoagulation in aprotinin treated patients during heart operations. *Ann Thorac Surg* 1994;58:774–777.
26. Taylor KM. Perioperative approaches to coagulation defects. *Ann Thorac Surg* 1993;56:S78–82.
27. Edmunds LH Jr. Surface-bound heparin—panacea or peril? *Ann Thorac Surg* 1994;58:285–286.
28. von Segesser LK, Garcia E, Turina MI. Low-dose heparin versus full-dose aprotinin during cardiopulmonary bypass. A preliminary report. *Texas Heart Inst J* 1993;20(1):28–32.

Part III
Postoperative Bleeding and Management

19
Blood Salvage After Cardiac Surgery

JOSEPH A. DEARANI AND HARTZELL V. SCHAFF

Public awareness of the risks associated with administration of homologous blood has increased dramatically since the discovery of the acquired immunodeficiency syndrome (AIDS) and the fact that the human immunodeficiency virus (HIV) could be transmitted by transfusion.[1] This concern has had a salutary effect in reducing the rate of blood usage, although some risks have been exaggerated. For example, in 1989 slightly less than half of the adults in the United States believed that blood transfusions were safe,[2] and a 1991 report indicated 10% of adults believed that a patient was "very likely" to contract AIDS after a blood transfusion.[3]

In fact, donor screening and serologic testing of blood have reduced the risk of transmission of HIV to very low levels. Cumming and associates[4] estimated the risk as 1 per 153,000 units (0.00065%), and Donahue et al[5] reported an incidence of 1 per 60,000 units (0.0017%). These infectious risks of homologous blood transfusion are far lower than the risks of acquiring non-A, non-B hepatitis, or cytomegalovirus. Other potential sequelae of blood transfusions range from transient fevers to hemolytic reactions,[6] transfusion-related acute lung injury,[7] and fatal graft-versus-host disease.[8,9]

Patient inquiries about these risks and their personal request to avoid transfusions have led to the practice of various blood conservation techniques including reinfusion of the patient's own blood both during and after operative procedures. Since the mid-1980s, the National Institutes of Health consensus conferences[10–12] and publication of transfusion practice guidelines[13,14] have recommended autologous blood as the blood of choice when transfusion is necessary.

Reinfusion of shed blood after surgical procedures or trauma was first reported in the early 1800s.[15,16] From that time until the early 1970s, this technique was reported only sporadically, and the method was employed mainly for reinfusion of shed blood during operations.[17] With an increase in the number of open-heart operations for coronary artery disease in the mid-1970s, the demand for blood product availability rose dramatically. By the late 1970s, autotransfusion of shed mediastinal blood after cardiac surgical procedures was reported to be safe and effective in reducing the need for homologous blood transfusions.[18] In current practice, autotransfusion of shed blood is a routine and standard component of intraoperative and postoperative management of patients undergoing open-heart surgery.

Efficacy of Postoperative Autotransfusion of Shed Mediastinal Blood

The usefulness of autotransfusion of shed mediastinal blood seems self-evident; retransfusion of a sufficient volume of homologous red blood cells should reduce the need for blood bank transfusions. In fact, some investigations of postoperative autotransfusion have not shown significant reductions in homologous blood transfusions, and these findings may be due to different study designs as well as to variations in transfusion protocols.[18–25]

The first report of autotransfusion from the Johns Hopkins Hospital[19] described a randomized trial of 114 patients who received autotransfusion of unwashed shed mediastinal blood or transfusion of homologous blood as dictated by standard practice. Several important points about this trial and subsequent ones require explanation. First, the indication for banked blood transfusion was a postoperative hematocrit of less than 0.35, a value notably higher than that which would be accepted in current practice. Also, the investigators retransfused shed blood only when the collected volume was 400 ml or greater during the first 4-hour period. This resulted in 52% of patients actually receiving autotransfusion, and the average volume was approximately 800 ml of shed blood for each patient who received autotransfusion.

The thresholds were chosen arbitrarily because the hemoglobin content of shed mediastinal blood is approximately one half that of fresh whole blood; infusing lesser volumes of shed blood would have little impact on systemic hemoglobin levels and would not be economical because of the cost of disposable liners in the autotransfusion canisters. Collecting blood for longer periods at room temperature would increase the hazard of bacterial contamination and growth. With these criteria for autotransfusion, the investigators demonstrated a 50% reduction in the amount of banked blood administered in the autotransfusion group.

It is apparent, then, that multiple factors determine the efficacy and cost of postoperative autotransfusion. First is the volume of postoperative blood loss, which is surprisingly difficult to estimate. Mean blood loss after elective cardiac surgery ranges from 760 to 1250 ml per patient[19,20,25] and may be higher in reoperations with vascular adhesions. Of note, however, is the fact that one study of multiple preoperative variables that might affect postoperative bleeding suggests that only low preoperative red cell mass predicts the need for postoperative blood transfusion.[26]

Adan and colleagues[21] reported a 50% reduction in the amount of banked blood transfused in a randomized study of 50 patients, and the criteria for transfusion of collected shed blood or banked blood were blood loss exceeding 500 ml in 12 hours and hemoglobin <5 mmol/L within the first 24 hours postoperatively. Eng and coworkers[24] demonstrated a 39% decrease in homologous blood use among randomized patients receiving autotransfusion, and the average volume of shed mediastinal blood autotransfused in the initial 6 hours postoperatively was 371 ml. Banked blood transfusion was reduced from a mean value of 760 ml in the control group to a mean value of 466 ml in the autotransfused group ($p < .05$).

In a more recent study, Page and colleagues[22] showed no reduction in the amount of banked blood requirements when the autotransfused volume was less than 500 ml, but when mediastinal blood loss was greater than 500 ml banked blood requirements were decreased by 50%.

Other investigators have not been able to identify reductions in homologous blood requirements in patients receiving autotransfusion of shed mediastinal blood. In the randomized study by Turer et al[20] of 113 patients undergoing primary coronary artery bypass operations, there was no minimal criterion for reinfusion of shed blood, and of the 54 patients in the autotransfusion group, 83% actually received autotransfused blood. Among patients receiving autotransfusion of shed blood, the average volume was 436 ml, and this did not result in a significant reduction in the amount of banked blood transfused or in the number of patients requiring transfusion. It should be noted that the threshold for transfusion in this study was also relatively low, a hematocrit of less than 0.30.

One explanation for the lack of efficacy in postoperative autotransfusion in the smaller randomized trials reported by Ward and associates[23] and Axford et al[25] is that protocols for patient care in the current era reduce bleeding and make collection of shed mediastinal blood inefficient. Our own data, however, do not support this. Morris and Tan[27] prospectively analyzed a series of 155 consecutive adult cardiac surgical procedures at the Mayo Clinic from 1991 to 1992; approximately half underwent operation before and half after the addition of postoperative autotransfusion. All surgical procedures were performed by one surgeon; operative technique, postoperative patient management, and transfusion practice remained constant throughout the study period with the exception of the addition of postoperative autotransfusion. Mean blood loss in the first 24 hours was 1278 ml and 1721 ml in the nonautotransfused and autotransfused groups, respectively ($p < .03$). The mean volume reinfused in the autotransfusion group was 1122 ml, and this resulted in a significant reduction in banked blood requirements for patients in this group.

Morris and Tan[27] also analyzed risk factors for postoperative banked blood requirements. Multivariate analysis identified advanced preoperative angina class and heart failure class, smaller body surface area, and greater postoperative blood loss as predictors of need for transfusion (Table 19.1).

TABLE 19.1. Multivariate logistic regression analysis of the determinants of postoperative banked blood requirement in all patients.

Variable	χ^2	p value	Estimated risk ratio (95% confidence intervals)
Angina class (one class increment)	12.1	<.01	2.0(1.3–2.8)
Blood loss (250 ml increment)	10.4	<.01	1.2(1.1–1.4)
Body surface area (0.1 m^2 decrement)	7.2	<.01	1.3(1.1–1.6)
Non-ATS group CHF class (one class increment)	6.9	<.01	1.3(1.1–1.6)

ATS, autotransfusion with shed mediastinal blood; CHF, congesitve heart failure.
From Morris and Tan,[27] with permission.

In addition, after controlling for these factors, the authors found that nonuse of postoperative autotransfusion was an additional significant incremental risk factor for homologous blood requirement. Because it is impossible to predict which patients will have substantial postoperative blood losses after cardiac surgery, we believe that the *routine use of postoperative autotransfusion in addition to other blood conservation techniques affords a significant decrease in the use of banked blood products.*

Hematologic Effects of Reinfused Mediastinal Blood

It is clear that there are compositional differences between shed mediastinal and banked blood (Table 19.2). Numerous studies have been undertaken to investigate the effects of autotransfusion on the blood elements and the coagulation profile.[20,21,28,29] Axford et al[25] examined in a prospective randomized trial whether the use of shed mediastinal blood exacerbated platelet and related hematologic dysfunction after cardiopulmonary bypass compared with homologous, liquid-preserved red blood cells. Despite significantly greater amounts of fibrin degradation products and D-dimer present in shed blood, patient bleeding times were not significantly different between the groups at any time interval postoperatively, and the total postoperative blood loss was not different between the groups. This study also demonstrated that levels of protein C (a natural anticoagulant and a fibrinolytic agent) were increased in patients receiving shed mediastinal blood, but the functional significance of this finding is not clear as it did not precipitate any apparent bleeding tendencies. Finally, the investigators found no evidence of activation of fibrinolytic pathways, i.e., no consumption of clotting factors, plasminogen, or antiplasmin in patients receiving shed mediastinal blood.

Similarly, Schaff et al,[19] Johnson et al,[17] and Hartz and associates[28] found no evidence for disseminated intravascular coagulation, increased

TABLE 19.2. In vitro blood unit analysis.*

Hematologic variables	Shed blood†	Banked blood‡	p value
Hemglobin (g/dL)	7.9 ± 0.4	19.2 ± 0.9	.0001
Hematocrit (vol%)	19 ± 1	55 ± 3	.001
Plasma hemoglobin (mg/dl)	312 ± 32	198 ± 87	NS
White blood cells (× $10^3/\mu l$)	4.5 ± 0.4	7.3 ± 2.0	NS
Platelet count (× $10^3/\mu l$)	22 ± 9	118 ± 29	.005
Factor V11lc (%)	25 ± 4	0 ± 0	.001
Fibrinogen (mg/dl)	26 ± 11	42 ± 9	NS
Antithrombin III (%)	33 ± 4	19 ± 3	.01
Protein C (%)	71 ± 7	22 ± 3	.001
Fibronectin (μg/ml)	112 ± 16	89 ± 13	NS
Plasminogen (%)	57 ± 3	26 ± 1	.0001
Antiplasmin (%)	39 ± 2	20 ± 2	.001
White blood aggregates (Swank; mm Hg/b Hb)	16 ± 4	64 ± 23	NS

*Values expressed as mean ± standard error of mean.
†Nonwashed shed mediastinal blood.
‡Liquid preserved packed red blood cells.
From Axford et al.[25] with permission.

fibrinolysis, or evidence of bleeding complications attributable to transfusion of shed mediastinal blood. Fuller et al[29] demonstrated that collected shed mediastinal blood contains significant levels of fibrin degradation products, but the effects of these substances on prothrombin and partial thromboplastin times, activated clotting time, and thrombin clotting time is minimal and transient, and after 24 hours these elevated levels completely disappeared. Similar findings were also noted by Hartz and colleagues,[28] who showed no elevation in fibrinopeptide A- or B-beta 15-42 peptide, sensitive markers of systemic fibrinolysis, in postoperative patients receiving transfusions of shed mediastinal blood. Importantly, in all of these studies, the volume of transfused mediastinal blood was in the range of 300 to 1700 ml with a mean volume of 400 to 700 ml; transfusion of massive amounts of shed mediastinal blood (>2000 ml) has not been studied in a similar manner, and systemic fibrinolysis may develop with rapid transfusion of larger volumes of shed blood.

Complications of Postoperative Autotransfusion

Potential problems of autotransfusion include the coagulation abnormalities discussed above, renal impairment, microembolism, and infection. It seems clear from the preceding discussion that *transfusion of shed mediastinal blood in the range of 300 to 1700 ml causes no measurable bleeding complications and no disseminated intravascular coagulopathy or increased fibrinolysis.*

Concern about elevated plasma hemoglobin in shed mediastinal blood causing renal failure appears to be unfounded; in the absence of acidosis and oliguria, the slight increase in free hemoglobin associated with autotransfusion has no clinical significance.[20] Also, Axford et al[25] showed no significant differences in serum creatinine levels between autotransfused and nonautotransfused patients preoperatively, or at any time postoperatively.

Microemboli resulting from massive transfusion have been implicated in the pathogenesis of multisystem organ failure following severe trauma and major operative procedures.[30] These microaggregates consisting of platelets, white blood cells, fibrin, fat, and denatured proteins occur in both banked blood as well as shed mediastinal blood but are effectively removed by appropriate micropore filters. Our earlier studies showed no clinical evidence of systemic emboli in patients receiving shed mediastinal blood.[19] Most autotransfusion devices in current use contain two micropore filters, one that filters shed mediastinal blood as it drains *from* the patient and a second that filters blood as it is being transfused back *to* the patient.

The risk of contamination and subsequent infection from shed mediastinal blood has also been raised. In the first clinical study of postoperative autotransfusion, bacteriologic cultures were obtained from 36 separate units of collected mediastinal blood in 35 patients. Six cultures (16.7%) were reported positive; four of the six were felt to be contaminants, and none of the patients who received reinfusion of culture-positive mediastinal blood contracted postoperative infections.[19] Eng and colleagues[24] also obtained bacteriologic cultures from both the patient and the shed blood after priming of the autotransfusion system and after 6 hours following autologous transfusion. While there were no septic complications and all patients had negative venous blood cultures, 50% of the specimens of shed blood grew bacteria after 48 hours. *Other investigators have confirmed that the risk of sepsis with autotransfusion is very low.*[20,22]

Postoperative Autotransfusion Systems

The Sorenson Autotransfusion System (Sorenson Research, Salt Lake City, UT) was initially used as an intraoperative device and was later adapted for postoperative retrieval of shed mediastinal blood. The system consisted of a reusable rigid canister containing two disposable plastic bags, one a reservoir and the other a collection bag. Blood entering the system was filtered, and when sufficient blood was collected, the bag was pierced with a filtered blood administration set and then given back to the patient. Since the use of the Sorenson system in the late 1970s, newer systems have been developed. Many currently used systems now provide the ability for continuous autotransfusion.

The Atrium 2050 (Atrium Medical, Hollis, NH) blood recovery chest drainage system (Fig. 19.1) is presently used at the Mayo Clinic. In contrast

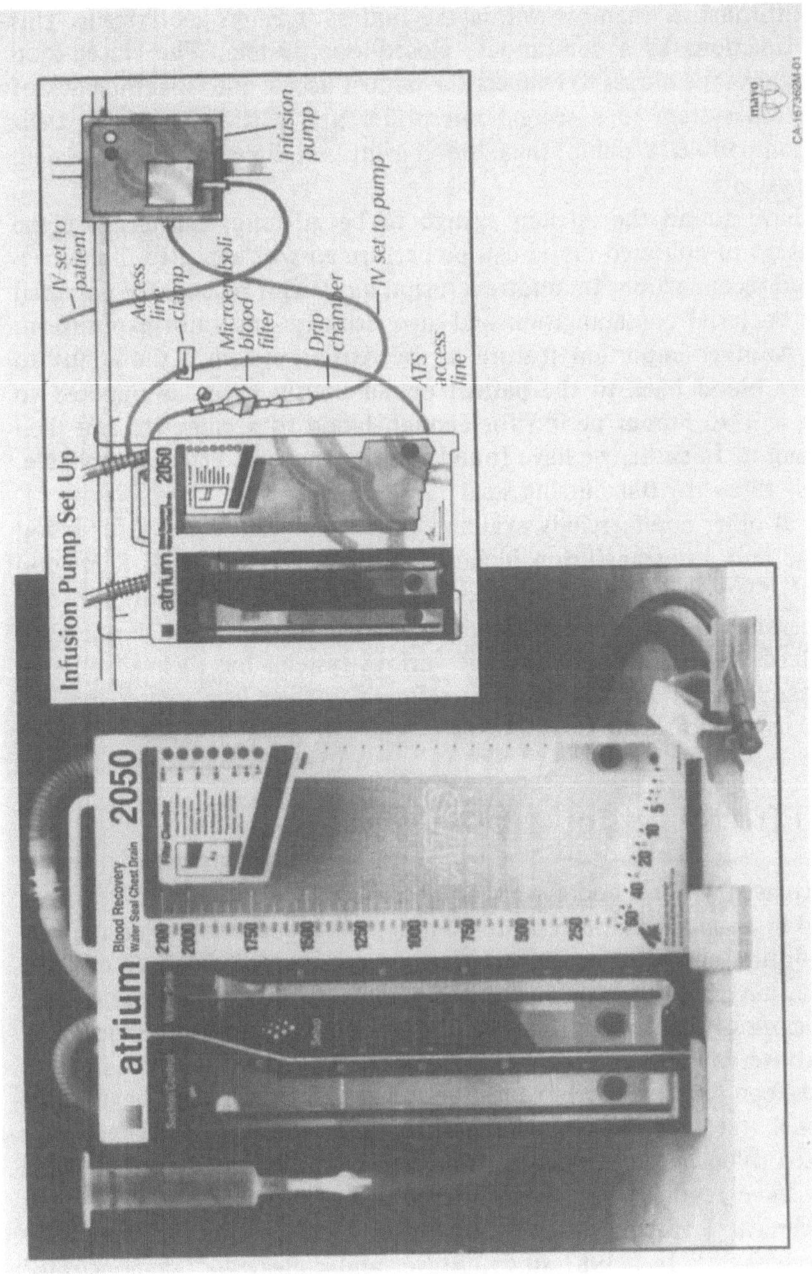

FIGURE 19.1. The Atrium 2050 blood recovery system. Inset: The infusion pump setup that provides "closed-loop" autotransfusion.

to the traditional chest drainage systems, the Atrium 2050 does not require the addition of an in-line blood bag in order to make the blood accessible for transfusion. Shed mediastinal blood is retrieved from the patient and is filtered through a chamber within the unit as it enters the system. This device functions as a continuous, closed-loop system. The closed-loop design allows the nurses to connect the patient access line from the back of the Atrium system to a second microfilter and a straight set for their blood-compatible IV pump; thus, blood is infused directly from the system to the patient.

We have found the Atrium system to be advantageous because the transfusion of collected blood can be performed with repeated disconnections and reconnections to autotransfusion bags. This reduces the potential risk of bacterial contamination and also decreases operator exposure to blood. Another important feature of the Atrium system is the ability to transfuse blood back to the patient on an hourly basis, as opposed to waiting a 3- to 5-hour period for enough blood to accumulate and then reinfusing it. In short, we have found this system to be effective, reliable, and easy to use by our nursing staff.

Several other commercially available devices appear effective for blood drainage and autotransfusion including systems by Deknatel, Sherwood Medical, Davol, and Sorenson Research. Systems that incorporate the intraoperative use of the cardiotomy reservoir include Gish Biomedical, C.R. Bard, and Baxter. Each of the various systems has their advantages and disadvantages and the reader is referred to their local representatives for details regarding these issues.

Cost-Effectiveness of Autotransfusion

The increased use of blood conservation techniques during recent years has resulted in a significant decrease in homologous blood transfusion requirements during and after cardiac surgical procedures.[18,26,31] Some of these practices have been described above. The intraoperative and postoperative transfusions of shed mediastinal blood are major components of successful blood conservation programs, and because the equipment for these last two methods can be costly, the question arises as to whether or not the additional resource requirements offset the savings associated with decreased blood utilization. Previous studies utilizing autotransfusion devices have reported decreased banked blood requirements,[19,20,32] but other clinical investigations have questioned their efficacy[32] and cost-effectiveness.[32,33] In a 1987 study, Breyer and colleagues[34] demonstrated that intraoperative use of the Cell Saver system was associated with substantial savings of banked blood, and the addition of postoperative autotransfusion of shed mediastinal blood resulted in further banked blood savings.

At the Mayo Clinic, we have examined the cost-effectiveness of postoperative autotransfusion. In 1995 charges or the cost to the patient of transfusion for the first unit of homologous packed red blood cells was $404.80, and this includes fees for compatibility testing, ABO/Rh typing, RBC antibody screening, and administration. The charge for each subsequent unit of packed red cell is $252.10. The charge for the Atrium Autotransfusion System is $72.02, and there is no blood administration fee. The charge for the alternative mediastinal chest tube system (Deknatel), which does not allow for autotransfusion, is $56.63. It is clear, then, that routine use of postoperative autotransfusion can result in cost saving even if the average reduction in homologous blood requirements is less than one unit per patient.

More importantly, the possible savings to patients and the health care system are even greater if one considers the potential cost in terms of morbidity or mortality associated with a transfusion-related complication. Thus, in a time of increasing financial constraints and malpractice litigation, utilization of all blood conservation techniques during cardiac surgical procedures should lead to a cost-effective reduction in banked blood use and transfusion-related risks.

Postoperative Autotransfusion at the Mayo Clinic

The blood conservation program at the Mayo Clinic begins in the preoperative phase. Patients undergoing elective open-heart surgery are advised to avoid aspirin products for 10 days prior to surgery[35] and to participate in autologous blood predonation programs.

Intraoperatively, hemodilution is minimized through conservative fluid replacement by the anesthesia staff, use of a membrane oxygenator (Bentley-Univox, Bentley Laboratories, Irvine, CA) with a small, bloodless prime volume (unless the estimated hematocrit of the mixed patient-pump oxygenator blood volume is calculated to be less than 0.20), and use of a hemoconcentration system (Hemocor, Minntech, Plymouth, MN) in the bypass circuit when the patient has preoperative renal failure and/or marked fluid retention due to congestive heart failure. Intraoperative hemodilution is tolerated to a hemoglobin level of 6 to 7 g/dl, and meticulous surgical hemostasis is practiced prior to sternal closure.

In the postoperative period, normovolemic anemia (hemoglobin ϵ7.0 g/dl) is accepted in asymptomatic and hemodynamically stable patients. Autotransfusion with the Atrium system as described above is begun within 4 hours of arrival at the cardiovascular surgical intensive care unit. Each hour, the mediastinal drainage is measured and the infusion pump is programmed to deliver that amount of blood during the next hour. Autotransfusion is continued as long as there is substantial chest tube drainage for the initial 12 to 18 hours postoperatively. Autotransfusion is discontinued if the core body temperature is greater than 39.5°C. Banked packed red blood cells are not administered unless the patient's hemoglobin level drops below 7.5 g/dl. Additional banked blood components such as fresh frozen plasma, platelets, or cryoprecipitate are not administered unless chest tube output exceeds 150 ml/h for two consecutive hours and there is a specific coagulation defect identified by hematologic testing. Fresh frozen plasma is transfused if the international normalized ratio (INR) is >1.5 or the partial thromboplastin time is >40 seconds, or both; platelets are transfused if the platelet count is <100,000/μl, and cryoprecipitate is transfused if the fibrinogen level is less than 100 mg/dl.

Summary

The development of cardiac surgery over the past 20 years has been accompanied by various techniques and apparatuses for blood conservation in the pre-, intra-, and postoperative phases of open-heart operations. In our experience, postoperative autotransfusion is safe, confers a substantial benefit in reducing postoperative banked blood needs, and is cost-effective. Autotransfusion of shed mediastinal blood should be employed routinely in patients undergoing cardiac surgical procedures.

References

1. Ammann AJ, Cowan MJ, Wara DW, et al. Acquired immunodeficiency in an infant: possible transmission by means of blood products. *Lancet* 1983; 1:956–958.
2. Dawson DA. AIDS knowledge and attitudes for January-March 1989: provisional data from the National Health Interview Survey. *Advance Data from Vital and Health Statistics.* Hyattsville, MD: National Center for Health Statistics, 1989; no. 176.
3. American Association of Blood Banks. *Attitudes of US Adults Toward AIDS and the Safety of America's Blood Supply.* Bethesda, MD: AABB and the Gallup Organization, 1991.
4. Cumming PD, Wallace EL, Schorr JB, Dodd RY. Exposure of transfused patients to human immunodeficiency virus through the transfusion of blood components that test antibody negative. *N Engl J Med* 1989;321:917–924.
5. Donahue JG, Nelson KE, Munoz A, et al. Transmission of HIV by transfusion of screened blood. *N Engl J Med* 1990;323:1709.
6. Myhre BA. Fatalities from blood transfusion. *JAMA* 1980;244:1333–1335.
7. Malouf M, Glanville AR. Blood transfusion related adult respiratory distress syndrome. *Anaesth Intensive Care* 1993;21:44–49.
8. Thaler M, Shamiss A, Orgao S, et al. The role of blood from HLA-homozygous donors in fatal transfusion-associated graft versus host disease after open heart surgery. *N Engl J Med* 1989;321:25–28.
9. von Fliedner V, Higby DJ, Kim U. Graft-versus-host reaction following blood product transfusion. *Am J Med* 1982;72:951–961.

10. National Institutes of Health Consensus Conference. Perioperative red cell transfusion. *JAMA* 1988;260:2700–2705.
11. National Institutes of Health Consensus Conference. Fresh frozen plasma: indications and risks. *JAMA* 1985;253:551–553.
12. National Institutes of Health Consensus Conference. Platelet transfusion therapy. *JAMA* 1987;257:1777–1780.
13. Goodnough LT, Johnston MFM, Ramsey G, et al. Guidelines for transfusion support in patients undergoing coronary artery bypass grafting. *Ann Thorac Surg* 1990;50:675–683.
14. American College of Surgeons. Practice strategies for elective red blood cell transfusion. *Ann Intern Med* 1992;116:403–406.
15. Cuello L, Vasquez E, Rios R, et al. Autologous blood transfusion in thoracic and cardiovascular surgery. *Surgery* 1967;62:814–818.
16. Brown AL, Debenham MW. Use of blood from hemothorax. *JAMA* 1931; 96:1223–1225.
17. Johnson RG, Rosenkrantz KR, Preston RA, et al. The efficacy of postoperative autotransfusion in patients undergoing cardiac operations. *Ann Thorac Surg* 1983;36:173–179.
18. Schaff HV, Hauer J, Gardner TJ, et al. Routine use of autotransfusion following cardiac surgery: experience in 700 patients. *Ann Thorac Surg* 1979; 27:493–499.
19. Schaff HV, Hauer JM, Bell WR, et al. Autotransfusion of shed mediastinal blood after cardiac surgery. *J Thorac Cardiovasc Surg* 1978;75:632–641.
20. Thurer RL, Lytle BW, Cosgrove DM, et al. Autotransfusion following cardiac operations: a randomized, prospective study. *Ann Thorac Surg* 1978; 27:500–507.
21. Adan A, Brutel R, Haas F, et al. Autotransfusion of drained mediastinal blood after cardiac surgery: a reappraisal. *Thorac Cardiovasc Surg* 1988;36:10–14.
22. Page R, Russell GN, Fox MA, et al. Hard-shell cardiotomy reservoir for reinfusion of shed mediastinal blood. *Ann Thorac Surg* 1989;48:514–517.
23. Ward HB, Robin RR, Landis KP, et al. Prospective, randomized trial of autotransfusion after routine cardiac operations. *Ann Thorac Surg* 1993; 56:137–141.
24. Eng J, Kay PH, Murday AJ, et al. Postoperative autologous transfusion in cardiac surgery: a prospective, randomized study. *Eur J Cardiothorac Surg* 1990;4:595–600.
25. Axford TC, Dearani JA, Ragno G, et al. Safety and therapeutic effectiveness of reinfused shed blood after cardiac surgery. *Ann Thorac Surg* 1994;57:615–622.
26. Cosgrove DM, Loop FD, Lytle BW, et al. Determinants of blood utilization during myocardial revascularization. *Ann Thorac Surg* 1985;40:380–384.
27. Morris JJ, Tan YS. Autotransfusion: Is there a benefit in a current practice of aggressive blood conservation? *Ann Thorac Surg* 1994;58:502–508.
28. Hartz RS, Smith JA, Green D. Autotransfusion after cardiac operation. Assessment of hemostatic factors. *J Thorac Cardiovasc Surg* 1988;96:178–182.
29. Fuller JA, Buxton BF, Picken J, et al. Haematological effects of reinfused mediastinal blood after cardiac surgery. *Med J Aust* 1991;154:737–740.
30. Aaron RK, Beazley RM, Riggle GC. Hematologic integrity after intraoperative autotransfusion. Comparison with bank blood. *Arch Surg* 1974;108:831–837.
31. Utley JR, Moores WY, Stephens DB. Blood conservation techniques. *Ann Thorac Surg* 1981;31:482–490.

32. Winton TL, Charrette EJP, Salerno TA. The cell saver during cardiac surgery: Does it save? *Ann Thorac Surg* 1982;33:379–381.
33. Carter RF, McArdle B, Morritt GM. Autologous transfusion of mediastinal drainage blood: a report of its use following open heart surgery. *Anaesthesia* 1981;36:54–59.
34. Breyer RH, Engelman RM, Rousou JA, et al. Blood conservation for myocardial revascularization. Is it cost effective? *J Thorac Cardiovasc Surg* 1987; 93:512–522.
35. Ferraris VA, Ferraris SP. Limiting excessive postoperative blood transfusion after cardiac procedures. A review. [Review] *Texas Heart Inst J* 1995; 22:216–230.

20
Assessment and Control of Postoperative Bleeding

Robert E. Helm and Karl H. Krieger

Use of the cardiopulmonary bypass (CPB) apparatus generates varying degrees of coagulopathic bleeding in all patients. In addition, open-heart procedures provide ample opportunity for incomplete mechanical hemostasis. These two factors lead to an often realized potential for increased bleeding during the postoperative period. The true incidence of increased postoperative bleeding is difficult to determine because of the inherent variability in the surgeon and institutional definitions of what constitutes above-normal or "excessive" blood loss. At one institution excessive blood loss might be "microvascular" bleeding after separation from bypass; at another, bleeding above a predetermined quantity or rate; at a third, the need for platelet and coagulation factor transfusion. Regardless of the way in which it is defined, because allogeneic transfusion has served as the "gold standard" for the treatment of postoperative bleeding, such bleeding has traditionally been directly and indirectly responsible for a large portion of the allogeneic blood used in cardiac surgery. This situation still largely exists today, despite evidence that platelet and coagulation factor transfusion during the early postoperative period has limited effect, and despite the increasing availability of nontransfusion strategies to prevent and control postoperative bleeding. It is these nontransfusion strategies, combined with a rational and informed approach to the transfusions that are administered, that provides the key to decreasing both postoperative bleeding *and* allogeneic transfusion.

Nontransfusion strategies for the control of postoperative bleeding fall under four general categories, (1) prevention of the development of coagulopathic bleeding through appropriate technical and pharmacologic interventions, (2) normalization of homeostatic and hemostatic function through immediate and optimal application of nontransfusion supportive measures, (3) tolerance to bleeding that does not exceed normal limits by adhering to appropriate transfusion guidelines, and (4) delineation and timely correction of inadequate mechanical hemostasis.

It is rapidly becoming apparent that the optimal approach to controlling excessive postoperative coagulopathic bleeding is the prevention of its development in the first place. Cardiopulmonary bypass leads to a massive inflammatory response in all patients, and the amount of postoperative bleeding in any given patient that is not mechanical in origin, is simply a variation of the extent to which the coagulation limb of this inflammatory response is expressed. By preventing or attenuating this inflammatory response, the incidence of excessive postoperative bleeding can be significantly decreased. Blood conservation modalities falling under the heading of prevention include intraoperative autologous donation, improved biocompatibility of CPB circuitry, and the various blood anesthesia techniques.[1] Prominent among the latter are the antifibrinolytic agents and aprotinin. When appropriately applied, through risk factor recognition, these modalities can markedly attenuate the coagulopathy of CPB, and therefore reduce the incidence of excessive postoperative bleeding requiring additional treatment measures.

Despite optimal application of preventive measures, a significant number of patients demonstrate increased blood loss during the early postoperative period. In a majority of these patients this increased bleeding will spontaneously resolve, given appropriate time for normalization of homeostatic and hemostatic function. Essential in optimally treating this group of patients is providing for the maximum rate and degree of normalization. This can be achieved without allogeneic transfusion through the immediate application of a comprehensive set of technical and pharmacologic nontransfusion supportive measures, and then by allowing time for these measures to work. Supportive technical measures include adequate patient warming, blood pressure control, and minimizing unnecessary hemodilution. Pharmacologic strategies, aimed at either suppressing or eliminating coagulopathic processes, include the insurance of adequate heparin reversal, the suppression of pathologic fibrinolysis, mobilization of endogenous coagulation factor stores, and protection and restoration of platelet function. By applying a comprehensive set of nontransfusion strategies at the first manifestation of increased postoperative blood loss, the incidence of postoperative bleeding progressing to the level of requiring transfusion or other more serious intervention can be minimized.

Despite optimal application of nontransfusion therapies to patients exhibiting increased postoperative bleeding, this bleeding will continue or progress in a certain percentage of patients. A third basic strategy for reducing allogeneic transfusion while at the same time optimally treating this bleeding, is to *withhold* transfusion, reserving its use for only those patients who achieve a clinically significant excessive level of bleeding. A rational set of transfusion guidelines, based on analysis and understanding of each institution's normal postoperative blood loss, is therefore required. These guidelines must ensure that only a safe level of bleeding is allowed to occur, and must be closely linked to the institution of a full set of nontransfusion measures that accelerate spontaneous resolution of coagulopathic bleeding. These guidelines must also ensure that appropriate laboratory testing is performed in a timely manner, so that specific blood product support can be given should bleeding fail to resolve with supportive measures only.

Inadequate mechanical hemostasis typically results in a critical level of postoperative bleeding. This rate and quantity of blood loss can lead to hemodynamic instability as well as the need for large-volume allogeneic transfusion of both red cells and hemostatic factors. The keys to controlling critical hemorrhage attributable to inadequate hemostasis are (1) early recognition, (2) early operative intervention. While it is important to institute supportive and transfusion measures early in these patients, the primary treatment for critical bleeding is expeditious return to the operating room. Prompt recognition and early return to the operating room for correction of the offending defect can decrease and even eliminate the use of allogeneic transfusion,[2] and can markedly reduce overall morbidity. Early recognition and reoperation serve as the fourth and final method of optimally controlling both postoperative bleeding and excessive transfusion.

This chapter delineates the optimal manner in which to control postoperative bleeding while minimizing allogeneic blood exposure. It begins by defining and determining the incidence of increased postoperative bleeding, based on analysis of the literature as well as our own clinical experience. This information is essential for accurate clinical identification and classification of increased postoperative bleeding, the first steps in implementing appropriate and timely interventions. The next section addresses risk factors for bleeding, delineating these risk factors so that preventive measures can be instituted in appropriate patients. An algorithm that we use for bleeding prophylaxis, based on preoperative risk factor analysis, is provided. The final section focuses on the treatment of postoperative bleeding. It begins by reviewing presently available technical and pharmacologic measures for the treatment of increased postoperative bleeding. These measures are then drawn together into a comprehensive protocol for optimal control of increased postoperative bleeding in the cardiac surgical patient.

Definition and Scope of the Problem

Definition of Increased Postoperative Bleeding

At the New York Hospital–Cornell Medical Center we have developed a simple method of grading increased postoperative bleeding based on both the relative quantity of blood lost, as well as the treatment necessary to control this loss. Three basic levels of increased postoperative bleeding are described using this classification scheme: (1) accelerated bleeding, (2) excessive bleeding, and (3) critical bleeding. *Accelerated* bleeding is bleeding within a predetermined range that can be predicted to resolve spontaneously with institution of supportive nontransfusion measures only. *Excessive* bleeding is bleeding beyond this level that requires transfusion intervention for resolution to occur. *Critical* postoperative bleeding is rapid or massive blood loss, excessive blood loss that fails to respond to transfusion therapy, or bleeding that leads to hemodynamic instability. Typically this level of bleeding requires prompt return to the operating room for surgical correction of inadequate mechanical hemostasis. Table 20.1 outlines this classification scheme for increased postoperative bleeding, according to both the rate of blood loss and the intensity of necessary treatment. It can be seen that as the level of bleeding increases, so does the number of treatment modalities invoked. Adopting such a graded approach allows prompt recognition and rapid and appropriate intervention. Institution of lesser measures should never delay definitive therapy. This is particularly important when a critical level of bleeding is reached. While it is important to initiate nontransfusion supportive therapy and transfusion therapy as rapidly as possible, these should not delay return to the operating room for definitive surgical correction. Of note is that associated abnormalities (e.g., laboratory values) do not play a role in delineating the severity of bleeding according to this scheme, underscoring the general feeling that patients should not be treated for laboratory value abnormalities alone.[3] Classification of bleeding as well as choice of primary treatment modality—supportive, transfusion, or reoperative—is based on quantitative measures only. Laboratory values are used only to help guide the type of transfusion therapy applied.[3] Our numerical criteria for resternotomy are in alignment with those put forth by Kirlin and Barratt-Boyes.[4] As discussed in the next section, expected bleeding rates vary with surgeon, institution, and type of procedure performed. The rate of blood loss criteria outlined in Table 20.1 are those that we have found to lead to clinically acceptable results with respect to bleeding and transfusion reduction in our own clinical practice.

Incidence of Increased Postoperative Bleeding

The incidence of level I or accelerated bleeding—bleeding significant enough to invoke application of nontransfusion supportive therapy, but not severe enough to warrant transfusion therapy or return to the operating room—is difficult to assess because of significant variation in expected or normal mediastinal bleeding. Mediastinal drainage varies considerably according to procedure type, surgeon, and institution.[5,6] These differences have been compounded by the inconsistent application of newer pharmacologic and technologic preventive measures, which can markedly decrease the mean chest tube output, as well as the incidence of increased chest tube output. It is equally difficult to define the incidence of accelerated bleeding by identifying how often nontransfusion treatment strategies are initiated. There are no set indications in the literature for when to increase positive

TABLE 20.1. Classification of postoperative bleeding by quantity of blood loss and treatment.

Level of increased postoperative bleeding	Quantity of bleeding	Associated abnormalities	Treatment
I. Accelerated bleeding	1. Microvascular bleeding prior to chest closure 2. Drainage >200 cc first hour or any hour thereafter 3. Drainage >150 cc second hour 4. Drainage >100 cc over any 2 consecutive hours after the first hour	1. Plt count >50 K 2. PT ± nl 3. PTT ± nl	1. Rapid application of nontransfusion supportive therapy
II. Excessive bleeding	1. Severe microvascular bleeding with suspected or documented quantitative platelet or coagulation factor deficiency 2. Drainage >300 cc during first hour (order products, do not give unless #3 occurs) 3. Drainage >250 cc second hour 4. Drainage >200 cc during any 2 consecutive hours after the first hour 5. Drainage >100 cc over any 4 hours after the first postoperative hour	1. Plt count ± nl 2. PT ± nl 3. PTT ± nl	1. Rapid application of nontransfusion supportive therapy 2. Transfusion therapy (guided by laboratory values)
III. Critical bleeding	1. 500 ml first postop hour 2. 400 ml/hr first 2 postop hours 3. 300 ml/hr first 3 postop hours 4. 1000 ml total during first 4 hours 5. 1200 ml total first 5 hours 6. Excessive bleeding that restarts 7. Sudden massive bleeding	1. Plt count ± nl 2. PT ± nl 3. PTT ± nl	1. Rapid application of nontransfusion supportive therapy 2. Rapid transfusion therapy (if mixed or unclear picture) 3. Early return to operating room for surgical hemostasis*

*Early and prompt return to the operating room should never be delayed by institution of nontransfusion and transfusion supportive measures. It is, however, always important to implement these measures as rapidly as possible while preparation for prompt return to the operating room is made.

end-expiratory pressure (PEEP), initiate aggressive blood pressure control, or start epsilon amino caproic acid (EACA), and institutions differ widely in their approaches to these supportive maneuvers. At our own institution these nontransfusion maneuvers are instituted when increased microvascular-type bleeding is encountered in the operating room following protamine reversal of heparin, or when bleeding exceeds the quantitative criteria listed in Table 20.1. In a review of 250 primary coronary artery bypass graft (CABG) patients operated on after the institution of treatment guidelines based on the quantity of bleeding, we found the incidence of accelerated bleeding to be approximately 13% (Table 20.2).[7]

The incidence of level II or excessive postoperative bleeding—that amount of bleeding necessitating platelet and/or coagulation factor transmission—is an equally difficult number to quantitate. This difficulty is again attributable to variability in expected normal chest tube drainage according to procedure, cardiopulmonary bypass technique, surgeon, and institution, but also to extreme differences in platelet and coagulation factor transfusion practices.[6,8–13] Table 20.3 lists 18 recent blood conservation studies that provided criteria for platelet and coagulation factor transfusion, as well as the incidence of transfusion using these criteria. These transfusion results suggest that the incidence of excessive postoperative bleeding, as defined by the need for hemostatic transfusion, is as high

TABLE 20.2. Incidence of increased postoperative bleeding in 250 primary CABG patients.

Level of increased postoperative bleeding	Quantity of bleeding	Incidence (n = 250)
I. Accelerated bleeding	1. Microvascular bleeding prior to chest closure	33 (13.2%)
	2. Drainage >200 cc first hour or any hour thereafter	
	3. Drainage >150 cc second hour	
	4. Drainage >100 cc over any 2 consecutive hours after the first 2 hours	
II. Excessive bleeding	1. Drainage >300 cc during first hour (order products, do not give unless #2 occurs)	12 (4.8%)
	2. Drainage >250 cc second hour	
	3. Drainage >200 cc during any 2 consecutive hours after the first 2 hours	
	4. Drainage >100 cc over any 3 consecutive hours after the first 2 hours	
III. Critical bleeding	1. 500 ml first postop hour	5 (2.0%)
	2. 400 ml/hr first 2 postop hours	
	3. 300 ml/hr first 3 postop hours	
	4. 1000 ml total during the first 4 hours	
	5. 1200 ml total first 5 hours	
	6. Excessive bleeding that restarts	
	7. Sudden massive bleeding	

as 47% (repeat CABG population, with tranexamic acid), with a mean incidence of approximately 10% to 20%. Using the incidence of transfusion in the literature to define the incidence of excessive postoperative bleeding assumes, however, that (1) transfusion guidelines were appropriate, and (2) that these guidelines were actually followed. Results of studies with more restrictive guidelines—such as those applied by us and delineated in Table 20.1—suggest that many investigators adopt inappropriate guidelines that result in the systematic overtransfusion of patients. Multiinstitutional comparison studies have confirmed that such overtransfusion occurs.[6,14] In these studies transfusion of platelets and coagulation factors ranged from 3% to 75%, despite similar postoperative chest tube drainage volumes. In our analysis of the bleeding patterns of 250 primary CABG patients operated on after the institution of the quantitative treatment guidelines listed in Table 20.1, we found the incidence of hemostatic blood product transfusion to be approximately 6.8%.[7] As stated, however, the degree to which institutional transfusion policies are actually followed, regardless of where they are set, also makes estimation of the incidence of excessive bleeding as defined by the need for postoperative allogeneic transfusion difficult to quantify. For example, in our analysis of bleeding and transfusion patterns in 250 primary CABG patients, we found a transfusion and therefore perceived excessive bleeding incidence of 6.8% (Table 20.4). Further analysis reveals, however, that if the preset transfusion guidelines had been adhered to, the rate of transfusion could have been decreased to as low as 3.2% (Table 20.4). For these reasons the actual incidence of excessive postoperative bleeding requiring transfusion is difficult to quantitate. A safe general estimate is that excessive bleeding requiring transfusion currently occurs in 3% to 20% of patients undergoing cardiac surgery—this number varying according to preoperative risk, intraoperative hemostatic interventions, procedure type, surgeon, and institution.[10]

In contrast to accelerated and excessive postoperative bleeding, the incidence of level III or critical postoperative bleeding, either from severe,frank coagulopathy or inadequate mechanical hemostasis, is readily identified because of its clearly defined end point—return to the operating room. Nonetheless, criteria for return to the operating room vary, and so too, therefore, does the incidence of resternotomy. Table 20.5 lists the criteria used by several authors for resternotomy, as well as the incidence of resternotomy when using these criteria (when available). Generally, the literature places the incidence of critical bleeding after cardiac surgery—as marked by the need for resternotomy—at between 1.5% and 18%, with variation occurring primarily by procedure type.[10,15,16] Using data from the Veterans Administration (25,000 mixed patients) and the Society for Thoracic Surgery (65,000 CABG patients), Grover placed the incidence of return to the operating room for bleeding, at 4.8% and 2.3%, respectively.[17] In our review of 250 primary CABG patients we found this incidence to be about 2%. Approximately two thirds of patients returned to

Table 20.3. Criteria used to identify excessive (Level II) postoperative bleeding as marked by the need for blood product transfusion.

		Criteria for platelet/FFP/cryoprecipitate transfusion				Study outcome						
			Laboratory value or other qualitative measures			Transfusion requirements			Postoperative bleeding			
Author	Study	Quantity or rate	Criteria for platelet transfusion	Criteria for FFP transfusion	Criteria for cryotransfusion	Platelet (% / units)	FFP (% / units)	Cryo (% / units)	6 hrs	8 hrs	12 hrs	24 hrs
Horrow (1991)[98]	TA	250 ml/hr	Thrombocytopenia	Prolonged PT	–	0	0	0			366	
						0	0	0				
Horrow (1995)[99]	TA	250 ml/hr	Thrombocytopenia	Prolonged PT	–	0.009%	0	0			363	
	DDAVP					0.052 U	0	0				
Shore-Lesserson (1996)[102]	TA	"Obvious bleeding"	Ct < 100K	<150% of nl	Fibrin < 100 mg/dl	47.1%	35.3%	0				
						5 U	–	0				
Lambert (1979)[61]	ECAC	>600 ml	None	>19 sec	PTT > 45, PT < 19	0	–	–				
		(in first 8 postop hrs)			Fibrin <225	0	0.9 U	2.5 U				
Karski (1993)[101]	TA	>300 ml/hr × 2 hrs	Ct < 60K	<150% of nl	PT < 1.5 × nl	0	0.9%	3.8%	250			
	EACAC	>750 ml in first 6 hrs				0	–	–				
Rousou (1995)[114]	TA	>300–400 ml/hr × 2 hrs	–	–	–	–	–	0				804
		>200 ml/hr × 2 hrs				0.03 U	0.024 U	0				
Karski (1995)[102]	TA	>200 ml/hr × 2 hrs	Ct < 50K	<150% of nl	PT < 1.5 × nl	2%	0	2%	287			
	ECAC	>400 ml × 1 hr				0.1 U	0	0.08				
		>750 ml in first 6 hrs										
Goodnough (1990)[103]	Review;	Clinically significant bleeding	Ct < 50K	>1.5 ×nl	Fribrinogen < 100	–	–	–				
	transfusion guidelines					–	–	–				
Katsaros (1996)[104]	TA	"Increased rate of" blood loss	Ct < 100K, and:	Abnormal PT		2.8%	3.8%	0				
			(1) ↑bleed or			0.12 U	0.05 U	0				
			(2) ASA or hep preop									
Casas (1995)[105]	Apr	Microvascular bleeding	Ct < 60K	>1.5 × nl		4.0%	4.0%	–				
	DDAVP			Fibrinogen < 100		–	–	–				

Despotis (1994)[106]	On-site coagulation monitoring	Microvascular bleeding	Plt Ct < 50K	PT/PTT > 1.5 × nl +	-	-	-	0		705		
		Diffuse bleeding without a surgical source	CT = 50–100K +	Plt Ct > 100 K		5.5 U	1.6 U	0				
			PT > 1.8 × nl	PT/PTT > 1.8								
			Plt Ct > 100K + PT nl									
Sandrelli (1995)[107]	Preoperative autologous donation	"Bleeding"	Plt Ct < 100K	PT > 1.5	-	-	-	-	338			
		Hemostatic unbalance		PTT > 40		-	-	-	-			
Ward (1993)[108]	Shed mediastinal blood	Excessive nonsurgical bleeding	Plt Ct < 100K	PT > 16	Never used	14%	15%	0			750	
						-	-	0				
Yau (1992)[109]	TA	>200 ml/hr	Plt Ct < 70K + bleed	PTT > 45	Elevated FSPs, decreased fibrinogen	7.5%	5.5%	7.5%			557	
	ECAC		Plt Ct < 50K			0.63 U	0.15 U	0.63 U				
Essell (1993)[110]	TEG monitoring	>1500 ml first 24 hrs	Abnl coag test results;	Abnl coag tests; clinical susp abnl coagulation	Abnl coag tests; clinical susp abnl coagulation	29%	25%	0				1010
		"need to transfuse plts," FFP to control hemorrhage	clinical susp abnl			3.1 U	0.89 U	0				
Nuttall (1995)[111]	Near patient testing	Microvascular bleeding (wet field);	Plt Ct < 50	PT > 1.5 × nl	Factor defic.	>13.5%	>14.2%	0				813
		"Bleeding patient"	"Plt dysfunction"		↑bleeding time fibrinogen < 100	2.0 U	1.2 U	0				
Woodman (1990)[112]	Review postop bleeding	≥100 ml/hr	-	-	-	-	-	-				
Helm (1996)[93]	Large volume	>550 after first 2 hours	Plt Ct < 50K	PT > 16 (1.3 × nl) *with* bleeding	Persistent bleed after 2 rounds plts/FSP	11%	14.5%	0	405	488	605	849
	IAD	>200 cc/hour × 2 hours after first 2 hours >100 cc × 4 hours after first 2 hours			(2) 2 rounds plt/FFP	0.67 U	0.4 U	0				

DDAVP = D-arginine amino vasopressin; TA = tranexamic acid; ECAC = ϵ-aminocaproic acid; TEG = thromboelastography; IAD = intraoperatin autologous donation; Plt = platelet; Ct = count; PT = prothrombintime; PTT = partial thromboplastin time; nl = normal; U = unit; FSP = fibrin split products; ASA = aspirin; hep = heparin.

TABLE 20.4. Adherence to transfusion guidelines in 250 CABG patients.

Level of postoperative bleeding	Percent meeting transfusion criteria	Actual percent transfused
I. Normal blood loss (n = 200)	9%	2.0%
II. Accelerated bleeding (n = 33)	0%	2.4%
III. Excessive bleeding (n = 12)	1.2%*	1.2%
IV. Critical bleeding (n = 5)	2.0%	1.2%
Total (n = 250)	**3.2%**	**6.8%**

*Most patients with an initial excessive (Level II) level of postoperative bleeding spontaneously resolved their bleeding with nontransfusion supportive therapy only, so that only 3 of 12 (1.2%) actually required transfusion.

the operating room will have a clear surgical source, although this number can vary between 50% and 100%. Newer rapid turnover testing modalities show the potential to increase specificity by demonstrating normal hemostatic function in the setting of critical hemorrhage.[15] The difficulty, however, lies in improving specificity in the patient group that constitutes the majority of patients with critical bleeding—those with mixed mechanical and hemostatic dysfunction. The essential components of successfully treating critical postoperative bleeding remain early recognition and early operative intervention.

Prevention of Increased Postoperative Bleeding

As stated in the introduction to this chapter, there are four general ways to decrease postoperative bleeding and platelet and coagulation factor transfusion: (1) prevention, (2) nontransfusion supportive therapy, (3) rational transfusion therapy, and (4) early reoperation. While all of these measures can act to decrease the quantity of blood lost, prevention is the only modality that can have impact on the incidence of excessive bleeding. This section briefly reviews the criteria that can be used to identify patients at increased risk for excessive postoperative bleeding, and then discusses appropriate bleeding prophylaxis in this increased risk population. For a more in-depth discussion of bleeding risk and prophylaxis, the reader is referred to Chapter 15.

The coagulopathy of CPB is multifactorial. While much has been learned about platelet and coagulation dysfunction during and following CPB, the breadth and depth of its inflammatory origins and sequelae leave an even greater amount still to be learned. Regardless of its etiology, its effects, or even its optimal treatment, it is clear that some patients are at increased preoperative risk for suffering the extremes of this coagulopathy.[14,17] Fortunately, investigations thus far have yielded several tools for protecting

TABLE 20.5. Excessive postoperative bleeding delineated by return to the operating room for bleeding.

Author	Population	Study Type	Criteria for Return to the Operating Room: Quantity of Bleeding	Criteria for Return to the Operating Room: Quality of Bleeding	% of Cases Requiring Reoperation
1. Kirklin/Barratt-Boyes (1993)[4]			>500 ml first postop hr	Excessive bleeding that re-starts	
			>400 ml/hr first 2 postop hrs >300 ml/hr first 3 postop hrs >1000 ml total during first 4 hrs >1200 ml total first 5 hours	Sudden massive bleeding	
2. Unswerht-White (1995)[115]		Reoperation for bleeding	Same as Kirklin/Barratt-Boyes	Excessive bleeding that restarts Sudden massive bleeding	3.8%
3. Moulton (1996)[119]	Mixed cardiac (n = 6015)	Resternotomy risk factors and outcome	Same as Kirklin/Barratt/Boyes	Sudden massive bleed Pericardial tamponade	4.2%
4. Lambert (1979)[113]	CABG	Postoperative bleeding	>600 ml (first 8 hrs)	nl PT/PTT and fibrinogen	0.65%
5. Edmunds (1987)[116]		Postoperative bleeding	10 ml/kg first hour 5 ml/kg avge over first 3 hrs	-	
6. Dietrich (1995)[117]	CABG (preop Hep)	Aprotinin (high dose)	300 ml/hr over first 2 hrs 200 ml/hr over first 2 hrs	-	0
7. Cicek (1996)[118]	Mixed cardiac	Aprotinin (preop, postop)	500 ml/hr over 2 consec hrs	No sign of decreasing bleeding despite appropriate treatment	2%
8. Cosgrove (1978)[120]	Mixed cardiac	Review	>500 ml × 1 hr >300 ml × 3 consec hrs	-	-
9. Speiss (1995)[15]	Mixed cardiac	Testing Algorithm	"hemorrhage"	Hemodynamic instability Normal thromboelastogram	5.7 % (No TEG) 1.5% (TEG)

TEG = thrombolestography; CABG = coronary artery bypass grafting; nl = normal; PT = prothrombin time; PTT = partial thromboplastin time.

these patients from the detrimental effects of cardiopulmonary bypass, thereby helping to offset their increased propensity to bleed.

A broad range of physiologic, pharmacologic, and operative variables place patients at increased risk for postoperative bleeding. These are listed in Table 20.6. Appropriate references are provided. In our own practice we have divided the risk factors for bleeding into three groups: low, moderate, and high. This classification is helpful in assigning relative risk so that optimal preparation—and prophylaxis—can be instituted prior to the planned procedure. Using this scheme, patients receive stepwise increments in protection from the inflammatory effects of cardiopulmonary bypass. Those with the most severe risk factors, or multiple risk factors, receive the highest level of protection. We feel that by applying this graded risk factor approach to bleeding prophylaxis, there is decreased chance of "overnormalization," with its potential thrombotic sequelae. This fear largely underlies present hesitation in application of the clearly effective agent aprotinin.[14,18] By applying this agent to only those patients who will likely

TABLE 20.6. Risk factors for postoperative bleeding and suggested prophylaxis.

Increased bleeding risk	Risk factor	Suggested prophylaxis
I. Low	1. Aspirin (<5 days before surgery)[121] 2. Age >70[123]	1. None
II. Moderate	1. Heparin <72 hours prior to surgery[124] 2. Warfarin with PT >15[124] 3. Thrombolytic therapy within 5 days 4. Reoperation[123] 5. ETOH abuse, liver dysfunction[124] 6. Anticipated CPB run >90 min[122,123] 7. Procedure type a. Valve-CABG[122] b. Double valve[122] c. Other complex procedure[122] 8. Uremic renal dysfunction[124] 9. Ongoing infection/sepsis[124] 10. Emergency procedure[123] 11. Preoperative bleeding disorder[123]	1. Amicar (full strength regimen) 2. Optional a. DDAVP (if uremic renal dysfunction)
III. High	1. Multiple low or moderate bleeding risk factors[123] 2. Jehovah's Witness	1. Aprotinin (1/2 strength Hammersmith regimen) 2. Optional a. Full Hammersmith regimen aprotinin b. Heparin bonded circuit c. If contraindication to aprotinin give Amicar d. White cell filtration

suffer severe coagulopathic response to CPB, for reasons of preexisting disease or severity of procedure, the tendency toward thrombosis is minimized. Our clinical experience has confirmed theoretical safety and efficacy of this approach.[2]

Before proceeding to the topic of treatment, it important to discuss another form of prophylaxis that should be instituted for all patients undergoing cardiac surgery—optimal cardiopulmonary bypass and surgical technique. While these topics have received in-depth attention elsewhere in this text, their importance in minimizing postoperative blood loss cannot be overemphasized. Length of cardiopulmonary bypass time, for example, has clearly been associated with increased postoperative blood loss. Intuitively, this makes sense, as longer CPB times lead to more prolonged foreign surface exposure, greater blood element damage and loss, and a higher overall likelihood of autologous component depletion or inactivation. To minimize such damage and loss, operations must be performed quickly, with minimal procedural losses requiring salvage, and with maximum and dependable mechanical hemostasis. In addition, physiologic supportive measures, such as adequate patient warming and blood pressure control, should be instituted prior to and during separation from bypass. By combining such optimized techniques, with appropriate risk factor-based pharmacologic prophylaxis, the number of patients experiencing increased postoperative bleeding requiring intervention should be minimized.

Treatment of Postoperative Bleeding

There are three principal means of treating increased postoperative bleeding that arises despite appropriate prophylaxis: (1) immediate institution of all appropriate nontransfusion strategies, (2) application of rational transfusion guidelines based on understanding the normal limits of clinically acceptable postoperative blood loss, and (3) early return to the operating room for definitive repair of surgical bleeding. These three strategies are typically applied in an additive stepwise progression that parallels the severity of bleeding (Table 20.1, Fig. 20.1). This section focuses on these treatment strategies, delineating the full range of interventions available, as well as the optimal way in which to apply each of these interventions.

Nontransfusion Therapy for Increased Postoperative Bleeding

Techniques available for nontransfusion control of postoperative bleeding can be divided into physiologic and pharmacologic groupings. Each technique seeks in some way to return postoperative patient as rapidly as possible to the "normal" homeostatic and hemostatic state. The role of each

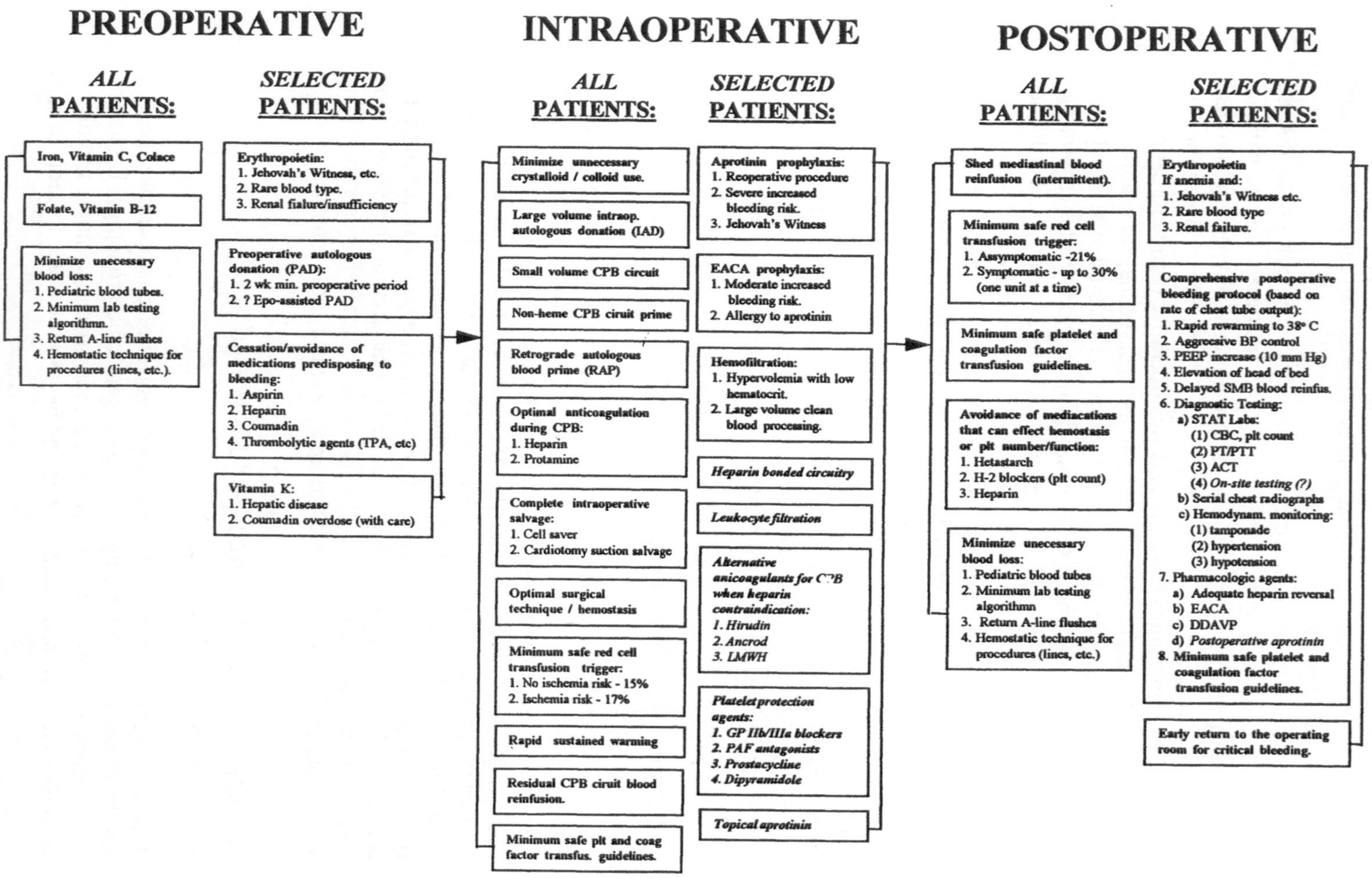
PREOPERATIVE
ALL PATIENTS:
Iron, Vitamin C, Colace
Folate, Vitamin B-12
Minimize unecessary blood loss: 1. Pediatric blood tubes. 2. Minimum lab testing algorithmn. 3. Return A-line flushes 4. Hemostatic technique for procedures (lines, etc.).
SELECTED PATIENTS:
Erythropoietin: 1. Jehovah's Witness, etc. 2. Rare blood type. 3. Renal fialure/insufficiency
Preoperative autologous donation (PAD): 1. 2 wk min. preoperative period 2. ? Epo-assisted PAD
Cessation/avoidance of medications predisposing to bleeding: 1. Aspirin 2. Heparin 3. Coumadin 4. Thrombolytic agents (TPA, etc)
Vitamin K: 1. Hepatic disease 2. Coumadin overdose (with care)
INTRAOPERATIVE
ALL PATIENTS:
Minimize unnecessary crystalloid / colloid use.
Large volume intraop. autologous donation (IAD)
Small volume CPB circuit
Non-heme CPB ciruit prime
Retrograde autologous blood prime (RAP)
Optimal anticoagulation during CPB: 1. Heparin 2. Protamine
Complete intraoperative salvage: 1. Cell saver 2. Cardiotomy suction salvage
Optimal surgical technique / hemostasis
Minimum safe red cell transfusion trigger: 1. No ischemia risk - 15% 2. Ischemia risk - 17%
Rapid sustained warming
Residual CPB ciruit blood reinfusion.
Minimum safe plt and coag factor transfus. guidelines.
SELECTED PATIENTS:
Aprotinin prophylaxis: 1. Reoperative procedure 2. Severe increased bleeding risk. 3. Jehovah's Witness
EACA prophylaxis: 1. Moderate increased bleeding risk. 2. Allergy to aprotinin
Hemofiltration: 1. Hypervolemia with low hematocrit. 2. Large volume clean blood processing.
Heparin bonded circuitry
Leukocyte filtration
Alternative anicoagulants for CPB when heparin contraindication: 1. Hirudin 2. Ancrod 3. LMWH
Platelet protection agents: 1. GP IIb/IIIa blockers 2. PAF antagonists 3. Prostacycline 4. Dipyramidole
Topical aprotinin
POSTOPERATIVE
ALL PATIENTS:
Shed mediastinal blood reinfusion (intermittent).
Minimum safe red cell transfusion trigger: 1. Assymptomatic -21% 2. Symptomatic - up to 30% (one unit at a time)
Minimum safe platelet and coagulation factor transfusion guidelines.
Avoidance of mediacations that can effect hemostasis or plt number/function: 1. Hetastarch 2. H-2 blockers (plt count) 3. Heparin
Minimize unecessary blood loss: 1. Pediatric blood tubes 2. Minimum lab testing algorithmn 3. Return A-line flushes 4. Hemostatic technique for procedures (lines, etc.)
SELECTED PATIENTS:
Erythropoietin If anemia and: 1. Jehovah's Witness etc. 2. Rare blood type 3. Renal failure.
Comprehensive postoperative bleeding protocol (based on rate of chest tube output): 1. Rapid rewarming to 38° C 2. Aggressive BP control 3. PEEP increase (10 mm Hg) 4. Elevation of head of bed 5. Delayed SMB blood reinfus. 6. Diagnostic Testing: a) STAT Labs: (1) CBC, plt count (2) PT/PTT (3) ACT (4) On-site testing (?) b) Serial chest radiographs c) Hemodynam. monitoring: (1) tamponade (2) hypertension (3) hypotension 7. Pharmacologic agents: a) Adequate heparin reversal b) EACA c) DDAVP d) Postoperative aprotinin 8. Minimum safe platelet and coagulation factor transfusion guidelines.
Early return to the operating room for critical bleeding.

FIGURE 20.1. Algorithm for the treatment of increased postoperative bleeding.

of these measures in the treatment of the postoperative patient demonstrating increased (accelerated, excessive, critical) bleeding is discussed in the following subsections. Our comprehensive nontransfusion supportive therapy protocol for the treatment of increased postoperative bleeding delineated in Table 20.7.

Physiologic Modalities

Rapid and Sustained Patient Warming

This fundamental blood conservation measure should be applied to all patients, not just those exhibiting increased bleeding. Platelet and coagulation enzyme function is optimized at normothermia—the range in which these systems were designed to work. Hypothermic platelet dysfunction has been clearly documented by a number of investigators.[19,20] Such dysfunction is largely if not wholly reversible given appropriate warming. Likewise coagulation factor activity is diminished at hypothermia. This dysfunction is commonly overlooked, however, as prothrombin and partial thromboplastin time testing is typically performed under normothermic conditions in the hospital hematology laboratory, revealing normal values for these parameters.[21] It is clear that platelet and coagulation function is optimal at normothermia, and it is therefore essential to return all cardiac surgical patients to this state prior to separation from bypass, and to maintain this condition during the entire postoperative period. In our review of 250 primary CABG patients we found that although the degree of hypothermia did not correlate significantly with the level of chest tube output, virtually all patients arrived in the ICU with some degree of hypothermia (Table 20.8). Normothermia, defined as temperature ≥37°C, was typically achieved only during the third postoperative hour—generally the time by which most increased postoperative bleeding resolves. Although from a retrospective standpoint it is not statistically possible to prove a link between such warming and cessation of bleeding, as multiple other factors are obviously at work during this period, the parallel nature of the two suggests that such a relationship exists. Whether this relationship holds true is not a debate worth arguing, however, as nothing is lost by returning the patient as rapidly as possible to normothermia. Based on the results of this analysis, we have instituted a specific warming protocol at our institution (Table 20.9). This protocol begins prior to CPB when a water warming blanket is placed beneath the patient, and an upper extremity convection air warming blanket is placed over the head and upper extremities. During CPB moderate hypothermia (mean low core temperature = approximately 30°-31°C) is typically employed. Prior to separation from CPB, a core temperature (bladder and esophageal) of at least 37°C is achieved. All fluids and autologous and allogeneic blood products are given through a warming device once patient warming has been initiated, and the room temperature is elevated to the highest tolerable level. Upon arrival in the ICU postop-

Table 20.7. Nontransfusion supportive therapy algorithm for the treatment of increased (accelerated, excessive, and critical) bleeding during the intraoperative post-CPB and postoperative periods.

Quantity of bleeding	Treatment
I. Intraoperative post-CPB period A. Microvascular bleeding with low to moderate suspicion of severe coagulopathy (based on characteristics of CPB run and/or procedure performed) and/or documented normal platelet and/or coagulation factor levels II. Postoperative period A. Immediate bleeding 1. Drainage > 250 cc first hour 2. Drainage > 150 cc second hour 3. If drainage < 150 ml/hr during second hour, patient is then assessed for delayed accelerated postoperative bleeding (below) B. Delayed bleeding 1. Drainage > 150 cc over any single hour after the first postoperative hour during any 3 consecutive hours after the first hour (except after turning patient) 2. Drainage > 100 cc over any two consecutive hours after the first postoperative hour	I. Rapid application of nontransfusion therapy A. Physiologic 1. Rapid sustained warming to 38°C 2. Aggressive blood pressure control (SBP <110) 3. PEEP increase to 10 mm Hg (Caution: "tight" IMA) 4. Elevation of head or bed 5. STAT Labs: PT/PTT, CBC + plt count B. Pharmacologic 1. Adequate heparin reversal (100 mg additional protamine dose, then check ACT if continued bleeding) 2. EACA 3. DDAVP

TABLE 20.8. Core body temperature during CPB and at the start of the first four postoperative hours ($n = 250$).

Perioperative	CPB	Arrival	1 hour	2 hours	3 hours
Mean temperature (degrees C)	31.34	35.22	35.53	36.21	37.0
Standard deviation	1.37	0.66	0.68	0.65	0.71
Range (degrees C)	26.8–36.4	33.3–37.2	33.6–37.8	34.6–37.6	35.1–38.6
Change (degrees C/hour)	–	–	0.71	0.68	0.69

eratively the patient is placed on a water warming blanket, and a full body length air convection warming blanket (set at 39°C) is used to fully cover the patient. Several additional standard blankets are placed over the convection blanket. All fluid infusions continue to be administered through the Hot Line warming device. Room temperature is maintained at the upper acceptable range, and is increased in the event of increased postoperative bleeding. Applying such a protocol to every patient has proven to be cost-effective, and has markedly increased and accelerated our ability to achieve rapid and sustained rewarming in all patients.

Blood Pressure Control

Blood pressure control is an essential tool for reducing postoperative blood loss. Like adequate patient warming, however, it is a measure that should

TABLE 20.9. Warming interventions for the cardiac surgical patient.

Perioperative time period	Warming interventions
I. Pre-CPB	1. Water warming mattress placed beneath patient. 2. Air convection warmer for head and upper extremities.
II. CPB (Weaning)	1. Full patient rewarming to core temperature = 37°C. 2. Water warming blanket beneath patient warmed to 39°C. 3. Air convection warmer for head and upper extremities warmed to 39°C. 4. All IV fluids / blood through warming device once warming begun. 5. Room warming to 38°C.
III. Post-CPB (OR)	1. Water warming blanket beneath patient maintained at 39°C. 2. Air convection warmer for head and upper extremities maintained at 39°C. 3. All IV fluids / blood through warming device. 4. Room warmth maintained at 38°C.
IV. Post-CPB (ICU)	1. Water warming mattress placed beneath patient, maintained at 39°C. 2. Full length convection air warming blanket placed over patient; maintained at 39°C, covered with extra standard blankets. 3. All IV fluids / blood through warming device. 4. Room warmed if increased bleeding and patient <37°C.

be enacted regardless of the presence of increased postoperative bleeding. The presence of such bleeding simply serves to indicate that blood pressure control efforts must be accelerated and intensified. Typically, for reasons of both afterload reduction as well as bleeding prophylaxis, systolic blood pressure (SBP) is maintained below 100 to 120 mm Hg in the nonbleeding postoperative cardiac surgical patient. A number of agents, most commonly beta blockers, nitroglycerine, and nitroprusside, can be applied alone or in combination to achieve these pressure goals. When a patient is seen to exhibit excessive oozing at the time of chest closure, or if drainage meets or will be predicted to meet criteria for increased postoperative bleeding, then systolic pressure should be aggressively decreased to between 90 and 100 mm Hg, as tolerated by the patient.[22] Nitroprusside is particularly useful for manipulation of pressures in this range. When using controlled hypotension, patients must be monitored closely for adequacy of perfusion, particularly those with preexisting hypertension who are accustomed to higher perfusion pressures. Often urine outputs will reflect hypoperfusion under these circumstances. Immediate and aggressive control of blood pressure in the patient displaying accelerated bleeding is an essential component of nontransfusion therapy of postoperative bleeding.

Positive End Expiratory Pressure (PEEP) Increase

Theoretically, by increasing intrathoracic pressure and maintaining greater lung volumes, positive and expiratory pressure can serve to tamponade postoperative bleeding, particularly that which is venous in origin. Whether it achieves this effect clinically has been debated since the early 1980s. While initial studies suggested the benefit was provided to the patients with increased postoperative blood loss,[23–25] subsequent randomized controlled trials did not confirm this benefit.[26,27] Nevertheless, PEEP remains widely used as an initial nontransfusion supportive therapy for accelerated postoperative bleeding.[28,29] The widespread use of this unproven modality undoubtedly occurs because of the ease of application of the technique, as well as the very limited downside.[28] PEEP has been increased to as high as 20 mm Hg in the cardiac surgical literature for the control of hemorrhage,[24] although typically PEEP should not be elevated above 10 mm Hg with serial evaluation for potential hemodynamic compromise attributable to decreased venous filling.[30] We typically employ a baseline PEEP of 5 mm Hg for all of our postoperative cardiac surgical patients, and this number is increased to 10 mm Hg if accelerated bleeding is encountered. Rarely, PEEP is increased to 12.5 in patients with good cardiopulmonary performance status and continued bleeding. Caution is maintained in the population undergoing internal mammary artery grafting as the tension on an already tight mammary artery graft can be aggravated by increased lung and thoracic volumes.[31] Consultation with the operating surgeon regarding this matter should always be obtained prior to raising PEEP for increased bleeding. Likewise, serial hemodynamic evaluation is mandatory when increasing PEEP, to ensure that cardiac performance status is not compromised. When assessing volume status of the postoperative bleeding patient on PEEP, appropriate corrections for the influence of PEEP on pulmonary capillary wedge pressure (PCWP) and central venous pressure (CVP) must be performed.[26]

Other Supportive Measures

A final physiologic measure that has been suggested in the initial control of accelerated bleeding in the postcardiotomy patient is elevation of the head of the patient's bed to an angle of 30° to 45°. Theoretically, this serves to collapse the innominate vein and its branches, decreasing the tendency of these potential bleeding sites to continue bleeding.[29] No prospective trials have been performed to confirm the efficacy of this maneuver, but, in the absence of contraindication to head elevation, e.g., intraaortic balloon pump (IABP), it appears reasonable. Similar to increasing PEEP, ease of application, the absence of significant downside, and total absence of cost increase the attractiveness of this clinically unproven maneuver.

Pharmacologic Modalities

Protamine

Protamine sulfate, a small highly charged protein derived from fish sperm, is the primary agent used to reverse the anticoagulant effect of heparin following separation from CPB. While protamine clearly does bind and inactivate circulating heparin, controversy regarding the use of protamine has arisen with regard to (1) a mild anticoagulant effect, (2) activation of complement and other inflammatory mediators by protamine or heparin-protamine complexes, (3) diminution in platelet number and/or function by the heparin-protamine complex, and (4) heparin rebound. Protamine itself has a mild anticoagulant effect.[32] However, the short half-life of protamine likely precludes important clinical consequences (but supports allowing appropriate time for such effects to dissipate before institution of transfusion therapy, see Transfusion Strategies, below). Protamine and heparin protamine complexes have been shown to have proinflammatory effects mediated through the complement and other systems.[33,34] While these effects can be severe, particularly in presensitized individuals, such as insulin-dependent diabetics with prior exposure to neutral protamine Hagedorn (NPH) insulin, the relatively low incidence of severe reaction allows the use of protamine in a vast majority of patients. Reduction in platelet number and function immediately following the use of protamine has been reported,[35] and function may be affected as well.[11] But because of the large number of concurrent events at the time of protamine reversal of heparin, it is difficult to assign alterations to any single cause. Finally, the importance of the phenomenon of heparin rebound has been variably reported.[36,37] Clearly delayed release of heparin from multiple sources can occur, and additional unneutralized heparin can be introduced into the bloodstream through reinfusion of Cell Saver processed blood and unprocessed residual circuit blood.

Until more is known regarding the potential adverse effects of protamine, and until an alternative agent or anticoagulation scheme is available (e.g. recombinant platelet factor 4), protamine remains the sole agent clinically for reversing heparin anticoagulation following CPB. It therefore is essential to apply this agent in the most effective and least insulting manner. Two principles underlie the optimal application of protamine: (1) use of only enough heparin to achieve the necessary level of anticoagulation, (2) use of only enough protamine to reverse the anticoagulant effect of heparin. Our heparin-protamine protocol, outlined elsewhere in this text, includes the use of only enough heparin to maintain an activated clotting time (ACT) at or slightly above 400 seconds (750 seconds if aprotinin is used), and reverses heparin with only enough protamine to return the ACT to normal range (<180 seconds). Our standard protamine regimen is 1 mg per 100 mg heparin given. An ACT is then checked and additional protamine given as required to normalize the ACT. Prior to leaving the operating room, and following administration of residual circuit and Cell Saver blood, the ACT is rechecked and additional protamine given as required. Patients with increased postoperative bleeding (class I–III) are given an extra 50 mg protamine upon arrival in the ICU. If the bleeding continues and the partial thromboplastin time (PTT) and/or ACT is prolonged, then this supplemental dose is repeated.

DDAVP

D-8-Arginine vasopressin (DDAVP) is a synthetic analogue of vasopressin that is devoid of significant antidiuretic, vasopressor, and oxytocic effects. It exerts a hemostatic effect through three general mechanisms: (1) release of factor VIII from endothelial stores, (2) release of von Willebrand factor from endothelial stores, and (3) improvement in platelet function. In addition, and counter to these hemostatic effects, DDAVP acts as a fibrinolytic agent by releasing tissue plasminogen activator from endothelial stores.[38] These actions of DDAVP are summarized in Table 20.10).

The half-life of DDAVP is between 55 minutes and 4.5 hours, and a dose of 0.3 μg/kg has been found to result in maximum increases in factor VIII and von Willebrand factor.[38,39] Factor VIII levels increase to 3.1 to 3.7 times normal approximately 30 to 50 minutes after intravenous injection of DDAVP, and the half-life of this released factor VIII is 3 to 6 hours.[38,40] While useful in the treatment of hemophilia A (factor VIII deficiency), clinically significant reductions in levels of factor VIII are rare following CPB, and therefore this is not likely a primary mechanism for its effectiveness in improving hemostasis following CPB.[11,41–43]

Levels of von Willebrand factor (vWF) increase 2.5- to 3.1-fold by 1 to 2

TABLE 20.10. Hemostatic and antihemostatic functions of DDAVP in the cardiac surgical patient.

Hemostatic functions	Antihemostatic functions
1. Increases blood levels of factor VIII*	1. Increased blood levels of tissue plasminogen activator* (increased fibrinolytic activity)
2. Increases blood levels of von Willebrand factor*	
3. Improves platelet function (adhesion, aggregation)	

*Mobilized from endothelial stores.

hours after IV injection, and the half-life is between 5 and 9 hours. vWF is a very large multimeric protein (the largest known soluble protein[44]) that serves a primary role in platelet adhesion and aggregation, and also serves to protect factor VIII from degradation in the bloodstream. Levels of vWF have been shown to be normal in uremia, the primary population in which DDAVP has shown hemostatic efficacy, and levels are elevated following CPB, consistent with vWF's status as an acute-phase protein. The extent to which improved hemostasis in these populations is related to augmentation of serum levels of vWF is, therefore, unclear. It is likely that improved hemostasis is attributable to a shift in the ratio of larger multimeric forms of vWF, rather than to the absolute increase of vWF levels.[44] Several disease states, most notably systemic lupus erythematosus (SLE), are associated with an acquired form of von Willebrand's disease, and DDAVP is indicated when performing cardiac surgery on patients with these disorders.[38]

DDAVP is also believed to improve platelet function in certain disease or platelet disorder states.[38] This enhancement in platelet function appears to be independent of increases in serum levels of vWF induced by DDAVP, as vWF levels are normal or elevated in many of the states in which DDAVP has shown effectiveness (e.g., uremic bleeding; excessive bleeding associated with CPB).[45] The mechanism(s) behind this platelet functional preservation are not fully understood, however. Postulated mechanisms include modification of endothelial and subendothelial surfaces, thereby allowing enhanced adhesion,[46] and increases in the number and ratio of large vWF multimers, leading to enhanced platelet adhesion and aggregation.[44] These larger vWF multimers may help to overcome the decreased platelet vWF adhesiveness attributable to plasmin-mediated loss of vWF receptors (GP1b) on the platelet surface.[47] Whatever the mechanism, it has now been convincingly established that DDAVP is useful in decreasing the increased postoperative bleeding associated with cardiopulmonary bypass.[45,48,49] This benefit may only be provided in the immediate early post-CPB period when coagulopathic bleeding is at its highest levels.[50–51] When used in low bleeding risk patients or those who do not actually develop CPB-associated coagulopathy, DDAVP provides little or no clinical benefit.[51–55] Its use, therefore, should be limited to only those patients at very high risk for, or who actually develop, increased postoperative bleeding. It has been recommended that these patients be identified thromboelastographically.[48] However, because not all patients with thromboelastographic platelet abnormalities bleed excessively, we prefer to utilize the much more direct and therefore specific and cost-effective measure of the actual presence of increased postoperative bleeding.

The final activity of DDAVP is release of tissue plasminogen activator (tPA) from endothelial stores. The peak in tPA activity occurs 20 to 60 minutes following intravenous injection of DDAVP, levels increase between 3.5- and 76-fold.[38] The half-life of released tPA is between 15 and 50 minutes. The implications of this tPA release are not well understood, particularly with regard to its role in the control of increased postoperative bleeding following cardiac surgery.[56] Intuitively, however, it would appear counterproductive to administer an agent that stimulates fibrinolysis when treating a state in which enhanced fibrinolysis is a distinct problem. In fact, early use of DDAVP in mild hemophiliacs was usually accompanied by the use of tranexamic acid in an effort to counter DDAVP's fibrinolytic effects (concomitant antifibrinolytic therapy has since been found to be unnecessary as the half-life of the fibrinolytic effect of DDAVP is very short).[38] Nevertheless, it is fortuitous and perhaps of benefit that our comprehensive nontransfusion supportive therapy bleeding protocol (Table 20.7) automatically counters the potential fibrinolytic activity of DDAVP by concurrently instituting EACA therapy at the time that increased bleeding is encountered.

The cost of a standard 0.3 μg/kg dose of DDAVP in the United States is approximately $65. To this must be added blood bank or pharmacy administrative fees, which at our institution are $22.50. The total cost of DDAVP is, therefore, approximately $90 per patient.[57] This cost, of course, must be viewed in a relative manner.

When assigning a role to DDAVP in the treatment of the cardiac surgical patient, all of the above information must be carefully considered. Based on such consideration, we have integrated the use of DDAVP into our bleeding control algorithm in two general situations. First, patients with inherited or acquired coagulation factor deficiencies (factor VIII and vWF) are given DDAVP prophylactically (pre-CPB) in conjunction with exogenous factor supplementation as required. These rare patients should be closely followed by a hematologist. The second situation in which DDAVP is applied is in the treatment of increased postoperative bleeding. We feel that there is no role for prophylactic DDAVP in the patient who is not demonstrating increased postoperative bleeding, although occasionally in the appropriate clinical setting (e.g., very long bypass time with large blood losses, extensive blood salvage, and large-volume blood transfusion) we administer DDAVP prior to actual recognition of anticipated increased bleeding. We maintain a low threshold for administering DDAVP to patients with uremic renal failure as well. In all other patients, DDAVP is applied only when increased bleeding—either intraoperatively as "microvascular" bleeding, or postoperatively as chest tube output above our established clinical guidelines—is encountered following cardiopulmonary bypass. When such bleeding is established, DDAVP is given immediately as part of a full bleeding protocol. We administer 0.3 μg/kg over 15 minutes as soon as increased blood loss is recognized. We feel that it is clear that DDAVP provides a yet to be fully understood benefit in patients with platelet dysfunction, and when such dysfunction becomes clinically manifest during the postoperative period, that its use is warranted. Its relative low cost and good safety profile support the empiric application of DDAVP in the bleeding patient. It is of importance to note that, as stated above, our protocol also initiates antifibrinolytic therapy using EACA at the time that increased bleeding is first identified, as we feel that it is important to address the potential fibrinolytic component of increased postoperative bleeding at this early time point as well. Theoretically, this serves the additional purpose of helping to counteract the fibrinolytic activity of DDAVP, as discussed previously.

Antifibrinolytic Therapy

Excessive fibrinolytic activity constitutes one arm of the inflammatory coagulopathy of CPB. While its relative importance as an etiology of increased postoperative bleeding is still debated, there is no doubt that activation of the fibrinolytic cascade occurs.[58–61] Plasmin, the primary mediator of fibrinolysis, is activated during CPB by release of tPA from endogenous stores, and by activation of factor XIIa from the contact activation system. Additional fibrinolysis may occur through cellular mechanisms whereby neutrophils act to locally degrade fibrin via release of enzymes such as elastase.[62–65] The fibrinolytic cascade has been linked to other coagulopathic mechanisms as well, particularly the plasmin-linked degradation of platelet receptors responsible for adhesion (GPIb).[47,66]

Three agents are available clinically to block fibrinolytic activity during or following cardiopulmonary bypass: (1) EACA, (2) tranexamic acid, and (3) aprotinin. Tranexamic acid differs from EACA primarily in its potency (7–10 times more potent) and half-life. Both agents block the binding of plasminogen to fibrin through reversible competitive blockade of the active lysine binding site of the plasminogen molecule.[67] EACA and tranexamic acid have been shown in multiple studies to reduce the postoperative bleeding in cardiac surgical patients. Both are most effective when begun prophylactically prior to CPB, presumably through blockade of profibrinolytic activity.[68–74] The antifibrinolytics, and more recently aprotinin, have also been shown to be effective, although relatively less so, when begun postoperatively once excessive bleeding has been identified.[61,75–77] This postoperative benefit is obtained through inhibition of the fibrinolytic component of post-CPB bleeding. Because of tranexamic acid's significant added expense, we routinely utilize EACA when applying antifibrinolytic therapy to the bleeding patient, and therefore the following discussion focuses on the use of this agent. Postoperative use of aprotinin, a much broader acting serine protease antifibrinolytic agent, is discussed in the following section. Preoperative (pre-CPB) prophylactic use of EACA, tranexamic acid, and aprotinin has been discussed previously, both in this and other chapters.

The very short half-life of EACA requires a 10-g loading dose and a continuous intravenous infusion of 1 g/hr to achieve and maintain a minimum effective plasma concentration of 0.01 mg/L.[67] The standard dosing regimen for postoperative bleeding in the cardiac surgical patient is a 5-10 gram load, followed by 1-2 gram/hr for 4 hours, but other regimens have been applied. Lambert et al,[61] in an early study of EACA, found that once significant fibrinolysis had developed post-CPB, 60 g of EACA was required for complete fibrinolytic suppression. Because no adverse sequelae were noted with these higher doses, it is likely that if bleeding persists a second loading dose (10 mg) can be administered. The cost of a typical 30-g course of EACA is approximately $10.

Concern has been expressed regarding the safety of the use of antifibrinolytic agents in cardiac surgery. While concern has been most directed at aprotinin and its effects on graft patency and renal function, the prothrombotic potential of blocking fibrinolytic activity (e.g., inhibition of clot modification, and/or excessive clot propagation) using EACA and tranexamic acid has directed criticism toward these agents as well.[68,73] It is our feeling that the prothrombotic potential of these agents is minimized when they are applied correctly, that is, to only restore systems to normal. Prophylactic use of the antifibrinolytics in only those patients with increased coagulopathic risk, or postoperative use in only those with actual bleeding, are strategies that seek only to counteract predicted or actual excessive fibrinolysis. Theoretically, it is primarily when these agents are used in patients who do not have coagulopathic excess of fibrinolytic activity that significant prothrombotic activity is possible.

Aprotinin

The efficacy of the anti-inflammatory antifibrinolytic agent aprotinin in decreasing postoperative bleeding is well established. A nonspecific serine protease inhibitor, aprotinin inhibits or attenuates the activity of a majority of the inflammatory and coagulation cascades, as well as the far-reaching and intricate consequences of these cascades. While the prophylactic use of aprotinin has been discussed in detail elsewhere in this text, it recently has been applied to patients following CPB with encouraging results.[78-80] In 1990 Agnelli et al[78] reported a reduction in bleeding following administration of postoperative aprotinin in six patients with severe post-CPB coagulopathic hemorrhage refractory to other treatment modalities. Review of the literature reveals that aprotinin has been used empirically to treat excessive bleeding prior to this time in patients with coagulopathic obstetrical hemorrhage.[81,82] In 1994 Kallis et al[80] performed a prospective randomized placebo-controlled trial evaluating the effects of postoperative aprotinin in 60 patients with increased postoperative bleeding. The authors found that bleeding was significantly decreased in the aprotinin group, and that other measures of coagulopathic bleeding were improved as well. Specifically, tPA activity was decreased, the fibrinogen, von Willebrand factor, and platelet surface glycoprotein GPIb receptor expression (the vWV receptor mediating platelet adhesion) all were significantly increased in the aprotinin-treated patients. The authors suggested that inhibition of plasmin-mediated GPIb cleavage by aprotinin might allow for enhanced GPIb receptor expression, and improved platelet adhesion function. Such rapid platelet recovery following plasmin neutralization has been demonstrated.[83] The findings of Kallis et al prompted a recent prospective randomized trial of postoperative aprotinin versus standard prophylactic aprotinin therapy and no aprotinin.[79] The authors found a significant reduction in bleeding in both aprotinin groups relative to controls, but no difference between the two aprotinin groups. This is a significant finding, with important implications. If aprotinin can provide efficacy in attenuating the coagulopathy of CPB without the need for prophylactic dosing, then the morbidity associated with nonspecific use of aprotinin can be avoided. Similar to our use of EACA and desmopressin, it can be used only in those patients who actually develop coagulopathic bleeding—acting only to normalize their coagulopathic state, and markedly diminishing the chance of thrombotic sequelae.

Postoperative aprotinin was given in these studies as a single 2 million unit intravenous bolus. This dose is insufficient to fully inhibit kallikrein, but high enough to inhibit plasmin activity and therefore preserve platelet GPIb receptor function. Further studies in different cardiac surgical populations are needed to more fully delineate the effects of postoperative aprotinin, and to determine optimal dosing regimens should its benefit be confirmed.

Other Agents

Several other pharmacologic agents have been applied experimentally and clinically during the perioperative period in efforts to prevent or control the coagulopathy of CPB, primarily through preservation of platelet number and function. Although theoretically well grounded, none of these agents has yet proven itself effective in the clinical arena. Included in this group of agents are dipyramidole,[84] prostacyclin,[85] several prostacyclin analogues,[86] thromboxane synthetase inhibitor,[87] platelet membrane glycoprotein receptor blocking agents, and platelet activating factor receptor antagonist.[88] All of these agents are targeted as prophylactic agents, and none has yet proven clinically useful in the treatment of established increased postoperative bleeding.

Transfusion Strategies for Excessive Postoperative Bleeding

Bleeding that progresses despite appropriate application of nontransfusion modalities requires either platelet and coagulation factor transfusion, return to the operating room, or both of these measures. As stated multiple times previously, the essential first step in delineating appropriate treatment is to allow bleeding to occur, based on knowledge of the upper limit of clinically acceptable chest tube output. This period of observation must be undertaken, however, only after institution of the full set of nontransfusion supportive measures delineated in the previous section. Serving to return homeostasis and hemostasis to normal as rapidly as possible, these measures ensure that only those cases of true, severe coagulopathy and/or inadequate mechanical hemostasis progress to the point of requiring transfusion or operative intervention. Which intervention is chosen, or whether both of these modalities are employed, then depends on the rate and character of the bleeding that is present.

If the key to minimizing transfusion is to only transfuse for bleeding rates that exceed clinically acceptable limits, then it is essential to accurately define these limits. We feel strongly that these limits can and should be defined at each individual institution by simple objective clinical assessment. While prospective randomized controlled trials delineating the extent to which it is safe to withhold transfusion would ethically be difficult to perform, analysis of bleeding and treatment patterns at hospitals that generally apply high triggers for platelet and coagulation factor transfusion reveals that a remarkable amount of initially excessive postoperative blood loss resolves spontaneously. Data from multiinstitution comparison studies, which found large variation in the percentage of patients transfused with platelets and coagulation factors despite equivalent chest tube drainage, support the fact that most platelet and coagulation factor transfusions are unnecessary.[6,8,14] Additional evidence supporting a decreased need for platelets and coagulation factors during the postoperative period is found in multiple prospective randomized studies that have found no reduction in bleeding following the prophylactic transfusion of these products in the early postoperative period.[89-96] These data confirm that it is quite safe for programs currently overaggressive with such transfusion to slowly but progressively elevate their transfusion thresholds and observe the clinical outcome. By doing this at our own institution, we were able to markedly decrease the use of platelets, FFP, and cryoprecipitate, without concomitantly increasing mean chest tube output, or the incidence of excessive chest tube output. This was achieved without an increase in morbidity or mortality, and in fact, our risk-adjusted mortality rate for 1100 CABG procedures was the second lowest in New York State in 1994, the year after these guidelines were instituted.

Discussion of the transfusion of blood products for suspected or actual coagulopathic bleeding is best performed according to perioperative period, of which there are three to consider: (1) intraoperative during CPB, (2) intraoperative post-CPB, and (3) postoperative. The following sections address each of these periods individually, with specific focus on delineating characteristics affecting bleeding and the need for platelet and coagulation factor transfusion.

Intraoperative CPB Period

We feel that platelets and coagulation factors should only very rarely be administered during CPB, as this degrades and destroys a portion of these products unnecessarily (as anticoagulation, not coagulation, is required during CPB), while still exposing the patient to the same number of blood donors. Only in cases of massive blood loss, salvage, and allogeneic red cell transfusion, when numerical deficits in platelets and coagulation factors are measured or anticipated, do we consider the use of platelets and coagulation factors during CPB. If these are to be given, it is only done immediately prior to separation from bypass, so that circuit exposure and mechanical trauma are minimized.

Intraoperative Post-CPB Period

Most early increased bleeding resolves spontaneously, without transfusion intervention. This includes "microvascular" bleeding often seen in the early post-CPB period following protamine reversal of heparin. Such bleeding has been described in 15% to 35% percent of patients undergoing cardiac surgery, and often leads to platelet and coagulation factor transfusion.[16,97] Our analysis of bleeding and transfusion patterns in 250 primary CABG patients revealed that only two of a total of 250 patients received platelets in the operating room during the post-CPB period for perceived excessive bleeding, and that no patients received FFP or cryoprecipitate. This is consistent with our general feeling that platelets and coagulation factors should be utilized in the operating room only under clinical circumstances consistent with the most severe frank coagulopathy (e.g., CPB time >2 hours, large-volume blood loss, and/or salvage with likely significant numerical platelet and coagulation depletion), when quantitative depletion of platelets and coagulation factors is anticipated or measured. Our practice of closing the chest in the setting of "microvascular" bleeding, after full mechanical hemostasis has been ensured, and while full nontransfusion supportive therapy is instituted, has revealed that in a majority of cases such initial microvascular bleeding will resolve without transfusion intervention.

It is this portion of our postoperative bleeding protocol that is perhaps most difficult to accept. It is against human, and particularly surgical, nature to not immediately intervene when a problem is identified. It must be remembered, however, that the coagulopathy of CPB is in a large majority of cases not attributable to quantitative deficiencies in platelets and coagulation factors. Rather it is the result of a massive stress and inflammatory response to the act of cardiopulmonary bypass, coupled with the effects of systemic hypothermia. The consequences of this response are far-reaching and only partially understood. While undoubtedly qualitative platelet defects and modest reductions in coagulation factor levels contribute to initial coagulopathic bleeding, there clearly exist other equally if not more important abnormalities, such as fibrinolysis, a majority of which are only beginning to be understood. Proof of the relative importance of these abnormalities to the coagulopathy of CPB can be found in the simple effectiveness of the drug aprotinin. When used prophylactically, this drug blocks a significant portion of the coagulopathy of CPB from occurring. In addition, as discussed above, postoperative administration of aprotinin has the ability to "shut down" coagulopathic bleeding after it has developed.[78–80] Conversely, prophylactic transfusion of platelets, FFP, fresh homologous blood, and large volumes of fresh autologous blood following CPB have not been shown to have any impact on coagulopathic bleeding.[89–96] Clearly events refractory to the simple quantitative addition of even fresh autologous platelets and coagulation factors are at work during the early post-CPB period, and when the relative importance of these intrinsic elements is appreciated, the need to automatically transfuse the bleeding patient becomes less powerful. Rather, it becomes clear that efforts should be directed toward shutting down coagulopathic processes, and returning the whole body to its normal state as rapidly as possible. It is likely that if platelets and coagulation factors are quantitatively sufficient, the rapid transfusion of never fully antigen-matched donor blood products does little to advance this goal of homeostatic normalization. Armed with this perspective, we feel comfortable in closely following the patient with increased "microvascular" bleeding in the early post-CPB period, transfusing blood products only for measured or strongly suspected quantitative abnormalities. We concentrate our efforts on rapidly and aggressively instituting a comprehensive set of nontransfusion supportive strategies (Table 20.7), for it is these physiologic and pharmacologic measures that address the underlying problem. Our criteria for intraoperative post-CPB transfusion are listed in Table 20.11.

Given our approach to the patient with early intraoperative post-CPB "microvascular" bleeding, it is necessary to address the issue of "near patient" or "on-site" testing during this period. It is difficult for us to accept as necessary the routine laboratory testing of patients during the early intraoperative post-CPB period, or even the testing of patients with increased bleeding in whom a severe quantitative deficiency of hemostatic factors is not suspected.[16] New cost-efficiency standards dictate that laboratory testing should be performed only when results of those tests will affect subsequent treatment. It is our protocol to observe all patients (except those with suspected quantitative platelet and coagulation factor deficiencies) during the early post-CPB intraoperative period, allowing time for the coagulopathy of CPB to resolve spontaneously. Abnormal prothrombin times, either alone or in conjunction with simple microvascular bleeding, would, therefore, not affect our use of FFP during this time.

TABLE 20.11. Treatment algorithm for excessive bleeding during the intraoperative post-CPB and postoperative periods.

Quantity of bleeding	Treatment
I. Intraoperative post-CPB period A. Severe "microvascular" bleeding with suspected (based on characteristics of CPB run and/or procedure performed) or documented quantitative platelet or coagulation factor deficiency II. Postoperative period A. Immediate bleeding 1. Drainage > 300 cc during first hour (*order* products, but do not give unless #2 occurs) 2. Drainage > 250 cc second hour (actually *give* ordered products) 3. If drainage < 250 ml/hr during second hour, patient continuous to be then assessed for delayed postoperative bleeding (below) B. Delayed bleeding 1. Drainage > 200 cc during any 2 consecutive hours after the first 2 postoperative hours (plts and/or factors ordered after the first > 200 cc hours) 2. Drainage > 100 cc over any 4 hours after the first 2 postoperative hours (plts and/or factors ordered after the third of these hours)	I. Rapid application of nontransfusion therapy (see Table 20.7) II. Transfusion therapy A. Transfusion 6 units platelets: 1. Plt count < 100 K 2. Plt count > 100 K, with nl PT (<15.0 sec [i.e. for persumed severe plt dysfunction]) B. Transfusion 2 units FFP: 1. PT > 15.0 sec 2. PTT > 1.5 × control, ACT wnl or no correction with 100 mg extra protamine dose C. Transfuse 10 units cryoprecipitate if 12 units platelets + 4 units FFP and still coagulopathic bleeding (PT/PTT > 1.5 × nl, fibronogen < 100)

PH = platelet; K = thousand; ACT = activated clotting time; PT = prothrombin time; PTT = partial thromboplastin time; FFP = fresh frozen plasma.

Likewise, platelets would only be administered during this time for counts less than 50–80 thousand. While this can occur in up to 20% of patients with severe microangiopathic bleeding,[16] it is typically only in those patients in whom a high index of suspicion for platelet and factor depletion *already* exists based on clinical parameters alone (long CPB times, etc.). As this is the only patient group in which we would act with transfusion, this is the only group that would benefit from such testing at our institution. Cost considerations do not allow us the luxury of maintaining near patient testing capability for this very small patient group, a group that is likely to be transfused appropriately with platelets based on clinical suspicion alone.

Postoperative (ICU) Period

During the postoperative period bleeding can occur early as a continuation of bleeding first appreciated during the intraoperative post-CPB period, or it can occur in a delayed fashion. Transfusion criteria listed in the literature generally recognize these two types of bleeding—early and delayed—as do our own (Tables 20.3 and 20.11). Our treatment of early postoperative bleeding is identical to that applied during the intraoperative post-CPB period. The primary difference is that while increased bleeding in the operating room is typically delineated by a wet surgical field ("microvascular" bleeding), during the postoperative period it is delineated strictly by chest tube output. Criteria for transfusion intervention must therefore be based on this output. Table 20.11 lists our transfusion criteria during the early postoperative period. They are consistent with our general philosophy that most bleeding will resolve on its own, and that transfusion should be reserved for clinically suspected or documented quantitative deficiencies in platelets and coagulation factors. It is reemphasized that this degree of bleeding is allowed to occur only after institution of a comprehensive set of physiologic and pharmacologic supportive measures. In addition, while this bleeding is occurring, preparation is made for immediate transfusion, should bleeding not resolve. When criteria for excessive early bleeding are initially met (e.g., chest tube output greater than 300 cc after the first hour), a set of laboratory values is obtained (hematocrit, platelet count, prothrombin time, partial thromboplastin time), and blood products are *ordered* from the blood bank (Table 20.11). If bleeding over the subsequent hour meets quantitative criteria (e.g., output >250 cc), then these laboratory values are assessed and appropriate blood products transfused. We apply an algorithm similar to that applied by "near patient testing" or "on site testing" advocates for microvascular bleeding in the operating room.[15,16] We generally agree with their qualitative transfusion criteria, just not with the timing of their application of these criteria.

The treatment of *delayed* excessive postoperative bleeding is theoretically identical to that for early excessive bleeding. By the time that bleeding has been identified as excessive, the full set of nontransfusion supportive measures will have been instituted (as the criteria for accelerated bleeding will have been met). When the criteria for excessive delayed bleeding are met (e.g., bleeding > 100 cc for 3 consecutive hours after the first 2 hours, > 200 cc for any single hour after the first 2 postoperative hours, Table 20.11), then the standard set of stat laboratory values is obtained, and blood products are ordered. If over the subsequent hour bleeding continues at an equivalent or higher rate, these blood products are given based on laboratory data (Table 20.11). Applying this ordered regimen for all transfusions ensures optimal supportive therapy, allows time for these measures to take effect, and applies transfusion therapy to correct specific hemostatic defects.

It should be understood that the development and application of appropriate transfusion criteria is an evolving process. As pharmacologic and other bleeding control methods improve, expected or normal chest tube outputs will decrease. Serious coagulopathic bleeding requiring transfusion, therefore, may be signified by a lower rate of bleeding. Similarly, the percentage of coagulopathic versus mechanical bleeding cases will likely shift, with a higher percentage of cases of inadequate mechanical hemostasis. These shifts must be considered, bleeding patterns monitored, and transfusion criteria appropriately adjusted.

It could be argued that allowance of increased bleeding may eventually lead to red cell transfusion, and donor exposures via this indirect mechanism. Several points can be made against this, however. First, the hematocrit of mediastinal blood is typically lower than that of blood found in the intravascular space. One unit of mediastinal blood does not equal one unit of banked blood, unless bleeding is severe (level III or critical bleeding). Second, if shed mediastinal blood is reinfused, a significant portion of lost red cell mass is returned to the patient. Third, one "round" of platelets and coagulation factors constitutes eight donor exposures (unless single-donor products are utilized). The loss of 500 to 800 cc of mediastinal blood during the first several hours necessitates atmost *two* units of red cell mass replacement, and this will be needed only if the patient's hematocrit lies in the range of the institution's stated red cell transfusion trigger, which in most cases it is not. Clearly, an automatic eight donor exposures are far worse than an unlikely one to two unit donor exposure. Fourth and finally, until a prospective randomized trial comparing the effects of transfusion versus no transfusion in the patient with moderately increased postoperative bleeding is performed, there exists no data to prove that transfusion therapy improves bleeding attributable to coagulopathic or mechanical causes when hemostatic factors (platelets and coagulation factors) are quantitatively sufficient. Until such data are available, we feel justified in allowing clinically safe levels of increased bleeding to occur.

Reoperative Strategy for Critical Postoperative Bleeding

Critical postoperative bleeding, at rates delineated in Table 20.12, mandates immediate return to the operating room unless severe overwhelming

TABLE 20.12. Treatment algorithm for critical (Level III) postoperative bleeding.

Quantity of bleeding	Associated abnormalities	Treatment
I. Intraoperative post-CPB period Do not leave operating room until complete mechanical hemostasis and/or correction of severe frank coagulopathy	1. Active clotting of blood in chest tubes and or collecting system (indicates rapid rate) 2. Pulsatile flow of blood from chest tubes	I. Rapid application of nontransfusion therapy II. Rapid transfusion therapy (unless normal lab values obtained) III. Early return to operating room for surgical hemostasis*
II. Postoperative period 1. 500 ml first postop hour 2. 400 ml/hr first 2 postop hours 3. 300 ml/hr first 3 postop hours 4. 1000 ml total during first 4 hours 5. 1200 ml total first 5 hours 6. Excessive bleeding that restarts 7. Sudden massive bleeding		

*Early and prompt return to the operating room should never be delayed by institution of nontransfusion and transfusion supportive measures. It is, however, always important to implement these measures as rapidly as possible while preparation for prompt return to the operating room is made.

coagulopathy is felt to be the cause of bleeding based on clinical circumstances and laboratory data. While resternotomy for bleeding is the topic of another chapter in this text, it is useful to also outline the accessory clinical markers that can be used to help delineate the patient who is bleeding from a mechanical (vs coagulopathic) source (Table 20.12). When assessment for these clinical markers is combined with close monitoring of the rate of blood loss and analysis of hemostatic defects, the presence of a mechanical source of blood loss can be accurately predicted. Critical bleeding in the setting of normal hematologic values dictates immediate return to the operating room. In most cases of level III critical hemorrhage a mixed coagulopathic/mechanical picture is present. In this setting it is essential to institute nontransfusion and transfusion therapy as rapidly as possible, typically prior to laboratory data being available, and while rapid preparation for resternotomy is made. Reoperation should never be delayed for implementation of lesser measures, however.

Summary

This chapter outlined methods for accurate assessment and control of increased postoperative bleeding. Accurate assessment of blood loss is essential in order to institute timely and appropriate therapy, and, just as importantly, to withhold therapy from those who do not require it. Therapy for increased bleeding includes both prevention and treatment. By optimizing preventive measures, the number of patients experiencing increased postoperative bleeding can be minimized. Despite appropriate prophylaxis, however, some patients will bleed. Whether this bleeding is the result of coagulopathy, inadequate mechanical hemostasis, or both, the key to controlling this bleeding is prompt and appropriate treatment. There are three levels of therapy for increased postoperative bleeding: (1) nontransfusion supportive therapy, (2) transfusion therapy, and (3) return to the operating room for mechanical hemostasis. The rate of bleeding is the primary determinant of the level of intervention that is required. Figure 20.1 provides a summary of our bleeding protocol, which recognizes the rate of bleeding, and, based on this quantity, assigns an appropriate level of therapeutic intervention.

References

1. Gorman JH, Edmunds LH. Blood anesthesia for cardiopulmonary bypass. *J Cardiovasc Surg* 1995;10:270–279.
2. Helm RE, Rosengart TK, Klemperer JD, et al. 100 consecutive patients without transfusion using a comprehensive multimodality blood conservation program. *Ann Thorac Surg* (submitted for publication).
3. Goodnough LT, Johnston MFM, Ramsey G, et al. Guidelines for transfusion

support in patients undergoing coronary artery bypass grafting. *Ann Thorac Surg* 1990;50:675–683.
4. Kirklin JW, Barratt-Boyes BG. Postoperative care. In: Kirklin JW, Barratt-Boyes BG, eds. *Cardiac Surgery*. New York: Churchill Livingstone 1993;224.
5. Sobel M, Dyke CM. Hemorrhage and thrombotic complications of cardiac surgery. In: Baue AE, Geha AS, Hammond GL, Laks H, Naunnheim R, eds. *Glenn's Thoracic and Cardiovascular Surgery*. Stamford, CT: Appleton and Lange, 1996;1800.
6. Goodnough LT, Johnston MF, Toy PT, et al. The variability of transfusion practice in coronary artery bypass surgery. Transfusion Medicine Academic Award Group. *JAMA* 1991;265:86–90.
7. Helm RE, Rosengart TK, Klemperer JD, et al. Analysis of bleeding patterns in 250 primary CABG patients. (Submitted for publication).
8. Goodnough LT, Johnston MFM, Shah T, et al. A two institution study of transfusion practice in 78 consecutive adult elective open heart procedures. *Am J Clin Pathol* 1989;92:468–472.
9. Cosgrove DM, Loop FD, Lytle BW, et al. Determinants of blood utilization during myocardial revascularization. *Ann Thorac Surg* 1985;40:380–384.
10. Hardy JF, Perrault J, Tremblay N, et al. The stratification of cardiac procedures according to the use of blood products: a retrospective analysis of 1480 cases. *Can J Anesth* 1991;38(4):511–517.
11. Speiss BD. Coagulation dysfunction after cardiopulmonary bypass. In: Williams JP, ed. *Postoperative Management of the Cardiac Surgical Patient*. New York: Churchill Livingstone, 1996:175.
12. Goodnough LT, Johnstone MFM, Ramsey G, et al. Guidelines for transfusion support in patients undergoing coronary artery bypass grafting. *Ann Thorac Surg* 1990;50:675–683.
13. Harker LA. Bleeding after cardiopulmonary bypass. *N Engl J Med* 1986; 314(22):1446–1447.
14. Stover EP, Siegel LC, Parks R, et al. Variability in transfusion practice for coronary artery bypass persists despite national consensus guidelines: a 23-institution study. *Anesthesiology* 1994;81(3A):A1224.
15. Speiss BD, Gillies BSA, Chandler W, et al. Changes in transfusion therapy and reexploration rate after institution of a blood management program in cardiac surgical patients. *J Cardiothorac Vasc Anesth* 1995;9(2):168–173.
16. Despotis GJ, Santoro SA, Spitznagel E, et al. Prospective evaluation and clinical utility of on-site monitoring of coagulation in patients undergoing cardiac operation. *J Thorac Cardiovasc Surg* 1994;107:271.
17. Grover FL. Discussion of: Reexploration for bleeding is a risk factor for adverse outcome after cardiac operations (Moulton MJ, Creswell LL, Mackey ME, et al.). *J Thorac Cardiovasc Surg* 1996;111:1037–1046.
18. Cooper BE. A perspective on aprotinin. *Ann Pharmacotherapy* 1996; 30:407–409.
19. Michelson AD, MacGregor H, Barrard ML, et al. Reversible inhibition of human platelet activation by hypothermia in vivo and in vitro. *Thromb Haemost* 1994;71:633–640.
20. Valeri CR, Cassidy G, Khuri S, et al. Hypothermia induced reversible platelet dysfunction. *Ann Surg* 1987;205:175–181.
21. Rohrer MJ, Natale AM. Effect of hypothermia on the coagulation cascade. *Crit Care Med* 1992;20(10):1402–1405.

22. Postoperative bleeding. In: Elefteriades JA, Geha AS, Cohen LS, eds. *House Officer Guide to ICU Care. Fundamentals of Management of the Heart and Lungs.* New York: Raven Press, 1994;178.
23. Ilabaca PA, Ochsner JL, Mills NL. Positive end-expiratory pressure in the management of the patient with a postoperative bleeding heart. *Ann Thorac Surg* 1980;30(3):281–284.
24. Hoffman HS, Tomasselo DN, Mac Vaugh H. Control of postcardiotomy bleeding with PEEP. *Ann Thorac Surg* 1982;34(1):71–73.
25. Mills NL. Postoperative hemorrhage after cardiopulmonary bypass. *Ann Thorac Surg* 1982;34(6):607.
26. Zurick AM, Urzua J, Ghattas M, et al. Failure of positive end expiratory pressure to decrease postoperative bleeding after cardiac surgery. *Ann Thorac Surg* 1982;34(6):608–611.
27. Murphy DA, Finlayson DC, Craver JM, et al. Effect of positive end-expiratory pressure on excessive mediastinal bleeding after cardiac operations. *J Thorac Cardiovasc Surg* 1983;85(6):864–869.
28. Kerr G, Thomas SJ. Ventilatory management. In: Williams JP, ed. *Postoperative Management and Care of the Cardiac Surgical Patient.* New York: Churchill Livingstone, 1996;105.
29. Postoperative bleeding. In: Elefteriades JA, Geha AS, Cohen LS, eds. *House Officer Guide to ICU Care. Fundamentals of Management of the Heart and Lungs.* New York: Raven Press, 1994;178.
30. Dorinsky PM, Whitcomb ME. The effect of PEEP on cardiac output. *Chest* 1983;2:210–216.
31. Todd K. Rosengart, MD, personal communication.
32. Cobel-Geard RJ, Hassouna HI. Interaction of protamine sulfate with thrombin. *Am J Hematol* 1983;14:227–232.
33. Cavarocchi NC, Schaff HV, Orzulak TA, et al. Evidence for complement activation by protamine-heparin interaction after cardiopulmonary bypass. *Surgery* 1985;98:525.
34. Salama A, Hugo F, Heinrich H, et al. Deposition of terminal C5b-9 complement complexes on erythrocyte and leukocytes during cardiopulmonary bypass. *N Engl J Med* 1988;318:408–414.
35. Heynes A, Lotter MG, Badenhorst PN, et al. Kinetics and in-vivo redistribution of III Indium-labelled human platelets after intravenous protamine sulfate. *Thromb Hemost* 1980;44:65.
36. Kesteven PJ, Ahred A, Aps C, et al. Protamine sulphate and rebound following open-heart surgery. *J Cardiovasc Surg* 1986;27:600–603.
37. Gravlee GP, Rogers AT, Duidas LM, et al. Heparin management protocol for cardiopulmonary bypass influences heparin rebound but not bleeding. *Anesthesiology* 1992;76:393–401.
38. Schulman S. DDAVP—the multipotent drug in patients with coagulopathies. *Trans Med Rev* 1991;5(2):132–134.
39. Horrow JC. Desmopressin and antifibronlytics. *Int Anesth Clin* 1990; 28(4):230–236.
40. Mannucci PM, Vicente V, Alberca I, et al. Intravenous and subcutaneous administration of desmopressin (DDAVP) to hemophiliacs: pharmacokinetics and factor VIII responses. *Thromb Haemost* 1987;58:1037–1039.
41. Kalter RD, Saul CM, Wetstein L, et al. Cardiopulmonary bypass. Associated hemostatic abnormalities. *J Thorac Cardiovasc Surg* 1979;77:427–435.

42. Mammen EF, Koets MH, Washington BC, et al. Hemostasis changes during cardiopulmonary bypass surgery. *Semin Thromb Hemost* 1985;11:281–292.
43. Bachman F, McKenna R, Cole ER, et al. Hemostatic mechanism after open heart surgery. I. Studies on plasma coagulation factors and fibrinolysis in 512 patients after extracorporeal circulation. *J Thorac Cardiovasc Surg* 1975; 70:76–85.
44. Ruggeri ZM, Ware J. The structure and function of von Willebrand factor. *Thromb Haemost* 1992;67(6):594–599.
45. Salzman EW, Weinstein MJ, Weintraub, et al. Treatment with desmopressin acetate to reduce blood loss after cardiac surgery. *N Engl J Med* 1986; 314(22):1403–1406.
46. Barnhart MI, Chen S, Lusher JM, et al. DDAVP: Does the drug have a direct effect on the vessel wall? *Thromb Res* 1983;31:239–253.
47. Van Oeveren W, Harder MP, Roozendaal JK, et al. Aprotinin protects against the initial effect of cardiopulmonary bypass. *J Thorac Cardiovasc Surg* 1990;99:788–797.
48. Mongan PD, Hosking MP. The role of desmopressin acetate in patients undergoing coronary artery bypass grafting. *Anesthesiology* 1992;77(1): 38–35.
49. Czer LSC, Bateman TM, Gray RJ, et al. Treatment of severe platelet dysfunction and hemorrhage after cardiopulmonary bypass: reduction in blood usage with desmopressin. *J Am Coll Cardiol* 1987;9:1139–1147.
50. Rocha E, Llorens R, Paramo JA, et al. Does desmopressin acetate reduce blood loss after surgery in patients on cardiopulmonary bypass? *Circulation* 1988;77(6):1319–1323.
51. de Prost D, Barbier-Boehm G, Hazebroucq J, et al. Desmopressin has no beneficial effect on excessive postoperative bleeding or blood product requirements associated with cardiopulmonary bypass. *Thromb Haemost* 1992; 68(2):106–110.
52. Lazenby WD, Russo I, Zadeh BJ, et al. Treatment with desmopressin acetate in routine coronary artery bypass surgery to improve postoperative hemostasis. *Circulation* 1990;82(suppl IV):413–419.
53. Hackmann T, Gascoyne RD, Naiman SC, et al. A trial of desmopressin (1-desamino-8-D-arginine vasopressin) to reduce blood loss in uncomplicated cardiac surgery. *N Engl J Med* 1989;321:1437–1443.
54. Hedderich GS, Petsikas DJ, Cooper BA, et al. Desmopressin acetate in uncomplicated coronary artery bypass surgery: a postoperative randomized controlled trial. *Can J Surg* 1990;33(1):33–36.
55. Ansell J, Klassen V, Lew R, et al. Does desmopressin acetate prophylaxis reduce blood loss after valvular heart operations. *J Thorac Cardiovasc Surg* 1992;104:117–123.
56. Seear MD, Wadsworth LD, Rogers PC, et al. The effect of desmopressin acetate (DDAVP) on postoperative blood loss after cardiac operations in children. *J Thorac Cardiovasc Surg* 1989;98:217–219.
57. Carl Wolf MD, Director, Blood Bank, The New York Hospital–Cornell Medical Center, personal communication.
58. Kucuk O, Kwaan HC, Frederickson J, et al. Increased fibrinolytic activity in patients undergoing cardiopulmonary bypass operation. *Am J Hematol* 1986;23:223–229.
59. Gram J, Janetzko T, Jespersen J, et al. Enhanced effective fibrinolysis

following the neutralization of heparin in open heart surgery increases the risk of post-surgical bleeding. *Thromb Haemost* 1990;63:241–245.

60. Kongsgaard UE, Smith-Erichsen N, Geiran O, et al. Changes in coagulation and fibrinolytic systems during and after cardiopulmonary bypass surgery. *Thorac Cardiovasc Surg* 1989;37:158–162.
61. Lambert CJ, Marengo-Rowe AJ, Leveson JE, et al. The treatment of postperfusion bleeding using epsilon aminocaproic acid, cryoprecipitate, fresh frozen plasma, and protamine sulfate. *Ann Thorac Surg* 1979;28(5):440–444.
62. Plow EF. The major fibrinolytic proteases of human leukocytes. *Biochem Biophys Acta* 1980;630:47–56.
63. Hines RL, Rinder C. Perioperative coagulopathy. In: Lake CL, Moore RA, eds. *Hemostasis, Transfusion, and Alternatives in the Perioperative Period.* New York: Raven Press, 1995;469.
64. Hind CRK, Griffen JF, Pack S, et al. Effect of cardiopulmonary bypass on circulating concentrations of leukocyte elastase and free radical activity. *Cardiovasc Res* 1988;22:37–41.
65. Faymonville ME, Pincemail J, Duchateau J, et al. Myeloperoxidase and elastase as markers of leukocyte activation during cardiopulmonary bypass in humans. *J Thorac Cardiovasc Surg* 1991;102:309–317.
66. Marx G, Pokar H, Reuter H, et al. The effects of aprotinin on hemostatic function during cardiac surgery. *J Cardiothorac Vasc Anesth* 1991;5:467–474.
67. Verstraete M. Clinical application of inhibitors of fibrinolysis. *Drugs* 1985;29:236–261.
68. Daily PO, Lamphere JA, Dembitsky WP, et al. Effect of prophylactic epsilon-aminocaproic acid on blood loss and transfusion requirements in patients undergoing first-time coronary artery bypass grafting. *J Thorac Cardiovasc Surg* 1994;108:99–108.
69. Desmond J, Delphin E, Rose E. Prophylactic D-aminocaproic acid (EACA) administration minimizes blood replacement therapy during cardiac surgery. *Anesth Analg* 1995;80:827–829.
70. Del Rossi AJ, Cernaianu AC, Botros S, et al. Prophylactic treatment of post perfusion bleeding using EACA. *Chest* 1989;96:27–30.
71. Horrow JC, Hlavacek J, Strong MD, et al. Prophylactic tranexamic acid decreases bleeding after cardiac operations. *J Thorac Cardiovasc Surg* 1990;99:70–74.
72. Coffey A, Pittman J, Halbrook H, et al. The use of tranexamic acid to reduce postoperative bleeding following cardiac surgery: a double blind randomized trial. *Am Surg* 1995;61:566–568.
73. van Oeveren W, Harder MP, Roozendaal KJ, et al. Aprotinin protects platelets against the initial effect of cardiopulmonary bypass. *J Thorac Cardiovasc Surg* 1990;99:788–797.
74. Rousou JA, Engelman RM, Flack JE, et al. Tranexamic acid significantly reduces blood loss associated with coronary revascularization. *Ann Thorac Surg* 1995;59:671–675.
75. Sterns LP, Lillehei CW. Effect of epsilon aminocaproic acid upon blood loss following open-heart surgery: an analysis of 340 patients. *Can J Surg* 1967;10:304–307.
76. Vander Salm TJ, Ansell JE, Okike ON, et al. The role of epsilon-aminocaproic acid in reducing bleeding after cardiac operation: a double blind-randomized study. *J Thorac Cardiovasc Surg* 1988;95:538–540.

77. Ovrum E, Am Holen E, Abdelnoor M, et al. Tranexamic acid (Cyclapron) is not necessary to reduce blood loss after coronary artery bypass operations. *J Thorac Cardiovasc Surg* 1993;105:78–83.
78. Angelini GD, Cooper GJ, Lamarra M, et al. Unorthodox use of aprotinin to control life-threatening bleeding after cardiopulmonary bypass. *Lancet* 1990;355:799–800.
79. Cicek S, Demirkilic U, Kuralay E, et al. Postoperative aprotinin: effect on blood loss and transfusion requirements in cardiac operations. *Ann Thorac Surg* 1996;61:1372–1376.
80. Kallis P, Tooze JA, Talbot S, et al. Aprotinin inhibits fibrinolysis, improves platelet adhesion, and reduces blood loss and related variables after cardiopulmonary bypass. *J Thorac Cardiovasc Surg* 1994;108:1083–1091.
81. Sher G. Trasylol on the management of abruptio placentae with consumption coagulopathy and uterine inertia. *J Reprod Med* 1980;25(3):113–118.
82. Sher G. Trasylol in cases of accidental hemorrhage with coagulation disorder and associated uterine inertia. *S Afr Med J* 1974;48:1452.
83. Michelson AD, Barnard MR. Plasmin-induced redistribution of platelet glycoprotein Ib. *Blood* 1990;76:2005–2010.
84. Teoh KH, Christakis GT, Weisel RD, et al. Dipyramidole preserved platelets and reduced blood loss after double-blind study of 50 patients having coronary revascularization. *Ann Thorac Surg* 1984;38(5):515–519.
85. DiSesa VJ, Huval W, Shlomo L, et al. Disadvantages of prostacycline infusion during cardiopulmonary bypass: a double-blind study of 50 patients having coronary revascularization. *Ann Thorac Surg* 1984;38(5):515–519.
86. Bernabei A, Gikakis N, Kowalska MA, et al. Iloprost and echistatin protect platelets during simulated extracorporeal circulation. *Ann Thorac Surg* 1995;59:149–153.
87. Huddleston CB, Hammon JW, Wareing TH, et al. Amelioration of the deleterious effects of platelets activated during cardiopulmonary bypass. Comparison of a thromboxane synthetase inhibitor and a prostacycline analogue. *J Thorac Cardiovasc Surg* 1985;89:190–195.
88. Nathan N, Mercury P, Denizot Y, et al. Effects of the platelet-activating factor receptor antagonist BN 52021 on hematologic variables and blood loss during and after cardiopulmonary bypass. *Anesth Analg* 1994;79:205–211.
89. Swafford MWG, Yawn D, Wenker O, et al. Effect of adding fresh frozen plasma to the cardiopulmonary bypass machine on blood component requirements in complex CV procedures. *Anesth Analg* 1995;80:A128(abstract).
90. Martinowitz U, Goor DA, Ramot B, et al. Is transfusion of fresh plasma after cardiac operations indicated? *J Thorac Cardiovasc Surg* 1990;100:92–98.
91. Kaplan JA, Cannarella C, Jones EL, et al. Autologous blood transfusion during cardiac surgery: A re-evaluation of three methods. *J Thorac Cardiovasc Surg* 1977;74(1):4–10.
92. Shinfeld A, Zippel D, Lavee J, et al. Aprotinin improves hemostasis after cardiopulmonary bypass better than single-donor platelet concentrates. *Ann Thorac Surg* 1995;59:872–876.
93. Helm RE, Klemperer JD, Rosengart TJ, et al. Intraoperative autologous donation preserves red cell mass but does not decrease postoperative bleeding. *Ann Thorac Surg* 1996;62(5):1431–1441.
94. Harding SA, Shakoor MA, Grindon AJ. Platelet support for cardiopulmonary bypass surgery. *J Thorac Cardiovasc Surg* 1975;70(3):350–353.

95. Simon TL, Bechara FA, Murpht W. Controlled trial of routine administration of platelet concentrates in cardiopulmonary bypass surgery. *Ann Thorac Surg* 1984;37(5):359–364.
96. Consten EJC, Henny CHP, Eijsman L, et al. The routine use of fresh frozen plasma in operations with cardiopulmonary bypass is not justified. *J Thorac Cardiovasc Surg* 1996;112(1):162–167.
97. Nuttall GA, Oliver WC, Beynen FM, et al. Determination of normal vs abnormal activated partial thromboplastin time and prothrombin time after cardiopulmonary bypass. *J Cardiothorac Vasc Anesth* 1995;9(4):355–361.
98. Horrow JC, Van Riper DF, Strong MD, et al. Hemostatic effects of tranexamic acid and desmopressin during cardiac surgery. *Circulation* 1991; 84:2063–2070.
99. Horrow JC, Van Riper DF, Strong MD, et al. The dose-response relationship of tranexamic acid. *Anesthesiology* 1995;82(2):383–392.
100. Shore-Lesserson L, Reich DL, Vela-Cantos F, et al. Tranexamic acid reduces transfusions and mediastinal drainage in repeat cardiac surgery. *Anesth Analg* 1996;83:18–26.
101. Karski JM, Teasdale SJ, Norman PH, et al. Prevention of postbypass bleeding with tranexamic acid and E-aminocaproic acid. *J Cardiothorac Vasc Anesth* 1993;7(4):431–435.
102. Karski JM, Teasdale SJ, Norman PH, et al. Prevention of bleeding after cardiopulmonary bypass with high-dose tranexamic acid. *J Thorac Cardiovasc Anesthesia* 1995;110:835–842.
103. Goodnough LT, Johnstone MFM, Ramsey G, et al. Guidelines for transfusion support in patients undergoing coronary artery bypass grafting. *Ann Thorac Surg* 1990;50:675–683.
104. Katsaros D, Petricevic M, Snow N, et al. Tranexamic acid reduces postbypass blood use: a double blinded, prospective, randomized study of 210 patients. *Ann Thorac Surg* 1996;61:1131–1135.
105. Casas JI, Zvazu-Jausoro I, Mateo J, et al. Aprotinin versus desmopressin for patients undergoing operations with cardiopulmonary bypass. *J Thorac Cardiovasc Surg* 1995;110:1107–1117.
106. Despotis GJ, Santoro SA, Spitznagel E, et al. Prospective evaluation and clinical utility of on-site monitoring of coagulation in patients undergoing cardiac operation. *J Thorac and Cardiovasc Surg* 1994;107:271–279.
107. Sandrelli L, Pardini A, Lorusso R, et al. Impact of autologous blood predonation on a comprehensive blood conservation program. *Ann Thorac Surg* 1995;59:730–765.
108. Ward HB, Smith RR, Landis KP, et al. Prospective, randomized trial of autotransfusion after routine cardiac operations. *Ann Thorac Surg* 1993; 56:137–141.
109. Yau TM, Carson S, Weisel RD, et al. The effect of warm heart surgery on bleeding. *J Thorac Cardiovasc Surg* 1992;103:1155–1163.
110. Essell JH, Martin TJ, Salinas J, et al. Comparison of thromboelastography to bleeding time and standard coagulation tests in patients afte cardiopulmonary bypass. *J Cardiothorac Vascu Anesth* 1993;7(4):410–415.
111. Nuttall GA, Oliver WC, Beynan FM, et al. Determination of normal versus abnormal activated partial thromboplastin time and prothrombin time after cardiopulmonary bypass. *J Cardiothorac Vasc Anesth* 1995;9(4):355–361.

112. Woodman RC, Harker LA, et al. Bleeding complications associated with cardiopulmonary bypass. *Blood* 1990;76(9):1680–1697.
113. Lambert CJ, Marengo-Rowe AJ, Leveson JE, et al. The treatment of postperfusion bleeding using epsilon aminocaproic acid, cryoprecipitate, fresh frozen plasma, and protamine sulfate. *Ann Thorac Surg* 1979;28(5):440–444.
114. Rousou JA, Engelman RM, Flack JE, et al. Tranexamic acid significantly reduces blood loss associated with coronary revascularization. *Ann Thorac Surg* 1995;59:671–675.
115. Unswerht-White MJ, Herriot A, Oswaldo V, et al. Resternotomy for bleeding after cardiac operation: a marker for increased morbidity and mortality. *Ann Thorac Surg* 1995;59:664–667.
116. Edmunds LH, Addonizio VP. Extracorporeal circulation. In: Coleman RW, Hirsh J, Marder VJ, Salzman EW, eds. *Hemostasis and Thrombosis.* Philadelphia: Lippincott, 1987;901.
117. Dietrich W, Dilthey G, Spannagl M, et al. Influence of high-dose aprotinin on anticoagulation, heparin requirement, and celite and kolin-activated clotting time in heparin-retreated patients undergoing open-heart surgery. *Anesthesiology* 1995;83(4):679–689.
118. Cicek S, Demirkilic U, Kuralay E, et al. Postoperative aprotinin: effect on blood loss and transfusion requirements in cardiac operations. *Ann Thorac Surg* 1996;61:1372–1376.
119. Moulton MJ, Cresswell LL, Mackey ME, et al. Reexploration for bleeding is a risk factor for adverse outcome after cardiac operations. *J Thorac Cardiovasc Surg* 1996;111:1037–1046.
120. Cosgrove DM, Loop FD, Lytle BW, et al. Blood conservation in cardiac surgery. In: Vidt DG, Brest AN, eds. *Cardiovascular Therapy.* Philadelphia: F.A. Davis, 1978;171.
121. Ferraris VA, Ferraris SP, Lough FC, et al. Preoperative aspirin ingestion increases operative blood loss after coronary artery bypass grafting. *Ann Thorac Surg* 1988;45:71–74.
122. Moulton MJ, Cresswell LL, Mackey ME, et al. Reexploration for bleeding is a risk factor for adverse outcome after cardiac operations. *J Thorac Cardiovasc Surg* 1996;111:1037–1046.
123. Grover FL. Discussion of: reexploration for bleeding is a risk factor for adverse outcome after cardiac operations (Moulton MJ, Creswell LL, Mackey ME, et al.). *J Thorac Cardiovasc Surg* 1996;111:1037–1046.
124. Taylor KM. Perioperative approaches to coagulation defects. *Ann Thorac Surg* 1993;56:S78–S72.

21
Blood Conservation: A Critical Care Nursing Perspective

MAUREEN E. GOMEZ AND ROBERT E. HELM

Previous chapters have delineated the important contributions surgeons, anesthesiologists, and perfusionists can make toward the goal of optimal blood conservation in the surgical patient. Little has been written about the significant part that nurses play in a blood conservation program. Particularly during the postoperative period, nurses are on the front line and play a critical role in patient management.

The role of the nurse in blood conservation is described in this chapter. The first section gives a brief overview of the physiologic changes that occur in a patient from a nursing perspective. It is during this period of time that the intensive care nurse has the responsibility of restoring the physiology of the patient to a state of normalcy. A particular focus of the nurse is the volume status of the patient and the nurse's assessment will often direct fluid replacement and pharmacologic interventions. Using sound clinical judgment, nurses often dictate the early postoperative care, and at this time crucial decisions can be made that will minimize blood loss and promote blood salvage. The second section includes a description of the autotransfusion system (ATS) routinely used at New York Hospital and it emphasizes, from a nursing perspective, the critical importance of adhering to transfusion guidelines. The ATS device enables the nurse to reinfuse blood that has drained from the thoracic cavity. The fundamental principles behind the transfusion guidelines are examined and the nurse's responsibility in adhering to this protocol is emphasized. Monitoring the health care team to assure adherence to transfusion protocols has become a critical nursing responsibility in our blood conservation program.

General Review of Cardiac Procedure

Management of the patient in the early postoperative period is dictated by the multisystem insult imposed by cardiopulmonary bypass. These patients are in a special biologic and very unique situation.[1] The function of the bypass machine is to provide oxygenation, circulation, and hypothermia during bypass and during cardiac arrest. The pump is primed with crystalloid solution and is connected to the patient via venous and arterial cannulae. Heparin is administered to prevent clot formation prior to the blood entering the bypass machine. As the blood is pumped through the heart-lung machine, formed elements including red blood cells, white blood cells, and platelets, and unformed elements (plasma proteins) are traumatized by direct contact with the surface of the pump tubing, by turbulent flow, and by the intracardiac suction system. Free hemoglobin released by traumatized red blood cells is cleared via the kidneys. Administration of mannitol and Lasix may facilitate the clearance process. The oxygenated blood travels to the heat exchanger where it may be cooled to 25° to 30°C. The aorta is cross-clamped and the heart is cooled by an infusion of cold hyperkalemic, cardioplegic solution pumped directly into the aortic root or directly into the coronary ostia. A cold solution may be topically administered. The induced hypothermia reduces the oxygen requirements of the body as well as the myocardium. The mean arterial pressure is maintained by adjusting blood flow through the heart-lung machine and by infusing pharmacologic agents to regulate vascular tone.

Upon completion of the cardiac procedure, the heart is rewarmed and the cardioplegic solution is flushed from the heart. As blood circulates through the myocardium, the heart muscle regains its rate, rhythmicity, and strength of contraction. The patient is weaned from bypass and the heart resumes its normal pumping function. Protamine sulfate is given to counteract the effect of heparin.[2]

Physiologic Changes

The physiologic changes experienced by the postoperative patient were discussed in Chapter 11. A number of hormonal changes take effect during bypass such as a marked increase in serum levels of epinephrine and norepinephrine. Hypoglycemia and impaired insulin response are present. Lipid metabolism is augmented and carbohydrate metabolism may be decreased. A prolonged elevation (48 hours) in plasma-free cortical levels are seen in bypass patients. Increased secretion of vasopressin or antidiuretic hormone (ADH) is of immediate consequence. Its elevation is marked and far exceeds the elevation seen after most major general surgical procedures. Serum complement is activated and through its "kinin-like" activity increases vascular permeability. These changes, in combination with numerous other alterations in homeostasis, result in a marked increase in interstitial edema and in total body water. It should be understood, however, that most of these changes are unavoidable and some may actually be desirable.[3]

Volume Control

As a result of these changes, most patients retain fluid in the early postoperative period. The patient's total body water may be increased by

8%to 10%. Early fluid replacement therefore should consist of minimal mounts of free water and sodium (typically 25 to 30 cc per hour of 0.2% sodium chloride and 5% dextrose, and moderate amounts of potassium 40 meq per liter).[3] It is important to keep maintenance fluids at a minimum, but some patients during warming may vasodilate and volume loading and the usage of vasopressors may be required. A Swan-Ganz catheter can effectively serve as an adjunct by allowing accurate elevation of the patient's volume status and hemodynamic function. Continuous bedside monitoring by an intensive care nurse allows accurate assessment of vascular tone, myocardial contractility and fluid levels.

Minimizing Discard Volume

While carefully monitoring the fluid status of the postoperative patient, it is also important to minimize iatrogenic blood loss. This can be safely achieved by minimizing the amount of blood discarded during diagnostic sampling, by reinfusing discard volume via the arterial line, and by implementing the use of pediatric-size blood sample tubes during the postoperative course. All three methods will be described.

In the critical care setting an arterial line is utilized to continuously monitor hemodynamics. In addition, this catheter provides easy access for blood specimens and minimizes patient discomfort by eliminating the need for venipuncture. Patency of the arterial line is maintained by the continuous infusion of heparinized saline solution. The premixed heparin solution contains 25,000 units per 500 cc of saline and is delivered by a pressurized system at 3 cc per hour. For accurate diagnostic specimens, one must first clear the heparinized saline from the patient's tubing. This is referred to as the *discard volume.* In most intensive care units, the discard volume accounts for an average of 30% of the volume withdrawn from the patient during standard diagnostic testing.[4]

The discard volume, which is a mixture of crystalloid solution and blood, should be quantified by *the amount of dead space in the pressurized tubing.* The dead space is measured from the tip of the arterial catheter to the proximal port where a syringe is placed for blood removal. Although pressurized arterial line tubing comes in varying lengths, a 10- to 12-inch link is placed between the arterial catheter and the stopcock. This is standard in most hospitals throughout the United States.[5] When drawing blood specimens the amount of discard volume should double the length of this dead space. The dead space for a 12-inch tubing is 1 cc[5] and therefore 2 cc should be removed. When obtaining tests such as arterial blood gases, glucose levels, coagulation levels, daily laboratory specimens (CBC, biochemistry profile, electrolytes), and specific medication levels, the absolute minimum rule should apply (i.c., the absolute minimum amount of discard volume should be used when clearing a line for blood drawing). Discarding excess blood undermines the basic tenets of a blood conservation program. Preusser and Lash,[5] in a study to define the minimum amount of discard volume necessary for the accurate recording of arterial blood gases (ABGs), found that ABGs are the most commonly ordered test in a postoperative cardiac patient. They found that a 2-mL discard was sufficient to guarantee accurate blood gas analysis when withdrawing blood from an arterial catheter with 1 mm of dead space.

Serum glucose and potassium levels are frequently ordered tests in the postoperative period. When using a glucometer only one drop of blood is placed on the measuring level. A common misconception is that one must discard 5 cc of blood before obtaining a specimen when only 1.6 cc of discard volume is needed to assure accurate levels.[6] An accurate prothrombin time can be achieved with a 3-cc discard and a partial prothrombin time necessitates 5.3 cc.[7] Since these tests are usually obtained simultaneously and in one specimen tube, 6 cc of discard is a sufficient amount.

To summarize, for accurate diagnostic sampling, clear only a minimal amount of discard from the arterial line. This entails doubling the amount of space in the arterial line between the arterial catheter and the specimen port. This is a 2-cc volume for most radial arterial lines and 6 cc for most femoral lines. The first specimen should be used for blood gas analysis. From this sample, a glucose level can also be obtained. When sampling for daily lab specimens a CBC should be first (2.5 ml of blood), followed by a biochemistry profile and electrolytes. The later two samples can be analyzed from one 4-ml serum tube. The coagulation studies should be the last specimen drawn. At this point 6.5 ml have been removed and an accurate sample is assured.

An alternative technique to minimize discard volume utilizes a closed arterial line system. Three commonly used systems have been examined. The first system requires blood to be withdrawn through the heparin flush tubing into a distal reservoir syringe. This clears the line of heparinized saline and blood (Fig. 21.1). A sample is taken through a three-way stopcock placed proximal to the reservoir syringe. The blood and saline discard volume is then returned to the patient after the laboratory sample is drawn. The cost of this system is the price of one 10-cc plastic syringe. No data regarding infection control are available.[8]

The second device maintains a closed arterial line circuit. The venous arterial blood management protection (VAMP) system is produced by Baxter Healthcare, Irvine, CA (Fig. 21.2). The advantage of the VAMP system is that it does not alter pressure waveform. A preliminary study suggests that blood can be conserved with this system when compared with conventional blood sampling. Surprisingly, hemoglobin concentrations in the blood conservation group (VAMP catheters) did not reach statistical significance until a patient had been maintained in the critical care unit for a period of 9.5 days.[9]

A third device studied in our intensive care unit is Safeset manufactured by Abbott Laboratory, North Chicago, IL. This product contains two

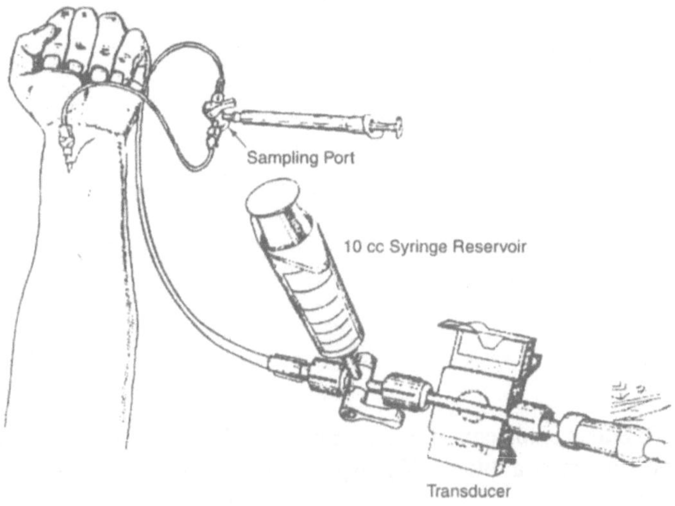

FIGURE 21.1. Conversion of conventional arterial tubing for blood conservation. (Artist: R. Neill. Reprinted with permission, Abbott Critical Care Systems. Mountain View, California.)

permanently placed rubber sealed sampling ports for needle puncture and blood withdrawal. The ports have been incorporated into the arterial line pressure tubing (Fig. 21.3). The first sampling port is proximal to the patient and serves as a blood withdrawal site. The second port is mounted closer to the transducer and serves as an aspiration port to withdraw fluid. The second port is therefore used to draw blood into the tubing and past the

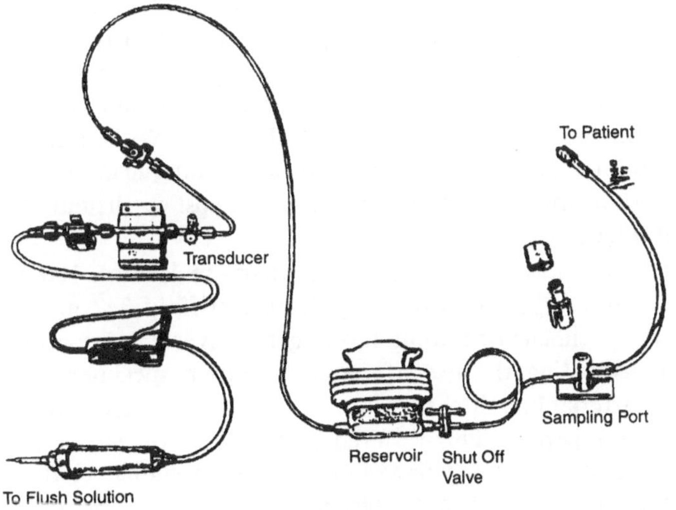

FIGURE 21.2. VAMP blood conservation tubing. (Artist: R. Neill. Reprinted with permission, Abbott Critical Care Systems. Mountain View, California.)

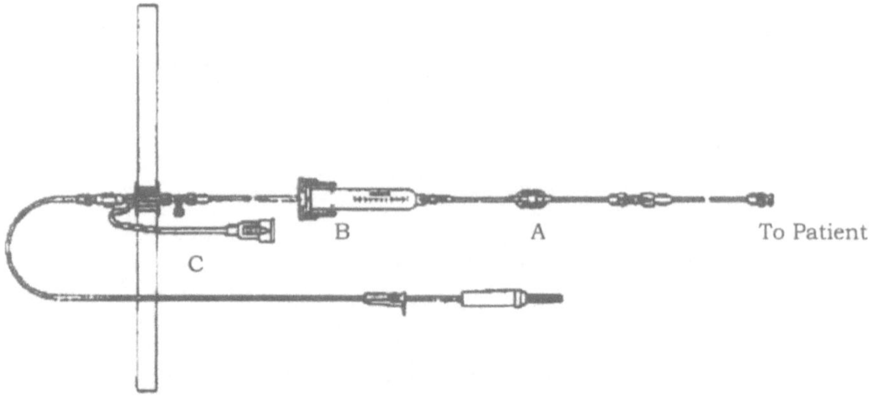

FIGURE 21.3. Safest blood conservation device. (A) Rubber seal for removing blood. (B) Reservoir for arterial blood. (C) Aspiration port to withdraw fluid.

proximal sampling site. After sampling, the blood is flushed back into the patient with saline from the tubing flush system. Each port has a rubber multiple puncture seal that permits withdrawal of fluid or blood following aseptic preparation with providone/iodine 10%. Because the circuit remains closed throughout the sampling procedure, not only is blood conserved, but this system also is associated with a low risk of nosocomial infections.[10]

Minimize Blood Volume Removal for Diagnostic Testing

Reducing the volume of blood sent to the laboratory for routine laboratory testing can be accomplished through the use of pediatric tubes. This technique is widely practiced at a variety of tertiary hospitals. In addition, adult-sized tubes manufactured with a reduced vacuum are also available from Becton and Dickenson (Franklin Lakes, NJ). With either type of tube a smaller sample of blood is collected. Either technique minimizes the blood sample withdrawn from the patient and the cost is virtually the same as standard tubes.

At our institution, a retrospective chart review of 100 post-bypass patients revealed that the average patient sacrificed 347 ml of blood for laboratory specimens (including blood gases) over a 7-day hospitalization. After implementing the use of reduced-volume specimen tubes and by reinfusing arterial line discard volumes, this figure decreased to 103 cc for the same time period. This resulted in a savings of 244 cc of blood per patient per hospital stay. This volume savings is similar to the amount of blood in one unit of packed red blood cells, which is approximately 300 cc (Fig. 21.4). Additionally, there is an economic bonus to using the reduced-

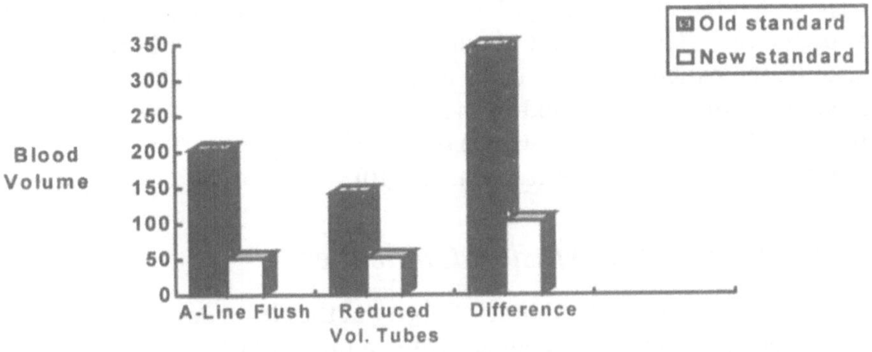

FIGURE 21.4. The difference in blood volume removed after implementing closed arterial line system and reduced volume tubes.

volume tubes. Refuge costs are based on weight, and because the tubes weigh less they are less expensive for hospital disposal.

In summary, nurses and nurse practitioners can contribute to a broad-based blood conservation program through the minimizing of discard volume by removing the absolute minimum amounts of blood for diagnostic testing, by utilizing small-volume or pediatric tubes for laboratory samples, and by using a closed arterial line system that reinfuses discard volume.

Salvaging Postoperative Blood Loss

The autologous transfusion system (ATS) is a technique of reinfusing a patient's blood that has drained from the thoracic or the mediastinal cavities into a Pleurevac collection system. Because this blood is defibrinated and sterile, it can be reinfused without washing or heparinization. This system is reviewed in greater detail in Chapter 19. Contraindications to ATS are (1) pericardial, mediastinal, and pleural infections or malignancies; (2) documented or suspected bacteremia; (3) renal insufficiency/failure, with creatine > 4.0; (4) chest or abdominal trauma with suspected enterocontamination; and (b) interoperative use of fibrin glue.

When using an ATS system it is important to carefully assess the rate of bleeding, starting with the patient's arrival in the intensive care unit. During the first hour and a half, bleeding is assessed in the collection system every 15 minutes. In the second hour it is reviewed every 30 minutes. If the drainage is less than 100 cc of blood, it is then followed hourly. If after the third hour the blood collected is greater than 100 cc,it should be reinfused. If it is less, reinfusion is not mandated.

During reinfusion the collected blood is filtered through a 40-μm aggregate filter. A large gauge (greater than 20) peripheral intravenous site is preferred.[11] The flow rate should be determined by the hemodynamic state of the patient, but 250 cc of blood can usually be infused within 30 minutes. Although the blood in the ATS bag often has a low hematocrit (between 10 and 20) it is a valuable source of homologous blood and poses minimal risk to the patient (see Chapter 10).

Adherence to Transfusion Guidelines

The Department of Cardiothoracic Surgery at the New York Hospital–Cornell Medical Center recently implemented a protocol of postoperative care with specific transfusion guidelines. Observed bleeding parameters and appropriate clinical interventions have been printed on a pocket card and distributed to all members of the cardiothoracic team. These guidelines were formulated after a roundtable discussion among cardiac surgeons, cardiac anesthesiologists, intensive care nurses, and blood bank physicians. The guidelines are listed in Table 21.1.

It has become the primary responsibility of the nursing staff to maintain adherence to the transfusion guidelines. Physicians may have slightly different personal guidelines for the transfusion of red blood cells, fresh frozen plasma (FFP), platelets, and other factors. This is affected by interoperative observations of the patient's heart, the surgeon's attention to hemostasis, his past experience with bleeding, and by other factors such as the fatigue level of the ordering physician, and the time of day. The overworked resident who has just finished closing a case at midnight, once informed that his patient has bled 300 cc in the first hour, is very apt to order six units of platelets and two units of FFP. It often becomes the responsibility of the nurse at the patient's bedside to remind the resident that the initial burst of bleeding usually slows and the coagulation factors should not be given until continued bleeding occurs in the second hour. Most often when a careful, unhurried surgical closure has been completed, early bleeding will stop under the watchful eye of the bedside nurse. Careful adherence to the transfusion guidelines has significantly decreased factor and blood utilization in our intensive care unit over the past 3 years. *Nurse-mandated careful adherence to the transfusion guidelines has become a key component of our blood conservation program.*

Nursing Care of the Bleeding Patient

Nursing care of the bleeding patient is a critical responsibility and may determine the success or failure of a patient's early postoperative course. These patients pose a significant challenge to the nursing staff, and expeditious decision making may be required to avoid hemodynamic compromise.

The first priority is to determine if the source of bleeding is surgical or

TABLE 21.1. Guidelines for postoperative blood transfusion.

Red blood cells
- Transfuse one unit PRBC for Hct <22% or clinically symptomatic anemia.
- All Cell Saver blood remaining from the OR should be reinfused regardless of chest tube output.
- Autotransfusion blood should be reinfused for all eligible patients.

Platelet/FFP/cryoprecipitate
- Treatment of the patient with clinically significant postoperative bleeding
  - Chest tube output > 300 cc in the first postoperative hour (early bleeding)
  - Chest tube output > 100 cc/hr × 3 consecutive hours after the first 2 postoperative hours (delayed bleeding)
  - Chest tube output > 200 cc/hr × 1 hour after the first 2 postoperative hours, except after turning the patient (delayed bleeding)

Treatment protocol
1. Send a stat CBC/PLT and PT/PTT
2. Warm the patient as rapidly as possible to 38°C
3. Maintain systolic BP < 120 mm Hg
4. Increase PEEP to 7.5 or 10 mm Hg, if there are no contraindications
5. Give one dose of protamine if within the postoperative hour (one dose maximum)
6. Order (but do not administer) one round of factors: six units of platelets (preferably single donor) and two units of FFP
7. Amicar 5 g/hr × 1 hr, then 1 g/hr × 5 hr (if patient did not receive aprotinin)
8. DDAVP for patient with history of renal disease and/or bleeding disorder
9. If bleeding continues at the same or higher rate over the next postoperative hour, then give:
   - Platelets: 6 units, preferably single donor
   - FFP: if PT > 15, two units
   - Cryoprecipitate: 10 units after two rounds of factors administered and suspect that a coagulopathic state is cause of bleeding
10. Consider returning to OR for persistent heavy bleeding or rapid increase in the rate of bleeding to control potential surgical source.

FFP, fresh frozen plasma; Hct, hematocrit; PEEP, positive end-expiratory pressure; PRBC, packed red blood cells; PT, prothrombin time; PTT, partial thromboplastin time.

nonsurgical. Surgical bleeding is usually associated with early significant blood loss and usually reflects bleeding from a leaking suture line or a specific anatomical site. Bleeding greater than 300 cc in the first hour, greater than 250 cc in the second hour, and greater than 150 cc thereafter is often surgically correctable. Bleeding at this rate usually mandates a return to the operating room and reexploration.

Nonsurgical bleeding is expected in the patient with significant hypothermia, prolonged cardiopulmonary bypass, and postoperative coagulopathies. The causes of nonsurgical bleeding include heparin rebound, qualitative and quantitative platelet deficiencies, dilutional thrombocytopenia and factor deficiency, local and systemic fibrinolysis, disseminated intravascular coagulation (DIC), and preexisting coagulopathies. Nursing goals in postoperative bleeding include the efficient and prompt rewarming of the patient, the reinfusion of autologous blood retrieved from the operating room, the infusion of warm blood products as defined by the transfusion guidelines, and the implementation of homeostasis-promoting pharmacologic agents. Additional goals include careful attention to the vital signs and the maintenance of hemodynamic output with a cardiac index greater than 2 L/m^2. The systolic blood pressure is maintained between 100 and 120 mm Hg. The institution of positive end-expiratory pressure (PEEP) to levels of 7.5 or 10 mm Hg may be helpful.

Efficient rewarming occurs with the implementation of a forced-air warming device (Bair Hugger, Augustine Medical Corp., Eden Prairie, MN). An airflow sheath is placed over the patient and connected to the warm air generator. A thermal blanket or sheet may be sandwiched on top of the air sheath to weigh it down, and the air temperature is set at 46°C. The mean time needed to reach normothermia in most patients is less than 30 minutes.[12] No complications with the air warming sheath have been encountered. Adequate reversal of heparin should be ensured especially if heparin rebound is suspected. Careful monitoring of the activated clotting time (ACT) in the ICU and additional protamine administration may be required.[1]

Obtaining blood products from the blood bank requires a collaborative effort between ancillary staff and the ICU nurses. The blood bank staff should be informed that a specific patient is bleeding and they may need to recheck compatibility so that the supply is always four units ahead of the patient's requirements.

The transfusion of red blood cells is guided by hematocrit, rate of blood loss, the underlying medical problems of the patient, and the indications of oxygen delivery. The infusion of packed red blood cells will replace twice the hemoglobin as the same volume of whole blood. Hemoglobin will increase about 1 g % per unit of packed red blood cells, and hematocrit rises 2% to 3% per unit depending on the blood volume of the patient. The infusion of red blood cells should be warmed using a conduction blood warming device; at our institution we use a device called Hot Line (Level 1 Technologies, Inc., Rockland, MA). This device warms the blood by surrounding the patient's transfusion line with warm circulating water. The blood temperature reaches 37°C in approximately 4 minutes of exposure to the warm water. The circulating water in the bath is controlled at 40°C and the pump will automatically stop with an audible alarm if the temperature reaches 41°C.[13]

Once the decision to transfuse platelets, FFP, or other factors has been made in accordance with the transfusion guidelines, the factors should usually be given as soon as possible. Single-donor platelets are preferred but are usually not available. We normally recommend six units of platelets be given simultaneously. The platelet count will increase approximately 10,000 units of platelets per square centimeter for each unit transfused divided by the patient's body surface area[14] (six units of platelets in a patient with a body surface of 2 m^2 will result in an increase in platelet count of approximately 30,000 cm^2).

Verifying the patient's postoperative coagulation status is further enhanced by reviewing the prothrombin time (PT), partial thromboplastin time (PTT), and fibrinogen levels. These results are usually available within an hour of the patient's arrival in the ICU and will help guide further factor replacement. Prolongation of the PT and PTT may prompt infusion of FFP. This contains all clotting factors except platelets. Stored at $-30°C$ to preserve factors V and VII, FFP takes 20 minutes to thaw. Low fibrinogen levels may be corrected with cryoprecipitate infusion, which contains factors VII, fibrinogen, and factor XIII.[15]

Initial volume replacement should be accomplished with autologous blood retrieved from the operating room. Often 500 to 1,000 cc of hemoconcentrated blood from the pump is available. This blood is heparinized and usually will require additional protamine administration. Hematocrit of this fluid ranges between 30% and 50% when it has been hemoconcentrated. Further autologous blood from the ATS retrieval system can also be infused. The reinfusion of up to 1,000 cc of mediastinal shed blood has been shown to be safe and effective.[16] Other products that can be used in volume replacement include hespan, albumin, and plasma protein fraction (Plasmanate).

Pharmacologic interventions include the use of protamine sulfate, and amino caproic acid (Amicar), an inhibitor of fibrinolysis. Tranexamic acid (Cyclokapron) is an isomer of amino caproic acid with a 7- to 10-fold increase in inhibitory activity on fibrinolysis. Desmopressin acetate (DDAVP) has been used to help attenuate bleeding, especially in patients with renal insufficiency. Aprotinin, a protease inhibitor, may have a role when administered in high doses before and during cardiopulmonary bypass.[17]

Other interventions that may be initiated by the nursing staff to help minimize bleeding include careful attention to blood pressure. Maintaining the systolic pressure between 100 and 120 mm Hg can be achieved with alpha blockers like nitroprusside. Its immediate action and short half-life make it an ideal choice for the postoperative setting. Its principal action is on the prearteriolar smooth muscle, but it may also cause pulmonary and systemic venous dilatation. The effective circulating volume may be decreased and fluid infusion (preload restoration) may be necessary. Increasing the PEEP to greater than 7.5 mm Hg creates positive intrathoracic pressure and may decrease mediastinal bleeding. The patient must have sufficient cardiac output because the pressure generated by the PEEP is applied to the intrathoracic great veins and the pulmonary vasculature and may reduce venous return.[2]

Conclusion

The critical care nurse plays a pivotal role in the implementation of a blood conservation program. The bedside nurse is the "gatekeeper" for the

TABLE 21.2. How to implement a blood conservation protocol.

Delegate specific individuals to the blood conservation liaisons.
Conduct multidisciplinary meetings among surgeons, anesthesiologists, perfusionists, and nurses to create tailored departmental guidelines that will work for your institution.
Meet with the director of laboratory services to determine the specimen tube manufacturer for the institution. Next, determine what type of analyzer is used; is it automated or manual? How much blood is needed for an accurate specimen?
In-service staff members regarding the actual amount of blood needed for diagnostic testing.
Contact representatives from different manufacturers who make blood sparing arterial line tubing. Ask for samples and conduct your own research project.
Once guidelines and protocols are created; post the information where the staff can review it.
Every 6 months review the transfusion guidelines for the department.

therapeutic interventions that will dictate a patient's care and ultimate survival. The creation of a cardiovascular program's transfusion guidelines should be a collaborative effort involving the same nurses, cardiac anesthesiologists, intensive care physicians and cardiac surgeons. This creative undertaking and the active participation of the nursing staff is mandatory for the successful implementation of a blood conservation program (Table 21.2).

References

1. Jacobs M. Postoperative intensive care of the cardiac surgical patient. CUMC & The New York Society for Thoracic Surgery. Postgraduate course in cardiothoracic surgery. A state of the art review. 1996;3.
2. Dolan J. *Critical Care Nursing. Clinical Management Through the Nursing Process.* Philadelphia: F.A. Davis, 1991.
3. Moreno-Cabral C, Mitchell R, Miller D. *Manual of Postoperative Management in Adult Cardiac Surgery.* Baltimore: Williams & Wilkins, 1988.
4. Garner HM, Fabri P. Iatrogenic anemia. *Am J Surg* 1986;151:362–363.
5. Preusser B, Lash J. Quantifying the minimum discard sample required for accurate arterial blood gases. *Nurs Res* 1989;38(5):277–278.
6. Wallace H. Obtaining reliable plasma glucose and potassium values from intraarterial catheters. *Heart Lung* 1987;1:20–23.
7. Konopad E. Comparison of PT and a PTT values drawn by venipuncture and arterial line using three discard volumes. *Am J Crit Care* 1992;1(3):99.
8. Lopez S, Wheat D. How we draw arterial blood without bleeding the patient. *RN* 1987;50:34–37.
9. Peruzzi WT, Parker MA. A clinical evaluation of a blood conservation device in medical intensive care unit patients. *Crit Care Med* 1993;21:501–506.
10. Crow S. Microbial contamination of arterial infusions used for hemodynamic monitoring. *Infect Control Hosp Epidemiol* 1989;10(12):558.
11. Peterson K. Nursing management of autologous blood transfusion. *Am J Nurs* 1992;15(3):131.
12. Biasi C, Mastropasqua D, et al. Comparison between two postoperative

warming systems in cardiac surgery. Unpublished study, Verona: Oespedale Civile Maggiore Borgo Trento.
13. The New York Hospital Division of Nursing. *Critical Care Practice Manual,* 1993.
14. Alspach J, Williams S. *Core Curriculum for Critical Care Nursing.* 3rd ed. Philadelphia: W.B. Saunders, 1985.
15. Harker LA, Malpass TW, Branson HE, et al. Mechanisms of abnormal bleeding in patients undergoing cardiopulmonary bypass: acquired transient platelet dysfunction associated with selective-granule release. *Blood* 1980;56(5):824.
16. Cosgrove DM, Amiot DM, Meserko JJ. An improved technique for autotransfusion of shed mediastinal blood. *Ann Thorac Surg* 1985;40(5):519.
17. Kirklin JW, Barratt-Boyes BG. *Cardiac Surgery.* 2nd ed. New York: Churchill Livingstone, 1993.
18. Dech Z. Blood conservation in the critically ill. *AACN Clinical Issues in Critical Care Nursing,* 1994;5(2):172–175.
19. Neill R. Blood conservation in the critically ill. *AACN Clinical Issues in Critical Care Nursing* 1994;5(2):172–175.

22
Reoperative Strategies for the Bleeding Cardiovascular Patient

Samuel J. Lang

Although progress in cardiac surgery has been extensive, and mortality rates for most procedures continue to decline, postoperative bleeding has remained a potentially life-threatening complication of heart surgery. Management frequently results in excessive blood product administration and reoperation is necessary in 3% to 5% of all open-heart procedures.[1–3] Excessive bleeding may be the result of inadequate surgical hemostasis, preexisting coagulopathic states, or coagulopathy related to cardiopulmonary bypass.

Whatever the reason for excessive postoperative bleeding, management is complex and the decision to return to the operating room is a difficult one. A fatigued surgeon who is confident that the suture lines were "dry" may be reluctant to return a patient to the OR for exploration. At times the surgeon is the last member of the surgical team to concede that the reexploration is indicated. Supporting the surgeon's reluctance is the knowledge that in over half of reexplorations, no specific bleeding site will be identified. Supporting the concept of every reexploration is the observation that a patient's coagulopathy often resolves after control of a bleeding point on the mammary pedicle or chest wall. Regardless of the etiology of the bleeding, we favor early exploration in an effort to reduce the requirements for blood product administration and, one hopes, lower perioperative morbidity and mortality.

Indications for Reoperation for Bleeding

Mediastinal exploration for bleeding is usually done for excessive blood loss in stable patients or when there is suspicion of tamponade in hemodynamically compromised patients (Fig. 22.1). Fortunately, the majority of patients fall into the former category and have few sequelae. Our criteria for reexploration include 500 ml in the first hour, greater than 250 ml/hr for the first 3 postoperative hours, or a total of 1000 ml during the first 12 postoperative hours.

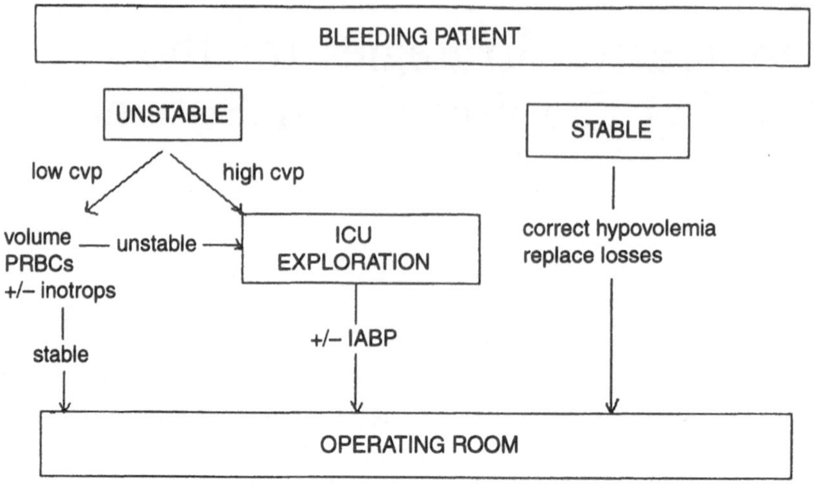

FIGURE 22.1. Algorithm to determine treatment for a bleeding patient.

In pediatric patients we consider >10 ml/kg in 1 hour or >5 ml/kg/hour for 3 consecutive hours to be indications for returning to the OR. Sudden increased drainage from the chest tubes of a patient who has not been bleeding excessively may indicate bleeding from a surgical site and could be considered an indication for reexploration. A chest x-ray showing an obvious mediastinal or pleural collection in the first 24 hours is an indication for reoperation to evacuate the clot and irrigate the chest.

Patients with signs of tamponade require exploration regardless of the amount of chest tube drainage. We consider any patient with hypotension, borderline cardiac output, or unexplained acidosis, in the setting of elevated filling pressures (specifically a [central venous pressure] CVP >20), to have tamponade until proven otherwise. Although echocardiography may be helpful in confirming a diagnosis of tamponade, we have often found emergency echoes misleading and time-consuming. We will not delay returning a patient to the OR while waiting for an echo if the patient's hemodynamic data are diagnostic of tamponade.

Protocol for Transport

Once the decision to return the patient to the OR is made, efforts must concentrate on maintaining patient stability and avoiding delays. As arrangements for the operating room are being made, packed red blood cells (PRBCs), fresh frozen plasma (FFP), and platelets are ordered. Cryoprecipitate is also ordered if we anticipate diffuse bleeding at exploration.

Autotransfusion of shed blood or administration of PRBCs is continued to replace volume losses and to maintain an acceptable hematocrit.

Correction of a low hematocrit may improve bleeding following cardiopulmonary bypass by increasing the blood viscosity and by reducing platelet-mediated bleeding tendencies. Duke[4] first reported in 1910 that the bleeding time was prolonged in anemic patients, independent of the platelet count, and that the abnormality was corrected by transfusion. Subsequent experimental evidence suggest "transport enhancement" of platelets by red cells, and that the extent of platelet deposition on the subendothelial surface is proportional to the hematocrit.[5,6] In addition, it is postulated that adenosine diphosphate (ADP) release by erythrocytes at the site of vessel injury enhances platelet aggregation and formation of the hemostatic plug.[7] Red cell infusion studies have shown that hematocrits of 30 are usually sufficient to correct the bleeding time and there is little further improvement with higher values.[8]

We routinely administer DDAVP, which may be of benefit in patients with excessive bleeding postcardiopulmonary bypass through its effect on von Willebrand factor and the antifibrinolytic agent Amicar (Lederle Laboratories).[9,10] Although hyperfibrinolysis is not the principal cause of postoperative coagulopathy, cardiopulmonary bypass does reduce both fibrinogen and plasminogen levels primarily due to hemodilution.[9]

We do not have a pump standby for routine explorations for postoperative bleeding. However, if there is reason to suspect bleeding from friable aortic suture lines, arteriovenous (AV) groove injuries, or other inaccessible locations, the pump team should be notified and on standby. Rarely, patients will be returned to the OR with uncontrollable bleeding, or requiring internal cardiac massage, and immediate institution of cardiopulmonary bypass will be required for resuscitation.

The majority of bleeding postoperative patients remain stable and can be uneventfully transported to the operating room. Unstable patients must be stabilized prior to transport. Hypovolemia is aggressively treated with volume and red blood cells (RBCs). Vasoconstrictors and/or inotropic support may be necessary until the patient's volume status improves. Profound low cardiac output or severe refractory hypotension in the setting of elevated filling pressures suggest acute tamponade and an emergent exploration in the ICU should be performed. Opening of the inferior portion of the sternotomy incision may relieve the tamponade and allow the patient to be safely transported to the operating room for a more formal exploration. More often, full sternotomy in the ICU will be necessary to allow evacuation of a clot within the pericardium. Exsanguinating hemorrhage or a cardiac arrest in a bleeding patient requires immediate full ICU sternotomy. An obvious source of massive hemorrhage may be temporarily controlled by direct pressure on the bleeding site or placement of sutures. Internal cardiac massage may be necessary until the patient is resuscitated or arrives in the operating room. Insertion of an intraaortic balloon pump may be beneficial or even lifesaving, but could worsen bleeding from aortic suture lines. Although rarely required, emergency ICU sternotomy can be carried out with a low complication rate,[11] and is much preferred over the high-risk transport of an unstable patient.

Intraoperative Protocol

Stable patients undergo a full chin to toes prep, and draping to allow for harvesting of saphenous vein, or insertion of an intraaortic balloon pump (IABP). Pericardial sutures should be placed and the chest should be thoroughly irrigated with removal of all clot. If pleural spaces are open, the chest cavities must be irrigated and evacuated as well.

Every effort should be made to prevent hypothermia in the operating room. The coagulopathy observed in hypothermic patients is in part independent of clotting factor levels, and may result from inhibition of the enzymatic activation necessary for the coagulation cascade.[12,13]

It has also been suggested that hypothermia induces reversible platelet dysfunction by impairing synthesis of platelet thromboxane A_2, a potent platelet aggregating agent.[14] The room temperature should be raised, and blood warmers should be used for intraoperative infusion of cold blood products. The pleural spaces can be filled with warm saline to facilitate rewarming. Rarely, cardiopulmonary bypass for rewarming of a critically ill hypothermic patient could become necessary.

A meticulous search for bleeding points is carried out that includes all cannulation sites, suture lines, and coronary anastomoses. All vein grafts should be circumferentially examined throughout their entire lengths. Special attention should be given to internal mammary artery pedicles and the chest wall mammary bed, as these are common sites for small bleeders. When a coagulopathy is present, specific bleeding points may be obscured by the continuous diffuse hemorrhage. It may be helpful to pack all four quadrants of the chest with dry lap pads, which are then removed one at a time for inspection.

Small bleeding points may be readily controlled with cautery. Larger vessels or side branches off vein grafts or the mammary artery pedicle must be clipped or ligated. Most suture line bleeding points can be controlled by accurately placed sutures on the beating heart. At times the location of bleeding from a distal coronary anastomosis may make placement of hemostatic sutures difficult because of the movement of the heart. Bleeding from aortotomy incisions or left ventricular vent sites may worsen with attempts at repair under arterial pressure. It may be helpful to use a brief period of induced ventricular fibrillation to facilitate precise placement of sutures, or to temporarily reduce the aortic pressure. In extreme circumstances, up to 5 minutes of ventricular fibrillation may be possible without neurologic sequelae if bypass is not available.[15] Some distal coronary anastomotic leaks, for example at the heel of an internal mammary artery graft, are best managed by use of cardiopulmonary bypass and a brief period of aortic cross-clamping. Bleeding related to injuries to the left ventricle, significant leaks in very friable aortic suture lines, and bleeding from the aortic root after valve replacement are best managed using cardiopulmonary bypass and aortic cross clamping. AV groove injuries complicating mitral valve replacement uniformly require bypass, aortic cross-clamping, and usually removal of the valve to attempt repair of the injury.

Rarely, a patient will arrive in the OR with massive bleeding or in cardiac arrest. Resuscitation usually requires immediate heparinization and cannulation of the aorta for cardiopulmonary bypass. Venous return can be established using the pump suckers until cannulation can be accomplished. The nature of the bleeding and the status of the heart will determine the operative strategy and usually the outcome in these difficult cases.

Local application of topical hemostatic agents may sometime be useful in improving hemostasis, and include such products as Oxycel cotton (oxidized cellulose, Becton Dickinson), thrombin-soaked Gelfoam (bovine thrombin, GenTrac), and fibrin glue. The Oxycel cotton adheres to bleeding surfaces and forms an artificial clot on contact with blood. It does not interact with the normal clotting mechanism. Thrombin-soaked Gelfoam promotes clotting by its action on the fibrinogen of the patient's blood at the site of bleeding.

Fibrin glue has had widespread use in Europe, Canada, and Japan, and its effectiveness has been documented in several review articles.[16–19] It has recently been advocated as the ideal operative sealant in cardiovascular surgery.[20] Commercial fibrin glue is not available in the United States, but a satisfactory alternative method involves the simultaneous application of cryoprecipitate and reconstituted topical thrombin (100 u/ml) to bleeding surfaces. The sealant mimics the final state of the coagulation cascade with the conversion of fibrinogen to the monomer fibrin by the action of thrombin. Ionized calcium and factor VIII contribute to the cross-linking of the fibrin into a stable clot. The tensile strength and adhesiveness are proportional to the concentration of fibrinogen. The process is independent of the internal clotting mechanisms and is therefore effective even in the presence of coagulopathy.[20] It does not require a dry surface to adhere. It is biodegradable and may promote local healing.[21] Our experience has been similar to that reported in studies showing fibrin glue to be useful in controlling diffuse oozing, synthetic graft leakage, and needle hole bleeding, but of little value in controlling brisk arterial hemorrhage. We have found it especially useful in patients with severe coagulopathy who undergo reoperation for bleeding. The cryoprecipitate and thrombin are drawn into separate 600-cc syringes and applied to all suture lines and points of diffuse bleeding just prior to sternal closure. There are theoretic risks for transmission of viral infection from single-donor or pooled cryoprecipitate used for glue, but the risk may be less than that of receiving additional blood product if the bleeding is not controlled.

Complete closure of the chest with sternal wiring is routinely carried out. If the patient does not tolerate sternal bone closure, an attempt to close the subcutaneous layer and the skin should be made. In addition to maintaining sterility, we feel that the tissue apposition provided by chest closure is beneficial for hemostasis. If necessary, the chest can be left open, with or without a sternal retractor in place and covered by placement of a Steri-drape. The Steri-drape can be easily removed and replaced if repeat evacuations of the chest are required in the ICU. Delayed sternal closure has been shown to be an effective approach to patients who are too unstable to safely close at the time of exploration.[22,23]

Conclusion

The risk for early repeat sternotomy for bleeding is small. Our experience has been similar to that reported by others in that we have found that stable patients explored early for bleeding have a postoperative course that does not differ significantly from similar patients who don't bleed.[24] Although there have been reports of increased morbidity and mortality with reoperation for excessive bleeding,[25] we feel that the risk is primarily related to the bleeding and not to the sternotomy procedure itself. Bleeding patients are more likely to be unstable, require inotropic support, or sustain injury from end-organ hypoperfusion. The reported incidence of sternal wound infection following resternotomy for bleeding ranges from 0% to 11%.[11,22,23,25] The basic cause of sternal infection is contamination of the surgical wound, which is not procedure specific. The risk of delay in returning the bleeding patient to the operating room far outweighs the risk of reexploration.

References

1. Mills NL. Postoperative hemorrhage after cardiopulmonary bypass. *Ann Thorac Surg* 1982;34:607.
2. Salm T. Two techniques for the control of cardiac bleeding. *Ann Thorac Surg* 1994;57:762–764.
3. Harker L. Bleeding after cardiopulmonary bypass (editorial). *N Engl J Med* 1988;314:1446–1447.
4. Duke W. The relation of blood platelets to hemorrhagic diseases. *JAMA* 1910;60:1185–1192.
5. Turrito V, Baumgartner H. Platelet interactions with subendothelium in a perfusion system: physical role of red blood cells. *Microvasc Res* 1975; 9:335–344.
6. Turrito V, Weiss H. Red blood cells: their dual role in thrombus formation. *Science* 1980;207:541–543.
7. Blajchman M, Bordin J, Bardossy L, et al. The contribution of haematocrit to thrombocytopenic bleeding in experimental animals. *Br J Haematol* 1994; 86:347–350.

8. Anand A, Feffer S. Hematocrit and bleeding time: an update. *South Med J* 1994;87:299–301.
9. Woodman R, Harker L. Bleeding complications associated with cardiopulmonary bypass. *Blood* 1990;76:1680–1697.
10. Salzman E, Weinstein M, Weintraub R, et al. Treatment with desmopressin acetate to reduce blood loss after cardiac surgery. *N Engl J Med* 1986; 314:1402–1406.
11. Kaiser G, Naunheim K, Fiore A, et al. Reoperation in the intensive care unit. *Ann Thorac Surg* 1990;49:903–908.
12. Reed R II, Bracy A Jr, Hudson J, et al. Hypothermia and blood coagulation: dissociation between enzyme activity and clotting factor levels. *Circ Shock* 1990;32:141–152.
13. Valeri C, Hhabbaz K, Khuri S, et al. Effect of skin temperature on platelet function in patients undergoing extracorporeal bypass. *J Thorac Cardiovasc Surg* 1992;104:108–116.
14. Valeri C, Cassidy G, Khuri S, et al. Hypothermia-induced reversible platelet dysfunction. *Ann Surg* 1987;205:175–181.
15. Cooley D. *Techniques in Cardiac Surgery*. 2nd ed. Philadelphia: W.B. Saunders, 1984;4–5.
16. McCarthy P. Fibrin glue in cardiothoracic surgery. *Transf Med Rev* 1993; 7:173–179.
17. Borst H, Haverich A, Walterbusch G, et al. Fibrin adhesive: an important hemostatic adjunct in cardiovascular operations. *J Thorac Cardiovasc Surg* 1982;84:548–553.
18. Jessen C, Sharma P. Use of fibrin glue in thoracic surgery. *Ann Thorac Surg* 1985;39:521–524.
19. Tawes R, Sydorak G, DuVall T. Autologous fibrin glue: the last step in operative hemostasis. *Am J Surg* 1994;168:120–122.
20. Gibble J, Ness P. Fibrin glue: the perfect operative sealant? *Transfusion* 1990;30:741–747.
21. Sierra DH. Fibrin sealant adhesive systems: a review of their chemistry, material properties and clinical applications. *J Biomat Appl* 1993;7:309–352.
22. Johnson J, Gundersen E, Stickney I, et al. Selective approach to sternal closure after exploration for hemorrhage following coronary artery bypass. *Ann Thorac Surg* 1990;49:771–774.
23. Bouboulis N, Rivas J, Juo J, et al. Packing the chest: a useful technique for intractable bleeding after open heart operation. *Ann Thorac Surg* 1994; 57:856–861.
24. Hill J, Rodvien R, Mielke C. Bleeding and hemorrhagic complications. In: Litwak R, Jurado R, eds. *Care of the Cardiac Surgical Patient*. Norwalk, CT: Appleton-Century-Crofts, 1982;380–381.
25. Unsworth-White M, Herriot A, Valencia O, et al. Resternotomy for bleeding after cardiac operation: a marker for increased morbidity and mortality. *Ann Thorac Surg* 1995;59:664–667.

23
Blood Transfusion Reaction, Diagnosis, and Treatment

KATHLEEN A. LEONARD

Adverse reactions to blood transfusions occur with 0.5% to 4% of all transfusions. The exact incidence varies by patient population, but in general transfusion reactions are more common in multiply transfused patients. In Table 23.1 reactions are grouped by the approximate frequency of occurrence. The two most common reactions, febrile nonhemolytic and urticarial, are also the most benign. Potentially life-threatening acute transfusion reactions, including acute hemolysis, anaphylaxis, bacterially contaminated units causing sepsis, and transfusion-related acute lung injury (TRALI), are far more unusual.[1–3]

Although there are major exceptions, in general, severe and life-threatening reactions are most likely to occur quickly, often within 50 ml of starting a transfusion. Whenever possible, the first 15 ml should be infused slowly, at a rate on the order of 1 ml per minute for an average 70-kg adult. If there is any doubt as to whether a clinical sign or symptom is a manifestation of a transfusion reaction, the transfusion should be stopped immediately.

Transfusion reactions, being diverse in etiology and clinical presentation, do not lend themselves readily to simple classification. One practical classification system divides the disorders based on time of clinical presentation, whether acute or delayed, as shown in Table 23.2. This chapter discusses each type of reaction in terms of its pathophysiology, clinical manifestations, diagnosis, and management, with an emphasis on acute reactions likely to be seen in the perioperative period. Where applicable, preventive measures are included. Before covering each reaction type in detail, the general approach to evaluation of transfusion reactions is reviewed.

General Approach to the Patient

Overview

The standard transfusion reaction evaluation sent to the blood bank is made up of tests that primarily rule out an acute hemolytic reaction. It does not

TABLE 23.1. Transfusion reactions: risk per unit transfused.

Common	
Febrile nonhemolytic	1–3/100
Urticarial	1–3/100
Unusual	
Delayed hemolytic	1/1700
Transfusion-related acute lung injury	1/5000
Acute hemolytic	1/12,000–1/19,000
Rare	
Anaphylactic	
Sepsis/bacterially contaminated unit	
Transfusion-associated graft-versus-host disease	

address the other acute life-threatening reactions: anaphylaxis, bacterially contaminated units causing sepsis, or transfusion-related acute lung injury. For these reactions, there are several other tests that may need to be pursued depending on the initial transfusion reaction evaluation results and the clinical picture. Additional testing will often be pursued only if the blood bank is aware of the clinical situation and the exact reaction manifestations; hence, the importance of communication on the patient status. This is especially applicable for a negative reaction report in a patient for whom the clinical impression is that a serious transfusion reaction took place.

Clinical Manifestation and Diagnosis

Conscious Patients

Table 23.3 lists the wide variety of possible signs and symptoms that may indicate the occurrence of an acute hemolytic transfusion reaction (AHTR).

TABLE 23.2. Transfusion reactions: acute and delayed.

Acute reactions: occur during transfusion, or up to 4 hours posttransfusion
Acute hemolytic
Transfusion-related acute lung injury
Anaphylactic/immediate generalized reactions grade II–IV
Bacterial contamination/sepsis
Febrile nonhemolytic
Urticarial
Mimics of AHTR: thermal, mechanical, or osmotic hemolysis
Volume overload
Delayed reactions: occur days to weeks posttransfusion
Delayed hemolytic
Transfusion-associated graft-versus-host disease
Posttransfusion purpura
Alloimmunization to erythrocyte, leukocyte, or platelet antigens

TABLE 23.3. Clinical manifestations of major acute hemolytic transfusion reactions.

Fever	With or without chills
Subjective complaints	Dyspnea
	Pain in back, chest, or IV site
	Restlessness
	Nausea
	Flushing
	Malaise
	Feeling of impending doom
Change in vital signs	Tachypnea
	Tachycardia
	Hypotension/shock
	Oliguria/anuria with renal failure
Bleeding/hemolysis	Generalized bleeding
	Disseminated intravascular coagulation
	Hemoglobinuria/hemoglobinemia
Lab test findings	Direct Coombs' positive (ABO/alloantibody incompatibility)
	Indirect Coombs' positive (alloantibody incompatibility)
	Total bilirubin, indirect bilirubin elevated
	Lactage dehydrogenase elevated
	Haptoglobin reduced or absent

Most of these clinical manifestations of an AHTR are relatively nonspecific and could be due to a number of other factors, particularly in an acutely ill patient in the perioperative period. There is also considerable overlap with other severe transfusion reactions, including anaphylaxis, TRALI reactions, and sepsis from a contaminated blood unit. On a purely statistical basis, the vast majority of patients who develop a fever and/or chills during transfusion are found to have a febrile, nonhemolytic transfusion reaction. Most patients who develop mild dyspnea, especially in the elderly population, have mild volume overload. In an unstable patient, hypotension may be due to the underlying clinical condition. However, there is no way to be certain that the fever, or any of the other clinical manifestations on the list, do not represent the early signs of acute hemolysis without stopping the transfusion and sending of a transfusion reaction workup. Despite lists of clinical manifestations signifying a potential reaction, there is no substitute for direct patient evaluation and good clinical judgment. In a patient febrile at baseline, prior to transfusion, another fever spike may or may not be related to the blood products being given. Although strictly speaking stopping the transfusion is the safest approach, that is not always clinically practical and a firsthand evaluation of the patient is necessary.[4]

Anesthetized or Obtunded Patients

In the anesthetized patient, subjective symptoms cannot be assessed, and fever, the most common presenting sign of a true AHTR, may be masked. Development of hemoglobinuria, otherwise unexplained hypotension, and bleeding at line sites are the three findings most commonly used as markers of serious reactions in this setting. Diagnosis depends on a high index of suspicion following detection of any of these findings. Many of the same cautions also apply to the detection of transfusion reactions in neonates.[5–7]

Differential Diagnosis of Common Presenting Signs and Symptoms

Table 23.4 lists some of the more common signs of serious transfusion reactions, along with a differential diagnosis. This list is not meant to be comprehensive, but illustrates the overlapping nature of reaction manifestations and the importance of clinical evaluation and appropriate laboratory testing.

Immediate Management Issues

Table 23.5 lists the initial steps to take in the event a patient develops any signs or symptoms that clinically might represent a transfusion reaction. With the exception of simple urticaria, for any other manifestation the transfusion should be stopped. For urticaria, it is almost universally considered acceptable medical practice to interrupt the transfusion, admin-

TABLE 23.4. Acute tranfusion reactions: differential diagnosis.

Transfusion should be discontinued	
Fever/chills	Acute hemolytic transfusion reaction
	Sepsis/bacterially contaminated blood unit
	Febrile, nonhemolytic transfusion reaction
	Transfusion-related acute lung injury (but not anaphylaxis/systemic allergic)
Dyspnea	Transfusion-related acute lung injury
	Acute hemolytic transfusion reaction
	Sepsis/bacterially contaminated blood unit
	Anaphylaxis/systemic allergic
	Volume overload
	Febrile, nonhemolytic transfusion reaction
Dyspnea, delayed	Transfusion-related acute lung injury
Hemoglubinuria	Acute hemolytic transfusion reaction
	Sepsis/bacterially contaminated blood unit
	In vitro hemolysis: thermal, oncotic or mechanical lysis
Hypotension	Anaphylaxis/systemic allergic
	Sepsis/bacterially contaminated blood unit
	Acute hemolytic transfusion reaction
	Transfusion-related acute lung injury
Nausea/gastrointestinal distress	Acute hemolytic transfusion reaction
	Sepsis/bacterially contaminated blood unit
	Anaphylaxis/systemic allergic
Transfusion may be interrupted for treatment with antihistamine	
Urticaria, pruritus	Urticarial reaction

ister antihistamines intravenously, and continue the transfusion with close observation of the patient. Also, at most institutions, for urticarial reactions no samples are drawn and transfusion reaction testing is not done.

Otherwise, following any reaction, the transfusion should be stopped immediately, clamping off the blood line at the infusion hub. Intravenous access should be maintained at all times, by replacing the tubing setup or starting a new line. Particularly when the presenting signs and symptoms indicate a serious reaction (profound hypotension or dyspnea, hemoglobinuria, or unexplained bleeding at line sites), it is critical that no additional blood be infused; fatal reactions have been reported following infusion of as little as 30 ml of blood.[8] A quick check of the patient identity and the information on the blood bag and paperwork should be performed at the bedside, to confirm that the unit was not given to the wrong patient.

Acute patient management depends on the individual situation and clinical manifestations. Pending results of diagnostic testing, it may be unclear exactly which type of catastrophic reaction is occurring, and broad-based empiric therapy is reasonable. This might include aggressive hydration with normal saline and pressor support together with renal dose dopamine to maximize renal blood flow for fulminant hypotension, starting antibiotics to cover for sepsis in a patient who appears to develop fulminant septic shock, or epinephrine and corticosteroids for clinically apparent anaphylaxis. Continuous monitoring; frequent lab testing to monitor for acidosis, renal insufficiency, and coagulopathy; serial urine examination to monitor for hemoglobinuria; and pressor and ventilatory support as needed are all important considerations.

Lab Testing: Transfusion Reaction Evaluation

Generally, the blood bank's main lab should be notified by telephone. The purpose of this notification is to prevent delays in therapy; if the reaction workup is delayed in transit, or sent to the wrong lab, there can be follow-up prior to an urgent request for additional blood. As soon as is practical given the patient condition, the transfusion reaction workup should be sent. The exact protocol may vary by institution, but generally involves collecting both a clotted and an ethylenediaminetetraacetic acid (EDTA)-preserved blood sample, and a urine sample. The samples, together with some type of written description of the reaction, are sent to the blood bank. In addition, for all blood products given within the past 4 hours, the empty blood bags (numbered in the order of transfusion, indicating which was infusing at the time of reaction) should be sent to the blood bank. It may not always be feasible to retrieve already discarded blood bags, but this is critical if the reaction is suspected to be due to a sepsis/bacterial contamination type of event. For this reaction, it is the actual remaining blood component in the bag that is needed for evaluation and definitive testing with gram stain and culture.

TABLE 23.5. Management of acute transfusion reactions.

Reaction type	Signs/symptoms	Transfusion reaction workup	Other diagnostic testing	Management
Acute hemolytic	Fever/chills Dyspnea Pain Hemoglobinuria Nausea/vomiting Hypotension DIC Renal failure Bleeding (See Table 23.3)	Positive direct Coombs', due to red cell sensitization with incompatible antibody Positive for free hemoglobin in plasma/urine, with intravascular hemolysis Positive for clerical error, if patient was given incorrect unit blood	Total/indirect bilirubin LDH Haptoglobin Plasma free hemoglobin BUN/creatinine PT/PTT Urinalysis	1. Consider nephrology/hematology consultation 2. Supportive therapy as indicated: IV hydration Furosemide Renal dose dopamine Vasopressor Oxygen/ventilatory support Treatment for DIC 3. Discuss further transfusion needs with blood bank attending
In vitro hemolysis: thermal, oncotic damage	Hemoglobinuria Hemoglobinemia May resemble AHTR on occasion	Positive for hemolysis, due to red cell destruction in the blood bag Negative direct Coombs' Negative for clercial error	Total/indirect bilirubin LDH Haptoglobin Plasma free hemoglobin BUN/creatinine PT/PTT Urinalysis	As above: 1. Consider nephrology/hematology consultation 2. Supportive therapy as indicated: IV hydration Furosemide
Transfusion-related acute lung injury	Dyspnea Tachycardia Hypoxemia Fever Hypotension	Negative	Chest x-ray Arterial blood gas Leukocyte antibody testing on donor blood and patient	1. Supplemental oxygen 2. Pulse oximetry 3. Ventilatory support as needed 4. Leuko-reduced red cells and platelets, at least until acute episode resolves

Anaphylaxis	Hypotension Flushing, rash Nausea/vomiting Dyspnea (no fever)	Negative	Quantitative IgA level on pretransfusion specimen Anti-IgA	1. Epinephrine 2. Corticosteroids 3. IV fluids, vasopressor support 4. Discuss further transfusion needs with blood bank attending; (IgA deficient; WRBC or FTC) 5. Consider premedication regimen
Sepsis/bacterially contaminated unit	High fever/chills Hypotension Dyspnea Nausea/vomiting Hemoglobinuria DIC	Negative Hemolysis may be seen with contaminated red cell unit	Gram stain of remaining blood component Culture of remaining blood component Patient blood cultures	1. Supportive therapy as indicated: Broad-spectrum antibiotics IV hydration Vasopressor support Oxygen/intubation Treatment for DIC 2. Further transfusion with standard blood products
Febrile, nonhemolytic	Fever/chills Dyspnea Headache Myalgia Malaise	Negative		1. Further transfusions with standard blood products 2. Premedicate for future transfusions with antipyretics 3. If recurrent, leuko-reduced products

Management procedure:

1. Stop transfusion. Maintain IV access: change IV tubing or place new line.
2. Call blood bank to report reaction. Draw posttransfusion specimens and send to blood bank along with remaining blood product: clotted sample, EDTA sample, urine.
3. Further transfusions should generally be delayed until transfusion reaction workup results are known. If urgent transfusion is needed, discuss with blood bank's attending physician; use O negative red cells and AB plasma.

BUN, blood urea nitrogen; DIC, disseminated intravascular coagulation; EDTA, ethylenediaminetetraacetic acid; typically lavender-top tube; FTC, frozen, thawed (deglycerolized) red cells; IV, intravenous; LDH, lactate dehydrogenase; PT/PTT, prothrombin time/partial thromboplastin time; WRBC, washed red blood cells.

The blood bank lab can quickly rule out an acute hemolytic transfusion reaction by performing three procedures on a stat basis. First, a record check is done to look for evidence of a clerical error: all labels, blood bags, and blood tags are examined for correct identification and assignment to the proper patient. Second, the patient's posttransfusion samples are examined for evidence of hemolysis, looking for free hemoglobin in serum and/or urine. Third, testing is done to check for evidence of serologic incompatibility. Pretransfusion testing is repeated, but now done in parallel with the posttransfusion patient sample. The exact tests done may vary by institution, but at a minimum includes a direct Coombs' test to check for red cell sensitization by incompatible antibodies. If there are any testing irregularities, then additional testing would include repeat ABO/Rh typing of the patient and the blood units administered, the patient antibody screen, and the cross-match.

If all three components of the transfusion reaction evaluation are negative, it is safe to assume that an AHTR has not occurred. In the sections that follow, specific diagnostic tests for each type of reaction is discussed. Briefly, for a suspected sepsis reaction due to a bacterially contaminated unit, a gram stain and culture of the remaining blood from the blood bag must be done. Blood cultures should be done on the patient as well. For a suspected anaphylactic reaction, immunoglobulin A (IgA) deficiency should be ruled out. For a suspected TRALI/pulmonary reaction, testing for leukocyte antibodies should be done on the donor blood, as well as the patient.

Decisions Regarding Further Transfusions

Generally, no additional red cells should be transfused until a new posttransfusion sample has been drawn and an AHTR due to red cell incompatibility is ruled out with blood bank testing. The reason for this delay, usually on the order of 20 to 30 minutes, is that any units cross-matched from the initial sample may be just as incompatible as the unit that caused the reaction, and may worsen the clinical situation. If there is a desperate clinical need for transfusion before a transfusion reaction workup is completed, this should be discussed with the blood bank's attending physician. In this situation, O negative red cells and AB plasma products may be given under close observation of the patient. It is worth keeping in mind that if the reaction was an AHTR due to a red cell alloantibody even with use of O negative red cells, the reaction may recur with serious adverse consequences. O negative red cells are the universal donor, and will satisfy ABO compatibility requirements, but if the patient has an alloantibody, then red cells negative for the alloantigen would have to be given to avoid hemolysis.

Once an AHTR has been ruled out, with a few exceptions, it is safe to give additional blood products immediately. For patients who have had an urticarial or benign febrile reaction, transfusion can be given immediately, with premedication with antihistamine or acetaminophen. There is no need to delay further transfusion following a sepsis reaction due to a bacterially contaminated blood product, as this reaction is due to infection of an individual unit of blood, and will not be seen with additional transfusions given. For TRALI-type reactions with severe pulmonary manifestations, there is also no need to delay further transfusion, but it would be prudent to request filtered, leuko-reduced blood products at least until leukocyte antibody testing can be performed. The vast majority of TRALIs are due to a single blood component taken from a donor with large quantities of white cell antibody, and will not be seen with other units of blood. Rarely, TRALI is due to a patient having large quantities of white cell antibody,and in this setting leuko-reduced blood products should be used.

For patients who have had a severe reaction with anaphylaxis or fulminant hypotension without fever, the decision to transfuse again is somewhat more difficult and there are a few points to keep in mind. Hypotensive reactions (immediate generalized reactions grades II to III) are often idiosyncratic, of unknown etiology, and will happen only once to a patient even if multiply transfused. In these patients, future transfusions will not be a problem and should not be delayed. Immediately following such a reaction, however, there is no way to predict how a patient will react to the next transfusion. Obviously, the patient should receive additional blood products only if necessary, and should be observed closely during the transfusion. This is less of a dilemma for a patient in the operating room or intensive care unit, but for a patient in a nonmonitored setting, transfer should be considered. Consideration should also be given to allergy premedication regimen including corticosteroids and antihistamines. Plasma-poor red cell products (washed platelets and washed or frozen-thawed red cells) may help prevent recurrent allergic reactions, and fresh-frozen plasma should be avoided if possible. At most hospitals, plasma-poor products will take several hours to prepare or obtain from a blood center, and the decision to delay transfusion or proceed with premedication and monitoring is a judgment call. Although rare, if the reaction was due to anaphylaxis in an IgA-deficient patient, any standard blood product would cause a second reaction. IgA negative products or frozen-thawed red cells would have to be provided, as discussed below in the description of anaphylaxis

Finally, it is worth keeping in mind that identification errors leading to true hemolytic transfusion reactions may involve two patients, if type and cross-match samples were switched by the phlebotomist. Until the situation is clarified, caution should be used in transfusing other patients in the same patient care unit.

Diagnostic Lab Testing for Hemolysis

Red Cell Antigens and Antibodies

The red cell membrane contains several hundred different red cell antigens, the presence of which is genetically determined. Blood group systems are comprised of closely related blood group antigens, the most familiar being the AB and Rh systems. Other examples of blood group antigen systems include Kell, Kidd, and Duffy, which are important in AHTR and delayed hemolytic transfusion reactions due to alloantibody reactions. A limited number of the 400 red cell antigens are involved in hemolytic reactions.

Red cell antibodies may be classified as naturally occurring, alloantibody, or autoantibody. The naturally occurring antibodies anti-A and anti-B develop during the first 6 to 12 months of life, and are directed against the red cell antigens not present on the red cells. Type AB individuals have no naturally occurring antibodies, and type O individuals have both anti-A and anti-B. Red cell antigens and naturally occurring antibodies provide the basis for blood typing procedures.

Alloantibodies are circulating antibodies present in plasma, produced in response to foreign red cell alloantigens introduced into the circulation by either blood transfusion or pregnancy, such as when an Rh(D) negative mother produces anti-D during pregnancy with an Rh(D) positive fetus. Antibody formation usually begins 2 to 4 weeks after transfusion. The development of alloimmunization is unpredictable. Some patients never develop alloantibodies, while others quickly develop multiple antibodies. The incidence of red cell alloimmunization is approximately 1% overall, but varies by patient population and can be as high as 20% in some multiply transfused groups.[9] These antibodies are directed against specific red cell antigens, and the specificity of such antibodies can be determined by serologic testing with commercial panels of red cells of known antigenic type. Alloantibodies are detected with the antibody screen, also referred to as the indirect Coombs' or indirect antiglobulin test, routinely performed as part of the type and screen or type and cross procedure. If detected in pretransfusion testing, appropriate antigen negative blood is provided by the blood bank and there are no clinical consequences to having red cell antibodies. Otherwise, as discussed previously, red cell alloantibodies may play a role in acute or delayed hemolytic transfusion reactions or hemolytic disease of the newborn.

Types of Hemolysis

Hemolysis may be intravascular or extravascular. Intravascular hemolysis, in which red cells are rapidly destroyed in the circulation, occurs in the setting of red cell antibodies capable of complement fixation, typically those in the ABO system and certain alloantibodies such as those of the Kidd (Jk^a, Jk^b) and Duffy (Fy^a, Fy^b) blood groups. Extravascular hemolysis, in which sensitized red cells are destroyed more slowly by the reticuloendothelial system of the spleen and liver, is seen with antibodies that do not fix complement, such as those of the Rh group (D, C, c, E, e).[10]

Lab Tests for Hemolysis

Several serum, plasma and urine tests are helpful in confirming the presence of hemolysis, by providing evidence of hemoglobin catabolism. Lab test results vary, depending on the site of hemolysis, the rate of hemolysis, and the amount of blood destroyed.

With intravascular and extravascular hemolysis, serum levels of both the released red cell enzymes lactate dehydrogenase (LDH) and serum glutamate oxaloacetate transaminase (SGOT), and the metabolic product of released hemoglobin, unconjugated bilirubin, are often elevated, usually peaking 5 to 8 hours after an acute event. The degree of elevation is variable, particularly with extravascular hemolysis. With both intravascular and extravascular hemolysis, in the absence of hepatobiliary disease, serum levels of conjugated or direct bilirubin are normal. Additionally, because the unconjugated bilirubin circulates bound to albumin, and cannot be filtered through the glomeruli, even with severe intravascular hemolysis bilirubin is not present in the urine, a helpful differential diagnostic finding.[11,12]

Intravascular Hemolysis

With intravascular hemolysis, hemoglobin is released into plasma, causing hemoglobinemia. The free hemoglobin is bound by haptoglobin, an α_2-globulin. The haptoglobin-hemoglobin complex is rapidly cleared by the liver reticuloendothelial system. With significant hemolysis, haptoglobin synthesis in the liver lags behind haptoglobin clearance, and haptoglobin levels fall and may become undetectable. Intravascular lysis of as little as 20 ml of whole blood or 10 ml of packed red cells may decrease the serum haptoglobin level significantly. Haptoglobin is an acute-phase reactant protein; very high levels seen with stress states may mask increased hemoglobin binding in hemolysis, and may not be diagnostically helpful. Conversely, extremely low levels may be present with severe liver disease, and are not diagnostically helpful.[13]

When haptoglobin levels are depleted, hemoglobin may be visible in the plasma, serum, and urine. Even with severe intravascular hemolysis, hemoglobinemia may be present only transiently, and urine hemoglobin and urine hemosiderin tests may be diagnostically helpful after an acute episode. At plasma hemoglobin levels 20 ml/dl, the plasma is amber in color; at levels of 50 to 100 mg/dl it is reddish brown; and at levels above 200 mg/dl plasma is cherry red. If the hemoglobinemia is present for more than 1 hour, free hemoglobin will be oxidized to methemoglobin, and methem albumin, with a characteristic brown color, will appear. Free plasma hemoglobin will be filtered by glomeruli, absorbed by the cells of the renal tubule, and metabolized to hemosiderin. Tubular epithelium is gradually sloughed off, and urine hemosiderin can be detected for up to 5 to 10 days following hemolysis by staining the urinary sediment with a Prussian blue dye, and noting intracellular hemosiderin granules. After haptoglobin stores are depleted, and the tubular cells have been saturated by hemoglobin, free urinary hemoglobin is detectable. Hemoglobinuria, like hematuria, is generally visible as red or cola-colored urine. Hemoglobinuria can be distinguished from hematuria by the absence of intact red cells on urinalysis.[11–13]

Extravascular Hemolysis

With extravascular hemolysis, there generally is no hemoglobinemia, hemoglobinuria, or urine hemosiderinuria. The affected red cells are removed from the circulation by the liver and spleen, and destroyed in situ. Although no significant hemoglobin is released directly into the circulation, haptoglobin levels may be reduced, particularly with ongoing hemolysis. With severe extravascular hemolysis, plasma hemoglobin levels may be minimally elevated.[11]

Acute Transfusion Reactions

Acute Hemolytic Transfusion Reactions

Pathophysiology

AHTRs occur when incompatible red cell units are transfused in the setting of a preformed antibody. Most commonly, transfusion of ABO-incompatible blood, e.g., giving A blood to an O patient (with anti-A) is seen. Less common is AHTR due to alloantibody in patient plasma reacting with corresponding antigen or donor red cells. The most severe AHTRs are generally seen with ABO incompatibility, due to complement fixation resulting in intravascular hemolysis.[14]

True acute hemolytic transfusion reactions are uncommon, but the exact incidence is unclear. A large retrospective study at the Mayo Clinic showed one reaction for every 11,167 transfusions given. Similar results were found in a summary of reported incidents by the New York State Department of Health, with a rate of between 1 in 12,000 and 1 in 18,000 units transfused. Statistically, there is a female preponderance, largely due to sensitization during pregnancy and the presence of preformed alloantibodies. The fatality rate of AHTR is 17%, mostly in cases of ABO incompatibility. The overall risk of fatal AHTR appears to be low, with 158 cases reported to the Food and Drug Administration (FDA) in over 100 million transfusions given during a 10-year period, but it is likely that the true number is underreported.[8,15–19]

Clinical Manifestations

Table 23.3 lists the wide variety of possible signs and symptoms that may indicate the occurrence of an AHTR. AHTR is among the most dreaded of transfusion reactions, as it can result in disseminated intravascular coagulation (DIC), acute and chronic renal failure, and death. Fatal reactions have been noted to occur after transfusion of as few as 30 ml of blood. Clinically, the most common manifestations of AHTR are fever, chills, back pain, and dyspnea, followed by hemoglobinuria, hypotension/shock, and possibly DIC and renal failure. In the anesthetized, comatose or severely ill intubated patient, many of the signs and symptoms may be obscured, and the diagnosis depends on a high index of suspicion following detection of otherwise unexplained hypotension, hemoglobinuria, or bleeding at line sites.[8,20] The pathophysiology behind the multisystem manifestations of a major AHTR is complex, mediated by direct or indirect activation of a number of interrelated systems by the antigen-antibody complexes formed due to the red cell incompatibility. These systems include the kinin system, complement system, and coagulation cascade along with cytokine mediators. This topic has recently been reviewed in detail.[21]

Not all true AHTRs have such dramatic presentations; AHTRs have been categorized as major, minor, or insignificant in clinical severity. Major AHTRs generally are seen with intravascular hemolysis, in the setting of complement fixing antibodies, such as anti-A and anti-Jk^a. In addition to the manifestations listed above, major AHTRs may also include nausea, malaise, a feeling of impending doom, generalized bleeding, or cardiac arrest. In contrast, a minor AHTR is usually seen with extravascular hemolysis, caused by antibodies not capable of complement fixation. Minor AHTRs may manifest with only a falling hematocrit or a failure to increase the hematocrit posttransfusion, serologic evidence of incompatibility, and lab abnormalities indicative of hemolysis with an elevated LDH and bilirubin. Intermittent fever may be present, but generally there is no pain, and no significant change in blood pressure, heart rate, or respiratory rate. The patient may note increasing fatigue, as the transfused red cells are destroyed and the hematocrit falls. Along with a rising bilirubin level, jaundice/icterus may result.

Insignificant AHTRs, which may occur even with ABO-incompatible blood, are among the most puzzling and difficult to explain. Occasionally an AHTR occurs with few, if any, signs or symptoms. Possible explanations are related to the quantity and binding avidity of the antibody present, which may be reduced in elderly patients, and the amount of red cells given. In other rare instances, massive hemoglobinemia and hemoglobinuria occur, without other symptoms or sequelae, and extensive serologic workup fails to reveal any evidence of detectable antibodies. Red cell survival studies demonstrate rapid hemolysis of red cells with certain antigen compositions, typically in the Rh group.[15,20,22–27]

Laboratory Diagnosis and Evaluation

For major AHTR, laboratory findings indicate massive intravascular hemolysis, with hemoglobinemia and hemoglobinuria, with peak total bilirubin and LDH values usually occurring 5 to 8 hours posttransfusion. The peripheral smear may show spherocytosis. Evidence of DIC and thrombocytopenia may be noted as well. For a minor AHTR, lab findings will generally not show evidence of intravascular hemolysis or DIC but will otherwise be similar.

Serologic investigation includes a direct Coombs' test, which is usually positive as residual surviving red cells are coated by the offending antibody. For ABO incompatibility, the direct Coombs' is positive because of either anti-A or anti-B, and for alloantibody incompatibility, the direct Coombs' test is positive because of the corresponding alloantibody. Rarely, all transfused incompatible red cells may be almost immediately destroyed, and the direct Coombs' test will be negative. For alloantibody incompatibility, in addition to the positive direct Coombs' test, the indirect Coombs' test or antibody screen is also positive, revealing evidence of the circulating alloantibody.

Management and Prevention

The immediate management is the same as that described above for any serious reaction—stopping the transfusion as soon as possible, sending a reaction workup, and aggressive patient management with continuous monitoring. In discontinuing the transfusion, the entire tubing set should be replaced, without removing the catheter, so that venous access is maintained at all times but no additional blood is infused.[28] The patient identity and the patient information on the blood bag and paperwork should be performed at the bedside, to confirm that the unit was not given to the wrong patient.

Treatment of an acute hemolytic transfusion reaction, or any case of massive intravascular hemolysis, is largely supportive, and based on demonstrated toxicity, whether renal, hemodynamic, hematologic, or pulmonary. Due to the rarity of AHTR, few individuals have extensive experience with management of such patients, and there have been no controlled studies to compare treatment regimens. Early consultation with the nephrology and hematology departments may be helpful. Emphasis should be placed on maintaining renal blood flow and urine output by hydration with normal saline, along with renal dose dopamine and furosemide. DIC should be treated with platelets and plasma as needed. Heparin has been recommended for posttransfusion DIC, but this remains controversial. Mannitol is no longer recommended for diuresis.[21,28]

It is important that no additional red cell products be transfused until a new posttransfusion sample has been drawn and an AHTR is ruled out. The reason for this delay, usually on the order of 20 to 30 minutes, is that any units cross-matched from the initial sample may be just as incompatible as the unit that caused the reaction, and may worsen the clinical situation. As noted above (see Decisions Regarding Further Transfusion), if there is a desperate clinical need for transfusion, this should be discussed with the blood bank's attending physician. In this situation, O negative red cells and AB plasma products may be given under close observation of the patient. It is worth keeping in mind that if the reaction was due to a red cell alloantibody, even with use of O negative red cells, the reaction may recur with serious adverse consequences. O negative red cells are the universal donor, and they satisfy ABO compatibility requirements, but if the patient has an alloantibody, then red cells negative for the alloantigen would have to be given to avoid hemolysis. Finally, it is worth keeping in mind that identification errors leading to ABO hemolytic transfusion reactions may involve two patients if type and cross-match samples were switched. Until the situation is clarified, use caution in transfusing other patients in the same patient care unit.

In terms of prevention, avoiding errors in identifying the cross-match sample and the patient will prevent the vast majority of AHTR. Proprietary systems, to provide an additional level of security in verifying blood unit and patient identification, are available.[29]

Although unusual, it should be noted that acute intravascular hemolysis has also occurred following transfusion with ABO incompatible platelets, usually due to the presence of high titer anti-A present in the plasma. Removal of most of the plasma from such out-of-group platelet transfusions minimizes the risk of such a reaction.[30-32]

Mimics of AHTR: In Vitro Hemolysis Due to Thermal or Oncotic Damage to Red Cells

Pathophysiology

Red cells can be hemolyzed within the blood bag itself, giving rise to what clinically appears to be a true acute hemolytic transfusion reaction, but with the standard transfusion reaction workup being completely negative. This in vitro hemolysis may be oncotic or thermal in etiology, resulting in the infusion of large quantities of free hemoglobin into the circulation.

Although uncommon overall, there are multiple different reported causes of this type of event. Thermal mishaps are the most common, and include many instances of improper blood warming, due to malfunctioning conventional heat transfer blood warmers, water baths, and microwave blood warmers. Frozen red cells, improperly processed by blood centers, as well as the accidental freezing of liquid whole blood or packed red cells also have caused severe red cell destruction with subsequent acute renal failure. Accidental freezing has usually been the result of storing units of packed cells in standard refrigerators used for medications, where the temperature can cycle below 0°C, causing red cell lysis. Oncotic causes of in vitro hemolysis are less common, usually due to administration of packed cells with hypotonic solutions such as 5% dextrose or 0.45% half-normal saline, which can cause a clinical picture of an acute hemolytic transfusion reaction.[33–43]

Clinical Manifestations, Laboratory Diagnosis, and Evaluation

Signs and symptoms may mimic an acute hemolytic transfusion, with severe symptoms and renal insufficiency, but more commonly the patient may be relatively asymptomatic but with the rapid onset of hemoglobinuria with hemoglobinemia.

Any transfusion in progress should be stopped immediately, and a reaction workup sent to the blood bank. This type of reaction has a fairly typical pattern of testing: no clerical error, no serologic incompatibility problems, a negative direct antiglobulin/Coombs' test, all ruling out a true AHTR, but evidence of significant intravascular hemolysis with both hemoglobinemia and hemoglobinuria. Patient testing will also be typical for intravascular hemolysis, with elevated LDH, total and indirect bilirubin, and decreased or absent haptoglobin.

Examination of residual blood still in the blood bag shows substantial hemolysis of red cells, demonstrating the in vitro site of the red cell damage, with a negative Gram stain for bacteria ruling out a contaminated/septic unit. Although it is fairly easy to identify a case of in vitro hemolysis, determination of exactly which physical agent was responsible may be difficult.

Prevention

There is no specific preventive measure, other than proper handling of red cell units. Red cell components should be warmed only with systems that have been designed specifically for that purpose and are routinely quality controlled. Unused blood units should be placed only in certified, quality-controlled refrigerators designed for blood storage. Normal saline (0.9%) is the only fluid that should be used for transfusion of blood products.

Mimics of AHTR: Hemolysis Due to Mechanical Red Cell Damage and G6PD Deficiency

Recently, there have been several reports of hemoglobinuria occurring in red cells leuko-reduced by filtration while being infused with a pressure infusion device. It is thought that the filter web acts as a narrow bone cannula, with shear stress and red cell membrane damage. In all reports to date, the only clinical manifestation has been asymptomatic, transient hemoglobinuria with an AHTR ruled out by a negative transfusion reaction evaluation. When leukodepletion filters are used at the bedside, pressure infusion devices should be used with caution.[44–46]

Mechanical causes of red cell destruction are rare but include intravenous catheters and extracorporeal blood circuits. Although not a transfusion reaction, these events can cause a confusing clinical picture if the patient is transfused simultaneously. In these cases, the picture of intravascular hemolysis develops during or shortly following the procedure, and the peripheral smear shows schistocytes and irregular red cell fragments. No evidence of serologic problems is found. Technical difficulties with intraoperative autologous transfusion blood processors have caused traumatic intravascular hemolysis with acute renal failure. Single-needle hemodialysis and exchange transfusion with catheter trauma have also been associated with acute mechanical hemolysis.[47–50]

Finally, nonimmune hemolysis has also been noted in the setting of glucose-6-phosphate dehydrogenase (G6PD) deficiency, present in either the patient or the blood donor. Acute intravascular hemolysis occurring intraoperatively has been reported as the initial manifestation of G6PD deficiency, without any specific drug precipitant having been given to the patient. In the second type of G6PD-related hemolysis, patients receiving red cell units collection from blood donors with G6PD deficiency have demonstrated a milder form of hemolysis, without hemoglobinuria. Clinical manifestations included substantial elevations in bilirubin and LDH. This hemolysis has been reported both in patients receiving drugs known to precipitate G6PD hemolysis and in patients not receiving such drugs. Blood donors are not screened for G6PD deficiency. It has been suggested that the differential diagnosis of posttransfusion hemolysis, particularly in areas of high G6PD prevalence, include G6PD-related hemolysis. Confirmatory testing in that situation would include G6PD testing of the patient and/or donor.[51–53]

Transfusion-Related Acute Lung Injury

Pathophysiology

Transfusion-related acute lung injury (TRALI), also sometimes referred to as noncardiogenic pulmonary edema or pulmonary-type reaction, is estimated to occur in 1 in 5000 units transfused.[54] There are two possible etiologies, both related to the presence of antibodies directed against leukocytes; these antibodies can be granulocyte antibodies, lymphocytotoxic antibodies, or human leukocyte antigen (HLA)-specific antibodies. In the most common form of the reaction, the white cell antibodies are of donor origin, present in the plasma of a blood product, and upon transfusion react with the circulating patient leukocytes. Less commonly, the leukocyte antibodies are present in the patient, and react with white cells present in the transfused unit, usually only with granulocyte transfusions. With both mechanisms, large quantities of leukocyte aggregates are formed, and become trapped in pulmonary capillaries, with subsequent leukocyte and complement activation and immune response. TRALI has been reported following transfusion of whole blood, packed red cells, fresh-frozen plasma, cryoprecipitate, and platelets, but not with plasma derivatives such as albumin.[55]

Clinical Manifestations

Pulmonary symptoms predominate, with acute respiratory insufficiency in the setting of noncardiogenic pulmonary edema, usually within 1 to 2 hours posttransfusion. Dyspnea, tachycardia, and hypoxemia are present; fever and hypotension may be seen as well. The characteristic chest x-ray shows a "bat-wing" central distribution of pulmonary congestion. It is important to note that even severe TRALI reactions may be delayed in their clinical presentation, occurring up to 4 hours after completion of transfusion.

Laboratory Diagnosis and Evaluation

The standard transfusion reaction evaluation is negative, with no evidence of clerical error, hemolysis, or red cell serologic incompatibility. Additional special testing would include sending both patient blood and a sample of blood from the donor for antileukocyte antibody testing.

Management and Prevention

The immediate management is the same as described above for any serious reaction—stopping the transfusion as soon as possible, sending a reaction workup, and aggressive patient management. In the largest reported study to date, all patients required supplemental oxygen and over 70% required intubation, with ventilatory support for an average of 40 hours. For most patients, the pulmonary infiltrates and respiratory insufficiency are cleared within 48 to 96 hours, and there are no long-term sequelae to this type of reaction. However, fatalities are estimated to occur in 5% of cases.[54] Usually these are idiosyncratic reactions, and tend not to recur. In cases in which the donor is shown to have the leukocyte antibodies, this should be reported to the blood center supplying the blood unit, and the donor should be prevented from giving blood again. In cases where the patient has the leukocyte antibodies, additional granulocyte transfusions should be given only if absolutely necessary, and should be HLA matched to the patient. For other cellular transfusion needs, TRALI reactions are unlikely to occur because of the relatively low number of leukocytes present in the blood bag. Even given the unlikelihood of another reaction, leukocyte depletion filters should be used, which will remove 99.9% to 99.99% (3 to 4 log reduction) of leukocytes present in a red cell or platelet transfusion. Although the patient leukoagglutinating antibodies are still present, the removal of donor leukocytes makes further TRALI reactions unlikely. The various types of blood filters are discussed below (see Febrile, Nonhemolytic Transfusion Reactions).[56-60]

Systemic Allergic/Immediate Generalized Reactions

Pathophysiology

Immediate generalized reaction (IGR) is the term that has been used to cover the spectrum of reactions with allergic features, but of unclear etiology not necessarily due to immunoglobulin E (IgE) and not necessarily resulting in full anaphylaxis. True anaphylactic reactions to blood are rare, with the clinically cited etiology related to IgA-deficient patients who have preformed anti-IgA antibody of IgE specificity. Upon infusion of blood products containing IgA, this IgE mediates an immediate anaphylactic reaction.[61] Given the prevalence of IgA deficiency in the general population of 1 in 675 individuals,[62] anaphylactic reactions should be far more common. Investigation of many cases of clinically classic anaphylaxis have failed to show any evidence of IgA deficiency in the patients. Other mechanisms may be operative in these anaphylactoid reactions with severe clinical manifestations, including sensitivity to the Chido blood group antigens,[63,64] and unpredictable bradykinin generation during leukocyte reduction filtration of platelet concentrates.[65,66] Severe allergic reactions, with bronchospasm or hypotension, occur at a rate of approximately 0.1% to 0.2%. Anaphylactic shock is much less common, although the exact incidence is unclear, with a range of once per every 20,000 to 50,000 units transfused to once per 150,000 units transfused.[60,67]

Clinical Manifestations

With true anaphylaxis, typically within the first 30 ml of transfusion, anaphylactic shock develops, with profound hypotension, and often skin changes including flushing or rash. Both respiratory and gastrointestinal changes may be present, with coughing and respiratory distress, or abdominal cramping, vomiting, and diarrhea. Loss of consciousness may be seen. Fever and hemoglobinuria do not accompany the reaction.

For immediate generalized reactions, the severity of the reaction can be graded. Grade I reactions include skin manifestations only, with urticaria, erythema, or pruritus. Such reactions, discussed below, are the most common type of allergic reaction with an incidence of 1% to 3%. Grade II includes mild to moderate hypotension, respiratory distress, and nausea. Grade III includes severe hypotension or shock and bronchospasm, and grade IV is used to describe cardiac or respiratory arrest.[68]

Laboratory Diagnosis and Evaluation

The standard transfusion reaction workup is negative, with no evidence of clerical error, hemolysis, or serologic incompatibility. Given the hypotension and multisystem nature of the clinical manifestations, the blood unit bag should be returned to the blood bank and a Gram stain and culture should be performed to eliminate a sepsis/bacterial contamination type of reaction. Currently, there are no other tests that can be done acutely to aid in diagnosis. If an anaphylactic reaction is suspected, testing for IgA deficiency can be arranged. A pretransfusion patient specimen can be examined for the absence of IgA, and the presence of preformed anti-IgA antibody. Such testing is most reliably done at a large reference center for immunohematology, such as the American Red Cross.[69] Posttransfusion specimens should not be used for IgA testing, as these will contain donor IgA. At this time, there are no other specific tests for evaluation of an IGR.

Management and Prevention

The immediate management is the same as described above for any serious reaction—stopping the transfusion as soon as possible, sending a reaction workup, and aggressive patient management. The blood bag and attached tubing should be sent to the blood bank for evaluation. The absence of fever is an important differential sign, and if the anaphylactic nature of the reaction is realized, definitive therapy includes epinephrine and intravenous corticosteroids.

If IgA deficiency is documented as the cause of anaphylaxis, the patient will require IgA-deficient products for all future transfusions. IgA-deficient products can be obtained several ways, but all require advance planning. For eligible patients, autologous blood products can be collected and stored as frozen units. Otherwise, larger blood centers and reference centers keep an inventory of IgA-deficient blood components, including red cells, platelets, and fresh frozen plasma. Frozen-thawed red cells may be used as well, with premedication regimens and close observation of the patient.

For patients in whom no specific cause of anaphylaxis is documented, subsequent transfusions may prove more difficult. Although recurrent anaphylactoid reactions may occur, these reactions are often idiosyncratic, and the patient may do well with standard blood components for all future transfusions. However, caution should be exercised for at least the next several transfusions, with an aggressive premedication regimen and transfusion in a monitored setting. Autologous products are ideal, but usually not possible given the patient condition. Otherwise, the patient should receive blood products from which plasma has been removed. Washing packed red cells and platelets removes approximately 90% to 95% of plasma, and may be tried for patients who have had IGR, grade II. After an episode of full anaphylaxis or a grade III or IV IGR, frozen thawed red cells (FTC-deglycerolized) products should be used, as FTC units have 99% of plasma removed. Washed platelets are also appropriate in this setting. All subsequent transfusions should be monitored carefully, with advanced life support available. For fresh frozen plasma (FFP), there is no component modification to reduce the likelihood of an allergic reaction (other than IgA-deficient FFP for patients documented to be IgA deficient). The patient may be premedicated with antihistamines as well as corticosteroids, in a regimen similar to that used for allergy to radiographic contrast dye.[60,70]

Sepsis/Bacterially Contaminated Blood Unit Reactions

Pathophysiology

Sepsis-type reactions are rare. These reactions are caused by infusion of blood units that have been contaminated with bacteria, due to bacteremia in an apparently healthy donor, residual bacteria at the donor skin venipuncture site, or contamination in processing.[71] Subsequent growth in the dextrose storage solution results in infusion of large quantities of bacteria, and, with gram-negative organisms, endotoxin. Platelet concentrates, which must be stored at room temperature to maximize platelet function, are the blood product most likely to cause this type of reaction, with an estimated risk of 1 in 19,519 units transfused overall.[72,73] The exact incidence of this type of reaction is unknown, but thought to be underestimated particularly in acutely ill patients for whom other explanations are sought when sepsis develops.[74] Of note, this is the one type of transfusion reaction that may be seen with use of autologous blood.[75]

Clinical Manifestations

With a septic-type reaction caused by contaminated blood products, the clinical manifestations can be profound and occur quickly, often within 30 minutes of starting transfusion. High fever, with or without chills, may accompany hypotension, giving a picture of acute septic shock. Respiratory distress may also be seen. Nausea and vomiting may occur in the conscious patient. Approximately 20% of patients develop a rapid onset of hemoglobinuria after transfusion of contaminated red cells. The hemoglobinuria is not due to an immune hemolysis, but rather the result of red cell membrane damage in the blood bag itself, caused by overgrowth of bacteria depleting the nutrient solution of dextrose and other necessary substrates. Upon infusion, the bacteria cause the clinical reaction, and the free hemoglobin present in the transfusion leads to the development of hemoglobinuria. DIC with generalized bleeding may also be seen as the systemic effects of the infection are established. When contamination is due to gram-positive organisms, the clinical presentation may be somewhat less severe, with signs and symptoms developing during or following the transfusion. Overall mortality for sepsis-type reactions, including all organisms, is approximately 35%.[76-78]

Laboratory Diagnosis and Evaluation

As there are no specific signs or symptoms of the septic-type reaction, the clinical impression often is that an acute hemolytic transfusion reaction has occurred. The transfusion reaction evaluation results can be quite confusing. Reaction reports in the setting of septic reactions can be completely negative, or show a mix of positive and negative results. If there was red cell lysis in the blood bag, free hemoglobin present in the blood bag during infusion can be detected in the posttransfusion serum as free hemoglobin. Although there may be evidence of red cell destruction, the other two parts of the evaluation will be negative; there will be no evidence of a clerical error, and no evidence of serologic problems, with a negative direct Coombs' test and antibody screen. This essentially rules out AHTR, and additional testing is necessary to establish the cause of the reaction.

Gram stain and culture of the residual blood product are the essential diagnostic tests in this setting, particularly the Gram stain. The possible range of organisms is wide, including *Yersinia enterocolitica, Escherichia coli, Serratias* sp., *Pseudomonas* sp., *Klebsiella* sp., *Staphylococcus aureus,* and *S. epidermidis.* With sepsis/bacterially contaminated units, the Gram stain is typically positive, with high concentrations of bacteria. Occasionally, the blood culture is negative, either because of bacterial overgrowth resulting in nonviable organisms, or because of special temperature requirements of the organism. It has been recommended that any culture of donor blood or platelet products be carried out at 4°C, 20°C, and 37°C to maximize the yield.[79,80] DNA typing can be used for cases in which it is necessary to prove that a patient isolate is of the same strain as the blood bag culture isolate.[81]

Management and Prevention

The immediate management is the same as described previously—stopping the transfusion as soon as possible, sending a reaction workup, and aggressive patient management. The blood bag and attached tubing should be sent to the blood bank for evaluation. Blood cultures should be drawn and the patient should be treated empirically for sepsis based on the Gram stain results. The only even remotely possible preventive measure that has been suggested is observation of the unit of blood for clotting or color changes prior to starting the transfusion. Contaminated units of blood have been noted to show a darker, purplish discoloration of the bag contents, especially in comparison to the attached tubing segments, which typically are not contaminated and remain normal in color.[82,83]

Febrile, Nonhemolytic Transfusion Reactions/Benign Febrile Reactions

Pathophysiology and Incidence

Overall, febrile, nonhemolytic transfusion reactions (FNHTR) or benign febrile reactions are the most common reaction, occurring in up to 2% of all transfusions; they are somewhat more likely to be seen following transfusion of red cells than platelets.[3] The etiology was once thought to be entirely related to antibodies directed against donor leukocytes or platelets, but cytokines have now been shown to play a major role.[84] These reactions are often seen in the setting of prior blood exposure, both in multiply transfused patients and in women who have had several pregnancies.

Clinical Manifestations, Laboratory Diagnosis, and Evaluation

A febrile reaction to transfusion is defined as a rise in temperature of at least 1°C during or within up to 4 hours after transfusion. Such reactions may be accompanied by mild chills or severe rigors, headache, tachycardia, mild hypertension, or myalgia. Mild dyspnea and chest discomfort may also be present. As fever is also the most common presenting sign of a true acute hemolytic transfusion reaction, it is not possible to accurately determine the cause of a fever during transfusion without sending a transfusion reaction workup.[60] In most centers the unit of blood is discontinued when a fever occurs during transfusion, but in others the transfusion is only interrupted long enough for a transfusion reaction workup to be done.[4] If the lab testing, as discussed previously, shows no evidence of a clerical error, hemolysis, or serologic incompatibility, then the fever may be safely ascribed to an FNHTR. No other testing is routinely done for an FNHTR, but patients with such reactions may have positive HLA antibody screens or evidence of granulocyte specific antibodies.[4,60,85]

Management and Prevention

After stopping the transfusion, an antipyretic such as acetaminophen (500–1000 mg) should be administered. In the event of severe rigors, meperidine 25 mg IV may be required. For future transfusions, the patient may be premedicated 1 hour in advance with acetaminophen. If the patient has a second FNHTR, leuko-reduced red cells and platelets should be requested. Leuko-reduction filtration is far more effective than washing blood products, and is indicated to prevent febrile, nonhemolytic reactions in patients with a history of multiple such reactions.[86] Because only 15% of patients who experience one febrile reaction will have a second reaction, and because filters add substantially to the cost of each transfusion, leuko-reduction is generally recommended only after a patient has two or more such reactions.[87]

The most commonly used method for white cell removal involves the use of specialized leuko-depletion filter devices. There are three major types of filters used in transfusion practice.[88] First-generation filters are found in standard blood product infusion sets, which contain a 170-μm screen filter to remove particulate debris. This basic filter must be used with transfusion of all blood and blood components, but has little or no effect on the number of individual leukocytes removed. Second-generation filters include woven polyester mesh microaggregate filters, commonly produced in a 40-μm size, which will remove white cell aggregates but not individual cells. Although their efficacy is subject to question,[89] these filters are still used in some hospitals in the setting of multiple transfusion to prevent pulmonary complications. The newest filters are specialized third- and fourth-generation leukocyte reduction filters, consisting of nonwoven webs of synthetic microfibers. These filters are capable of a 3 to 4 log, or 99.9% to 99.99%, reduction in white cell content, which effectively prevents most FNHTRs.[90]

Filtration may take place at the bedside while the transfusion is occurring, or may be performed during processing in the blood bank. Current studies are evaluating the potential advantages of leukocyte reduction at the time the unit of blood is drawn.[91] Prestorage filtration has been shown to reduce levels of cytokines in the transfused product.[92] These cytokines in donor units play an important role in febrile transfusion reactions, and repeated febrile reactions in patients receiving leuko-reduced products are generally attributed to residual cytokine effects.[93-99]

Urticarial/Mild Allergic/Dermal Reactions

Pathophysiology

Simple urticaria, or IGR grade I, is the second most common transfusion reaction, with an incidence of approximately 2%. These reactions are caused by an allergic sensitivity to foreign donor plasma proteins, which are not well characterized, but are thought to include drug allergens, food allergens, and aero-allergens such as pollen.[100] Urticarial reactions have been shown to be more likely to occur in patients with a history of an allergy diagnosis. Urticarial reactions are also more likely to occur with fresh frozen plasma and platelets than with packed red cells.[3,101]

Clinical Manifestations, Laboratory Diagnosis, and Evaluation

Clinical manifestations usually include urticaria, often with skin erythema and pruritus. Occasionally, erythema and pruritus are predominant, and no urticarial wheals develop. The transfusion should be temporarily stopped, and antihistamines, typically diphenhydramine 25 to 50 mg IV, should be given. If the manifestations subside, the transfusion can be restarted slowly with careful observation of the patient. Although such progressions are not common, in this setting the patient should always be closely observed for development of systemic allergic signs, indicating progression to an IGR of at least type II.

Prevention

There is no diagnostic lab testing routinely used for urticarial transfusion reactions. Many urticarial reactions are thought to be idiosyncratic, related to a specific offending plasma protein present in the blood of a particular donor, and will not recur. Other patients seem to have a more broad-based sensitivity, with repeated urticarial reactions. Premedication with antihistamines, typically diphenhydramine 25 to 50 mg IV, is usually effective. For persistent reactions, a plasma-poor product such as washed red cells can be used.[60,100]

Volume Overload

Volume overload is a reaction not to a blood product itself, but to administration of fluids at too rapid a rate, often seen in the elderly or in the setting of congestive heart failure. There are several preventive measures for patients prone to volume overload. If not already provided, the clinician can request from the blood bank packed cell units processed with the nutrient solution Adsol, or AS-1. These units, although having approximately 40 ml greater volume than traditional CPDA-1 stored blood, have a much lower viscosity and can be administered without a concurrent normal saline drip. Slowing the infusion rate is often helpful, although the transfusion should still be completed in 4 hours or less. If slowed infusion is not adequate, a loop-type diuretic may be administered immediately prior to the start of transfusion. Finally, for the patient with persistent volume overload, split-volume units can be requested from the blood bank. A unit of packed cells can be divided into two or three aliquots of 80 to 120 ml, with each given over 4 hours.

Delayed Transfusion Reactions

Delayed Hemolytic Transfusion Reactions

Pathophysiology

Delayed transfusion reactions may be of two types, delayed serologic transfusion reactions (DSTR), with only a positive direct Coombs', or the more clinically important delayed hemolytic transfusion reaction (DHTR), with clinical or laboratory evidence of hemolysis. DHTR and DSTR are estimated to occur at a rate of between 1 in 1605 and 1 in 1899 red cell units transfused; the true incidence is unknown as prospective studies have not been performed due to logistical difficulties in a comprehensive, large-scale follow-up of transfusion recipients. DHTR may go unrecognized in patients with nonspecific complaints if diagnostic blood bank lab testing is not performed.[102,103]

Both DSTR and DHTR are mediated by red cell alloantibodies. Most common is an anamnestic immune response occurring within days after transfusion, in which a preformed antibody present in undetectable amounts is produced in quantities capable of red cell sensitization and destruction. Also possible is a new production of alloantibody as a result of sensitization to transfused red cells, resulting in hemolysis beginning several weeks to 3 months after transfusion.

Clinical Manifestations

Clinical manifestations of delayed transfusion reactions vary considerably. DSTR is clinically silent, with only lab test evidence of the positive antibody screen indicating presence of the alloantibody, and a positive direct Coombs' test indicating red cell sensitization. DHTRs are characterized by the presence of hemolysis, which is typically extravascular, but on occasion intravascular. The red cell destruction can be clinically apparent, with a falling hematocrit, fatigue, fever, and jaundice, or silent except for lab evidence of red cell destruction with elevated LDH and bilirubin and decreased haptoglobin. Other symptoms depend on the alloantibody involved. With antibodies capable of complement fixation, one can get hemoglobinenemia. Because the hemolysis is not acute or fulminant, the renal threshold for hemoglobin is not exceeded, and therefore hemoglobinuria is generally not seen. This syndrome of delayed, clinically evident intravascular hemolysis is characterized of alloantibodies of the Duffy and Kidd groups.

Laboratory Diagnosis and Evaluation

If a DHTR is suspected, a repeat type and screen specimen should be sent to the blood bank, along with a request for a direct Coombs' test. Indicating to the blood bank that a DHTR is suspected is helpful, because special enhancement techniques can be used to increase the chance of antibody detection. With a DSTR, the antibody screen is positive, indicating the presence of an alloantibody, and the direct Coombs' test is positive, indicating red cell sensitization. With a DHTR, again both the antibody screen and direct Coombs' are positive, but there is also evidence of hemolysis on other lab test results, with elevated LDH and bilirubin and decreased haptoglobin.

Management and Prevention

The patient should be followed for progression of anemia with serial hematocrits. Additional transfusion, with antigen negative units, may be needed. Renal insufficiency and DIC are rare. Fatalities have been reported with DHTR between 6 and 16 days posttransfusion, but are rare.[8] Future transfusions must be with antigen-negative blood.

Transfusion-Associated Graft-Versus-Host Disease

Pathophysiology

Transfusion-associated graft-versus-host disease (TA-GVHD) is a rare complication of transfusion most often seen in severely immunocompromised patients. In TA-GVHD, blood donor lymphocytes, which are viable and immunocompetent, are able to engraft in the bone marrow of the patient and multiply. This causes an immune response in which proliferating donor lymphocytes recognize the host/patient tissue as foreign, causing an immune rejection reaction.

TA-GVHD may also be seen in immunocompetent patients who have been exposed to blood from a patient with a very similar HLA type, involving an HLA match known as a "homozygous haplotype." This far less common form of TA-GVHD has been reported in over 40 such cases of immunocompetent patients, in the settings of surgery and trauma.[104–110] This form of TA-GVHD is the basis for irradiating directed donor blood given by first-degree family members, even when the patient is immunocompetent.

Clinical Manifestations, Laboratory Testing, and Management

The signs and symptoms of TA-GVHD are systemic, with fever, pancytopenia, diarrhea, liver dysfunction, rash, and hepatosplenomegaly developing 1 to 4 weeks posttransfusion. Diagnosis may be confirmed by a skin biopsy showing characteristic histologic features. HLA typing of the patient, to show evidence of both the patient and donor HLA types, may also be useful. Unlike bone marrow transplant GVHD, which is often manageable, the prognosis for TA-GVHD is exceedingly poor with a mortality rate in excess of 80%. Attempts at treatment have included high-dose steroids and intravenous immunoglobulin.[111]

Prevention

Prevention of TA-GVHD is of paramount importance, and requires gamma irradiation of blood for patients at risk. Leuko-reduction by filtration is not considered a safe method of preventing TA-GVHD, because the exact number of lymphocytes required to cause TA-GVHD is not known. Gamma irradiation of each cellular blood product must be used. Gamma irradiation damages cellular DNA, thus rendering the donor lymphocytes unable to multiply and engraft in the recipient.

There are five major risk groups for TA-GVHD: congenital immunodeficiencies, certain subsets of neonates, bone marrow transplant recipients and patients with other hematologic disorders, patients with immune suppression induced by chemotherapy and/or radiation therapy, and immunocompetent individuals transfused with HLA haplo-identical leukocytes or blood from first-degree family members. The definition of immunocompromised patients varies somewhat by local practice, but patient groups commonly receiving irradiated blood products include those with Hodgkin's disease, non-Hodgkin's lymphoma, congenital immunodeficiency syndrome, and leukemia, as well as recipients of organ transplants, and premature newborns. The necessity to irradiate blood for most solid tumor patients is still under review. No risk of TA-GVHD has been defined for AIDS patients and full-term neonates. Blood donated by a blood relative of the patient must be irradiated[60] because of the higher incidence of HLA homozygous haplotypes among family members.[112–117]

Posttransfusion Purpura

Pathophysiology

Posttransfusion purpura (PTP) is characterized by the development of severe thrombocytopenia approximately 1 week after blood transfusion. The exact mechanism is not fully understood, but is related to an immune reaction in which a high-titer platelet alloantibody is formed, with subsequent destruction of platelets. In more than 85% of cases, the patients are negative for the platelet antigen Pl^{A1} with formation of anti-Pl^{A1}. Passive transfer of the platelet specific antibody from donor to patient, with subsequent clinical PTP, has been reported.[118]

Clinical Manifestations, Laboratory Testing, and Management

Six to 8 days posttransfusion, the platelet count rapidly drops, typically to less than 10,000/μl, with development of petechiae and risk of spontaneous bleeding. Serologic testing is used to detect the antiplatelet antibody, and define the specificity (anti-Pl^{A1}, anti-Bak^a, etc.). Treatments have included intravenous immunoglobulin, plasma exchange to reduce the antibody burden, and steroids. The platelet count generally normalizes within several weeks. For the acute thrombocytopenic phase, the use of Pl^{A1}-negative platelets is controversial, but recently has been shown to improve the platelet count. For immediate and future transfusion needs, although not all patients will have a recurrence of PTP, frozen thawed red cells (FTC) have been recommended. FTCs are used because this product essentially is free of all platelet antigens, but may not prevent relapse in all cases.[119–121]

References

1. Walker RH. Special report: transfusion risks. *Am J Clin Pathol* 1987; 88:374–378.
2. Nicholls MD. Transfusion: morbidity and mortality. *Anaesth Intensive Care* 1993;21:15–19.
3. Dzieczkowski JS, Barrett BB, Nester D, et al. Characterization of reactions after exclusive transfusion of white cell-reduced cellular blood components. *Transfusion* 1995;35:20–25.
4. Oberman HA. Controversies in transfusion medicine: Should a febrile transfusion reaction occasion the return of the blood component to the blood bank? Con. *Transfusion* 1994;34:353–355.
5. Novak RW. Immediate transfusion reactions in the pediatric population. *Lab Med* 1987;18:388–390.
6. Holman P, Blajchman MA, Heddle N. Noninfectious adverse effects of blood transfusion in the neonate. *Transfus Med Rev* 1995;9:277–287.
7. DePalma L. Review: red cell alloantibody formation in the neonate and infant. Considerations for current immunohemorrhagic practice. *Immunohematology* 1992;8:33–37.
8. Sazama K. Reports of 355 transfusion-associated deaths: 1976 through 1985. *Transfusion* 1990;30:583–590.
9. Hoeltge GA, Domen RE, Rybicki LA, et al. Multiple red cell transfusions and alloimmunization. Experience with 6996 antibodies detected in a total of 159,262 patients from 1985 to 1993. *Arch Pathol Lab Med* 1995;119:42–45.
10. Garratty G. Mechanisms of immune red cell destruction, and red cell compatibility testing. *Hum Pathol* 1983;14:204–212.
11. Vilpo JA, Talvensaari KK, Mortensen E. Hemolysis—which laboratory investigations and when. *Scand J Clin Lab Invest Suppl* 1990;200:10–19.
12. Berlin NI, Berk PD. Quantitative aspects of bilirubin metabolism for hematologists. *Blood* 1981;57:983–999.
13. Fink DJ, Petz LD, Black MB. Serum haptoglobin. *JAMA* 1967;199:109–112.
14. Patten E. Immunohematologic diseases. *JAMA* 1987;258:2945–2951.
15. Pineda AA, Brizica SM, Taswell HF. Hemolytic transfusion reaction. Recent experience in a large blood bank. *Mayo Clin Proc* 1978;53:378–390.
16. Linden JV, Paul B, Dressler KP. A report of 104 transfusion errors in New York State. *Transfusion* 1992;32:601–606.
17. Murphy WG, McClelland DBL. Deceptively low morbidity from failure to practice safe blood transfusion: an analysis of serious blood transfusion errors. *Vox Sang* 1989;57:59–62.
18. Linden JV, Kaplan HS. Transfusion errors: causes and effects. *Transfus Med Rev* 1994;8:169–183.
19. Myhre BA. Fatalities from blood transfusion. *JAMA* 1980;244:1333–1335.
20. Greenwalt TJ. Pathogenesis and management of hemolytic transfusion reactions. *Semin Hematol* 1981;18:84–94.

21. Capon SM, Goldfinger D. Acute hemolytic transfusion reaction, a paradigm of the systemic inflammatory response: new insights into pathophysiology and treatment. *Transfusion* 1995;35:513–520.
22. Garratty G, Vengelen-Tyler V, Postoway N, et al. Hemolytic transfusion reactions associated with antibodies not detectable by routine procedures. *Transfusion* 1982;22:429.
23. Harrison CR, Hayes TC, Trow LL, et al. Intravascular hemolytic transfusion reaction without detectable antibodies: a case report and review of the literature. *Vox Sang* 1986;51:96–101.
24. Rosse WF. *Clinical Immunohematology: Basic Concepts and Clinical Applications.* Boston: Blackwell Scientific, 1990.
25. Davenport RD, Kunkel SL. Cytokine roles in hemolytic and nonhemolytic transfusion reactions. *Transfus Med Rev* 1994;8:157–168.
26. Cheng MS. Delayed reaction following ABO-incompatible transfusion (Letter). *Transfusion* 1995;35:791.
27. Lin CK, Wong KF, Mak KH, et al. Hemolytic transfusion reaction due to Rh antibodies detectable only by manual polybrene and polyethylene glycol technique. *Am J Clin Pathol* 1995;104:660–662.
28. Brecher ME, Taswell HF. Hemolytic transfusion reactions. In: Rossi EC, Simon TL, Moss GS, eds. *Principles of Transfusion Medicine.* Baltimore: Williams & Wilkins, 1991;619–634.
29. Wenz B, Burns ER. Improvement in transfusion safety using a new blood unit and patient identification system as part of safe transfusion practice. *Transfusion* 1991;31:401–403.
30. Conway LT, Scott EP. Acute hemolytic transfusion reaction due to ABO incompatible plasma in a platelet pheresis concentrate. *Transfusion* 1984; 24:413–414.
31. Murphy MF, Hook S, Waters AH. Acute haemolysis after ABO incompatible platelet transfusions. *Lancet* 1990;335:974–975.
32. Reis MD, Coovadia AS. Transfusion of ABO incompatible platelets causing severe haemolytic reaction. *Clin Lab Haematol* 1989;11:237–240.
33. Vaughan RL. Morbidity due to exchange transfusion with heat-hemolyzed blood. *Am J Dis Child* 1982;136:646–648.
34. Phillips WA, Pottenger LA, DeWald RL. Extracorporeal hemolysis in orthopedic patients. Report of two cases. *Clin Orthop Rel Res* 1989;238:241–244.
35. Staples PJ, Griner PF. Extracorporeal hemolysis of blood in a microwave blood warmer. *N Engl J Med* 1971;285:317–319.
36. McCullough J, Polesky HF, Nelson C, et al. Iatrogenic hemolysis: a complication of blood warmed by a microwave device. *Anesth Analg* 1972; 51:102–106.
37. Iserson KV, Huestis DW. Blood warming: current applications and techniques. *Transfusion* 1991;31:558–571.
38. Linko K, Hynynen K. Erythrocyte damage caused by the Haemotherm microwave blood warmer. *Acta Anaesth Scand* 1979;23:320–328.
39. Valeri CR, Pivacek LE, Gray AD. The safety and therapeutic effectiveness of human red cells stored at −80°C for as long as 21 years. *Transfusion* 1989;29:429–437.
40. Bechdolt S, Schroeder LK, Samia C, et al. In vivo hemolysis of deglycerolized red blood cells. *Arch Pathol Lab Med* 1986;110:344–345.
41. Cregan P, Donegan E, Gotelli G. Hemolytic transfusion reaction following

transfusion of frozen and washed autologous red cells. *Transfusion* 1991; 31:172–175.
42. Lanore JJ, Quarre Mc, Audibert G, et al. Acute renal failure following transfusion of accidentally frozen autologous red blood cells. *Vox Sang* 1989;56:293–297.
43. Whitelaw JP. Hemolysis caused by half-physiologic strength saline (letter). *Transfusion* 1990;30:78.
44. Gambino C, Craig D, Stiles M, et al. The effect of Pall RC-50 filtration under pressure on red cell hemolysis (abstract). *Transfusion* 1992;32(suppl):S98.
45. Carson TH, Bloom J, Ferguson DB, et al. Delayed hemolysis of white cell-reduced red cells (letter). *Transfusion* 1994;34:86.
46. Ma SK, Wong KF, Siu L. Hemoglobinemia and hemoglobinuria complicating concomitant usage of a white cell filter and a pressure infusion device (letter). *Transfusion* 1995;35:180.
47. Hemolysis and renal dysfunction associated with autotransfusion. *Health Dev* 1990;19:25.
48. Dhaene M, Gulbis B, Lietaer N, et al. Red blood cell destruction in single needle dialysis. *Clin Nephrol* 1989;31:327–331.
49. Hombrouckx RO, De Vos JY, Larno LA, et al. Atypical symptoms during single needle dialysis. *ASAIO Trans* 1990;36:M335–M337.
50. Bowman JM, Pollock JM. Haemolysis of donor red cells at fetal transfusion due to catheter trauma (letter). *Lancet* 1980;2:1190.
51. Shalev O, Manny N, Sharon R. Posttransfusional hemolysis in recipients of glucose-6-phosphate dehydrogenase-deficient erythrocytes. *Vox Sang* 1993; 64:94–98.
52. Beauregard P, Blajchman MA. Hemolytic and pseudo-hemolytic transfusion reactions: an overview of the hemolytic transfusion reactions and the clinical conditions that mimic them. *Transfus Med Rev* 1994;8:194–199.
53. Sazama K, Klein HG, Davey RJ, et al. Intraoperative hemolysis. The initial manifestation of glucose-6-phosphate dehydrogenase deficiency. *Arch Intern Med* 1980;140:845–846.
54. Popovsky MA, Moore SB. Diagnostic and pathogenetic considerations in transfusion-related lung injury. *Transfusion* 1985;35:573–577.
55. Popovsky MA. Transfusion-related acute lung injury. *Transfusion* 1995; 35:180–181.
56. Malouf M, Glanville AR. Blood transfusion related adult respiratory distress syndrome. *Anaesth Intensive Care* 1993;21:44–49.
57. Seeger W, Schneider U, Kreusler B, et al. Reproduction of transfusion-related acute lung injury in an ex vivo lung model. *Blood* 1990;76:1438–1440.
58. Popovsky MA, Chaplin HC, Moore SB. Transfusion-related acute lung injury: a neglected, serious complication of hemotherapy. *Transfusion* 1992; 32:589–592.
59. Eastlund T, McGrath PC, Britten A, et al. Fatal pulmonary transfusion reaction to plasma containing donor HLA antibody. *Vox Sang* 1989;57:63–66.
60. Walker RH. *Technical Manual.* 13th ed. Bethesda, MD: American Association of Blood Banks, 1993.
61. Pineda AA, Taswell TF. Transfusion reactions associated with anti-IgA antibodies: report of four cases and review of the literature. *Transfusion* 1975;15:10–15.
62. Paglieroni TG, Holland PV. Effects of serial plasmapheresis on serum IgA

levels in IgA-deficient blood donors with IgA-suppressor T cells. *Transfusion* 1992;32:139–144.

63. Westhoff CM, Sipherd BD, Wylie DE, et al. Severe anaphylactic reactions following transfusions of platelets to a patient with anti-Ch. *Transfusion* 1992;32:576–579.
64. Wibaut B, Mannessier L, Horbez C, et al. Anaphylactic reactions associated with anti-Chido antibody following platelet transfusions. *Vox Sang* 1995; 69:150–151.
65. Takahashi TA, Abe H, Hosoda M, et al. Bradykinin generation during filtration of platelet concentrates with a white cell-reduction filter (letter). *Transfusion* 1995;35:967.
66. Adverse reactions to platelet transfusions reported. *Blood Bank Week* 1993;10:1-2.
67. Greenberger PA. Plasma anaphylaxis and immediate type reactions. In: Rossi EC, Simon TL, Moss GS, eds. *Principles of Transfusion Medicine.* Baltimore: Williams & Wilkins, 1991;635–639.
68. Isbister JP. Adverse reactions to plasma and plasma components. *Anaesth Intensive Care* 1993;21:31–38.
69. Sandler SG, Eckrich R, Malamut D, et al. Hemagglutination assays for the diagnosis and prevention of IgA anaphylactic transfusion reactions. *Blood* 1994;84:2031–2035.
70. Greenberger PA, Patterson R. Adverse reactions to radiocontrast media. *Prog Cardiovasc Dis* 1988;31:239–248.
71. Heltberg O, Skov F, Gerner-Smidt P, et al. Nosocomial epidemic of *Serratia marcescens* septicemia ascribed to contaminated blood transfusion bags. *Transfusion* 1993;33:221–227.
72. Morrow JF, Braine HG, Kickler TS, et al. Septic reactions to platelet transfusions: a persistent problem. *JAMA* 1991;266:555–558.
73. Ciavarella D. Sepsis after platelet transfusions. *JAMA* 1992;267:1206.
74. Barrett BB, Andersen JW, Anderson KC. Strategies for the avoidance of bacterial contamination of blood components. *Transfusion* 1993;33:228–233.
75. Richards C, Kolins J, Trinidade CD. Autologous transfusion-transmitted *Yersinia enterocolitica. JAMA* 1992;268:1541–1542.
76. Barbara JAJ, Contreras M. Infectious complications of blood transfusion: bacteria and parasites. *Br Med J* 1990;300:386–389.
77. Morduchowicz G, Pitlik SD, Muminer D, et al. Transfusion reactions due to bacterial contamination of blood and blood products. *Rev Infect Dis* 1991;13:307–314.
78. Chiu EKW, Yuen KY, Lie AKW, et al. A prospective study of symptomatic bacteremia following platelet transfusion and of its management. *Transfusion* 1994;34:950–954.
79. Prentice M. Transfusing *Yersinia enterocolitica. Br Med J* 1992;305:663–664.
80. Napier JAF. *Handbook of Blood Transfusion Therapy.* 2nd ed. New York: John Wiley, 1995.
81. Muder RR, Yee YC, Rihs JD, et al. *Staphylococcus epidermidis* bacteremia from transfusion of contaminated platelets: application of bacterial DNA analysis. *Transfusion* 1992;32:771–774.
82. Kim DM, Brecher ME, Bland LA, et al. Visual identification of bacterially contaminated red cells. *Transfusion* 1992;32:221–225.

83. Woodfield DG. Transfusion acquired *Serratia liquefaciens* septicaemia. *NZ Med J* 1991;104:141.
84. Heddle NM, Klama L, Singer J, et al. The role of the plasma from platelet concentrates in transfusion reactions. *N Engl J Med* 1994;331:625–628.
85. Widmann FK. Controversies in transfusion medicine: Should a febrile transfusion reaction occasion the return of the blood component to the blood bank? Pro. *Transfusion* 1994;34:356–358.
86. Brittingham TE, Chaplin H Jr. Febrile transfusion reactions caused by sensitivity to donor leukocytes and platelets. *JAMA* 1957;165:819–825.
87. Menitove JE, McElligott MC, Aster RH. Febrile transfusion reaction: what blood component should be given next? *Vox Sang* 1982;42:318–321.
88. Dzik S. Leukodepletion blood filters: filter design and mechanisms of leukocyte removal. *Transfus Med Rev* 1993;7:65–77.
89. Snyder EL, Bookbinder M. Role of microaggregate blood filtration in clinical medicine. *Transfusion* 1983;23:460–470.
90. Freedman JJ, Blajchman MA, McCombie N. Canadian Red Cross Society Symposium on Leukodepletion: report of proceedings. *Transfus Med Rev* 1994;8:1–14.
91. Pietersz RNI, Steneker I, Reesink HW. Prestorage leukocyte depletion of blood products in a closed system. *Transfus Med Rev* 1993;7:17–24.
92. Sirchia G, Wenz B, Rebulla P, et al. Removal of white cells from red cells by transfusion through a new filter. *Transfusion* 1990;30:30–33.
93. Dzik WH. Is the febrile response to transfusion due to donor or recipient cytokine? (letter). *Transfusion* 1992;35:594.
94. Muyelle L, Joos M, Wouters E, et al. Increased tumor necrosis factor alpha (TNF alpha), interleukin 1 and interleukin 6 (IL-6) levels in the plasma of stored platelet concentrates: relationship between TNF alpha and IL 6 levels and febrile transfusion reactions. *Transfusion* 1993;33:195–199.
95. Heddle NM, Klama LN, Griffith L, et al. A prospective study to identify the risk factors associated with acute reactions to platelet and red cell transfusions. *Transfusion* 1993;33:794–797.
96. Sacher RA, Boyle L, Freter CE. High circulating interleukin 6 levels associated with acute transfusion reaction: cause or effect? *Transfusion* 1993;33:962–963.
97. Stack G, Snyder EL. Cytokine generation in stored platelet concentrates. *Transfusion* 1994;34:20–25.
98. Goodnough LT, Riddell J, Lazarus H, et al. Prevalence of platelet transfusion reactions before and after implementation of leukocyte-depleted platelet concentrates by filtration. *Vox Sang* 1993;65:103–107.
99. Aye MT, Palmer DS, Giulivi A, et al. Effect of filtration of platelet concentrates on the accumulation of cytokines and platelet release factors during storage. *Transfusion* 1995;35:117–124.
100. Contreras M, Mollison PL. Immunological complications of transfusion. *Br Med J* 1990;300:173–176.
101. Wilhelm D, Kluter H, Kouche M, et al. Impact of allergy screening for blood donors: relationship to nonhemolytic transfusion reactions. *Vox Sang* 1995; 69:217–221.
102. Ness PM, Shirey RS, Thoman SK, et al. The differentiation of delayed serologic and delayed hemolytic transfusion reactions: incidence, long-term serologic findings and clinical significance. *Transfusion* 1990;30:688–693.
103. Vamvakas EC, Pineda AA, Reisner R, et al. The differentiation of delayed

hemolytic and delayed serologic transfusion reactions: incidence and predictors of hemolysis. *Transfusion* 1995;35:26–32.
104. Shivdasani RA, Halusk FG, Dock NL, et al. Brief report: graft-versus-host disease associated with transfusion of blood from unrelated HLA-homozygous donors. *N Engl Med* 1993;328:766–770.
105. Capon SM, DePond WD, Tyan DB, et al. Transfusion-associated graft-versus-host disease in an immunocompetent patient. *Ann Intern Med* 1991; 114:1025–1026.
106. Otsuka S, Kunieda K, Kitamura F, et al. The critical role of blood from HLA-homozygous donors in fatal transfusion-associated graft-versus-host disease in immunocompetent patients. *Transfusion* 1991;31:260–264.
107. Kobayashi H, Kitano K, Kishi E, et al. Transfusion-associated graft-versus-host disease in an immunocompetent patient following accidental injury. *Am J Hematol* 1993;43:51–53.
108. Burdick JF, Vogelsang GB, Smith WJ, et al. Severe graft-versus-host disease in a liver-transplant recipient. *N Engl J Med* 1988;318:689–690.
109. Thaler M, Shamiss A, Orgad S, et al. The role of blood from HLA-homozygous donors in fatal transfusion-associated graft-versus-host disease after open heart surgery. *N Engl J Med* 1989;321:25–28.
110. Petz LD, Calhoun L, Yam P, et al. Transfusion-associated graft-versus-host disease in immunocompetent patients: report of a fatal case associated with transfusion of blood from a second-degree relative, and a survey of predisposing factors. *Transfusion* 1993;33:742–750.
111. Anderson KC, Weinstein HJ. Tranfusion-associated graft-versus-host disease. *N Engl J Med* 1990;323:315–321.
112. Anderson KC. Clinical indications for blood component irradiation. In: Baldwin ML, Jeffries LC, eds. *Irradiation of Blood Components.* Bethesda, MD: American Association of Blood Banks, 1992;31–50.
113. Anderson KC, Goodnough LT, Sayers M, et al. Variation of blood component irradiation practice: implications for prevention of transfusion-associated graft-versus-host disease. *Blood* 1991;77:2096–2102.
114. McMilin KD, Johnson RL. HAL homozygosity and the risk of related-donor transfusion-associated graft-versus-host disease. *Transfus Med Rev* 1993; 7:37–41.
115. Grishaber JE, Birney SM, Strauss RG. Potential for transfusion-associated graft-versus-host disease due to apheresis platelets matched for HLA class I antigens. *Transfusion* 1993;33:910–914.
116. Rosen NR, Weidner JG, Boldt HD, et al. Prevention of transfusion graft-versus-host disease: selection of an adequate dose of gamma irradiation. *Transfusion* 1993;33:125–127.
117. Lowenthal RM, Challis DR, Griffiths AE, Chappell RA, Goulder PJR. Transfusion-associated graft-versus-host disease: report of an occurrence following the administration of irradiated blood. *Transfusion* 1993; 33:524–529.
118. Scott EP, Moilan-Bergeland J, Dalmasso AP. Posttransfusion thrombocytopenia associated with passive transfer of a platelet-specific antibody. *Transfusion* 1988;28:73–76.
119. Brecher ME, Moore SB, Letendre L. Posttransfusion purpura: the therapeutic value of PL^{A1}-negative platelets. *Transfusion* 1990;30:433–435.

120. Vogelsang, G, Kickler TS, Bell WR. Post-transfusion purpura: a report of five patients and a review of the pathogenesis and management. *Am J Hematol* 1986;21:259–261.
121. Godeau B, Fromont P, Bettaieb A, et al. Relapse of posttransfusion purpura after transfusion with frozen-thawed red cells. *Transfusion* 1991;31:189–190.

24
Blood Substitutes

JOHN D. KLEMPERER AND O. WAYNE ISOM

The development of an effective substitute for homologous blood transfusion has been pursued for decades.[1,2] Of the numerous functions performed by whole blood, only those of the erythrocyte can realistically be performed by synthetic, cell-free substitutes. Research into oxygen carrying solutions has focused primarily on hemoglobin- and perfluorocarbon-based preparations. Despite considerable progress in this area, clinical application has been limited because of marginal efficacy as well as recognized and potential side effects. However, as research efforts continue to intensify due to the diminishing supply of blood products and the fear of viral illness transmission, it is likely that safe and effective substitutes will ultimately become available for routine use in a variety of clinical situations. In addition to the obvious benefits that intravenous fluids with oxygen transport capability could offer in trauma or perioperative blood loss resuscitation, unique opportunities exist for use in the cardiac surgery patient. An understanding of the metabolic and rheologic differences between the synthetic solutions and human blood is necessary to formulate a rational approach to their administration. This chapter reviews the properties of and problems associated with the major available agents, the relevant experimental data, the limited clinical experience, and potential applications in cardiac surgery.

Requirements for Blood Substitutes

An effective red blood cell (RBC) substitute must first and foremost contribute significantly to oxygen transport and delivery. Requirements related to the support of cardiovascular hemodynamics and the duration of intravascular persistence vary depending on the clinical indication for which treatment is initiated.[3] For example, the optimal blood substitute for rapid volume replacement in hemorrhagic shock may differ from the best agent for suppling oxygen to an ischemic region of myocardium during percutaneous transluminal coronary angioplasty (PTCA). Likewise, the utility of a specific blood substitute in the setting of cardiac surgery depends on whether it is intended for use during cardiopulmonary bypass or in the postoperative period, as well as whether it is targeted for systemic or regional distribution. Intelligent application of blood substitute therapy depends on appropriately matching the agent to a given clinical situation. While hemoglobin-based solutions have an obvious physiologic appeal, the perfluorocarbons are better suited for certain applications. The two classes differ dramatically in their oxygen carrying characteristics and rheologic properties. If red cell substitutes are to have advantage over homologous transfusion, they must be nontoxic, free of transmissible illnesses, and easy to administer. Ideally, they would remain stable during long periods of storage and be universally compatible.[3]

Physiology of Oxygen Transport

In blood, the majority of oxygen (98–99%) is carried reversibly bound to hemoglobin, and only a minimal amount is dissolved in plasma. The red blood cell is a highly efficient oxygen transport system. It contains about 35 g/dl of hemoglobin, and at normal hematocrits whole blood has an oxygen carrying capacity of approximately 18 vol%.[4] A detailed description of the structure and function of hemoglobin is beyond the scope of this chapter, but several important concepts are particularly relevant. The oxygen equilibrium curve (OEC) of hemoglobin is shown in Figure 24.1. The characteristic sigmoidal shape reflects the cooperative binding of oxygen by hemoglobin where small changes in oxygen tension result in large changes in the amount of oxygen bound in the lungs or released in the tissues.[4] At atmospheric pressures within human alveoli, hemoglobin rapidly becomes fully saturated. Oxygen is normally unloaded in the capillaries at partial pressures of approximately 40 mm Hg, a level sufficient to avoid venous hypoxia.[4] The P-50 of hemoglobin, the partial pressure of oxygen at which the molecule is half saturated, is 26 mm Hg in the human RBC. If the oxygen affinity increases, the OEC shifts to the left, lowering the P-50, and less oxygen is released at physiologic partial pressures. The principal modifiers of the OEC within the erythrocyte are shown in Figure 24.1. Rheologic factors also influence oxygen delivery by altering microcirculatory flow. Indeed, the optimal hematocrit in the cardiac surgery patient has been the subject of debate, and it is recognized that isovolumic hemodilution can enhance myocardial and other organ perfusion.[5] In certain clinical situations, the infusion of low-viscosity solutions may offer significant advantage over blood administration.[6]

Hemoglobin Solutions

Development

Cell-free hemoglobin-based solutions have been studied for over a century,[1] yet introduction into clinical use has been disappointing. Attempts to

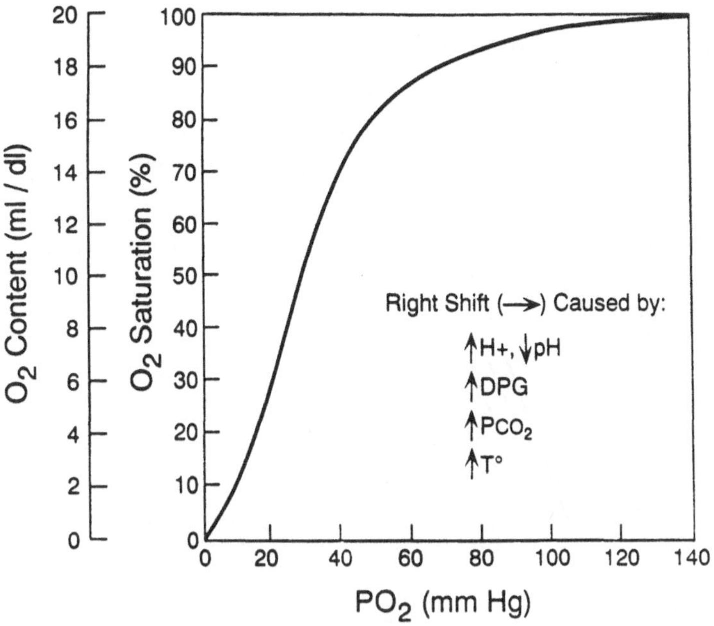

FIGURE 24.1. Oxyhemoglobin dissociation curve for normal human blood. The y-axis shows the relation of oxygen saturation to oxygen content. The principal effectors that alter the position and shape of the curve are indicated. A shift in the curve to the right or left will affect the amount of oxygen available for extraction at tissue if $PMVO_2$ remains normal (40 mm Hg). (From Greenberg,[91] with permission.)

develop an effective compound have evolved through several stages. Early unmodified hemoglobin solutions were derived by washing red cells obtained from outdated banked blood and lysing them in hypotonic solution. Administration of these preparations was characterized by rapid disappearance from the circulation and deterioration of renal function.[7-9] In the 1960s, researchers determined that residual red cell stroma was a major source of nephrotoxicity and intravascular coagulation.[10] Subsequently, stroma-free hemoglobin (SFH) preparations were produced via several methods.[11,12] Unmodified SFH solutions do not require cross-matching[13] and can be easily stored for up to 2 years.[14] SFH has successfully supported oxygenation and hemodynamic requirements in experimental animals that underwent total exchange transfusion to zero hematocrit.[15] Studies with SFH have also exhibited rheologic benefit in ameliorating the hyperviscosity state that develops early in myocardial ischemia.[16] However, important limitations and toxicities associated with these solutions mandate their modification. A major disadvantage of unmodified hemoglobin solutions is the strikingly lower P-50 than in human blood, typically in the range of 12 to 14 mm Hg[13] (Fig. 24.2). In contrast to the sigmoidal relation of human erythrocyte suspensions, SFH demonstrates an exponential relation between hemoglobin oxygen saturation and oxygen partial pressure. At

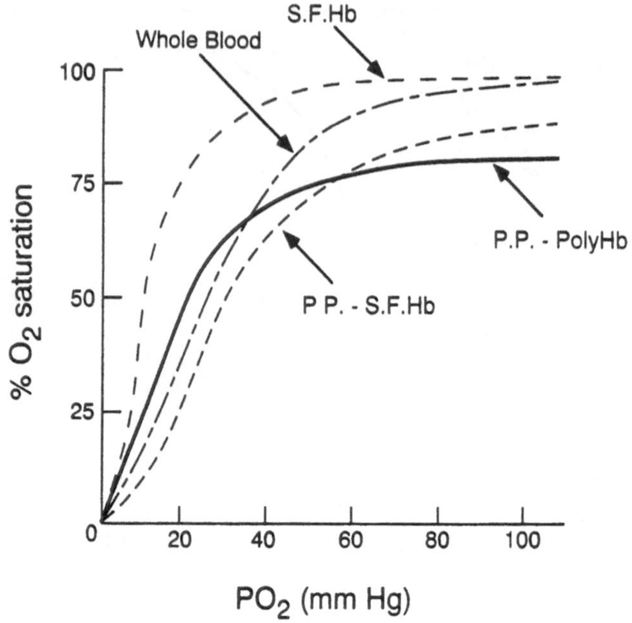

FIGURE 24.2. Oxyhemoglobin dissociation curves of modified hemoglobin solution with various oxygen affinities. Stroma-free hemoglobin (S.F.Hb), pyridoxated human hemoglobin (P.P.-S.F.Hb), pyridoxylated, polymerized human hemoglobin (P.P.-PolyHb). (From Keipert and Chang,[27] with permission.)

normal mixed venous oxygen tension (40 mm Hg), only about 4% of SFH bound oxygen is available for release. This increased oxygen affinity results primarily from lack of 2,3-diphosphoglycerate (2,3-DPG),[17] and severely limits oxygen delivery even to hypoxic tissues.[6] If used for resuscitation purposes, problems also arise because of the substantial oncotic pressure these solutions exert, effectively limiting the hemoglobin concentration to about 7 g/dl.[18] The unmodified solutions also have short half-lives (4 hours or less) due to rapid renal clearance following the dissociation of the free hemoglobin tetramers into dimers.[19,20] Most importantly, unacceptable renal toxicity has been a uniform finding in tolerance trials involving administration to human volunteers.[21]

A number of biochemical modifications have improved the oxygen carrying capacity and have prolonged the plasma retention time of hemoglobin-based solutions. The high oxygen affinity of SFH can be decreased by covalent binding of the 2,3-DPG analogue, pyridoxal-5′-phosphate.[22] The resulting compound, pyridoxylated stroma-free hemoglobin (SFH-P) is associated with P-50 values of 22 to 26 mm Hg (Fig. 24.2).[23] Despite a significantly lower oxygen affinity following infusion of the pyridoxylated preparation, baboons that underwent total exchange transfusion still displayed severely depressed mixed venous oxygen (MVO_2) levels.[24] Gould and coworkers[24] determined that the depression of MVO_2, which indicated inadequate tissue level oxygen delivery, was more dependent on the reduction of hemoglobin concentration than the decline in P-50.[25] As described, the amount of SFH that can be administered is limited by oncotic considerations. Several laboratories have developed methods for producing polymerized hemoglobin solutions.[26,27] To attain physiologic oncotic pressures (20–25 torr), SFH preparations must be diluted to 7.0 to 7.5 g/dl in comparison to polymerized solutions, which are isooncotic with plasma at 14.0 to 15.0 g/dl (Fig. 24.3).[27] By combining pyridoxylation with covalent cross-linking, isooncotic hemoglobin solutions have been produced that have near normal oxygen binding curves and prolonged half-lives.[28,29] A greater contribution to total oxygen delivery and prolonged intravascular persistence was evident in primates that underwent exchange transfusion with polymerized SFH-P.[30,31] These studies achieved hemoglobin concentrations of 10 g/dl with a plasma half-life of about 46 hours.[31] Phase I clinical trials were completed with a similar product, but phase II trials were recently stopped because of safety concerns.[13]

Bovine-based hemoglobin solutions are theoretically attractive since they are associated with neither the risk of hepatitis or HIV transmission nor a shortage of supply. Stromal-free bovine hemoglobin does not require 2,3-DPG to lower its oxygen affinity, but instead utilizes chloride ion. The

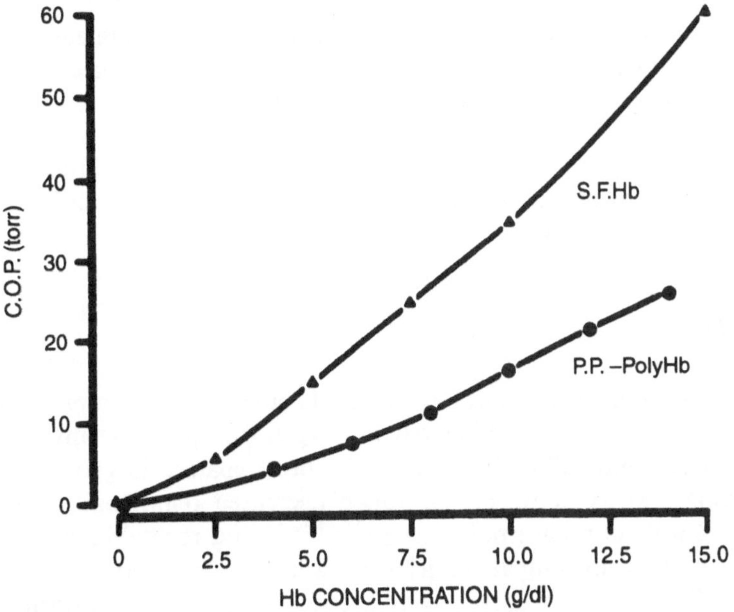

FIGURE 24.3. Colloid osmotic (oncotic) pressure measurements of stroma-free hemoglobin solution (S.F.Hb) and pyridoxylated polymerized human hemoglobin (P.P.-PolyHb). At normal physiologic oncotic pressures (20–25 torr), S.F.Hb solution concentration is approximately 7.0 g/dl while P.P.-PolyHb solution is approximately 15/dL. (From Keipert and Chang,[27] with permission.)

chloride ion concentration of human plasma is adequate to satisfactorily reduce the polymerized bovine hemoglobin P-50 to approximately 28 torr.[32,33] Polymerized bovine hemoglobin preparations have effectively supported oxygen consumption requirements and maintained hemodynamic stability following total exchange transfusion in sheep. A final arterial oxygen content of 7.6 vol% was obtained, corresponding to approximately 1.0 vol% oxygen carried per gram of bovine hemoglobin.[34] In another study, volume resuscitation with a polymerized bovine Hb solution permitted preoperative autologous blood donation of up to 80% of red cell mass with minimal renal toxicity.[35] A recent clinical trial using a highly purified polymerized bovine Hb was performed in severely anemic children suffering from aplastic sickle cell crisis.[36] Improvement in symptoms and erythropoietic recovery were documented. No adverse reactions were noted.

A novel strategy to reduce oxygen affinity and prevent side effects is to encapsulate free hemoglobin within liposomes. A circulation half-life of approximately 6 hours and P-50 values between 26 and 28 mm Hg have been reported.[37] Although liposomes are avidly taken up by the reticuloendothelial system, modification of the phospholipid composition can decrease this process and prolong intravascular retention time.[38] Perhaps the most important development in hemoglobin solution technology involves the production of recombinant human hemoglobin molecules.[39] Recombinant products may ultimately eliminate existing concerns related to purity, oxygen affinity, and in vivo stability.[40] A genetically engineered recombinant human hemoglobin molecule, consisting of a mutant β-globin chain that decreases oxygen affinity and fused α-globin subunits that prevent dissociation, had a prolonged half-life and no effect on renal function when administered to dogs.[41] Phase I clinical trials of recombinant hemoglobin solution are in progress.[40]

Safety

As discussed above, several modified hemoglobin solutions have been developed that function effectively as oxygen transport systems. However, introduction into clinical practice has been sparse, largely because of persisting toxicity concerns. Although decreased renal toxicity has been reported with ultrapure polymerized[33,34,36,42] and recombinant[41] preparations, there is no animal model that accurately predicts potential renal dysfunction in man.[43] Early experience suggested that the uniform finding of nephrotoxicity was related to impurities in production, and that removal of all traces of phospholipid and endotoxin would eliminate this problem.[10,33] In addition, the large size of the linked molecules in polymerized hemoglobin solutions further attenuated direct renal toxicity by precluding glomular filtration. However, the existence of an unidentified vasoactive substance within hemoglobin solutions that can adversely affect renal blood flow has been suggested.[6,17,44]

Recently, investigators have questioned whether hemoglobin itself may be intrinsically toxic, regardless of the degree of its purity. Accumulating evidence suggests that hemoglobin-based solutions may induce vasoconstriction via interference of the hemoglobin molecule with endothelial nitric oxide release.[6,44,45] Coronary vasoconstriction has been demonstrated in vitro[46] and in isolated heart models,[47,48] but the evidence for in vivo vasoconstriction is less clear.[16,49,50] Further work is needed to clarify this important issue. Others have focused on the occurrence of autoxidation and the generation of toxic free oxygen radicals.[51] In the clinical trial of Feola and colleagues,[36] mannitol was coadministered with the bovine hemoglobin preparation.

An advantage of bovine and recombinant hemoglobin solutions is the absence of any human pathogens. However, it will be necessary to ensure that these preparations are free of animal viruses and endotoxin.[40] Another concern is the potential downregulation of immune function following infusion of hemoglobin-based solutions.[17,20,52] Free hemoglobin was found to act as an adjuvant when injected into the peritoneal cavity in a rat model of experimental peritonitis.[53] When injected intravenously as a volume expander, however, no alteration in host immune function was detected.[53,54] Effects of polyhemoglobin solutions on recipient immunocompetence will need to be carefully delineated before widespread clinical use could be advocated in patients who are at risk for septic complications.

Perfluorocarbon Solutions

Chemical Properties

Extensive research has been directed toward the potential application of perfluorocarbons (PFC) as oxygen transport fluids. PFCs are a class of compounds derived from cyclic or straight-chain hydrocarbons in which hydrogen atoms have been replaced with fluorine (or bromine) atoms.[55–58] Compounds of varying complexity have been synthesized. These liquids are highly stable due to the presence of strong carbon-fluorine bonds and are essentially chemically inert.[55–58] They have attracted great attention as potential red blood cell substitutes because of their high solubility for gases and stability within biologic systems. PFCs, however, are hydrophobic and immiscible in aqueous solution. Therefore, to allow intravenous administration, the preparations must be emulsified in an electrolyte solution with a surfactant/emulsifier that stabilizes the PFC particles and prevents their coalescence.[58,59] Specific additives or oncotic components can be included as indicated. The average particle diameter in PFC emulsions is approximately 1/80 that of the RBC and the emulsions have a significantly lower viscosity than blood.[13,55–58]

Oxygen Transport by Perfluorocarbons

The high solubility of gases (O_2 and CO_2) within PFCs provided the rationale to investigate their usefulness as blood substitutes. Oxygen solubility within PFCs is typically in the range of 40 to 50 vol% for 100% pure oxygen under atmospheric pressure.[57] PFC-based solutions transport oxygen in a fundamentally different manner from hemoglobin. Oxygen simply dissolves in the PFC, resulting in a linear relation between the oxygen content and the partial pressure[13,57,58] (Fig. 24.4). Carbon dioxide solubility is about three to four times greater.[57] The quantity of gas that can be dissolved is dependent on the PFC concentration. The concentration of the perfluorocarbon component in an emulsion is generally expressed in weight percent. The corresponding volume percent of the PFC component is lower due to the high density of the PFCs. At physiologic oxygen partial pressures, the PFC-based solutions possess a limited oxygen carrying capacity, yet as evident in Figure 24.4, clinically meaningful oxygen delivery could be achieved at the high partial pressures present during mechanical ventilation with high inspired FiO_2. The solubility of oxygen and other gases is inversely related to temperature.[60] The small size of the PFC particles may facilitate oxygen delivery to tissues inaccessible to RBCs. In addition, it has been suggested that the presence of PFC particles may serve as a "high

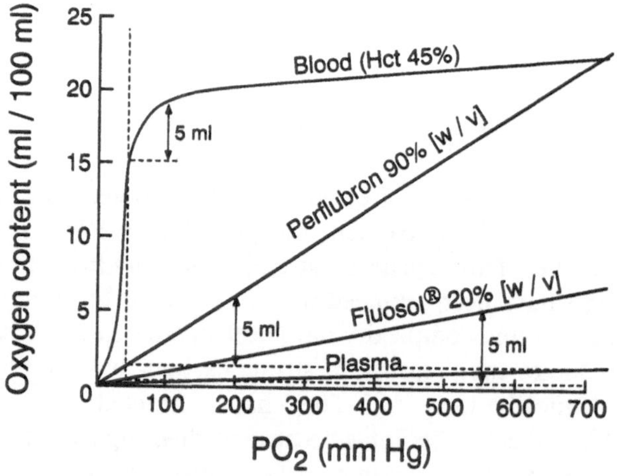

FIGURE 24.4. Oxygen content and release of normal blood, 90% w/v Perflubron emulsion, Fluosol-DA 20%, and plasma. Between 100 mm Hg (normal arterial oxygen tension) and 45 mm Hg (normal venous oxygen tension), whole blood with a hematocrit of 45% will release about 5 ml of O_2. (From Faithfull,[13] with permission.)

solubility pathway" and promote the transfer of oxygen from erythrocytes across the endothelial membrane.[61]

Development

Evidence that PFCs could support in vivo respiratory gas exchange was provided in the 1960s with the survival of liquid breathing mice.[62] PFC solutions containing pluronic emulsifiers were developed that could support oxygen requirements following total exchange transfusion in rats.[63] Subsequent research culminated in the development of Fluosol-DA 20% (Fluosol), the prototypical first-generation perfluorocarbon emulsion designed for intravenous use in man.[55–58] Fluosol contains a mixture of perfluorodecalin (FDC) and perfluorotripropylamine (FTPA) in a 7:3 molar ratio with an intravascular half-life of approximately 12 hours. Although FTPA was included to improve the stability of the base FDC emulsion, the preparation also required the addition of the surfactant Pluronic F-68.[64] The composition of Fluosol-DA 20% is shown in Table 24.1. After extensive testing in experimental animals,[55] Fluosol was administered to human subjects by investigators in Japan.[65] Mitsuno and colleagues[66] summarized the Japanese experience with Fluosol in 186 surgical patients who received, for a variety of indications including "bloodless surgery," an infusion of 20 ml/kg. Additional doses of 10 ml/kg were administered in nine patients. Although the investigators reported a definite contribution by the Fluosol infusion to total oxygen transport and to hemodynamic stability, the results of subsequent (and better controlled) trials were less favorable and pointed out important inadequacies and safety concerns. Clinical trials of Fluosol were initiated in the United States in 1979 and continued into the mid-1980s when they were discontinued. These studies were conducted primarily in severely anemic patients in need of surgery who

TABLE 24.1. Composition of Fluosol-DA 20% (Green Cross Corp., Japan).

Perfluorodecalin	14.0
Perfluorotripropylamine	6.0
Pluronic F-68	2.7
Yolk phospholipids	0.4
Glycerol	0.8
NaCl	0.600
KCl	0.034
$MgCl_2$	0.020
$Cacl_2$	0.028
$NaHCO_3$	0.210
Glucose	0.180
Hydroxyethyl starch	3.0

All values are w/v (%).
From Lowe.[56]

refused blood transfusion on religious grounds.[67–69] Patients received Fluosol in a 30-ml/kg dose and achieved fluorcrits (volume concentration of Fluosol) in the 3% to 5% range. Conclusions similar to those of the Japanese investigators were reached, including (1) Fluosol could be given safely to anemic patients following a test dose, (2) at high oxygen tensions Fluosol did contribute to oxygen delivery, and (3) the effect was short-lived and clinical benefit could not be documented. Safety was clearly an issue with consistent reports of adverse reactions to a 0.5-ml test dose.[67,68] The need to store the compound in a frozen state and a difficult thawing and reconstitution procedure were also disadvantages.[58]

The inability of Fluosol administration to have an impact on severe anemia is not surprising. The low PFC (10% by volume) content in Fluosol, as well as concerns related to the long-term consequences of FTPA retention in the reticuloendothelial system ($t_{1/2}$ of 65 days) that restricted administration to a single 30-ml/kg dose, made this an unreasonable treatment goal. Other first-generation PFC emulsions include the Chinese product Emulsion II,[70] which was tested in both civilian and military surgery, and Ftorosan, used exclusively in the Soviet Union.[13] The recognized limitations of Fluosol led to both the development of improved second-generation emulsions and a reassessment of potential applications for PFCs outside of major blood loss replacement. The use of Fluosol in settings where small doses and short-lived effects would be desirable prompted the investigation of a slightly modified product, renamed simply Fluosol-DA (Green Cross Corp., Japan) for use in PTCA. Studies in animal models demonstrated that the intracoronary administration of Fluosol attenuated reperfusion injury and preserved left ventricular function following experimental myocardial infarction.[71,72] In addition to rheologic properties that enhanced perfusion of the distal coronary bed, Fluosol was also shown to inhibit neutrophil chemotaxis and activation.[73] Several clinical trials in high-risk PTCA followed.[74,75] The combined experience from these trials suggested that transcatheter perfusion with oxygenated PFC emulsion during balloon occlusion reduced the incidence of angina and contractile dysfunction[74,75] and resulted in U.S. Food and Drug Administration (FDA) approval for this indication. In a recent trial studying the effects of intravenous Fluosol (15 ml/kg) in conjunction with thrombolytic therapy in acute myocardial infarction, a reduction in recurrent ischemic complications was detected in the Fluosol-treated group. However, no reduction in infarct size or improvement in left ventricular function was observed, and the Fluosol-treated group exhibited more episodes of transient pulmonary edema than placebo-treated controls.[76]

The first-generation Fluosol-type emulsions were characterized by low PFC concentrations, limited oxygen carrying capacity, short intravascular half-lives, and adverse reactions (probably related to the Pluronic F-68 surfactant). An improved, ready-to-use Fluosol-DA 20% emulsion was developed, replacing Pluronic F-68 with phospholipid emulsifiers.[57] This formulation, however, still has the same low PFC concentration. The most promising of the novel second generation PFC emulsions contain perfluoroctylbromide (PFOB/Perflubron). PFOB was initially developed as a radiologic contrast agent, but can be synthesized as a stable, highly concentrated oxygen carrying emulsion containing 90% to 100% perfluorocarbon by weight (47–52% by volume).[77] PFOB is readily emulsified with egg yolk lecithins (as used in lipid emulsions for parenteral nutrition).[57,77] The in vivo half-life of PFOB is approximately 4 days.[13] Commercial preparations that are stable at room temperature and easily administered are being developed under the trade names Oxygent and Imagent (Alliance Pharmaceutical Corp., San Diego, CA).[55–57] The major difference between Fluosol and Perflubron-type emulsions are shown in Figure 24.5.

Safety

Perfluorocarbons are biologically inert compounds that undergo no in vivo enzymatic degradation or metabolic processing. They are cleared from the intravascular compartment by the reticuloendothelial system (RES) much in the same way as fat emulsions or liposomes.[55,78] PFCs are slowly eliminated in vapor phase in expired air with a half-life dependent mainly on their molecular weight. Half-lives of some common PFCs are FDC, 6 days; PFOB, 4 days; and FTPA, 65 days.[55] Following intravenous administration in man and experimental animals, no increases in fluoride ion concentration have been reported.[13] Despite the apparent innocuous nature of these compounds, Fluosol administration was associated with transient elevations in transaminase levels and hepatosplenomegaly.[55,56] The long-term consequences of prolonged RES retention of PFCs has not been well characterized, but could potentially interfere with immune function.

Acute adverse reactions to PFC emulsions have also been widely reported. The occasional occurrence of acute, anaphylactic-type reactions necessitated the administration of a test dose (usually 0.5 ml) to patients before starting Fluosol infusion. The reactions were characterized by transient hypotension, increases in pulmonary artery pressures, leukopenia, and bronchospasm.[67,79] This prompted some investigators to routinely pretreat with corticosteroids.[69,79] Attention has focused on the role of complement activation in mediating these reactions,[79] and it appears that the surfactant used in the first-generation formulations, Pluronic F-68, was the inciting factor. The use of highly purified Pluronic fractions[80] and lecithin-based surfactants[77,81] in the second-generation emulsions may prevent the untoward effects. Egg yolk lecithins, although already used regularly in lipid emulsions for parenteral nutrition, are sensitive to degradation and contain potentially toxic contaminants such as lysophospholipids.[56] As with hemoglobin-based solutions, even trace amounts of toxic contaminants could have serious consequences when considering the doses given clinically, underlining the need for stringent quality control.

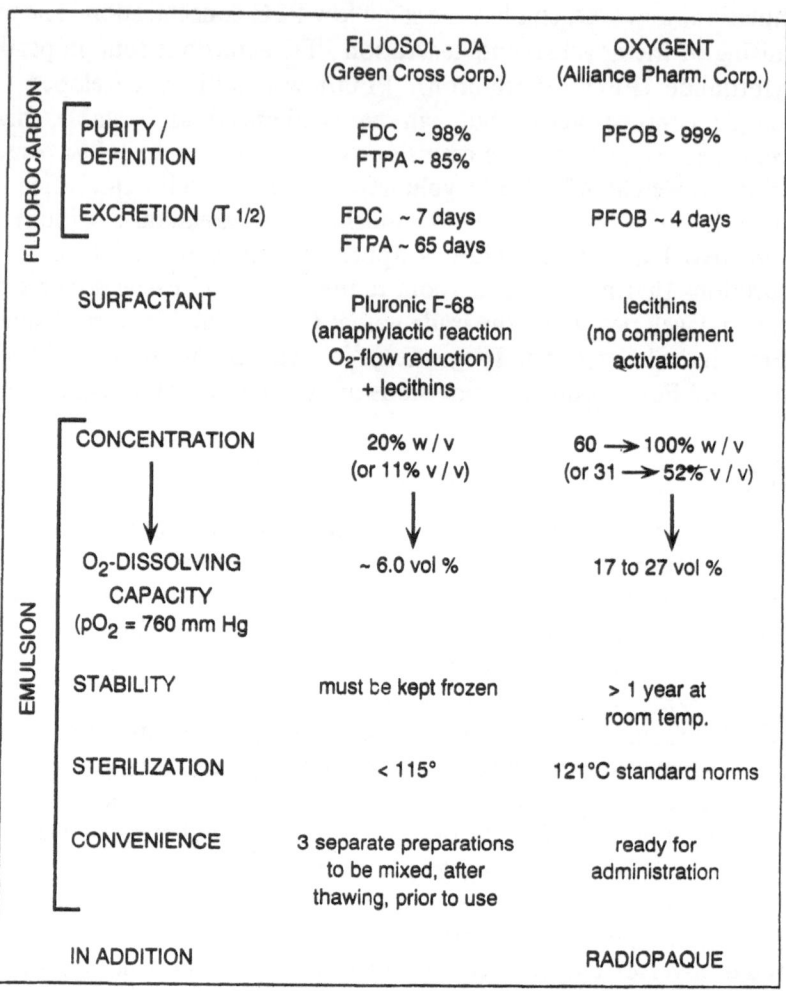

		FLUOSOL - DA (Green Cross Corp.)	OXYGENT (Alliance Pharm. Corp.)
FLUOROCARBON	PURITY / DEFINITION	FDC ~ 98% FTPA ~ 85%	PFOB > 99%
FLUOROCARBON	EXCRETION (T 1/2)	FDC ~ 7 days FTPA ~ 65 days	PFOB ~ 4 days
	SURFACTANT	Pluronic F-68 (anaphylactic reaction O_2-flow reduction) + lecithins	lecithins (no complement activation)
EMULSION	CONCENTRATION	20% w / v (or 11% v / v)	60 → 100% w / v (or 31 → 52% v / v)
EMULSION	↓ O_2-DISSOLVING CAPACITY (pO_2 = 760 mm Hg	↓ ~ 6.0 vol %	↓ 17 to 27 vol %
EMULSION	STABILITY	must be kept frozen	> 1 year at room temp.
EMULSION	STERILIZATION	< 115°	121°C standard norms
EMULSION	CONVENIENCE	3 separate preparations to be mixed, after thawing, prior to use	ready for administration
	IN ADDITION		RADIOPAQUE

FIGURE 24.5. Comparison between a first-generation perfluorocarbon oxygen carrying solution (Fluosol-DA) and a second-generation Perflubron-based solution (Oxygent). Perfluorodecalin (FDC), perfluorotripropylamine (FTPA), perfluoroctylbromide (PFOB). (From Reiss,[57] with permission.)

The reported increased incidence of pulmonary edema observed in the FDA-treated patients in the treatment of acute myocardial infarction (TAMI) trial,[76] was most likely related to the coadministration of a large amount of intravenous crystalloid.

Blood Substitutes and Cardiac Surgery

Clinical experience with erythrocyte substitutes has been limited, and to date they have had no impact on the conduct of cardiac operations.

However, the recent development of safer and more effective products may stimulate interest in their incorporation within blood conservation and myocardial protection strategies. Some potential applications, both during cardiopulmonary bypass and in the perioperative period, are discussed in this section.

Blood Replacement During Cardiopulmonary Bypass

Oxygen carrying solutions could be employed to maximize blood conservation at several points during the cardiac operation. Volume resuscitation with an erythrocyte substitute during intraoperative autologous blood donation could permit blood withdrawal to proceed to otherwise unacceptably low hematocrits. An experimental precedent has been reported, in which 80% of red cell mass was removed and preserved perioperatively in conjunction with polymerized bovine hemoglobin administration.[34] Priming of the cardiopulmonary bypass (CPB) circuit with both Fluosol[82,83] and bovine hemoglobin solution[84] has been reported in the experimental literature. In addition, an erythrocyte substitute could be infused if needed during CPB to avoid homologous transfusion or the premature reinfusion of autologous donated or Cell Saver blood. A short intravascular half-life would not be problematic.

Blood substitutes could theoretically enhance the benefits of isovolumic hemodilution. In particular, the small size of the particles in both hemoglobin and PFC solutions might optimize blood flow to the microcirculation while maintaining oxygen transport capacity. Advantages of PFC solutions, especially the second-generation preparations, are continued oxygen loading at the supraphysiologic oxygen tensions present during CPB and an increase in efficiency in hypothermia is employed.[60] Paramount in any discussion regarding the applicability of oxygen carrying solutions in CPB are safety issues. With respect to the hemoglobin-based solutions, it remains to be satisfactorily shown that no untoward renal effects or immunologic compromise will be encountered in the delicate perioperative period, especially in a patient population with many comorbid risk factors for such complications. Of concern was a recent study using polymerized bovine hemoglobin in the CPB priming solution. Although all animals were successfully weaned from bypass and ventilator support, significant increases in pulmonary vascular resistance and pressures were noted, suggesting vasoconstriction.[84] The effects of extracorporeal circulation on the stability of hemoglobin and PFC solutions will also have to be addressed.

Blood Replacement in the Postoperative Period

More information is available with respect to the treatment of perioperative anemia.[36,66–68] While early clinical experience was largely unsuccessful, novel agents with longer intravascular half-lives, better oxygen carrying capacity, and fewer associated side effects may produce more satisfactory results. Potential postoperative applications within a comprehensive blood conservation program are obvious. Erythrocyte substitutes could be employed instead of homologous transfusion while awaiting return of an endogenous or pharmacologically stimulated erythropoietic response.

Myocardial Protection

Small particle size, low viscosity, a linear oxygen dissociation curve, and increased solubility at low temperatures stimulated interest in the use of Fluosol as a cardioplegic agent. These qualities, combined with the absence of potentially detrimental neutrophils and platelets, suggested potential advantages over cold-blood cardioplegia. In the 1980s, several investigators reported that left ventricular functional recovery was improved with Fluosol cardioplegia compared with standard crystalloid or blood cardioplegia.[85–87] The differences were small and inconsistent, however, and clinical trials were not carried out. A more recent report[88] also failed to demonstrate a significant benefit over blood cardioplegia, but suggested that further studies were indicated.

Regional or Isolated Organ Perfusion

Oxygenated perfluorocarbon solutions are being investigated for the purpose of organ preservation in transplantation. They may also offer a means to improve oxygenation to ischemic organs during periods of surgical hypoxia. In one study, ex vivo isolated hearts were well preserved after 24 hours of PFC perfusion.[89] Intrathecal administration of Fluosol was also shown to prevent the development of paraplegia in an experimental model of prolonged thoracic aortic occlusion.[90] Other potential applications, such as retrograde cerebral perfusion during hypothermic circulatory arrest, can be envisioned.

Summary

Recently, important advances have been made in the production of hemoglobin- and perfluorocarbon-based oxygen carrying solutions. Many of the inadequacies and toxicity concerns associated with erythrocyte substitutes in the past have been ameliorated with the latest preparations. For the cardiac surgeon, effective substitutes could offer an additional margin of safety in aggressive blood conservation strategies, as well as unique rheologic benefits based on their composition. Indeed, uses for "blood substitutes" are likely to extend beyond the simple resuscitation of perioperative blood loss as initially envisioned. Ideally, specific products, each with its own unique physiologic characteristics, could be appropriately matched to a given clinical application. However, it will be necessary to carefully weigh the potential risks of a blood substitute in comparison to what is generally a very safe national blood supply. Additional research, in models designed to mimic the setting of cardiopulmonary bypass, is needed to establish the efficacy and safety of the novel formulations (especially with hemoglobin-based solutions). Successful introduction into cardiac surgery will depend on the results of such research as well as those of ongoing preliminary clinical trials.

References

1. Amberson WR. Blood substitutes. *Biol Rev* 1937;12:48–86.
2. Amberson WR, Mulder AG, Steggerda FR, et al. Blood substitutes. *Science* 1933;78:106–107.
3. Winslow RM. Clinical indications and properties. In: Winslow RM, ed. *Hemoglobin-Based Red Cell Substitutes*. Baltimore: Johns Hopkins University Press, 1992;18–36.
4. Nunn JF. *Applied Respiratory Physiology*. 2nd ed. London and Boston: Butterworths, 1977.
5. Guyton AC, Jones CE, Coleman TG. *Cardiac Output and Its Regulation*. 2nd ed. Philadelphia: W.B. Saunders, 1973.
6. Spahn DR, Leone BJ, Reves JG, et al. Cardiovascular and coronary physiology of acute isovolemic hemodilution: a review of nonoxygen-carrying and oxygen-carrying solutions. *Anesth Analg* 1994;78:1000–1021.
7. Pennell RB, Smith WE. Preparation of stabilized solutions of hemoglobin. *Blood* 1949;4:380–394.
8. Miller JH, McDonald RK. The effect of hemoglobin on renal function in the human. *J Clin Invest* 1951;30:33–40.
9. Hamilton PB, Hiller A, Van Slyke DD. Renal effects of hemoglobin infusions in dogs in hemorrhagic shock. *J Exp Med* 1948;85:477–487.
10. Rabiner SF, Helbert JR, Lopas H, et al. Evaluation of a stroma-free hemoglobin solution for use as a plasma expander. *J Exp Med* 1967;126:1127–1142.
11. Biro GP. Current status of erythrocyte substitutes. *Can Med Assoc J* 1983; 129:237–244.
12. Baldwin JE, Gill B. Approaches to the preparation of oxygen carriers for use as blood substitutes. *Med Lab Sci* 1982;39:45–51.
13. Faithfull NS. Artificial oxygen carrying blood substitutes. In: Erdmann W, Bruley DF, eds. *Oxygen Transport to Tissue XIV*. New York: Plenum Press, 1992;55.
14. De Venuto F. Stability of crystalline hemoglobin solution during extended storage. *J Clin Lab Med* 1978;92:976.
15. Moss GS, DeWoskin R, Rosen AL, et al. Transport of oxygen and carbon dioxide by hemoglobin-saline solution in the red cell-free primate. *Surg Gynecol Obstet* 1976;142:357–362.
16. Biro GP, Beresford-Kroeger D, Hendry P. Early deleterious hemorheologic changes following acute experimental coronary occlusion and salutary antihyperviscosity effect of hemodilution with stroma-free hemoglobin. *Am Heart J* 1982;103:870–878.

17. Gould SA, Seghal LR, Sehgal HL, et al. Artificial blood: current status of hemoglobin solutions. *Crit Care Clin* 1992;8:293–309.
18. Sehgal LR, Rosen AL, Gould SA, et al. An appraisal of polymerized pyridoxylated hemoglobin as an acellular oxygen carrier. In: Bolin RB, Geyer RP, eds. *Blood Substitutes.* New York: Alan R. Liss, 1983;19–28.
19. Bunn HF, Esham WT, Bull RW. The renal handling of hemoglobin. *J Exp Med* 1969;129:909–924.
20. DeVenuto F, Friedman HI, Neville JR, et al. Appraisal of hemoglobin solution as a blood substitute. *Surg Gynecol Obstet* 1979;149:417–436.
21. Savitsky JP, Doczi J, Black J, et al. A clinical safety trial of stroma-free hemoglobin. *Clin Pharmacol Ther* 1978;23:73–80.
22. Benesch RE, Kwong S. Bis-pyridoxal polyphosphates: a new class of specific intramolecular crosslinking agents for hemoglobin. *Biochem Biophys Res Commun* 1988;156:9–14.
23. Seghal LR, Rosen AL, Noud G, et al. Large volume preparation of pyridoxylated hemoglobin with high P_{50}. *J Surg Res* 1981;30:14.
24. Gould SA, Rosen AL, Sehgal LR, et al. The effect of altered hemoglobin-oxygen affinity on oxygen transport by hemoglobin solution. *J Surg Res* 1980;28:246–251.
25. Gould SA, Sehgal LR, Rosen AL, et al. Hemoglobin solution: Is a normal [Hb] or P_{50} more important? *J Surg Res* 1982;33:189–193.
26. Keipert PE, Adeniran AJ, Kwong S, et al. Functional properties of a new crosslinked hemoglobin designed for use as a blood substitute. *Transfusion* 1989;29:768–773.
27. Keipert PE, Chang TM. Pyridoxylated-polyhemoglobin solution: a low viscosity oxygen-delivering blood replacement fluid with normal oncotic pressure and long-term storage feasibility. *Biomater Artif Cells Artif Organs* 1988; 16:185–196.
28. DeVenuto F, Zegna A. Preparation and evaluation of pyridoxylated human hemoglobin. *J Surg Res* 1983;34:205.
29. Sehgal LR, Rosen AL, Noud G, et al. Large-volume preparation of pyridoxylated polymerized human hemoglobin with high P_{50}. *J Surg Res* 1981;30:14.
30. Lenz G, Junger H, van den Ende R, et al. Hemodynamic effects after partial exchange transfusion with pyridoxylated polyhemoglobin in chimpanzees. *Biomater Artif Cells Immob Biotech* 1991;19:709.
31. Gould SA, Sehgal LR, Rosen AL, et al. The efficacy of polymerization pyridoxylated hemoglobin solution as an O_2 carrier. *Ann Surg* 1990; 211:394–398.
32. Fronticelli C, Bucci E, Orth C. Solvent regulation of oxygen affinity in hemoglobin. *J Biol Chem* 1984;259:10841–10844.
33. Feola M, Gonzalez H, Canizaro PC, et al. Development of a bovine stroma-free hemoglobin solution as a blood substitute. *Surg Gynecol Obstet* 1983; 157:399–408.
34. Vlahakes GJ, Lee R, Jacobs EE, et al. Hemodynamic effects and oxygen transport properties of a new blood substitute in a model of massive blood replacement. *J Thorac Cardiovasc Surg* 1990;100:379–388.
35. Slanetz PJ, Lee R, Page R, et al. Hemoglobin blood substitutes in extended preoperative autologous blood donation: an experimental study. *Surgery* 1994;115:246–254.
36. Feola M, Simoni J, Angelillo R, et al. Clinical trial of a hemoglobin based blood

substitute in patients with sickle cell anemia. *Surg Gynecol Obstet* 1992; 174:379–386.

37. Hunt CA, Burnette RR, MacGregor RD, et al. Synthesis and evaluation of a prototypal artificial red cell. *Science* 1985;230:1165–1168.
38. Kibanov AL, Maruyama K, Torchilin VP, et al. Amphipathic polyethyleneglycols effectively prolong the circulation time of liposomes. *FEBS* 1990;268:235–237.
39. Hoffman SJ, Looker DL, Roehrich JM, et al. Expression of fully functional tetrameric human hemoglobin in *Escherichia coli. Proc Natl Acad Sci USA* 1990;87:8521.
40. Bunn HF. The use of hemoglobin as a blood substitute. *Am J Hematol* 1993;42:112–117.
41. Looker D, Abbott-Brown D, Cozart P, et al. A human recombinant haemoglobin designed for use as a blood substitute. *Nature* 1992;356:258–261.
42. Lee R, Atsumi N, Jacobs EE, et al. Ultra-pure, stroma-free, polymerized bovine hemoglobin solution: evaluation of renal toxicity. *J Surg Res* 1989;47:407–411.
43. Moss GS, Gould SA, Rosen AL, et al. Animal model for nephrotoxicity of haemoglobin tetramer. *Lancet* 1986;24:1219.
44. Vogel WM, Lieberthal W, Apstein CS, et al. Effects of stroma-free hemoglobin solutions on isolated perfused rabbit hearts and isolated perfused rat kidneys. *Biomater Artif Cells Artif Organs* 1988;248:653–661.
45. Martin W, Villani GM, Jothianandan D, et al. Selective blockade of endothelium-dependent and glyceryl trinitrate-induced relaxation by hemoglobin and by methylene blue in the rabbit aorta. *J Pharmacol Exp Ther* 1985;232:708–716.
46. Biro GP, Taichman GC, Lada B, et al. Coronary vascular actions of stroma-free hemoglobin preparations. *Artif Organs* 1988;12:40–50.
47. Macdonald VW, Winslow RM, Marini MA, et al. Coronary vasoconstrictor activity of purified and modified human hemoglobin. *Biomater Artif Cells Artif Organs* 1990;18:263–282.
48. Vogel WM, Dennis RC, Cassidy G, et al. Coronary constrictor effect of stroma-free hemoglobin solutions. *Am J Physiol* 1986;251:H413–420.
49. Feola M, Azar MD, Weiner L. Improved oxygenation of ischemic myocardium by hemodilution with stroma-free hemoglobin solution. *Chest* 1979;75:369–375.
50. Hodakowski GT, Page RD, Harringer W, et al. Greater maximal myocardial oxygen delivery after hemodilution with polymerized bovine hemoglobin substitute. *Surg Forum* 1991;43:304–306.
51. Faasen AE, Sundby SS, Panter RM, et al. Hemoglobin: a lifesaver and an oxidant. How to tip the balance. *Biomater Artif Cells Artif Organs* 1988; 16:93–104.
52. Otto BR, Verweij-van Vught AM, MacLaren DM. Blood substitutes and infection. *Nature* 1992;358:23–24.
53. Hau T, Simmons RL. Mechanisms of the adjuvant effect of hemoglobin in experimental peritonitis: III. The influence of hemoglobin on phagocytosis and intracellular killing by human granulocytes. *Surgery* 1980;87:588–592.
54. Hoyt DB, Greenberg AC, Peskin CW, et al. Resuscitation with pyridoxylated stroma free hemoglobin: tolerance to sepsis. *J Trauma* 1981;21:938–942.
55. Biro GP, Blais P. Perfluorocarbon blood substitutes. *Crit Rev Oncol Hematol* 1987;6:311–374.
56. Lowe KC. Synthetic oxygen transport fluids based on perfluorochemicals: applications in medicine and biology. *Vox Sang* 1991;60:129–140.

57. Reiss JG. Fluorocarbon-based in vivo oxygen transport and delivery systems. *Vox Sang* 1991;61:225–239.
58. Biro GP. Perfluorocarbon-based red blood cell substitutes. *Trans Med Rev* 1993;7:84–95.
59. Sharma SK, Lowe KC, Davis SS. Emulsification methods for perfluorochemicals. *Drug Dev Ind Pharmacol* 1988;14:2371–2376.
60. Reiss JG, LeBlanc M. Solubility and transport phenomena in perfluorochemicals relevant to blood substitution and other biomedical applications. *Pure Appl Chem* 1982;54:2383–2406.
61. Faithfull NS, Cain SM. Critical levels of O_2 extraction following hemodilution with Dextran or Fluosol-DA. *J Crit Care* 1988;3:14–18.
62. Clark LC, Gollan F. Survival of mammals breathing organic liquids equilibrated with oxygen at atmospheric pressure. *Science* 1966;152:1755–1756.
63. Geyer RP, Monroe RG, Taylor K. Survival of rats having red cells totally replaced with emulsified fluorocarbon. *Fed Proc* 1968;27:384.
64. Ohyanagi H, Toshima K, Sekita M, et al. Clinical studies of perfluorochemical whole blood substitutes: safety of Fluosol-DA (20%) in normal human volunteers. *Clin Ther* 1979;2:306–312.
65. Tremper KK, Anderson ST. Perfluorochemical emulsion oxygen transport fluids: a clinical review. *Annu Rev Med* 1985;36:309–313.
66. Mitsuno TM, Ophyanagi H, Naito R. Clinical studies of a perfluorochemical whole blood substitute (Fluosol-DA). *Ann Surg* 1982;19:60–70.
67. Tremper KK, Friedman AE, Levine EM, et al. The preoperative treatment of severely anemic patients with a perfluorochemical oxygen-transport fluid, Fluosol-DA. *N Engl J Med* 1982;307:277–283.
68. Gould SA, Rosen AL, Sehgal LR, et al. Fluosol-DA as a red-cell substitute in acute anemia. *N Engl J Med* 1986;314:1653–1656.
69. Spence RK, McCoy S, Constabile J, et al. Fluosol DA-20 in the treatment of severe anemia: randomized, controlled study of 46 patients. *Crit Care Med* 1990;18:1227–1231.
70. Chen HS, Yang ZH. Perfluorocarbon as blood substitute in clinical applications and in war casualties. In: Chang TM, Geyer RP, eds. *Blood Substitutes.* New York: Marcel Dekker, 1989;403–410.
71. Nunn G, Dance G, Peters J, et al. Effect of fluorocarbon exchange transfusion on myocardial infarction size in dogs. *Am J Cardiol* 1983;52:203–205.
72. Forman M, Bingham S, Kopelman H. Reduction of infarct size with intracoronary perfluorochemical in a canine preparation of reperfusion. *Circulation* 1985;71:1060–1068.
73. Bajaj A, Cobb M, Virmani R, et al. Limitation of myocardial reperfusion injury by intravenous perfluorochemicals: role of neutrophil activation. *Circulation* 1989;79:645–656.
74. Cowley MJ, Snow FR, DiSciascio G, et al. Perfluorochemical perfusion during coronary angioplasty in unstable and high-risk patients. *Circulation* 1990; 81(suppl 4):27–34.
75. Kent KM, Cleman MW, Cowley MJ, et al. Reduction of myocardial ischemia during percutaneous transluminal coronary angioplasty with oxygenated Fluosol. *Am J Cardiol* 1990;66:279–284.
76. Wall TC, Califf RM, Blankenship J, et al. Intravenous Fluosol in treatment of acute myocardial infarction. Results of the thrombolysis and angioplasty in myocardial infarction 9 trial. *Circulation* 1994;90:114–120.

77. Long DM, Long DC, Mattrey RF. An overview of perfluorooctyl bromide—application as a synthetic oxygen carrier and imaging agent for x-ray, ultrasound, and nuclear magnetic resonance. In: Chang TM, Geyer RP, eds. *Blood Substitutes.* New York: Marcel Dekker, 1989;411-421.
78. Faithfull NS. Fluorocarbons. *Anaesthesia* 1978;42:234-242.
79. Vercellotti G, Hammerschmidt DE, Craddock PR, et al. Activation of plasma complement by perfluorocarbon artificial blood: probable mechanism of adverse pulmonary reactions in treated patients and rationale for corticosteroid prophylaxis. *Blood* 1982;59:1299-1304.
80. Lane TA, Krukonis V. Reduction in toxicity of a component of an artificial blood substitute by supercritical fluid fractionation. *Transfusion* 1988; 28:375-378.
81. Mattrey RF, Hilpert PL, Loung CD, et al. Hemodynamic effects of intravenous lecithin-based perfluorocarbon emulsions in dogs. *Crit Care Med* 1989; 17:652-656.
82. Rousou JA, Engelman RM, Anisimowicz L, et al. Comparison of blood and Fluosol-DA for cardiopulmonary bypass. *J Cardiovasc Surg* 1985;26:447-453.
83. Holman WL, McGiffin DC, Viente WVA, et al. Use of current generation perfluorocarbon emulsions in cardiac surgery. *Artif Cells Blood Subs Immob Biotech* 1994;22:979-990.
84. Schistek R, Pohla G, Samhaber E, et al. Artificial blood and extracorporeal circulation (ECC). *Biomater Artif Cells Immob Biotech* 1992;20:731-734.
85. Kanter KR, Jaffin JH, Ehrlichman RJ, et al. Superiority of perfluorocarbon cardioplegia over blood or crystalloid cardioplegia. *Circulation* 1981;64(suppl II):75-80.
86. Flaherty JH, Jaffin JH, Magovern GJ, et al. Maintenance of aerobic metabolism during global ischemia with perfluorocarbon cardioplegia improves myocardial preservation. *Circulation* 1984;69:585-592.
87. Novick RJ, Stefaniszyn HJ, Michel RP, et al. Protection of hypertrophied pig myocardium. *J Thorac Cardiovasc Surg* 1985;89:547-566.
88. Pearl JM, Laks H, Drinkwater DC, et al. Fluosol cardioplegia results in complete functional recovery: a comparison with blood cardioplegia. *Ann Thorac Surg* 1992;54:1144-1150.
89. Kioka Y, Tago M, Bando K, et al. Twenty-four hour isolated heart preservation by perfusion method with oxygenated solution containing perfluorochemicals and albumin. *J Heart Transplant* 1986;5:437-443.
90. Maughan RE, Mohan C, Nathan IM, et al. Intrathecal perfusion of an oxygenated perfluorocarbon prevents paraplegia after aortic occlusion. *Ann Thorac Surg* 1992;54:818-825.
91. Greenberg AG. Life threatening acid-base disorders. In: Wilmore DW, et al., eds. *Care of the Surgical Patient,* vol. 1. New York: Scientific American, Inc.

25
Anemia During the Late Postoperative Period Following Cardiopulmonary Bypass Surgery

David J. Wolf

Owing to a variety of causes, most patients who undergo cardiopulmonary bypass (CPB) surgery develop anemia. Blood-loss anemia is related to the actual procedure; often delayed anemia follows. Causes range from common conditions such as poor nutrition and inadequate iron stores due to prior blood loss, and less common causes such as delayed hemolytic transfusion reactions (DHTR). This chapter discusses causation and treatment of delayed post-CPB anemia. Treatment of delayed anemia includes iron supplementation, subcutaneous (sc) recombinant human erythropoietin (rhEPO) injections, packed red cell transfusions (PRCT), folic acid, and diet. Less often, other types of anemia, such as hemolytic anemia, may need to be addressed from a specific perspective. The impact of perioperative blood product administration, the actual surgical procedure, and the individual patient's need for anticoagulation and/or antiplatelet drugs constitute additional considerations. Lastly, infectious complications of CPB surgery will be discussed with regard to the anemia such infections may engender. For the sake of clarity, the late post-CPB period will be considered to commence approximately 5 days after surgery.[1]

Causes of Anemia During the Late Postoperative Period

Anemia Preceding Surgery

Some patients requiring CPB surgery are relatively anemic on a subacute or chronic basis prior to surgical intervention. The causes for such preexisting anemia are varied and include chronic gastrointestinal blood loss anemia secondary to aspirin, oral anticoagulants, or heparin therapy.[2] Customarily, patients with ongoing coronary artery disease are maintained on some type of antithrombotic therapy. Patients may receive cardiac medications causing hemolytic anemias such as procainamide or quinidine.[3] Additionally, some patients may actually have underlying primary hematologic disorders causing anemia such as thalassemia, pernicious anemia, or anemia of chronic disease (ACD).[4] ACD stems from a combination of moderately increased red blood cell destruction secondary to an unknown extrinsic factor (probably a cytokine such as tumor necrosis factor, the interferons, and interleukin-1), as well as a failure of red blood cell production to compensate for the increased destruction. Restricted iron availability occurs during the ACD owing to failure of iron to be released from mononuclear cellular sites. Iron stores are invariably increased, and often the endogenous erythropoietin (EPO) response is inadequate.[5]

Blood Loss During Surgery

Blood loss during the perioperative period certainly has an impact on the degree of anemia during the postoperative period, particularly related to the extent to which the anemia is corrected within the first few days following surgery.[6]

Table 25.1[7–9] lists the causes of excessive bleeding following CPB. Patients receiving thrombolytic therapy prior to surgery are also at increased risk for postoperative bleeding.[10] Prophylactic transfusion should

TABLE 25.1. Potential causes of excessive blood loss following CPB surgery.

Definite	Probable		Possible
	Preoperative hemostatic dysfunction		
	Inherited	Acquired	
Localized bleeding site	von Willebrand's disease	Medication-related (aspirin, warfarin, fibrinolytics)	Protamine overdose
Acquired platelet dysfunction (alpha) degranulation)	Coagulation factor deficiency	Systemic disorders (uremia, hepatic dysfunction, vitamin K deficiency)	Free heparin (neutralized or rebound)
		Disseminated intravascular coagulation (DIC) associated with sepsis or low-output state	
		Primary fibrino(geno)lysis	
		Dilutional coagulopathy and thrombocytopenia	

See references 7–9.

not be used in uncomplicated primary cardiac surgery. Considering the risks of transmittable diseases and allergic complications, there is no rationale for attempts to circumvent bleeding problems with prophylactic transfusions unless the patient has a specific known hemostatic defect that will predictably cause increased blood loss. Standard practices to reduce the amount of postoperative blood loss include careful heparin reversal, employment of desmopressin acetate (DDAVP), and increasing use of aprotinin, a protease inhibitor that reduces bleeding after CPB by unknown mechanism(s).[11] Blood conservation, to minimize the number of allogenic PRCTs, is currently a major goal of CPB surgery owing to the large variety of infections[12–15] and potential adverse complications[14–19] that may follow the transfusion of blood products (Tables 25.2 and 25.3). Also, many of the

TABLE 25.2. Potential infections following blood product administration.

Variety	Microorganism	Frequency (per unit transfused)
Viral	HIV-1	1/225,000
	HTLV-1	1/50,000
	Hepatitis C	1/3,300
	Hepatitis B	1/200,000
	Hepatitis A	Rare
	EBV	Rare
	CMV	Rare
Parasitic	*Babesia microti*	$1/10^6$
	Plasmodium (malariae)	$1/10^6$
	Trypanosoma (Chagas' disease)	$1/10^6$
	Toxoplasma	Rare
	Filaria	Rare
	Leishmania (kala-azar)	Rare
Bacterial	*Yersinia enterocolitica*	$1/10^6$
	Staphylococcus	Rare
	Salmonella	Rare
	Pseudomonas	Rare
	Treponema pallidum (syphilis)	Rare
	Borrelia burgdorferi (Lyme disease)	Rare

See references 12–15.

TABLE 25.3. Potential adverse immunologic complications of blood product administration (noninfectious).

Red blood cell reactions	White blood cell reactions	Platelet reactions	Protein reactions
Hemolytic—immediate or delayed	Febrile Acute lung injury Graft vs. host	Posttransfusion purpura	Hypersensitivity Anaphylaxis
Alloimmunization	Alloimmunization	Alloimmunization	Alloimmunization

See references 14–19.

potentially transfusion-related infections themselves can cause anemia during the delayed postoperative period.

EPO is the major regulator of erythropoiesis.[20] Plasma levels of EPO increase within 6 hours of the appearance of an anemia following surgical bleeding. The magnitude of this increase correlates with the severity of the anemia. There is a considerable time lag between the onset of acute blood loss and responsive reticulocytosis driven by EPO despite a normal marrow's ability to increase red cell production to better than five times baseline, only if iron supply is adequate.[21] Although transfusion of whole blood or packed red cells (PRCs) is the obvious emergency therapy for blood-loss anemia of major severity, it is always to the patient's benefit to take full advantage of the normal endogenous mechanisms of compensatory red cell production. The patient's response can be predicted by the availability of iron and the ability to generate EPO. If either of these are impaired, as has been described for EPO following CPB surgery, then exogenous administration of both iron and recombinant human rhEPO will accelerate hematopoietic recovery.[22,23]

Anemia Related to Drugs and Infections

The post-CPB patient usually receives a variety of medications and is susceptible to infections, which in and of themselves may cause anemia. Often, several factors play a role causing anemia to be multifactorial and difficult to attribute to any one particular cause. For instance, *Escherichia coli,*[24] *Aspergillus,*[25] malaria,[24] and *Clostridium perfrigens* infection[26] have been reported to cause hemolytic anemia. Antibiotics often given prophylactically for CPB surgery, such as penicillin[27] and cephalosporins,[28] can cause immune hemolytic anemias. Patients who sometimes have occult hematologic abnormalities such as glucose-6-phosphate dehydrogenase (G6PD) deficiency and/or unstable hemoglobins can hemolyze following antibiotics (i.e., sulfonamides).[29,30] Although it is uncommon for cardiovascular medications usually employed during CPB surgery to cause anemia, sodium nitroprusside,[31] nitroglycerin,[32] propranolol,[33] and verapamil[34] may increase bleeding by interfering with platelet function. Propranolol has also been described to cause hemolysis following CPB surgery.[35]

Macroangiopathic Hemolysis

A specific variety of hemolysis, macroangiopathic hemolysis, may develop owing to shear-producing stress greater than the red cell membrane can withstand. Some cardiac and vascular disorders can cause intravascular hemolysis by actually fragmenting the red blood cell membrane.[36] Complications may cause turbulence in the blood flowing around or through a

TABLE 25.4. Potential causes of surgically related macroangiopathic hemolytic anemia.

Heart valve replacement		Patching procedures	Oxygenator
Outflow—too narrow	Ball variance	Ostium primum repair (especially if mitral regurgitation present)	Complement activation and mechanical shear stress related to tubing
Large area of exposed plastic	Regurgitation around seat	Aortic aneurysmal repair	
Cloth-covered struts	Strut rupture		
Multiple valves			

See references 36,37.

prosthetic heart valve and expose the red blood cells to very high shear stress.[37] The severe red cell destruction seen in some patients cannot be caused by hemodynamic turbulence alone,[37] but also requires that the turbulence occurs in a space enclosed by or bordered by a foreign surface (Table 25.4). Although red cell membrane damage is usually mild and compensated, severe hemolytic anemia sometimes occurs. A clinical diagnosis of intravascular hemolysis related to a prosthetic heart valve may be made by the appearance of schistocytes seen on the peripheral blood smear in concert with hemolytic parameters indicating hemolysis, e.g., elevated serum indirect bilirubin (SIB), elevated serum lactate dehydrogenase (LDH), low serum haptoglobin (HPT), and the presence of iron in the form of hemosiderin in the urine.

Methods of Treating Anemia During the Late Postoperative Period

Packed Red Cell (PRC) Transfusion

Analysis of 100 patients undergoing coronary artery bypass grafting (CABG) at the New York Hospital-Cornell University Medical Center (NYH-CUMC) demonstrated median total chest tube output of 1110 ± 440 ml (standard deviation) with a range of 390 to 2,650 ml. The use of the internal mammary artery, aspirin ingestion within 7 days of surgery, and preoperative platelet count were the only predictors of increased chest tube blood output by univariate or multivariate analysis. The mean number of allogenic units of PRCs was 2.3 ± 2.4 with 0.5 ± 1.1 occurring 24 hours or later postoperatively. Twenty-four percent of the patients who did not receive PRC within 24 hours following surgery, did receive at least one unit of PRCs thereafter. Twenty-five percent of patients received no transfusions whatsoever. By univariate analysis, the total PRC exposure was predicted by preoperative hematocrit (HCT) and postoperative chest tube output, as well as by age and gender. Multivariate analysis of all risk factors determined only chest tube output to be a significant predictor of the number of PRC transfusions.[23]

Owing to the multitude of potential adverse risks of blood product administration, general therapeutic principles for transfusions established by the American College of Physicians[38] have been adopted:

1. Avoid using an empiric, automated threshold for transfusion.
2. Avoid elective transfusion with allogenic blood.
3. Plan for the availability of autologous blood when acute blood loss can be predicted, if feasible.
4. Administer PRC transfusions on a unit-by-unit basis according to symptoms.
5. Consider rhEPO therapy to treat anemia when appropriate.

In surgical settings, such as CPB surgery, the concept of a "transfusion trigger" must be viewed with caution, because the HCT, even in combination with hemodynamic information, does not provide a precise estimate of erythrocyte deficits.[39] Clinicians, therefore, must judge the risk-to-benefit ratio of erythrocyte transfusions for each patient and adopt a conservative approach based on symptoms such as neurologic deficits (poor mentation), ischemic cardiac symptoms, and overall fatigue not related to other physiologic abnormalities or medications.

Although patients with impaired myocardial function require higher hemoglobin levels to maintain oxygen delivery during surgery, there are no current guidelines to determine when it is appropriate to transfuse surgical patients who have significant coronary artery disease.[40] Therefore, the development of transfusion guidelines based on observed cardiac function in patients with significant coronary artery disease undergoing major vascular procedures would be very valuable. The effects of preoperative volume loading on cardiac function, postoperative oxygen delivery, and hemoglobin levels necessary for adequate oxygen delivery to the heart in a high-risk population would be ideally studied to provide clinicians with guidelines.

In an era characterized by a high level of professional and public concern about infection, particularly the human immunodeficiency virus (HIV-1) and viral hepatitis, transfusion of blood products continues to be a major concern. Although special measures are important during and after cardiac surgery owing to the effects of CPB on the factors that normally maintain hemostasis to conserve homologous blood, immediate postoperative procedures to minimize blood loss as proper chest tube placement are clearly of great concern.[23] Johnson et al[41] compared two transfusion strategies following elective operations for myocardial revascularization. The more conservative strategy was to achieve and maintain HCT value of 32% or higher, and the more liberal strategy was to maintain HCT value of 25% or higher. As expected, the conservative group received larger numbers of PRC transfusions and a significant improvement in exercise endurance occurred during the fifth postoperative day. However, there was no significant difference in duration or degree of exercise demonstrated between the two groups thereafter. In comparing the two groups of anemic patients, there were no adverse consequences associated with a greater degree of hemodilution, and there was no correlation between HCT value and exercise capacity. The conclusion was that, although the limits of hemodilution may still be poorly defined, postoperative PRC transfusion in revascularized patients should be guided by clinical indications and not by specific hematocrit values. At NYH–CUMC, patients are often discharged from the hospital with HCT levels ranging from 22% to 25%.

Transfusion of PRCs can produce only transient improvement in a patient's overall condition. Furthermore, transfusions suppress the physiologic response to deficiency of a blood constituent. If a patient has a low red cell mass, tissue hypoxia results in an increase in EPO and the bone marrow responds with reticulocytosis. However, if the patient undergoes transfusion early in the sequence of events, then the reticulocyte response may be diminished and delayed.[42] In deciding when to order a packed cell transfusion, a series of questions should be considered:

1. Is blood transfusion really necessary?
2. What is the patient's particular clinical need?
3. Does the projected benefit justify the risks of blood transfusion?
4. What blood component will most effectively meet the special needs at the lowest cost?
5. Did the transfusion result in the anticipated benefit for the patient (after transfusion)?

Normal physiologic compensatory mechanisms protect tissue oxygenation and include increased blood flow to peripheral tissues mediated by cardiac or vascular mechanisms, increased oxygenation of arterial blood by pulmonary mechanisms, and shifting the oxygen dissociation curve to the right by metabolic mechanisms (2,3-biphosphoglycerate).[43] The most readily altered of these parameters is cardiac output, so tachycardia is an early sign of hemorrhage. For the physician, the most readily adjustable parameter is red cell mass, and this may be altered most quickly by PRC transfusion. Targeting an ideal hemoglobin (Hb) value of 10 g% is no longer acceptable. In certain settings, adequate oxygen-carrying capacity is provided by an Hb at a considerably lower level. Such guidelines have been endorsed by a National Institutes of Health Consensus Conference.[44] When considering whether to administer transfusions to a specific patient, the physician should consider age, duration of anemia, presence of coexisting cardiac, pulmonary and vascular conditions, and hemodynamic stability.

Some patients may require PRC transfusions at higher hemoglobin levels to meet oxygen delivery requirements. PRCs should not be transfused as a volume expander. Although the red cell mass may be low, oxygen delivery to tissues may be normal owing to compensatory mechanisms. The hematocrit of PRCs is 75% to 80% and thus is the most concentrated of all oxygen-carrying blood components. A bleeding patient may be better served by alternative blood components (i.e., platelets) to correct hemostatic defects, such as the acquired platelet storage pool deficiency generated by the CPB pump.[45]

Since transfusion of PRC is often determined by clinical judgment, it is not surprising that there is wide variability from institution to institution. Goodnough et al[40] evaluated 540 consecutive surgical patients undergoing CABG equally distributed among 18 centers in the United States. The proportion of patients transfused ranged from 28% to 100%. Hospitals where patients generally had high blood losses tended to transfuse most. But blood loss, estimated from the difference between admission and discharge HCTs and from PRCs infused, was not the only factor determining transfusion. Among the six hospitals showing very low mean red blood cell losses (<80 ml), the transfusion rate varied between 28% and 100%, closely reflecting the last hematocrit measured before discharge, which ranged between 29% and 38%. Variation of a similar magnitude applied to the infusion of plasma and platelets as well.

Owing to the risks and expense of packed cell transfusions, it should be the goal of every clinician to try to use the fewest units of PRCs as possible during the delayed postoperative period. Certainly, symptoms such as angina, cerebral ischemia, or syncope in concert with significant anemia warrant PRC transfusions. It should be noted, however, that in some instances such as syncope, volume depletion may be more significant, and treatment to induce hemodilution may be equally effective as giving PRCs. It has been shown by Rosengart et al[23] that a multimodality blood conservation program initially employed to permit Jehovah's Witnesses to benefit from CPB surgery, employing intraoperative administration of aprotinin, administration of high-dose rhEPO, preoperative autologous blood donation, intraoperative red cell salvage, low-prime CPB circuit, and continuous reinfusion of shed mediastinal blood can totally obviate the need for blood products including PRCs. Therefore, the administration of PRCs should be considered optional and relative only to the degree to which a concerted effort is made to obtain autologous blood for transfusion prior to surgery, as well as the degree of effort to achieve blood conservation during CPB surgery.[45,46] In addition, PRC transfusions should be leukocyte-depleted since this may help reduce the immunosuppressive effects of packed cell transfusion in addition to the more commonly observed acute febrile transfusion reaction.[47] Although such methods of sparing the use of all blood products are limited to Jehovah's Witnesses, it will be a challenge in the future for cardiovascular surgeons to apply such methods to the general population to minimize the amount of blood products administered for reasons of cost and safety.

Iron Therapy

The developing normoblast intrinsically possesses everything it needs to make hemoglobin except iron. A 70-kg man normally needs 21 mg of iron daily for hemoglobin synthesis. The plasma protein, transferrin, must deliver the iron to the normoblast. The primary source of iron released to transferrin from the breakdown of senescent red blood cells is derived from the mononuclear phagocyte system. Following sudden major blood loss, the kidney rapidly secretes EPO into the systemic circulation to stimulate erythropoiesis to replace the lost red blood cells. For the rate of erythropoiesis to increase threefold, the normoblast would need not 21 mg but 63 mg of iron daily. Although 21 mg of iron is readily available for the normal daily breakdown of senescent red blood cells, the additional 42 mg must come from body iron stores. If the stores are low, the rate at which iron can be mobilized will be insufficient to supply the full additional 42 mg. The lack of iron for increased hemoglobin synthesis would then limit the increase in erythropoiesis. Thus, in addition to EPO, whether it be exogenous or endogenous, the availability of iron ordinarily regulates the rate of red blood cell production.[48]

Iron stores in normal men are 500 to 2,000 mg, with the amount gradually increasing with age. Average iron stores for normal premenstrual women are estimated at 250 mg, but approximately 25% have no iron stores. In 2 ml of blood, there is approximately 1 mg of iron. If a patient is iron deficient prior to surgery (whether it be due to inadequate absorption owing to prior gastroduodenal surgery, occult gastrointestinal blood loss owing to aspirin or anticoagulation, or less likely iron loss in the urine as hemosiderin), it is clear that such patients will need oral iron postoperatively. Such patients can be identified by having a low mean corpuscular volume (MCV), transferrin saturation less than 15% and (if otherwise without liver or underlying inflammatory disease), a low serum ferritin level. Care should be taken to exclude a mild form of thalassemia or the anemia of chronic disease that may lower the MCV to less than 80 fl. If obtaining a serum ferritin level to demonstrate a value less than 12 μg/L is unavailable, a bone marrow to show absent iron stores may be obtained but usually is not necessary in the postoperative setting since a response to iron therapy would be sufficient. An adequate response can be assessed by obtaining a baseline reticulocyte count before initiation of oral iron and repeating the reticulocyte count 7 to 10 days after initiation of treatment to see if there is a rise owing to oral iron. Unless other factors are suppressing the marrow such as prior extensive blood transfusion or a chronic illness, then a reticulocyte response to iron is tantamount to demonstrating iron deficiency.[49]

The selection of an oral iron preparation and its dosage is based on the knowledge that ferrous iron is absorbed much better than ferric iron.[50] Approximately 180 mg of elemental iron should be given daily. This amount would raise the hemoglobin level by 0.2 g% daily. A 325-mg ferrous sulfate tablet contains 60 mg of elemental iron. Therefore, one tablet is given three times daily, preferably on an empty stomach to avoid the binding of iron with some food constituents. If the patient cannot tolerate this dosage of iron, then other iron preparations such as ferrous gluconate can be tried. A rise in hemoglobin level of 2 g% in 4 weeks is an acceptable response to oral ferrous sulfate therapy. Treatment should continue, not only until a hemoglobin level has returned to normal, but until iron stores measured by the serum ferritin level have been replaced. If the patient is truly iron deficient, then it usually takes approximately 6 months to totally replenish iron stores. If, for some reason, the patient continues to have occult gastrointestinal blood loss, then iron should be continued. It is seldom necessary to administer parenteral iron. Parenteral iron should be administered only when there is continued persistent blood loss requiring at least 100 to 250 mg of iron daily, such as constant gastrointestinal blood loss from a primary disorder of the gastrointestinal (arteriovenous malformations, telangiectasia, colitis, or ileitis) tract. Iron therapy should always be given in conjunction with parenteral (subcutaneous) exogenous rhEPO since iron availability and the precise uncertainty of its availability necessitate this practice.[51]

Recombinant Human Erythropoietin (rhEPO)

The development of rhEPO as a therapeutic agent will surely represent a major milestone in medical progress.[51] This glycoprotein offers many of the benefits of PRC transfusion without the need to transfuse blood. Coincidentally, the initiation of clinical trials with rhEPO coincided with the recognition that our blood supply is at risk from the lethal retrovirus HIV-1. It is also ironic that the "endogenous" transfusion trigger—the hemoglobin level below which EPO production unequivocally increases plasma EPO above the normal range—is 10.5 g%. This is below the level acceptable for autologous blood donation, which results in the inevitable deferral of some donors. Accordingly, rhEPO has been embraced for its potential to improve the efficiency of autologous blood donation. To date, there have been 20 published reports of experimental and clinical studies of the effect of rhEPO on autologous blood donation on erythropoiesis in the perioperative period. The data provide considerable insight into the potential role of rhEPO in transfusion medicine with respect to safety, efficacy, and cost.[52]

RhEPO has potential application in "nonelective" surgical settings in which preoperative autologous blood donation is not practical.[53] CABG procedures, in which blood loss is significant and blood transfusions are commonly required, constitute an example for which blood transfusion practices may be altered in the future owing to the availability of rhEPO. The majority of the 250,000 patients who undergo CABG are transfused, and these represent nearly 10% of the estimated 3.2 million recipients of PRC transfusions annually in the United States.[54] The effect of sc rhEPO on hematologic parameters has been assessed in normal volunteers. Doses of 150 units/kg cause significant, dose-related increases in serum EPO levels when administered. A peak serum level is observed approximately 12 hours after injection. Thereafter, the blood level of sc-injected rhEPO falls off slowly. Thus, preoperative and postoperative sc administration can be anticipated to promote erythropoiesis. Based on the study results of sc rhEPO therapy in autologous blood donors, reticulocytosis would be expected after 3.5 days, and a change in hematocrit by 7.2 days after sc rhEPO therapy. There is considerable promise in rhEPO as a pharmacologic alternative to allogenic blood transfusion in the surgical patient.

With regard to patients undergoing CPB specifically, preoperative rhEPO therapy and/or surgery does not adversely affect the postoperative EPO response to anemia. Following CABG procedures, administration of rhEPO to patients undergoing surgery could correct the EPO deficiency and accelerate postoperative erythropoiesis. Currently, the determination of the optimal dose, and interval of administration of rhEPO is the objective ongoing investigation in the striving toward bloodless, cardiac surgery. Until the optimal method of rhEPO administration has been developed, at NYH-CUMC those patients who require minimal blood component therapy receive 500 units/kg subcutaneously every other day until the time of CPB surgery. Operation has been delayed when possible until a minimum HCT of 36% is attained. Therapy with rhEPO has been continued through the fifth postoperative day or until discharge for patients with postoperative hematocrits lower than 30%.[23] Administration of sc rhEPO can theoretically minimize the immunosuppressive effects of packed cell transfusions.[54,55]

Folic Acid Administration

Natural folates are present in fresh green vegetables, many fruits, beans, nuts, liver, and kidney. The normal daily requirement is 50 to 100 μg. Folates found in food must be broken down to monoglutamates in order to be absorbed by the gastrointestinal tract, primarily the jejunum.[56] Relative or absolute lack of folic acid may occur during the postoperative period in those patients who have a relative increased need for folate owing to hemolysis, when jejunal mucosal absorption is impaired, when medications such as phenytoin are taken, or when there has been generally poor nutrition and/or excessive ethanol intake.[57] Following complete cessation of folate ingestion, serum folate level falls below 3 ng/ml within 3 weeks; tissue stores are exhausted several weeks thereafter. Alcoholics, particularly, have baseline decreased tissue folate stores and will require folic acid supplementation routinely postoperatively. Nutritional megaloblastic anemias often develop when a diet lacking folate is coupled with increased alcohol consumption. Patients who have primary chronic hemolytic disorders require increased folic acid owing to increased utilization of folate for red blood cell synthesis. Similarly, any patient who has abnormal jejunal absorption should receive folate supplementation as folic acid 1 mg parenterally during the postoperative period. In general, any patient who has had inadequate nutrition prior to surgery should be watched carefully for the development of more severe anemia postoperatively, which may require more intense treatment with any one of the modalities discussed above, such as PRC transfusion, sc rhEPO, oral iron, and/or oral or parenteral folic acid.

Vitamin K deficiency should also be prevented as a cause of excessive bleeding in patients with poor nutrition and/or receiving protracted courses of antibiotics.

Specific Considerations

Prosthetic Heart Valves and Anticoagulation

Thromboembolism and anticoagulated-related bleeding are the most frequent valve-related complications of both mechanical and bioprosthetic heart valves.[53,58] These complications represent approximately 75% of all valve-related complications in patients with mechanical aortic or mitral valves. Although complications related to durability are likely to exceed those related to thromboembolism in patients with bioprostheses, at present thromboembolism and anticoagulated-related bleeding cause approximately 50% of all valve-related complications in patients with aortic bioprostheses and 55% in those with mitral bioprostheses.[59,60] Patients with bioprostheses do not require long-term warfarin, although many are anticoagulated for 3 to 6 months after surgery when the incidence of thromboembolism is greatest. Although the incidence of thromboembolism in patients with mitral bioprostheses is greater than aortic bioprotheses, there is doubt whether or not warfarin is effective in reducing this incidence. There are data, however, to indicate that the incidence of thromboembolism is no higher in patients who take low-dose aspirin instead of warfarin. In an attempt to reduce thromboembolism without increasing bleeding, some have recommended both platelet inhibitors and warfarin. Aspirin (but not dipyridamole) with warfarin increases bleeding complications.[61]

Irrespective of the practice regarding the details of either the use of warfarin and/or antiplatelet drugs, clearly the late postoperative period is one during which the patient is at risk for increased bleeding and therefore may be more prone to anemia.[62] When using warfarin for bleeding prophylaxis with mechanical heart valves, the target international normalized ratio (INR) should be 2.5 to 3.5.[63] Occult blood in stool, Hb, HCT, and INR should be monitored carefully. If the patient appears to be anemic and not bleeding, then an attempt to demonstrate hemolysis owing to macrovascular shear stress destruction of the red cell membrane should be made. In such cases, patients often need continued oral iron and folate therapy. If the marrow cannot respond well enough, the addition of sc rhEPO may be of help in precluding or reducing the need of PRC transfusions.

Delayed Hemolytic Transfusion Reactions (DHTR)

Of particular note is the DHTR, which occurs days or weeks following transfusion and may result in jaundice and anemia due to hemolysis occurring some 4 to 14 days after the transfusion of apparently compatible PRCs.[64] The patient has usually been alloimmunized by a previous pregnancy or transfusion, and the concentration of antibody is below the level of serologic detection at the time of transfusion. When the transfused blood contains the corresponding antigen, an amnestic response occurs with formation of detectable antibody that coats the transfused red cells and leads to their hemolysis. As the patient becomes more anemic, the indirect Coombs' test and sometimes the direct Coombs' test become positive. In one report, the frequency of delayed hemolytic transfusion reactions was 1 in 4,000 units of PRCs transfused.[65,66] The treatment of a DHTR consists of identifying the specificity of the causative red cell antigen and avoiding transfusion of PRCs with the same specificity in the future.

Infectious Complications and Anemia

Since many patients undergoing CPB surgery receive blood products, namely PRCs, platelets, and fresh frozen plasma (Table 25.2), they are at risk of acquiring infections causing hemolytic anemia. Autoimmune hemolysis may typically occur with Epstein-Barr virus[67] or cytomegalovirus.[68] A careful examination of both the thick and thin blood smear in any patient who has postoperative fever with hemolytic anemia is essential (*Plasmodium, Babesia,* etc.). In addition, patients may have preoperative anemia owing to endocarditis.[25,26] For such patients, treatment of anemia is directed to treating the underlying infection. Support using PRCs may be required. The use of sc rhEPO for the treatment of chronic infections has not been well established. However, sc rhEPO may be indicated for anemia of pre- or postoperative renal failure.[69]

Anemia may also occur owing to antibiotic therapy. Cephalosporins, which are commonly used as prophylactic antibiotics for cardiothoracic surgical procedures, may induce autoimmune hemolytic anemia.[28] Such anemias are detected by the presence of a positive direct Coombs' test in concert with positive hemolytic parameters such as an elevated SIB, low serum HPT, increased reticulocyte count, and elevated serum LDH. Treatment of drug-induced hemolytic anemias is withdrawal of the drug, substitution of a pharmacologically different medication, and folic acid.

Cold-Related Autoimmune Hemolytic Anemia

Since CPB surgery requires systemic hypothermia and iced, cardioplegic solutions, complete preoperative screening for cold agglutinins should include testing for red blood cell agglutination in both saline at 10°C and albumin at 20°C. If significant cold-mediated autoagglutination is detected, such autoantibodies should be identified, classified, measured by titer, and characterized as to the critical temperature and thermal range of activity.[70] Although uncommon, patients with chronic cold hemoagglutinins can develop severe intraoperative hemolysis. Such patients may not be hemolyzing preoperatively if the thermal amplitude of their particular cold agglutinin is below room temperature. Treatment for the presence of such cold agglutinins may vary. Acute severe situations require plasmapheresis with removal of the usual immunoglobulin M (IgM) autoantibody. Such patients may continue to hemolyze during the late postoperative period if not kept in a warm environment. Special care should be taken to warm any blood products that may be administered,[71] and if necessary to warm the environment.

Refusal of Blood Products for Religious Reasons

As mentioned above, Jehovah's Witness patients may undergo CPB surgery. During the late postoperative period, employment of rhEPO, iron, and, if necessary, folic acid in conjunction with adequate volume repletion can obviate the need for blood components, which such patients' religious beliefs preclude. In concert with the aforementioned multimodality strategy of blood conservation, it is miraculous that bloodless CPB surgery can be performed safely.[23,72,73]

Summary

The major causes of anemia during the late CPB postoperative period have been described and indications for when to treat such anemias have been discussed. Methods of treating anemia include rhEPO, oral iron, PRC transfusion, folic acid, optimizing nutrition, and rarely parenteral iron. Specific surgical procedures such as heart valve replacement may result in complicating heart valve hemolysis requiring appropriate treatment, and bleeding owing to a variety of causes may also necessitate treatment of resultant anemia. Infectious complications due to transmission of infectious agents via blood products, infectious complicating surgical procedures, and medications may also contribute to anemia. Rarely, cold agglutinins and DHTRs may induce hemolysis. It is possible, owing to a multimodality strategy of blood conservation in conjunction with intense rhEPO and oral iron, to perform CPB surgery electively on patients whose religious beliefs preclude the use of any and all blood components.

References

1. Mora CT. *Cardiopulmonary Bypass–Principles and Techniques of Extracorporeal Circulation.* New York: Springer-Verlag, 1995.
2. Williams W. Approach to the patient. In: Beutler E, Lichtman M, Coller B, Kipps T, eds. *Williams' Hematology.* 5th ed. New York: McGraw-Hill, 1995;5.
3. Kleinman S, Nelson R, Smith L, Goldfinger D. Positive direct antiglobulin tests and immune hemolytic anemia in patients receiving procainamide. *N Engl J Med* 1984;311:809.
4. Means RT. Pathogenesis of the anemia of chronic disease: a cytokine-mediated anemia. *Stem Cells* 11995;13:32–37.
5. Ferguson BJ, Skikine BS, Simpson KM, et al. Serum transferrin receptor distinguishes the anemia of chronic disease from iron deficiency anemia. *J Lab Clin Med* 1992;19:385–390.
6. Cosgrove MD, Loop FD, Lytle BW, et al. Determinants of blood utilization during myocardial revascularization. *Ann Thorac Cardiovasc Surg* 1976; 72:714–726.
7. Ray MJ, Hawson GAT, Just SJE, McLachlan G, O'Brien M. Relationship of platelet aggregation to bleeding after cardiopulmonary bypass. *Ann Thorac Surg* 1994;57:981–986.
8. Kestin AS, Valeri CR, Khuri SF, Loscalzo J, et al. The platelet function defect of cardiopulmonary bypass. *Blood* 1993;82:107–117.
9. Salmerpera MT, Levy JH, Harker LA. Hemostasis and cardiopulmonary bypass. In: Mora CT, ed. *Cardiopulmonary Bypass–Principles and Techniques of Extracorporeal Circulation.* New York: Springer-Verlag, 1995;88–113.
10. Sane CD, Califf RM, Topel EJ, et al. Bleeding during thrombolytic therapy for acute myocardial infarction: mechanisms and management. *Ann Intern Med* 1989;111:1010–1022.
11. Cosgrove DM III, Heric B, Lytle BW, et al. Aprotinin therapy for reoperative myocardial revascularization: a placebo-controlled study. *Ann Thorac Surg* 1992;54:1031–1038.
12. Gillon J, Greenburg AG. Transfusion: infectious complications. *Blood* 1992; 81:19–28.
13. Waymack JP. Sequelae of blood transfusions. *Infect Surg* 1990;22:41–47.
14. Dodd RY. The risk of transfusion-transmitted infection (editorial). *N Engl J Med* 1992;327:419–421.
15. Selik RM, Ward JW, Buehler JW. Trends in transfusion-associated acquired immune deficiency syndrome in the United States, 1982 through 1991. *Transfusion* 1993;33:890–893.
16. Lostumbo MM, Holland PV, Schmidt PJ. Isoimmunization after multiple transfusions. *N Engl J Med* 1966;275:141–144.

17. Brunson ME, Alexander JW. Mechanisms of transfusion-induced immunosuppression. *Transfusion* 1990;30:651–658.
18. Anderson KC, Weinstein HJ. Transfusion-associated graft-versus-host disease. *N Engl J Med* 1990;323:315–321.
19. Vamvakas E, Moore SB. Preoperative blood transfusion and colorectal cancer recurrence: a qualitative statistical overview and meta-analysis. *Transfusion* 1993;33:754–765.
20. Erslev AJ, Beutler E. Production and destruction of erythrocytes. In: Beutler E, Lichtman M, Coller B, Kipps T, eds. *Williams' Hematology.* 5th ed. New York: McGraw-Hill, 1995;425.
21. Flaharty KK, Caro J, Erslev AJ, et al. Pharmacokinetics and erythropoietic response to human recombinant erythropoietin in healthy men. *Clin Pharmacol Ther* 1990;47:557.
22. Levine EA, Rosen AL, Sehgal LR, et al. Erythropoietin deficiency after coronary artery bypass procedures. *Ann Thorac Surg* 1991;51:759–763.
23. Rosengart TK, Helm RE, Klemperer J, et al. Combined aprotinin and erythropoietin use for blood conservation: results with Jehovah's Witnesses. *Ann Thorac Surg* 1994;58:1397–1403.
24. Dacie JV. Secondary or symptomatic hemolytic anemias. In: Dacie JV, ed. *The Haemolytic Anaemias.* New York: Grune & Stratton, 1967;908.
25. Robboy SJ, Salisbury K, Ragsdale B, et al. Mechanism of aspergillus-induced microangiopathic hemolytic anemia. *Arch Intern Med* 1971;128:790.
26. Suzuki A, Yamada A, Maruyama H. A case of acute haemolytic anemia due to *Clostridium perfrigens* septicemia. *Jpn J Clin Hematol* 1972;13:850.
27. Petz LD, Fudenberg HH. Coombs-positive hemolytic anemia caused by penicillin administration. *N Engl J Med* 1966;274:171.
28. Chamber LA, Donovan BA, Kruskall MS. Ceftazidime-induced hemolysis patient with drug-dependent antibodies reactive by immune complex and drug adsorption mechanisms. *Am J Clin Pathol* 1991;95:393.
29. Tishler M. Phenazopyridine-induced hemolytic anemia in a patient with G-6-PD deficiency. *Acta Haematol (Basel)* 1983;70:208.
30. Williamson D. The unstable haemoglobins. *Blood Rev* 1993;7:146.
31. Hines R, Barash PG. Infusions of sodium nitroprusside induces platelet dysfunction in vitro. *Anesthesia* 1989;70:611.
32. Schafer AI, Alexander RW, Handin RI. Inhibition of platelet function by organic nitrate vasodilators. *Blood* 1980;55:649.
33. Weksler B, Gillick M, Pink J. Effect of propranolol on platelet function. *Blood* 1977;49:185.
34. Barnathan E, Addonizio VP, Shattil SJ. Interaction of verapamil with human platelet alpha-adrenergic receptors (abstract). *Am J Physiol* 1982;242:H19.
35. Okita Y, Miki S, Kusukara K, et al. Propranolol for intractable hemolysis after open heart operation. *Ann Thorac Surg* 1991;52:1154-1157.
36. Rose JC, Hufnagel CA, Fries ED, et al. The hemodynamic alterations produced by plastic valvular prosthesis for severe aortic insufficiency in man. *J Clin Invest* 1954;33:8911.
37. Amidon TM, Chou TM, Rankin JS, Ports TA. Mitral and aortic paravalvular leaks with hemolytic anemia. *Am Heart J* 1993;125:266.
38. American College of Physicians. Practice strategies for elective red blood cell transfusion. *Ann Intern Med* 1992;116:403–406.
39. Cordts PR, LaMorte WW, Fisher JB, et al. Poor predictive value of hematocrit

and hemodynamic parameters for erythrocyte deficits after extensive elective vascular operations. *Surg Gynecol Obstet* 1992;175:243–248.

40. Goodnough LT, Johnston MFM, Toy PTCY, et al. The variability of transfusion practice in coronary artery bypass surgery. *JAMA* 1991;265:86–89.
41. Johnson RG, Thurer RL, Kruskall MS, et al. Comparison of two transfusion strategies after elective operations for myocardial revascularization. *J Thorac Cardiovasc Surg* 1992;104:307–314.
42. Goodnough LT. Clinical application of recombinant erythropoietin in the perioperative period. *Hematol Oncol Clin North Am* 1994;8:1011–1020.
43. Rapaport SJ. RBC metabolism: relations to RBC function and hemolytic anemias. In: Rapaport SI, ed. *Introduction to Hematology*. 2nd ed. Philadelphia: JB Lippincott, 1987;118–129.
44. Jain R. Use of blood transfusion in management of anemia. *Med Clin North Am* 1992;76:727–744.
45. Triulzi DJ, Gilmor GD, Ness PM, et al. Efficacy of autologous fresh whole blood or platelet-rich plasma in adult cardiac surgery. *Transfusion* 1995; 35:627–634.
46. LoCicero J III, Massad M, Gandy K, et al. Aggressive blood conservation in coronary artery surgery: impact on patient care. *J Cardiovasc Surg* 1990; 31:559–563.
47. Bordin JO, Heddle NM, Blajchmann MA. Biologic effects of leukocytes present in transfused cellular blood products. *Blood* 1994;84:1703–1721.
48. Finch C. Regulators of iron balance in humans. *Blood* 1994;84:1697–1702.
49. Rapaport SI. Iron deficiency anemia. In: Rapaport SI, ed. *Introduction to Hematology*. 2nd ed. Philadelphia: JB Lippincott, 1987;39–54.
50. O'Sullivan DJ, Higgins PG, Wilkinson JF. Oral iron compounds: a therapeutic comparison. *Lancet* 1955;2:482.
51. Spivak JL. Recombinant human erythropoietin and its role in transfusion medicine (editorial). *Transfusion* 1994;34:1–4.
52. Watanabe Y, Fuse K, Konishi T, et al. Autologous blood transfusion with recombinant human erythropoietin in heart operations. *Ann Thorac Surg* 1991;51:767–772.
53. Zuzza C, Ottino G, DiSumma M, et al. Porcine cardiac bioprostheses: evaluation of long-term results in 990 patients. *Ann Thorac Surg* 1985;39:243.
54. Rapaport SL. Transfusion therapy. In: Rapaport SI, ed. *Introduction to Hematology*. 2nd ed. Philadelphia: JB Lippincott, 1987;578–590.
55. Goodnough LT. Erythropoietin as a pharmacologic alternative to blood transfusion in the surgical patient. *Transfusion Med Rev* 1990;4:288–296.
56. Steinberg SE. Mechanisms of folate homeostasis. *Am J Physiol* 1984;246:G319.
57. Savage D, Lindenbaum J. Anemia in alcoholics. *Medicine (Baltimore)* 1986; 65:322.
58. Miller DC, Oyer PE, Mitchell RS, et al. Performance characteristics of the Starr-Edwards model 1260 aortic valve prosthesis beyond ten years. *J Thorac Cardiovasc Surg* 1984;88:193.
59. Cohn LH, Allred EN, DiSesa VJ, et al. Early and late risk of aortic valve replacement. *J Thorac Cardiovasc Surg* 1984;88:695.
60. Gonzalez-Lavin L, Tandon AP, Chi S, et al. The risk of thromboembolism and hemorrhage following mitral valve replacement. *J Thorac Cardiovasc Surg* 1984;87:340.
61. Chesebro JH, Fuster V, Elveback LR, et al. Trial of combined warfarin plus

dipyrimadole or aspirin therapy in prosthetic heart valve replacement: danger of aspirin compared with dipyrimadole. *Am J Cardiol* 1983;51:1537.
62. Levine MN, Hirsh J, Landefeld S, Raskob G. Hemorrhagic complications of anticoagulant treatment. *Chest* 1992;102(4):352S.
63. Hirsh J, Dalen JE, Deykin D, Poller L. Oral anticoagulants: mechanism of action, clinical effectiveness, and optimal therapeutic range. *Chest* 1992; 102(4):312S.
64. Pineda AA, Paswell HF, Brzica SM Jr. Delayed hemolytic transfusion reaction: an immunologic hazard of blood transfusion. *Transfusion* 1978;18:1.
65. Ness PM, Shirey RS, Thoman SK, Buck SA. The differentiation of delayed serologic and delayed hemolytic transfusion reactions: incidence, long-term serologic findings, and clinical significance. *Transfusion* 1990;30:688–693.
66. Pinkerton PH, Coovadia AS, Goldstein J. Frequency of delayed hemolytic transfusion reactions following antibody screening and immediate-spin cross-matching. *Transfusion* 1992;32:814–817.
67. Tonkin AM, Mond HG, Alford FP, Hurley TH. Severe acute haemolytic anaemia complicating infectious mononucleosis. *Med J Aust* 1973;2:1048.
68. Horwitz CA, Skradski K. Reece E, et al. Haemolytic anaemia in previously healthy adult patients with CMV infections: report of two cases and an evaluation of subclinical haemolysis in CMV mononucleosis. *Scand J Haematol* 1984;33:35.
69. Watson A, Gimerez L, Cotton J, et al. Treatment of anemia of chronic renal failure with subcutaneous rHEpo. *Am J Med* 1990;89:432.
70. Pruzanski W, Shumak KH. Biologic activity of cold-reacting autoantibodies. *N Engl J Med* 1977;297:583.
71. Taft EG, Propp RP, Sullivan SA. Plasma exchange for cold agglutinin hemolytic anemia. *Transfusion* 1977;17:173.
72. Ott DA, Cooley DA. Cardiovascular surgery in Jehovah's Witnesses. *JAMA* 1977;238:1256–1258.
73. Lee RB, Martin TD. Religious objections to blood transfusion. In: Mora CT, ed. *Cardiopulmonary Bypass—Principles and Techniques of Extracorporeal Circulation.* New York: Springer-Verlag, 1995;473–480.

26
Economics of Transfusion Medicine and Blood Conservation Practices

KARL H. KRIEGER, O. WAYNE ISOM, AND FERDINAND T. VELASCO

The health care industry today is undergoing radical changes in its economic architecture. Spiraling costs have prompted a widespread movement to reform the health care delivery system. In addition to legislative reform, there are significant market forces driving this process. Increasingly, the industry has shifted to a managed care model and a prospective payment system. Declining revenues have impelled hospitals to seek greater cost-effectiveness.

As is the case with other services, blood banks are under considerable pressure to contain and reduce costs. In the past, blood centers and transfusion services were able to compensate for increased costs with revenue growth. Wallace[1] reported that 40% of the growth in revenue during the early 1980s was attributable to increases in volume of components distributed. The remaining 60% came from component price increases. Recently, however, the declining volume of component transfusions and cutbacks in product price increases have constrained revenue growth. As a result, managers of blood centers and transfusion services must now achieve cost reduction through increases in efficiency or by reducing their services.

Strategies to limit the transfusion of blood products, therefore, are attractive from an economic viewpoint. However, the measures taken to accomplish blood conservation, particularly in cardiac surgery, are themselves costly. A careful analysis of the cost-effectiveness of a blood conservation strategy requires consideration of the cost of blood conserving techniques as well as the cost of blood products. Although the value of striving for blood conservation in cardiac surgery cannot be judged solely on the basis of this sort of cost analysis, in the present era of managed health care, one cannot afford to ignore the economic implications.

Cost of Blood Products

Calculating the cost of transfusing blood products is not a straightforward matter. Multiple factors must be taken into consideration and at best only an estimate can be derived. Much of the literature related to transfusion economics presents information based on patient charges.[2-4] Traditionally, cost calculations were made using the Medicare cost-to-charge ratio as an adjustment method to derive costs from patient charges. The relationship between patient charges and costs is not always clear-cut, however. As cost-accounting methodology has increased in sophistication, hospital administrators have shifted away from reliance on the cost-to-charge ratio to direct product costing.

Two recent articles have dealt with the issue of costing blood products and services. Forbes and associates[5] published the results of a large multicenter study aimed at determining the cost of delivering a unit of homologous whole blood or red cells. Lubarsky and associates[6] calculated the total hospital cost of a perioperative red blood cell blood transfusion at Duke University Medical Center. Despite the fact that the two studies employed significantly different accounting techniques, the results were surprisingly similar ($155 in the Forbes study, compared with $151 in the Lubarsky study). Much insight can be gained from an analysis of the costing methodologies used.

Forbes et al identified four components in the total cost of transfusing a unit of blood: acquisition, blood bank handling, laboratory tests, and blood administration (Table 26.1). The costs varied significantly among the 19 United States teaching institutions examined. Factors that were found to influence cost included geographic location of the blood supply source, type of red cell product transfused, prices charged by blood transfusion services, and frequency of laboratory tests.

The acquisition cost is the hospital cost of acquiring blood products from a blood center. Table 26.2 shows the 1994 price list for several blood products and services at the New York Blood Center.[7] Geographic location of the blood supply is a significant variable in the variation of acquisition costs among different institutions. The average acquisition cost of a unit of blood is $71 in the East, $68 in the Northeast, $58 in the Midwest, and $53 in the South.[5]

Specially treated blood products cost more than standard units. In New York City, washed red blood cells (RBCs) cost 46% more than standard RBCs. Irradiation adds 15% to the acquisition cost of a unit of RBCs. In the Forbes study, autologous units cost 21% more than bank blood.

Very little information has been published regarding the cost of handling

TABLE 26.1. Components of total hospital cost of one unit of homologous blood.

Description	Cost ($)	Percent
Acquisition	57	37
Handling cost	20	13
Laboratory cost	67	43
Administration cost	11	7
Total	155	

From Forbes et al.[5]

TABLE 26.2. Acquisition cost for selected blood products in New York City.

Description	Cost ($)
Components	
Red blood cells	106.25
Whole blood	122.00
Platelet concentrate	53.25
Fresh frozen plasma	53.75
Cryoprecipitate	51.25
Leukocyte concentrate	97.00
Apheresis	
Plateletpheresis	
Single donor	550.00
Referred donor	575.00
Human leukocyte antigen	750.00

From New York Blood Center Free Schedule.[7]

and testing blood products in the blood bank. Generally, this cost is estimated from the blood bank processing fee using the cost-to-charge ratio. However, processing fees are typically quite arbitrary and may bear only a marginal relationship to actual costs.

In the study at Duke University, the investigators studied the specific circumstance of perioperative blood transfusions, in which many more units are ordered than actually transfused. Lubarsky et al[6] noted a ratio of cross-matches to transfused units of 2.6:1 and a ratio of nontransfused patients who underwent ABO and Rh typing and antibody screening to transfused patients of 4.1:1. From these results, the total associated cost of testing for perioperative blood transfusion was estimated to be $17.91. In addition to the added cost of extra cross-matching and typing, there is the cost of handling nontransfused blood in the blood bank and the wastage of blood issued to the operating room that is unsuitable for reissue. These contributed an additional $7.67 to the transfusion service's costs. In the cardiac surgery population, since there is a higher proportion of patients undergoing surgery that receive blood, the cost of extra compatibility testing, typing and screening, handling, and wastage might be expected to be slightly lower. As strategies to achieve blood conservation during heart surgery improve, however, these "hidden costs" will become more significant. To remain cost-effective, transfusion services must compensate for improved blood conservation by reducing unnecessary testing and minimizing wastage.

The final consideration in assessing the cost of transfusing blood products is the cost associated with adverse outcomes resulting from blood transfusions. In the majority of cases, these costs are assumed by the hospital during the course of the patient's hospitalization. An example is the costs of treating a febrile reaction following a blood transfusion. In the Duke study, the direct hospital cost attributable to the most common adverse reactions was estimated at $3.32 per unit.[6]

In the case of infectious complications from transfused blood, the costs

TABLE 26.3. Cost-effectiveness of selected medical practices.

Medical practice	Cost per year of saved life ($)
CABG for left main coronary disease and severe angina, compared with medical therapy	6,000
Cervical cancer screening every 4 years compared with no screening	11,000
Adjuvant chemotherapy for node-negative breast cancer	18,000
Hemodialysis for end-stage renal disease	48,000
Autologous blood transfusion in hip surgery	40,000–1,470,000

From Birkmeyer et al.[8]

are much more difficult to measure. Long-term sequelae such as acquired immunodeficiency syndrome and chronic hepatitis often continue to consume health care dollars long after the period of the original hospital stay. In practice, these costs are not experienced by the hospital directly but are assumed by society in general. Consequently, they are defined as *external costs* and are not included in the hospital cost-accounting process.

Birkmeyer and associates[8] attempted to define the cost of transfusion-related complications in a cost-effectiveness analysis of preoperative autologous blood donation for orthopedic surgery. The authors used *quality-adjusted years of life saved* as a measure of benefit from autologous blood donation. The risk of hepatitis C infection, the primary cause of transfusion-related hepatitis, is approximately 0.03% per unit. Estimates of the risk of HIV transmission vary between 0.00065% and 0.0017% per unit. The mortality rate of infected patients above that predicted by age, gender, and race is 0.35% per year. In the study, the increased quality-adjusted life expectancy associated with autologous donation ranged from 0.04 to 0.26 days per patient. Cost-effectiveness was expressed as the ratio of cost to quality-adjusted year of life saved. Cost-effectiveness varied from $40,000 to $1,467,000 per year of life saved, which did not compare favorably with other selected medical practices (Table 26.3).

Cost of Blood Conservation Practices

Two studies have examined the cost-effectiveness of blood conservation techniques in cardiac surgery. A study by Scott and associates[9] reviewed the outcomes in 118 consecutive patients who underwent primary, elective cardiac operations at the Veterans Affairs Medical Center in Albuquerque, New Mexico, in 1989. Fifty-eight patients were operated on prior to institution of a comprehensive blood conservation program, while 60 patients underwent operation in the setting of the blood conservation program. This program consisted of attempts to limit preoperative aspirin use, intraoperative phlebotomy and hemodilution, use of a cell conservation device to concentrate residual oxygenator contents, reinfusion of chest drainage, and acceptance of a minimum hemoglobin level of 8.0 g/dl in stable patients.

The authors did not publish their methodology for deriving the cost of blood products. From the transfusion costs reported, the cost of a unit of red cells is calculated to be around $50. This suggests that the investigators used only the acquisition cost in making their cost comparisons, which presumably underestimated the transfusion costs in both groups.

The number of blood products transfused and the total cost for blood products were less in the postconservation group. The study reported that the cost of the various blood-saving techniques offset the cost savings (Table 26.4). Consequently, the cost per patient for each group was similar.

In calculating the costs associated with a blood conservation protocol, it is necessary to include the cost of the cell conservation (Cell Saver) system, the blood collection bags, postoperative chest drainage units, and other disposables, such as filters and solutions. At New York Hospital, the Cell Saver disposables and blood collection bag are packaged into a single kit costing $165. It is difficult to take into account the cost of the Cell Saver device itself, typically in the range of $20,000 to $25,000, since this equipment is often shared with other surgical services in the hospital.

Determining the cost of utilizing a cell conservation system is simplest when it is provided by an outside service that charges the hospital for the use of the equipment and disposables as well as for labor. Although this cost is typically higher than if the hospital purchased the equipment and hired the technician, it serves as a useful frame of reference. At New York Hospital, this cost is about $775 for a four hour case.

In the study by Scott et al,[9] only 62% of patients in the postconservation group received blood from the cell conservation unit. These patients had a mean of 809 ± 376 ml of blood returned after processing. Interestingly, there was no difference in the postoperative hematocrit in the two groups studied.

Since the study did not separately examine the contribution of the cell conservation device to the overall reduction in transfusion requirement, it is

TABLE 26.4. Comparison of costs between preconservation and postconservation groups.

Preconservation		Postconservation	
Description	Cost ($)	Description	Cost ($)
Cost of PRBCs	6,950	Cost of PRBCs	5,350
Platelets	1,792	Platelets	736
FFP	1,120	FFP	576
Miscellaneous costs	1,523	Miscellaneous costs	1,030
Chest drainage units	600	Cell conservation equipment	3,248
		Intraoperative blood collection bags	520
		Chest drainage units, blood recovery bags	2,760
		Miscellaneous (solutions)	84
Cost/patient	300		341

From Scott et al.[9]

not possible to evaluate its cost relative to the savings accrued in sparing the patient from a blood transfusion. However, it is possible to estimate a breakeven point at which use of the Cell Saver becomes cost-effective. Given that the average hematocrit of the blood returned to the patient from the Cell Saver after processing is about 55% and that the hematocrit of a unit of red blood cells is approximately 80%, one can assume that for every 360 ml of Cell Saver blood returned to the patient, the patient is spared a transfusion of one unit of red cells. The formula below expresses the volume at which use of the Cell Saver is cost-effective:

$$\text{Volume}_{\text{cell saver}} = \frac{\text{Cost}_{\text{cell save}}}{(0.0027)(\text{Cost}_{\text{blood}})}$$

where $\text{Cost}_{\text{cell saver}}$ is the total cost of a single use of the Cell Saver equipment and $\text{Cost}_{\text{blood}}$ is the total cost of a unit of red blood cells. Substituting these variables with $165 (the cost of using one Cell Saver kit at New York Hospital) and $150 (the average total cost of one unit of red cells reported in the Forbes study[5]), one arrives at a value of *400 ml of Cell Saver* blood that must be salvaged and returned to the patient. Clearly, this estimate varies depending on the value of the two cost variables.

Presently, the transfusion of shed mediastinal blood collected in a postoperative chest drainage chamber has become accepted as a standard practice following cardiac surgery. Scott et al[9] reported that 50% of the patients in the postconservation group received a mean of 287 ± 127 ml of chest drainage. The same logic applied to the analysis of the cell conservation equipment above can be used with this conservation technique. The average hematocrit of shed mediastinal blood collected in this setting and transfused back to the patient is approximately 20%. The formula that expresses the volume of transfused shed chest drainage at which use of the chest drainage collection system becomes cost-effective is expressed as follows:

$$\text{Volume}_{\text{chest drainage system}} = \frac{\text{Cost}_{\text{chest drainage system}}}{(0.0016)(\text{Cost}_{\text{blood}})}$$

where $\text{Cost}_{\text{chest drainage system}}$ is the cost of a single chest drainage collection system. At New York Hospital, this cost is $40. Using $150 as the cost of a unit of blood, the breakeven point is around *167 ml.*

While the study by Scott et al suggests that a comprehensive blood conservation strategy can be cost-effective, it does not provide sufficient evidence to support the routine use of a cell conservation system or of a postoperative chest drainage collection system for transfusing shed mediastinal blood. No cost analysis between subgroups (i.e., between those receiving blood from the Cell Saver unit or chest drainage unit and those that do not) within the postconservation group was performed. It is possible that employing a selective conservation strategy may be a more cost-effective approach. Further studies are needed to identify which preoperative and intraoperative risk factors are predictive of those patients most likely to benefit from the use of a Cell Saver device and postoperative drainage collection system.

In terms of cost, the most controversial aspect of a blood conservation program is the use of pharmacologic agents that improve hemostasis or increase the patient's red cell volume. Table 26.5 lists several agents that are commonly employed as part of a blood conservation strategy in cardiac surgery along with their cost. Drugs such as aprotinin and human recombinant erythropoietin are relatively expensive and their routine use in elective surgical patients at low risk for bleeding is difficult to justify using cost-benefit analysis.

A randomized controlled trial by Baele and associates[10] sought to examine the influence of systematic aprotinin use in elective cardiac surgery on total homologous exposure and hospital charges. The treatment group, which received a test dose of 2×10^4 kallikrein inactivator units (KIU), 2×10^6 KIU at incision, a maintenance dose of 0.5×10^5 KIU/hr (for a maximum of 5 hours), and 2×10^6 KIU following heparin administration but prior to extracorporeal bypass, experienced a statistically significant decrease in postoperative blood loss and transfusion requirement when compared with the control group. Despite the high cost of aprotinin, the total charges for the patients in the treatment group were 9% lower than the charges of the control group. The authors did not, however, examine the reasons for the lower charges associated with aprotinin therapy.

Because of the high cost of aprotinin ($600 for 4 million KIU), conservation of a relatively large amount of blood must be accomplished in order to achieve a positive savings to cost ratio. For example, in the elective patient undergoing primary cardiac surgery at New York Hospital, the average transfusion requirement is less than two units. Assuming that the routine use of aprotinin completely abolished the transfusion requirement in this group of patients, the transfusion costs saved would be only 50% of the cost of the drug. A patient would have to be spared the transfusion of at least four units of blood to compensate for the cost of aprotinin. From a cost-effectiveness standpoint, the use of aprotinin cannot be justified except in patients at high risk for a significant transfusion requirement during cardiac surgery.

TABLE 26.5. Costs of pharmacologic agents used in blood conservation.

Description	Unit dose	Cost ($)
Aprotinin	1 milion KIU*	150
Erythropoietin	2,000 units	18
	10,000 units	86
Desmopressin acetate	4 μg	18
Aminocaproic acid	5000 mg	0.60

*Kallikrein inactivator units.

To date, no analysis has been published showing the cost-effectiveness of recombinant human erythropoietin in cardiac surgical patients. Several studies have confirmed the cost-effectiveness of this drug in patients with anemia secondary to end-stage renal disease.[11,12] Hayashi and associates[13] presented data supporting the efficacy of preoperative subcutaneous doses of erythropoietin in cardiac surgery patients in a randomized controlled clinical trial. However, Strauss[14] argued that widespread use of large doses of erythropoietin in the cardiac surgery setting could not be justified from an economic standpoint. In the Japanese study, patients in the treatment group received 72,000 units of erythropoietin. The cost of erythropoietin at New York Hospital is approximately $9 per 1,000 units, yielding a cost per patient of $648. From a cost-benefit standpoint, the savings in transfusion cost match the cost of the drug when at least four units of allogeneic blood have been conserved.

Conclusion

Studying the cost-effectiveness of a blood conservation strategy requires analysis of many different factors, including the cost of blood products and the cost of the blood conservation techniques. Often these costs vary depending on geographic location, and an assessment of cost-effectiveness must always be performed using cost data pertinent to the particular medical center. As much as possible, true costs, rather than estimates based on hospital charges, should be used in performing calculations.

The literature that has been published devoted to blood conservation in cardiac surgery suggests that the use of a cell conservation device intraoperatively and the transfusion of shed mediastinal blood is cost-effective. However, it may be possible to identify low-risk patients in whom these techniques could be more selectively employed to achieve further cost savings.

The role of pharmacologic agents in a comprehensive blood conservation strategy is more controversial. Presently, insufficient data exist to justify the routine use of aprotinin or erythropoietin in elective surgical patients undergoing primary cardiac surgery.

References

1. Wallace EL. Costing blood products and services (editorial). *Transfusion* 1991;31:293–295.
2. Wallace EL, Wallace MA. *Hospital Transfusion Charges and Community Blood Center Costs, Prepared Under Contract with the National Heart, Lung, and Blood Institute.* Bethesda, MD: NHLBI, 1982.
3. Cumming PD, Wallace EL, Surgenor DM, et al. Public interest pricing of blood services. *Med Care* 1974;12:743–753.

4. Zuck TF. An hypothesis on the cost effectiveness of homologous blood transfusions in 1988. *Transfus Med Rev* 1988;2:245–249.
5. Forbes JM, Anderson MD, Anderson GF, et al. Blood transfusion costs: a multicenter study. *Transfusion* 1991;31:318–323.
6. Lubarsky DA, Hahn C, Bennett D, et al. The hospital cost (fiscal year 1991/1992) of a simple perioperative allogeneic red blood cell transfusion during elective surgery at Duke University. *Anesth Analg* 1994;79:629–637.
7. New York Blood Center Fee Schedule. New York, NY, 1993.
8. Birkmeyer JD, Goodnough LT, AuBuchon JP, et al. The cost-effectiveness of preoperative autologous blood donation for total hip and knee replacement. *Transfusion* 1993;33:544–551.
9. Scott WJ, Rode R, Castlemain B, et al. Efficacy, complications, and cost of a comprehensive blood conservation program for cardiac operations. *J Thorac Cardiovasc Surg* 1992;103:1001–1007.
10. Baele PL, Ruiz-Gomez J, Londot C, et al. Systematic use of aprotinin in cardiac surgery: influence on total homologous exposure and hospital cost. *Acta Anaesth Belg* 1992;43:103–112.
11. Stevens ME, Summerfield GP, Hall AA, et al. Cost benefits of low dose subcutaneous erythropoietin in patients with anaemia of end stage renal disease. *Br Med J* 1992;304:474–477.
12. Sheingold SH, Churchill DN, Muirhead N, Laupacis A. Recombinant human erythropoietin: factors to consider in cost-benefit analysis (editorial). *Am J Kidney Dis* 1991;17:86–92.
13. Hayashi J, Kumon K, Takanashi S, et al. Subcutaneous administration of recombinant human erythropoietin before cardiac surgery: a double-blind, multicenter trial in Japan. *Transfusion* 1994;34:142–146.
14. Strauss RG. Can the cost of erythropoietin for cardiac surgery patients be justified? (letter). *Transfusion* 1994;34:835.

Part IV

Algorithm for Bloodless Surgery at The New York Hospital–Cornell Medical Center

27
Development and Application of a Multimodality Blood Conservation Program

ROBERT E. HELM AND KARL K. KRIEGER

Efforts at reducing the use of homologous blood in cardiac surgery began almost 40 years ago. The impetus for these efforts has not changed over time. National blood shortages continue to surface periodically,[1,2] new infectious sequelae of transfusion continue to threaten both the quality and quantity of the blood supply,[3–6] and incompatibility and other immunologic reactions will remain a problem as long as allogeneic blood is utilized. The desire by both patients and their physicians to conserve blood during the perioperative period has led to many technical and pharmacologic advancements. These efforts have markedly decreased the need for allogeneic blood, and while doing so have affected virtually every aspect of the manner in which heart surgery and cardiopulmonary bypass (CPB) are performed. This book has focused on each of these techniques, with emphasis on their rationale, their track record of clinical effectiveness, and the optimal way in which each should be applied in order to obtain maximum benefit. While these measures are individually effective, there is perhaps no greater example than cardiac surgical blood conservation, where the whole is greater than the sum of its parts. Practiced in isolation or sporadically, these measures to varying degrees reduce the need for homologous blood. But practiced together and in concert, as part of an integrated comprehensive program, these measures can consistently decrease and even eliminate the need for homologous blood in a majority of cardiac surgical patients.

This chapter reviews the results of previous efforts at comprehensive blood conservation and the pursuit of bloodless cardiac surgery, analyzing both the types of measures combined as well as the results achieved. Having established this baseline of where blood conservation stands in 1996, our own experience in comprehensive multimodality blood conservation is then presented. Finally, a step-by-step guide to the application of our program is outlined, and an algorithm for its use provided.

Analysis of the Literature: Learning from the Past

Many reports have presented results of efforts to minimize the use of homologous blood in cardiac surgery. While a majority of clinical studies have focused on the use of one particular technique or pharmacologic agent, these techniques or agents invariably were applied in the context of an entire set of blood conservation measures that was the way that cardiac surgery was practiced at that institution at that time (the blood conservation "background"). Therefore, while reporting on the effectiveness of the particular technique or techniques under study, these reports also revealed the effectiveness of the investigator's overall approach to conserving blood. To this body of individual-technique literature can be added those studies that specifically stated as their goal the evaluation of a comprehensive or multimodality approach to blood conservation. Together, the results of these reports provide an important body of information that can be used as an aid to evaluating the relative effectiveness of various combinations of the presently available blood conservation measures. The understanding gained by this analysis is essential when attempting to construct a comprehensive integrated blood conservation program that can safely and cost-effectively minimize the use of homologous blood.

Table 27.1 summarizes the findings of 37 blood conservation studies performed on patients undergoing coronary artery bypass graft (CABG) surgery. Table 27.2 provides this same information derived from 31 studies performed on patients undergoing non-CABG or combined procedures requiring cardiopulmonary bypass. These 68 studies were selected from the relatively large body of blood conservation literature because they provided information about some or all of the techniques applied, and because they provided outcome measures of the percentage of patients receiving homologous transfusion and/or the average number of units transfused per patient. Several pieces of information can be gleaned from these tables. First, the extent to which each technique was applied can be seen. For example, while preoperative autologous donation was only sporadically applied (12/68 studies), non-blood prime was almost universally applied (65/68 studies). Second, because the studies are ranked with respect to transfusion outcome, the relative importance of each individual measure can be assessed. For example, in Table 27.1 a majority of studies achieving very low transfusion rates used low to low-moderate transfusion triggers both during and following CPB. Conversely, a majority of the studies reporting high rates of transfusion either used higher transfusion triggers, or the triggers were not stated, indicating that the investigators likely did not recognize, or place enough emphasis on, this essential blood conservation measure. Third and finally, the various *combinations* of procedures that were the most effective can be seen. For example, a majority of studies that achieved overall transfusion rates of less than 30% used a combination of pre- or intraoperative autologous blood donation, non-blood priming, return of residual circuit blood to the patient, low or moderately low intra- and postoperative transfusion triggers, and reinfusion of shed mediastinal blood.

Because coronary artery bypass surgery is the most commonly applied procedure that utilizes the heart-lung apparatus, and because CABG technique is fairly standardized, it provides the most useful body for evaluating the effectiveness of presently available blood conservation measures (Table 27.1). If a transfusion rate of 10% or less is used to delineate those programs that were maximally effective, and those studies that evaluated fewer than 25 patients are eliminated, a group of eight CABG studies are left to consider more closely. It is these programs that achieved consistent reductions in homologous transfusions, and it is these studies that should be used as the basis for the development of an optimal multimodality blood conservation program.

The first program to report rates of transfusion of less than 10% in non-Jehovah's Witness CABG patients was that of Cosgrove et al[15] at the Cleveland Clinic. Their 1978 report on 50 patients undergoing elective CABG surgery, which demonstrated transfusion of only 6% of patients with a mean of 0.06 unit per patient, stands as impressive when general transfusion rates at that time are considered. For example, Bayer[43] (1980), Schaff[39] (1979), and Zubiate[22] (1974), reported rates of 2.4, 2.6, and 3.8 units per patient, respectively, and Yeh[37] (1978) reported the transfusion of 77.8% of patients. Included in the program applied by Cosgrove et al was (1) intraoperative autologous donation, (2) non-blood prime, (3) return of all residual CPB circuit blood, (4) intraoperative salvage, (5) use of the lowest safe level of anemia during CPB and in the postoperative period, and (6) shed mediastinal blood reinfusion.* A 1985 study by Cosgrove,[16] applying this same general comprehensive program to a much larger group of primary CABG patients, reported similar low rates of transfusion (10% of patients; 0.3 unit per patient). Absent from these early but nevertheless very successful comprehensive efforts were the use of preoperative autologous donation, minimum volume CPB circuitry, and the application of pharmacologic adjuncts such as aprotinin, the antifibrinolytics, and erythropoietin. While this does not indicate that these additional measures are not important in current-day blood conservation, where sicker patients with more advanced cardiac disease are encountered, it does strongly suggest the effectiveness of the basic set of six core blood conservation measures applied by these investigators. This set of core measures can be summarized in three simple statements: (1) lose as little blood as possible, (2) give back what blood is lost, and (3) only transfuse banked blood if it is physiologically necessary.

In 1986 Belcher and Lennox[17] achieved similarly low transfusion rates

*It is important to note that implicit in this and presumably all studies of blood conservation is a seventh measure—maximum intraoperative surgical hemostasis. However, because its application is highly variable and typically not delineated as a specific technique that can be or is evaluated in these studies, it is not included as one of the six core techniques that may or may not be applied. Maximum surgical hemostasis should be applied to all patients, at all times.

TABLE 27.1. A survey of the technical and pharmacologic blood conservation measures applied to CABG patients in 37 selected studies. These studies were selected because they listed the blood conservation measures applied as well as the allogeneic transfusion outcome. The studies are ranked according to allogeneic transfusion requirement.

Year	Author	Number of patients	Preoperative autologous donation	Intraop. autologous donation	Non-blood prime	Volume CPB circuit	Circuit residual reinfusion	Intraop. salvage	RBC trigger CPB*	RBC trigger postop*	Shed mediastinal blood reinfusion	Pharm adjunct	Percent transfused	Units per patient
1996	Helm[7]	100	No	1450	Yes	1500	Yes	Yes	Low (15)	Low (22)	Yes	Apr/Epo	0	0
1997	Rosengart[8]	30	No	1300	Yes	1300	Yes	Yes	Low (15)	Low (22)	Yes	Apr/Epo	0	0
1992	Johnson[9]	18	Yes	750	Yes	NS	Yes	No	NS	Med (25)	Yes	No	0	0
1992	Watanabe[10]	26	Yes	NS	NS	NS	NS	NS	Med (18)	Low (21)	NS	Epo	0	0
1993	Kulier[11]	12	Yes	No	NS	NS	NS	NS	NS	NS	NS	Epo	0.08	0.33
1991	Ovrum[12]	500	No	799	Yes	2250	Yes	No	Low (15)	Med (25)	Yes	No	2.4	NS
1991	Ovrum[13]	121	No	815	Yes	2000	Yes	No	Low (15)	Med (25)	Yes	No	4.1	0.06
1994	Daily[14]	19	No	NO	Yes	1200	Yes	Yes	NS	Low (21)	Yes	Amicar	4.8	0.4
1979	Cosgrove[15]	50	No	675	Yes	NS	Yes	Yes	Low (15)	NS	Yes	No	6	0.06
1985	Cosgrove[16]	441	No	NS	Yes	NS	Yes	Yes	Low (15)	Low (22)	Yes	No	10	0.3
1986	Belcher[17]	90	No	550	Yes	NS	Yes	No	NS	Med (25)	No	No	10	0.18
1991	Jones[18]	100	No	1000 (PRP)	Yes	NS	Yes	Yes	Low (15)	Low (21)	Yes	No	18	0.31
1989	Owings[19]	107	Yes	1–2	Yes	NS	Yes	NS	NS	NS	Yes	No	27	0.8
1995	Helm[20]	45	No	1607	Yes	2200	Yes	Yes	Low (15)	Low (22)	Yes	No	28	1.2
1993	Karski[21]	75	NS	NS	Yes	2400	Yes	NS	Med (18)	Low (20)	Yes	Trax	28	NS

1974	Zubiate[22]	477	No	1000	Yes	1800	Yes	No	Low (15)	Low (22)	No	No	29	1.1
1988	Hartz[23]	21	NS	NS	NS	NS	NS	NS	NS	NS	NS	NS	30	NS
1990	LoCicero[24]	100	No	No	Yes	NS	Yes	Yes	NS	NS	Yes	No	31	0.7
1994	Paone[25]	314	No	No	Yes	2400	Yes	No	Med (18)	Low (20)	No	No	31.5	2.34
1990	Jones[26]	50	NS	1000 (PRP)	Yes	NS	Yes	No	High (21)	Low (23)	Yes	No	34	0.67
1993	Schoenberger[27]	50	No	799	Yes	2400	Yes	No	Med (18)	Med (25)	Yes	No	35	0.8
1995	Rousou[28]	206	NS	NS	Yes	NS	Yes	Yes	Med (18)	Low (22)	Yes	Apr	35	1.0
1994	Lemmer[29]	151	No	No	Yes	NS	Yes	Yes	Med (18)	Low (21)	Yes	Tranex	40	2.2
1987	Breyer[30]	43	No	No	Yes	NS	Yes	Yes	Med (18)	Med (25)	Yes	No	42	2.23
1984	Weisel[31]	13	No	NS	Yes	NS	Yes	NS	High (21)	Low (21)	No	No	50	1.4
1991	Parrot[32]	22	No	No	Yes	2000	Yes	Yes	Med (20)	High (30)	Yes	No	62	1.38
1994	Petry[33]	45	No	500–1000	Yes	1500	Yes	NS	Med (20)	High (30)	No	No	66	1.3
1989	Deitrich[34]	25	No	739	Yes	1400	Yes	No	Low (15)	High (30)	Yes	No	68	1.6
1993	Tobe[35]	24	No	750 (PRP)	Yes	NS	Yes	Yes	NS	NS	Yes	No	71	4.1
1989	Tyson[36]	52	No	Yes	Yes	NS	Yes	Yes	NS	Med (25)	Yes	No	74.5	4.5
1978	Yeh[37]	240	NS	NS	Yes	1800	Yes	NS	NS	High (33)	No	No	77.8	1.45
1993	Ward[38]	17	No	No	No	NS	Yes	Yes	No (24)	Med (24)	Yes	No	89	NS
1979	Schaff[39]	135	No	NS	NS	NS	NS	NS	NS	NS	Yes	No	100	2.4
1994	Arom[40]	100	NS	NS	Yes	NS	Yes	NS	NS	NS	No	Amicar	NS	1.4
1992	Davies[41]	32	No	857 (PRP)	Yes	NS	NS	NS	Med (20)	Med (24)	No	No	NS	1.6
1993	Sutton[42]	60	No	No	Yes	1500	Yes	No	NS	NS	No	No	NS	1.7
1980	Bayer[43]	1246	NS	NS	Yes	NS	Yes	NS	NS	NS	NS	No	NS	2.6

* = the number in parentheses is the hematocrit (90) used as the red cell transfusion trigger; PRP = platelet-rich plasmaphoresis; NS = not specified; Apr = aprotinin; EPO = erythropoietin; Tranex = tranexanic acid; med = medium.

TABLE 27.2. A survey of the technical and pharmacologic blood conservation measures applied to patients undergoing a variety of mixed procedures in 31 selected studies. These studies were selected because they listed the blood conservation measures applied as well as the allogeneic transfusion outcome. The studies are ranked according to allogeneic transfusion requirement.

Year	Author	Patient population	Number of patients	Preoperative autologous donation	Intraop. autologous donation	Non-blood prime	Volume CPB circuit	Circuit residual reinfusion	Intraop. salvage	RBC trigger CPB	RBC trigger postop	Shed mediastinal blood reinfusion	Pharm adjunct	Percent transfused	units per patient
1994	Rosengart[44]	Mixed	15	No	1180	Yes	1400	Yes	Yes	Low (15)	Low	Yes	Apr	0	0
1967	Beall[45]	Mixed	1818	No	No	Yes	2100	Yes	No	NS	NS	No	No	8.6	NS
1995	Sandrelli[46]	Mixed	348	Yes	Yes	Yes	NS	Yes	Yes	Med (18)	Med (24)	Yes	Apr	12.6	0.34
1993	Helm[47]	Mixed	35	No	1562	Yes	2200	Yes	Yes	Low (15)	Low (22)	Yes	No	17	1.0
1995	Parolari[48]	Mixed	1310	Yes	Yes	Yes	NS	Yes	Yes	NS	Med (24)	No	Apr	21.1	0.84
1994	Wong[49]	Mixed	20	No	1200 (PRP)	Yes	NS	Yes	Yes	Med (18)	Med (24)	No	No	30	0.45
1991	Horrow[50]	Mixed	77	NS	NS	Yes	NS	Yes	Yes	NS	Med (24)	Yes	Trax	32	NS
1992	Dzik[51]	AVR	79	Yes	NS	NS	NS	NS	NS	NS	NS	NS	NS	32	NS
1990	Horrow[52]	Mixed	18	No	No	Yes	NS	Yes	NS	NS	NS	Yes	Trax	NS	0.6
1989	Britton[53]	Mixed	104	Yes	1000	Yes	NS	Yes	Yes	NS	NS	No	No	34	0.7
1983	Johnson[54]	Mixed	168	NS	No	Yes	NS	Yes	NS	NS	NS	Yes	No	NS	1.0
1987	Love[55]	Mixed	58	Yes	No	Yes	NS	Yes	Yes	Low	Low	Yes	No	36	1.1

1995 Shinfeld[56]	Mixed	20	No	No	Yes	2000	Yes	No	No	NS	NS	Apr	50	1.1
1991 Carey[57]	Mixed	222	Yes	No	Yes	NS	Yes	Yes	High (21)	Med (24)	Yes	No	53	2.2
1979 Thurer[58]	Mixed	54	No	Some	Yes	NS	Yes	NS	NS	High (30)	Yes	No	59	1.6
1978 Schaff[59]	Mixed	63	NS	NS	NS	NS	NS	NS	NS	High (35)	Yes	No	NS	2.4
1989 DelRossi[60]	Mixed	170	NS	No	Yes	2500	Yes	NS	NS	High (30)	No	Amicar	NS	2.8
1992 Scott[61]	Mixed	60	Yes	575	Yes	NS	Yes	Yes	Med (18)	Low (24)	Yes	No	58	4.0
1994 Mukin[62]	Mixed	29	No	No	Yes	2000	Yes	Yes	NS	Low (20)	No	Apr	58.6	4.1
1994 Axford[63]	Mixed	16	No	No	Yes	NS	Yes	NS	NS	Med (25)	Yes	No	62	8.6
1979 Lambert[64]	Mixed	774	NS	NS	Yes	2000	Yes	Yes	NS	NS	No	Amicar	67	5.5
1992 Ikeda[65]	Mixed	3022	No	Yes	Yes	2250	Yes	Yes	High (21)	NS	Yes	No	72	9
1989 Lepore[66]	Mixed	67	No	NS	NS	NS	NS	NS	NS	NS	Yes	No	74.6	2.7
1976 Cove[67]	Mixed	44	Yes	No	Yes	1500	Yes	No	NS	NS	No	No	75	2.0
1995 Spiess[68]	Mixed	591	NS	NS	Yes	NS	NS	NS	NS	NS	No	No	78.5	6
1989 Page[69]	Mixed	50	No	Yes	Yes	NS	Yes	No	Low (17)	High (30)	Yes	No	88	3.15
1975 Cohn[70]	Mixed	400	No	500–1000	Yes	2200	Yes	No	Low (15)	NS	No	No	96.5	3.9
1977 Kaplan[71]	Mixed	60	No	750	No	2200	NS	No	NS	NS	No	No	100	5.5
1977 Lilleaasen[72]	AVR	30	No	855	No	2500	Yes	No	Yes	Yes	No	No	100	3.85
1988 Giordano[73]	Mixed	65	No	500 (PRP)	Yes	NS	Yes	Yes	NS	Med (25)	No	No	NS	6.32
1988 Giordano[74]	Mixed	50	No	No	NS	NS	NS	Yes	NS	NS	NS	No	NS	13.7

with a program that differed from Cosgrove's mainly in that shed mediastinal blood reinfusion was not employed. In 1990 Ovrum et al[29] confirmed the effectiveness of the simple "core" approach to blood conservation.[16] In 121 consecutive elective CABG patients the authors achieved a transfusion rate of 4.1% and 0.06 unit per patient. Ovrum's program differed from Cosgrove's only in that a dedicated intraoperative salvage device was not utilized (Cosgrove had used a heparinized cell centrifugation device). The authors did use standard cardiotomy suction—a form of intraoperative salvage—while the patient was on CPB, and so a significant amount of shed intraoperative blood was likely reclaimed. In 1991 Ovrum et al[28] applied this same program to 500 elective CABG patients and obtained similar low rates of transfusion (2.4% of patients; mean number of units per patient not stated).[12] The authors found the use of this simple six-step blood conservation approach to be simple, safe, and cost-effective.

By the early 1990s several pharmacologic adjuncts to blood conservation had become available. These could be divided into two groups: (1) those agents useful for the perioperative stimulation of red cell production (recombinant erythropoietin, iron), and (2) those agents useful in reducing postoperative bleeding (aprotinin, the antifibrinolytics, DDAVP). While typically adding significant cost to the procedure (erythropoietin, aprotinin, tranexamic acid), these pharmacologic adjuncts clearly helped to achieve their respective goals, and to reduce overall transfusion requirements. It remained, however, to appropriately and optimally integrate these pharmacologic measures with the technical blood conservation measures already in use.

Also by the early 1990s various technical modifications had become available to further advance blood conservation efforts. Oxygenator design improvements allowed a reduction in the volume of the CPB circuit, and, therefore, the amount of obligatory hemodilution that occurred during CPB. Circuit volume could be further reduced by replacing as much of the crystalloid circuit prime with autologous blood drained from the patient into the circuit immediately prior to CPB, a technique that we have termed "retrograde autologous priming" (RAP). Manipulations in global CPB circuit design and setup (tubing arrangement, optimal spatial relations) allowed further reductions in both the CPB circuit volume and the volume of crystalloid required to fill this circuit. Additionally, new devices and technical modifications, aimed at decreasing the body's inflammatory response to the standard CPB circuit, became available. Included in this group were improved leukocyte filters designed to selectively remove from the hematologic system the primary mediators of the inflammatory process. Likewise, pharmacology and technology were combined to create more biocompatible CPB circuitry—typified by the heparin bonded circuit. Finally, improvements in accessory equipment and technique allowed a significant decrease in ancillary blood use. "Near patient testing" apparatus required the use of only a single drop of blood to achieve results. Arterial lines became equipped with flush reinfusion devices to avoid the obligatory discard of the pre-laboratory sampling flush volume. Small-volume pediatric blood tubes allowed the use of significantly smaller blood volumes for those tests that could not be performed at the bedside.

Clearly by the early 1990s a variety of old and new technical and pharmacologic modalities were available to decrease the need for blood transfusion in cardiac surgery. Unfortunately, no attempt had been made to individually optimize and then logically integrate these measures into a single comprehensive program. Appropriate integration of newly available modalities into the proven "core" conservation programs of Cosgrove and Ovrum clearly had the potential to markedly reduce and even eliminate the need for transfusion, even in the face of the more difficult patient characteristics increasingly being encountered. This, therefore, became our goal: *the safe and cost-effective reduction or elimination of the need for homologous transfusion in a majority of cardiac surgical patients through the optimal and integrated application of all available blood conservation techniques* (Fig. 27.1).

Development of the New York Hospital Comprehensive Multimodality Blood Conservation Program

Meeting the Needs of the Jehovah's Witness Population

Our first efforts at the development and application of such a multimodality program were in response to the needs of the Jehovah's Witness

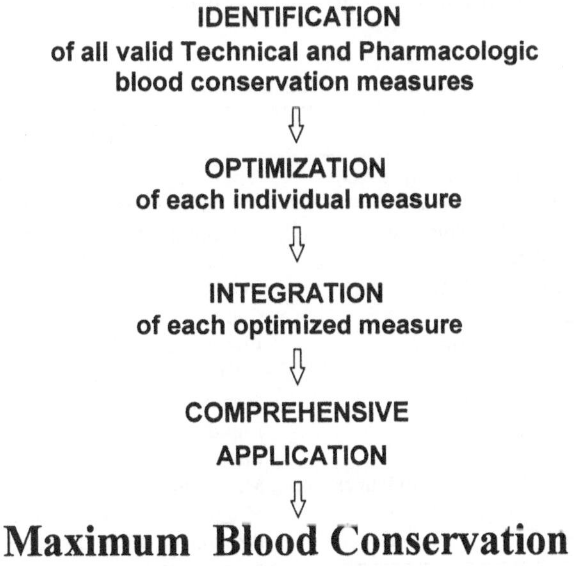

FIGURE 27.1. Conceptual development of a maximum blood conservation program.

population—patients referred to our institution because others refused to operate on them. Based on the results of Cosgrove and Ovrum, and equipped with the newly available pharmacologic adjuncts as well as our own technical modifications, we felt that we could safely and successfully perform even complex surgery on these patients without the need for transfusion. The multimodality program that was developed and applied to these patients had three basic components: (1) the six core conservation measures applied by Cosgrove and Ovrum, each one individually optimized and then fully integrated; (2) several additional supportive technical measures; and (3) full pharmacologic support.

Optimization and Integration of the Six Core Components

Central to the Jehovah's Witness program was application of the same set of core blood conservation measures applied by Cosgrove and Ovrum. Our application of these core measures differed, however, in that every effort was made to optimize the way in which each individual technique was applied (Table 27.3).

First, instead of removing the standard one to two units of blood during the pre-CPB period, an individually calculated maximum volume of blood was removed (a mean of 1300 ml per patient). This was approximately twice the volume removed by Cosgrove and Ovrum, and it was removed from patients of very small mean body size, a majority of whom had advanced disease. As discussed in Chapter 11, Intraoperative Autologous Blood Donation Practices, the removal of a maximum volume was essential to the preservation of as much autologous red cell mass as possible.

TABLE 27.3. Technical blood conservation measures.

Technique	Optimized form
Preoperative autologous donation (PAD)	Optimized donation schedule
Reduction in CPB circuit volume	Minimum CPB circuit volume (1200 cc)
Reduction in crystalloid/colloid use (decrease hemodilution)	Minimum safe crystalloid/colloid use (fluid guidelines, RAP)
Intraoperative autologous donation (IAD)	Maximum volume IAD (calculated)
Intraoperative salvage	Cell Saver "skin to skin"
Reduced RBC transfusion triggers	Lowest safe RBC transfusion trigger (15% CPB; 22% post op)
Hemostatic operative technique	Maximum
Adequate patient rewarming	Rapid and sustained to >37°C
Shed mediastinal blood reinfusion	Maximum SMB reinfusion
Platelet and coagulation factor guidelines	Minimum safe use guidelines
Reduced laboratory sampling	Minimum sampling (peds tubes, etc.)
Adjuvant therapies	BP control, PEEP increase, etc.

Second, not only was nonhomologous blood crystalloid priming of the circuit utilized, but the volume of the prime was minimized through the use of a small prime oxygenator, and by decreasing the length and size of all circuit tubing. A further reduction in CPB circuit prime volume was achieved by the technique of RAP, whereby immediately prior to the initiation of CPB the circuit's crystalloid prime was replaced by the patient's own blood drained into the CPB circuit retrograde from both the venous and arterial cannulas. By minimizing the CPB circuit volume and then minimizing the amount of crystalloid prime in this circuit, the amount of obligatory hemodilution that occurred as bypass was initiated was markedly decreased. Higher hematocrits during CPB in turn synergistically allowed the removal of more autologous blood during the pre-CPB period through intraoperative autologous donation (IAD), and so more autologous red cells could be saved from intraoperative loss and destruction.

Third, like Cosgrove and Ovrum, we reinfused all of the residual CPB circuit volume following CPB. But because we found that often patients required both volume and additional oxygen carrying capacity immediately after separation from CPB, and that IAD blood was not always available (sometimes IAD blood had already been returned during CPB, or had not been drawn in the first place because of insufficient pre-CPB red cell mass/hematocrit), we developed a method of rapidly returning *all* the red cell mass remaining in the circuit to the patient within 10 minutes of separation from CPB, while at the same time maintaining full circuit prime status and the ability to return to CPB should this be required. In effect, adequate overall autologous red cell mass was often available at the end of the bypass run, but part of this mass was in the wrong place (the CPB circuit) at the wrong time. To correct this situation, in the select group of patients with low post-CPB hematocrits and little or no IAD blood available, we would drain all the residual circuit blood into the Cell Saver immediately after separation from CPB, replacing this volume with crystalloid to maintain circuit prime status (in the rare event that return to CPB would be required). This reclaimed circuit blood could be processed and reinfusion begun within 5 to 10 minutes following separation of CPB.

Fourth, like Cosgrove, we chose to use intraoperative cell salvage to reclaim as much lost autologous red cell mass as possible. We extended the use of the Cell Saver, however, so that it was utilized from "skin to skin." Traditional lap pads, sponges, and discard suckers were eliminated from the operative field. This not only served to markedly increase the percentage of lost blood that was salvaged, but it also forced those operating to achieve maximum technical hemostasis. In addition, to enhance the quality of the salvaged product, suction pressure was reduced so that cellular trauma was minimized.

Fifth, our core program also incorporated the use of the lowest safe level of anemia during CPB as the trigger for the return of IAD blood. A hematocrit of 15% was chosen as this trigger, based on analysis of both clinical and physiologic data (see Chapter 16, Indications for Red Cell Transfusion).

Sixth and finally, like Cosgrove and Ovrum, we chose to maximally reclaim lost postoperative red cell mass through shed mediastinal blood reinfusion (the technique was modified to include the use of a continuous closed circuit in line with the requirements of the Jehovah's Witness faith).

Additional Technical Measures

In addition to optimizing and optimally integrating the six core components, we added several additional technical modifications. Like Cosgrove and Ovrum, we used the less traumatic membrane oxygenator, but in addition we were able to incorporate the use of the newly available and also less traumatic centrifugal pump. As stated, reverse autologous priming was performed on all patients at the initiation of bypass in order to minimize hemodilution. Hemofiltration was selectively used following separation from CPB to remove excess crystalloid (for patients judged to have a hypervolemic component to their hemodilution). Excessive blood loss through laboratory sampling was eliminated by using pediatric tubes for all blood draws, returning all arterial line flushes to the patient, and by minimizing the testing that occurred (see Chapter 21). Finally, meticulous surgical technique and hemostasis, in the tradition of Cooley, Beall, and Baily, was applied throughout each procedure.[75–77] By their excellent results in the Jehovah's Witness population, these two surgeons had demonstrated very early on in cardiac surgical blood conservation the power and importance of performing an operation quickly and well, with meticulous attention to hemostasis.

Maximum Pharmacologic Support

To augment these optimized technical aspects of the multimodality program, we integrated the use of each of the recently available pharmacologic blood conservation measures. As with the technical measures, an effort was made to optimize the application of each of these pharmacologic agents (Table 27.4). Four pharmacologic agents were incorporated into the multimodality program, each with a specific purpose: (1) *erythropoietin* to maximally and acutely stimulate perioperative red cell production, (2) *iron* to provide substrate for this increased red cell production, (3) *aprotinin* to ameliorate the inflammatory response to CPB and decrease postoperative coagulopathic bleeding, and (4) *DDAVP* to improve coagulopathic bleeding in patients with renal failure or insufficiency.

Erythropoietin (see Chapter 4, Erythropoietin in Cardiac Surgery) became available for the treatment of the anemia of chronic renal failure in 1987. Following immediate and overwhelming success in treating this form

TABLE 27.4. Pharmacologic blood conservation measures.

Agent	Optimized dosing
Erythropoietin	High-dose regimen (low preoperative Hct/RCM) (800 U/kg IV/SQ load, 500 U/kg SQ QOD)
Aprotinin	Full Hammersmith regimen (high bleed risk) Half Hammersmith regimen (moderate bleed risk)
Amicar	Standard dose (excessive postoperative bleeding) (nonaprotinin patients only)
DDAVP	Standard dose (excessive postoperative bleeding) (patients with renal insufficiency/failure only)
Iron	Standard dose (intravenous if iron deficiency, otherwise oral)
Adjuvant/other	Vitamin B_{12}, folate (intravenous if iron deficiency, otherwise oral)

Hct = hematocrit
IV = intravenous
SQ = subcutaneous
QOD = every other day
DDAVP = D arginine amino vasopressin

of anemia, its use was expanded to other areas, including perioperative applications. When we began using erythropoietin in 1992, its predominant perioperative use in the cardiac surgical setting was for the augmentation of autologous blood donation prior to elective cardiac surgery. The studies by Watanabe et al[26] and Kulier et al,[27] which achieved zero rates of homologous transfusion (Table 27.1), indicate the success of this approach. In the Jehovah's Witness population, however, long-term elective preoperative autologous donation was not permissible (because the blood is separated from the body), and so if erythropoietin were to be applied, alternative strategies needed to be developed. There existed three logical ways in which the drug could be applied: (1) correction of preoperative anemia, (2) acute stimulation of preoperative red cell production so that increased *intraoperative* autologous donation could be performed, and (3) correction of postoperative anemia.[78] For all of these applications it was theoretically and practically desirable to be able *to acutely* and *maximally* stimulate red cell production. Time was a luxury that could not be afforded, particularly in the Jehovah's Witness patient requiring urgent or emergent surgery. Unfortunately, however, at that time erythropoietin dosing regimens had been primarily aimed at the relatively gradual correction of anemia in the chronically uremic renal failure population. It became essential, therefore, to develop new methods for administering erythropoietin that would lead to a maximum rate of red cell production. By combining use of the intravenous and subcutaneous administration of the drug we found that we were able to recreate the natural maximum biphasic serum erythropoietin response (the response seen when the body is bled to a hematocrit of 10% to 12%). We were able to do this with amounts of the hormone that were not significantly larger than those often applied clinically previously,[79] and significantly less than the maximum amount that had been applied clinically.[80] An initial combined 300 U/kg IV and 500 U/kg SQ dose was given to all patients preoperatively. Administration was then continued at 500 U/kg SQ every other day until the time of surgery. When possible, surgery was delayed until the hematocrit had risen above 36%, and the red cell mass over 1600 ml. Erythropoietin was continued postoperatively only if the postoperative hematocrit was below 30%. We found this "natural maximum" erythropoietin dosing regimen to be safe and remarkably effective in stimulating a rapid and sustained increase in red cell generation.

The relationship between adequate iron stores and erythropoiesis had long been established (see Chapter 4, Erythropoietin in Cardiac Surgery). More recently the importance of adequate iron stores in ensuring the maximum bone marrow response to recombinant erythropoietin had also been demonstrated. Therefore, an essential part of the pharmacologic component of the multimodality program was the use of adequate iron supplementation. For patients without preoperative anemia and evidence of iron deficiency of preoperative testing, oral iron supplementation was immediately instituted, along with vitamin C therapy to aid in intestinal absorption of iron. If anemia was present, and iron deficiency documented, then intravenous iron therapy was implemented in order to provide larger amounts of iron more rapidly to support erythropoietin-generated red cell mass. Oral iron therapy was continued postoperatively until the time of discharge on all patients.

When the Jehovah's Witness program was developed, the remarkable effectiveness of aprotinin (see Chapter 15) in decreasing coagulopathic bleeding following CPB had already become apparent.[81–83] Incorporating the use of this third drug into the Jehovah's Witness program was relatively straightforward. To achieve maximum effect, we chose to use the full Hammersmith regimen (6 million units total). The activated clotting time was kept above 750 seconds in all patients to ensure adequate heparinization during CPB.

The fourth and final pharmacologic agent integrated into the multimodality protocol was DDAVP. While its efficacy in decreasing postoperative bleeding following routine cardiac surgery had largely been disproved, its usefulness in treating established severe coagulopathic bleeding following CPB, bleeding association with uremic renal failure, and bleeding associated with von Willebrand's disease, is generally accepted. We therefore reserved the use of this drug for the treatment of those Jehovah's Witness patients with either of these conditions predisposing to excessive bleeding, or to those demonstrating increased bleeding postoperatively.

Results of the First Comprehensive Multimodality Blood Conservation Program

In 1994 we first reported on the comprehensive multimodality approach that we had developed and applied to the Jehovah's Witness population.[44]

Fifteen patients, all at high risk for requiring perioperative transfusion, either because of preoperative risk factors and/or because of the complex nature of procedure performed (e.g., combined mitral-aortic valve replacement with two-vessel CABG, type I aortic dissection), were successfully operated on without the need for homologous transfusion. Results were compared to those obtained in a group of 100 contemporary primary CABG patients operated on with a more limited "standard" set of blood conservation measures. It was found that although the control CABG patients received 2.3 units of allogeneic red cells per patient, their postoperative hematocrits were four percentage points *lower* than those in the Jehovah's Witness group, indicating a significant improvement in generation and preservation of red cell mass in the Jehovah's Witness group. In addition, despite the variety of complex procedures and long bypass runs, postoperative bleeding in the Jehovah's Witness group was decreased by 65%. These remarkable results, in this very comorbid population, were obtained without an increase in either morbidity or mortality.

Additional Work with the Jehovah's Witness Population

Following our success in treating this initial group of patients, we continued to apply this multimodality program to all Jehovah's Witness patients referred to our institution. By 1996 we were able to report on the use of the program in 30 consecutive CABG patients, and 55 patients overall.[8] Included in this CABG population were six reoperative procedures and four combined CABG/valve procedures. As a whole the 30 CABG patients were at significant increased risk for requiring red cell transfusion according to several established criteria delineating transfusion risk. Seven patients were over the age of 80. Fifty-seven percent of patients were female. Ten patients had preoperative hematocrits less than 30%. Ten patients had a preoperative red cell mass less than 1400 cc, and a mean preoperative red cell mass of only 1690 ml. In addition, several patients presented with conditions or circumstances that would have absolutely precluded bloodless surgery prior to our institution of this program. For example, one patient presented status post–acute myocardial infarction and cardiac arrest, intubated, and on an intraaortic balloon pump for ongoing ischemia and congestive heart failure attributable to severe mitral regurgitation. The patient weighed only 63 kg, had a history of a recent lower gastrointestinal bleeding (and was passing melanic stools on admission), was in acute renal failure necessitating dialysis, was actively oozing blood from his balloon insertion site, and had a transfer hematocrit of 17%. Following stabilization and acute erythropoietin/iron therapy, on hospital day 19 the patient underwent a successful three-vessel CABG with combined mitral valve repair. His postoperative hematocrit was 44%, and he was discharged 1 week following operation with a hematocrit of 42%. A second patient was a 72-year-old woman admitted 3 months status post–three-vessel CABG with all three grafts occluded, severe mitral regurgitation, and unstable angina requiring

IV nitroglycerin and heparin. She weighed 45 kg, had a history of thalassemia trait, and her admission hematocrit was 30.9%. After 6 days of preoperative erythropoietin and intravenous iron therapy her hematocrit rose to 44%, and she underwent a successful reoperative three-vessel CABG (including use of the internal mammary artery) and mitral valve annuloplasty. Her postoperative hematocrit was 38%, and she was discharged 6 days later with a hematocrit of 35%.

A comparison between this subgroup of 30 Jehovah's Witness CABG patients and a group of 30 low to moderate risk control patients from one of our previous prospective randomized blood conservation trials further demonstrates the relative effectiveness of the program. Despite being at higher risk for requiring transfusion, the Jehovah's Witness group did not require any homologous or preoperatively donated autologous blood, compared with 1.8 units of allogeneic blood per patient per group in the control group. Even with this absence of transfusion, and red cell transfusion in particular, the postoperative hematocrits in the Jehovah's Witness group were significantly higher at all postoperative time points. There was only one death in the Jehovah's Witness group. This occurred in a male with a history of stroke, long-standing insulin-dependent diabetes mellitus (IDDM), and severe peripheral vascular disease, who suffered an intraoperative cerebral embolic event and died on the 42nd postoperative day.

We have operated on over 70 Jehovah's Witness patients requiring cardiopulmonary bypass in the 4 years since the first application of the multimodality program. Many of these techniques and strategies, including acute high-dose erythropoietin therapy, maximum-volume intraoperative autologous donation, the acceptance of the lowest safe level of anemia during and following surgery, and intraoperative salvage, have subsequently been extended to Jehovah's Witness patients undergoing other forms of surgery at our institution, with equally gratifying results.

Application of Multimodality Program to the General Population

Modification of the Jehovah's Witness Program

Our success in the Jehovah's Witness population prompted an extension of the multimodality program to our non-Jehovah's Witness cardiopulmonary bypass population as well. This extension necessarily required a reevaluation of the program with respect to (1) the ease with which various measures could be applied, and (2) the cost-effectiveness of the various measures and of the program in general (Fig. 27.2). We realized that the program would never be applied, either at our institution or elsewhere, if it were not user friendly. The program must not place significant additional burden on

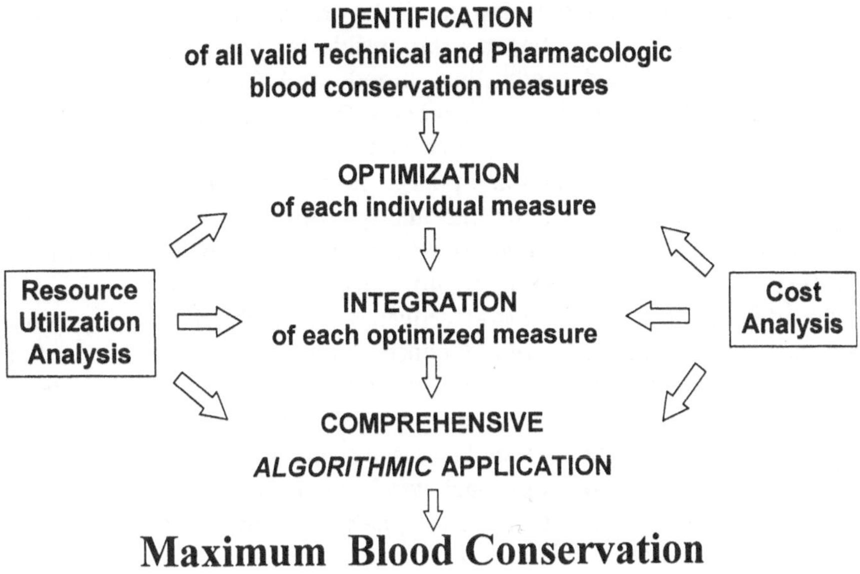

FIGURE 27.2. Development of a maximum cost efficient, blood conservation program.

those charged with its execution, and tasks must be rationally divided among those best equipped to perform them. Similarly, and particularly in today's health care environment, it was essential that the costs of the program not outweigh the savings in transfusion reduction.

To meet these two challenges several minor but important modifications were made to the comprehensive multimodality program. To help make the program simple to apply, we divided the components of the program into parts based on who would be most appropriately placed in charge of their execution. Therefore, the perfusionists were assigned the task of preparing the smallest-volume CPB circuit possible for each individual patient, for calculating the IAD volume, and for performing RAP at the initiation of CPB. In addition, they were charged with minimizing the use of crystalloid during CPB, and with the rapid and efficient processing of all blood salvaged from the operative field and from the CPB circuit. The anesthesiologists were charged with the administration of aprotinin (when used), removal of the appropriate IAD volume, minimization of perioperative fluid administration, and adherence to the stated intraoperative transfusion guidelines. The surgeons were charged with administering erythropoietin preoperatively and postoperatively when indicated, achieving maximum technical hemostasis, salvaging as much intraoperative blood loss as possible using both Cell Saver and cardiotomy suction devices where appropriate, adhering to the stated intraoperative and postoperative transfusion guidelines, and operating swiftly but accurately to minimize CPB time. The nursing staff was charged with minimizing blood loss through laboratory sampling by using pediatric blood tubes, returning arterial line flushes, and decreasing the amount of laboratory testing generally performed. In addition, they became responsible for reinfusion of the maximum amount of shed mediastinal blood, and for helping to ensure adherence to the postoperative protocols for treatment of the bleeding patient and the transfusion of all blood and blood products (the latter is a particularly important function at large teaching institutions with high resident turnover rates). The multimodality blood conservation was effectively transformed into a team approach, in which each of the parts worked together to achieve the whole in a simple organized fashion.

To address the issue of cost-effectiveness we realized that a selective approach to all expensive blood conservation measures was essential. Because a majority of the technical measures were very inexpensive (e.g., IAD), free (e.g., RAP), or even saved money (e.g., the new small-volume oxygenator was $50 less than the older large prime oxygenator), the primary area in which this selective approach would limit costs was in the application of the newer and more expensive pharmacologic blood conservation modalities (e.g., erythropoietin, aprotinin).

The first step in applying the selective approach was to identify the specific risk factor(s) for transfusion that were counteracted by each of the four drugs included in our program.[15] Patients with low preoperative hematocrit or red cell mass, a risk factor for red cell transfusion, were to be given erythropoietin preoperatively. To further contain the use of the drug, and therefore cost, erythropoietin would only be continued postoperatively if the hematocrit was beneath a critical level that would be expected to lead to red cell transfusion (if left untreated). Aprotinin use was reserved for any patient at increased risk for postoperative bleeding. Therefore, only patients with a history of aspirin use (within 5 days), preoperative heparin therapy, recent thrombolytic therapy, preoperative bleeding disorder, or significant hepatic disease or alcohol use were to be given aprotinin. In an effort to further contain costs, it was elected to apply the half-strength Hammersmith aprotinin regimen. We felt that the half-strength regimen would also help to limit any potential detrimental effects that the drug might have, such as transient renal insufficiency and graft thrombosis. Patients who experienced excessive bleeding postoperatively and who did not receive aprotinin, were given intravenous Amicar (standard 5-10 gm load, then 1 gm/hr over the next 5 hours) to combat the presumed fibrinolytic component of this bleeding. The use of DDAVP was limited to those patients with clinically significant increased postoperative bleeding, with a lower threshold for use in patients with preoperative (renal) disease or von Willebrand's disease. Because all patients lose a portion of their red cell mass and a large majority are rendered anemic following heart surgery, and because it is inexpensive, oral iron therapy was to be administered to all patients beginning on admission (except of course in the very rare instance of hemochromatosis or one of the iron overload states). We felt that the risk of anaphylaxis to intravenous iron, albeit small (1:30,000), precluded its use in the general cardiac surgery program. Its use therefore continued to be reserved for use in the preoperative Jehovah's Witness patients with severe anemia and iron deficiency who required urgent or emergent surgery. In this select patient population we felt that the potential lifesaving benefit of the drug outweighed the risk of anaphylaxis.

One Hundred Consecutive Patients Without Transfusion

Having assembled this modified selective but nevertheless maximum multimodality therapy program, we then evaluated its effectiveness prospectively in 100 consecutive primary CABG patients.[19] While previous combined programs had addressed primarily elective patients, we decided to include in our evaluation all patients except those in whom blood use could not likely be avoided even with use of the program. Excluded from enrollment in the protocol, therefore, were patients on intraaortic balloon pumps preoperatively, patients emergently operated on after arrest or other mishap in angiography/angioplasty, and patients with a preoperative hematocrit less than 34% or red cell mass less than 1500 cc. Because we also wanted to evaluate the safety of the program, we also excluded those patients with an increased likelihood of operative morbidity regardless of application of the multimodality program. If the program proved safe in this population, then it could be selectively expanded to these high-risk groups in the future. Patients excluded according to this criteria were those with a history of stroke, renal insufficiency or failure with a creatinine of >2.0, age >80, severe hepatic disease, or history of bleeding disorder.

We found the use of the multimodality program to be simple and remarkably effective. Transfusion requirement was not only reduced, but actually eliminated. One hundred consecutive elective and urgent primary CABG patients prospectively enrolled were operated on without the need for homologous blood, with the exception of one patient who received two units of directed donor blood on postoperative day 14. If the circumstances surrounding this transfusion are further elucidated, however, it is seen that even this patient successfully underwent heart surgery without the need for transfusion for reasons attributable to the heart surgery itself. The patient was a 65-year-old man with a history of endoscopically verified duodenal ulcer disease who had been admitted to the hospital twice in the past 2 years for gastrointestinal hemorrhage. The patient was placed on appropriate ulcer prophylaxis both pre- and postoperatively, but on postoperative day 8 his hematocrit was found to decrease from 34% to 24%. Stools were found to be guaiac positive and he was closely monitored. On postoperative day 13 his hematocrit acutely dropped from 26% to 17%. He was transfused two units of a family member's blood, and endoscopy subsequently revealed several duodenal ulcers, one of which was actively bleeding and able to be controlled endoscopically. The remainder of his hospital stay was uneventful, and no additional bleeding episodes or transfusions occurred.

The program also was found to be safe. There were two strokes, two patients experienced transient renal insufficiency (one with aprotinin, one without), there was one myocardial infarction, and one patient died. The first stroke occurred in a 79-year-old woman with a heavily calcified ascending aorta. In addition, loosely adherent pieces of plaque were seen by transesphaged echo to extend into the lumen and move with the blood flow. It was decided to proceed with the operation and all possible steps were taken to avoid embolization. The patient never awoke postoperatively, however, and subsequent computed tomography (CT) scan revealed massive bilateral infarcts. Her postoperative hematocrit was 35%. She was made DNR (do not resuscitate) on postoperative day 13, and can be considered as the single mortality in the 100 patients. The second stroke occurred in a 70-year-old man with a history of severe atherosclerotic disease. Two patients experienced transient renal insufficiency. The average length of time on respirator, ICU stay, infection rate, and length of postoperative hospital stay (mean = 6.5 days; median = 6 days) compared favorably to those seen in our general CABG population. Additionally, when these patients were stratified according to hospital Diagnostic Related Group (DRG), an actual cost savings of $1611 per patient was realized, the savings largely attributable to the decreased transfusion costs and the decrease in postoperative length of stay.

Following the successful application of the program to these 100 consecutive patients, its use was expanded to all patients undergoing cardiac surgery at our institution, with minor modifications according to procedure type and individual patient characteristics and morbidity risk factors. Nevertheless, the basic themes have remained the same: (1) apply each of the available technical and pharmacologic blood conservation measures in an optimized and integrated fashion, (2) selectively apply those measures that incur significant increases in cost or risk so that these specific measures are applied only to those most likely to benefit from their use, (3) utilize a simplified team approach in which all disciplines work in concert to achieve the whole. The following section provides a detailed outline of our multimodality program, as well as an algorithm that summarizes its use.[20–23]

The New York Hospital–Cornell Medical Center Multimodality Blood Conservation Program

Summary of the Technical and Pharmacologic Measures Employed

The following is a concise summary of each of the cardiac surgical blood conservation measures that are discussed in this text, and that serve as the components of the NYH multimodality based conservation program. Included for each technical or pharmacologic modality is (1) the rationale behind its use, (2) the selection criteria for its use, (3) the member(s) of the cardiac surgical team responsible for its execution, and (4) a description of the exact way in which the technique or pharmacologic agent is applied clinically. The technical and pharmacologic measures are listed in the order in which they are generally applied clinically during the perioperative period.

Technical Conservation Measures

Preoperative Autologous Blood Donation (PAD) (See Chapter 3)

This measure is reserved for strictly elective procedures when appropriate preoperative time is available for both blood donation and full red cell mass regeneration by the time of surgery. Allowing time for sufficient generation is essential, as otherwise no net gain in red cell mass is achieved at the expense of not being able to perform a directly proportional volume of intraoperative autologous donation on the day of surgery (i.e., PAD should not be performed in place of IAD, as IAD provides a superior autologous blood product, with far less expense and logistical and administrative complexity, and no waste). A good rule of thumb is that a 2-week regeneration period should be allowed for each unit of blood removed. Besides the requirement for sufficient time for red cell regeneration, the only criteria excluding the use of PAD are severe aortic stenosis and unstable angina/ongoing ischemia. PAD should typically be applied in a monitored setting, with appropriate interventions available. At our institution it is performed in the blood bank by blood bank technicians, with close physician availability. Oral iron therapy (with concomitant vitamin C therapy and an appropriate stool softener such as Colace) should be started at the time of the first donation.

Large-Volume Intraoperative Autologous Donation (IAD) (See Chapter 11)

All patients with adequate hematocrit and red cell mass should undergo intraoperative autologous donation. The maximum volume of autologous blood should be removed from each individual patient during the intraoperative pre-CPB period in order to preserve as much blood as possible from intraoperative loss and degradation, and to provide a volume of fresh red cells, platelets, and coagulation factors for reinfusion immediately following CPB. Patients with ongoing ischemia and severe aortic stenosis should have liberal volume replacement during blood removal to ensure adequate cardiac output, but these two disease states do not serve as contraindications to performing IAD. The only direct contraindications to IAD are (1) insufficient red cell mass and/or hematocrit as determined by the IAD calculation (see below), and (2) ongoing bacteremia/septicemia. The volume of blood to be removed is calculated by two equations that take into account the patient's estimated blood volume, the starting hematocrit in the operating room, the circuit prime volume, and a target hematocrit of 18% during CPB (Fig. 27.3). By dividing the calculation into two parts, the hematocrit that should be achieved after IAD blood removal, but before CPB, can be derived (Equation 1). A hematocrit should be checked after removal of the first two IAD units to gauge where the patient stands with respect to this number. If the patient is still more than 5 to 6 percentage points above this number, then an additional (third) unit of blood should be removed. Usually not more than three IAD units (1350–1500 cc) are removed. Four or more units are removed only from patients in whom a complex procedure and long CPB run are anticipated (and who have adequate initial hematocrit/red cell mass).

During CPB, IAD blood should be reinfused only for a hematocrit of 15% or less (17% or less if there is a history of stroke or cerebrovascular disease), and only after all available Cell Saver and PAD blood has been infused. All IAD blood should be reinfused before any homologous blood is used during CPB to prevent possible unnecessary homologous exposure. Following termination of CPB, IAD blood should be reinfused as rapidly as clinically possible through a blood-warming device. Reinfusion should be started *after* protamine reversal of heparin if a last hematocrit on CPB is 20% or greater. If it is 19% or less, or the patient is demonstrating instability or is difficult to wean from CPB, then IAD reinfusion should be initiated prior to protamine reinfusion in order to more rapidly restore

REQUIRED DATA:

HEIGHT = ________ cm. ________ inches
WEIGHT = ________ kg. ________ pounds
EBV = ________ ml
$HCT_{Initial}$ = ________ % (first hct in OR)
HCT_{Target} = 18 %

EQUATION 1: (STEP 1)

$$HCT_{Pre\,CPB} = HCT_{Target}\ (\,EBV + Prime\ Volume\,)\ /\ EBV$$

$$HCT_{Pre\,CPB} = 0.18\ (\ \_\_\_\_\ /\ \_\_\_\_\ )$$

$$HCT_{Pre\,CPB} = \_\_\_\_\ \%$$

EQUATION 2: (STEP 2)

$$IAD\ VOLUME = EBV\ (\,HCT_{Initial} - HCT_{Pre\,CPB}\,)\ /\ HCT_{Initial}$$

$$IAD\ VOLUME = \_\_\_\_\ (\ \_\_\_\_ - \_\_\_\_\ )\ /\ \_\_\_\_$$

CALCULATED IAD VOLUME = ________ ml.

FIGURE 27.3. Calculation of blood volume to be removed.

oxygen carrying capacity. All IAD blood should always be infused, regardless of the patient's hematocrit. Appropriate IAD blood labeling and record keeping should be performed. We assign this important task to the perfusion team.

Non-Blood CPB Circuit Prime (See Chapter 12)

Blood should rarely be used to prime the CPB circuit in adult patients. Homologous blood prime should be restricted only to those rare cases in which the on-CPB hematocrit is calculated to be less than 15% without performing IAD. The composition of the circuit prime is otherwise left to the individual cardiac surgical team and institution. Our prime consists of 1100 ml plasmacyte A solution, 0.3 mg Hg mannitol, and 100 ml 25% albumin. If aprotinin is used, this is also added to this basic CPB circuit prime solution.

Minimum Volume CPB Circuit (See Chapter 12)

This is one of the most important and yet often overlooked technical blood conservation measures. By minimizing the volume of the CPB circuit, the volume into which the patient's pre-CPB red cell mass must be distributed is reduced. This leads to less hemodilution during CPB, and in doing so, increases the volume of IAD that can be performed. In addition, it allows IAD to be performed in smaller patients and in those with lower hematocrits/red cell mass. There are three basic aspects of the CPB circuit that must be addressed when striving to maximally decrease circuit volume: (1) the oxygenator prime volume, (2) tubing diameter, and (3) tubing length and overall spatial configuration. The smallest prime volume oxygenator that can still provide adequate flow rates should be utilized for all cases. We have found that a 400 ml low prime volume oxygenator can adequately handle all but the very highest flow rates. For all patients weighing less than 75 kg, a ⅜" venous line is substituted for the standard ½" line. Smaller-diameter cardioplegia tubing can also be utilized. It is essential to place components of the CPB circuit in a spatial configuration that allows for maximum shortening of all tubing segments. The position of each component in relation to one another, as well as the overall position of the circuit with respect to the patient, must be taken into consideration. Performing these basic changes in our own circuit reduced our CPB circuit volume from 2200 cc to 1400 cc. This is one of the areas in both our program and in blood conservation in general where increased awareness and further technologic advancement will lead to additional savings in the future.

Minimization of Unnecessary Crystalloid Administration

To minimize the hemodilution that occurs first with IAD and then with CPB, only the amount of crystalloid required to maintain hemodynamic stability should be administered. During the pre-CPB/IAD period we have found that a 1.5–2:1 ratio of blood removed to crystalloid reinfused is typically adequate to maintain stable cardiovascular status. If the patient has unstable angina or severe aortic stenosis, then more traditional replacement with a ratio approximating 3:1 should be utilized. If systolic blood pressure decreases to less than 100 mm Hg during the pre-CPB period and the cardiac index (CI) is greater than 2.2–2.5, the use of alpha support (vs crystalloid reinfusion) should be considered. During CPB, crystalloid use can be minimized by maintaining minimum safe reservoir volumes, and by returning all available salvaged blood when reservoir volume drops below this minimum safe level. Postoperatively, crystalloid use/hemodilution can be minimized by ensuring the reinfusion of all autologous blood (IAD and Cell Saver) and through appropriate use of vasoconstrictive agents. The latter becomes particularly important in the postoperative patient with borderline low hematocrit (e.g., 23%). If such a patient were to become mildly hypotensive with an adequate cardiac output but low systemic vascular resistance (SVR), administration of crystalloid would likely cause the patient's hematocrit to drop below the transfusion trigger, leading to red cell transfusion. Conversely, initiation of alpha support might allow the avoidance of such a hemodilution-induced decrease in hematocrit/increase in transfusion. Minimization of crystalloid is the responsibility of the anesthesiologist during the pre-CPB period, the perfusionist during CPB, and the nursing/surgical staff during the post-CPB period.

Autologous Blood Circuit Prime (RAP) (See Chapter 11)

To further reduce the hemodilution that occurs during CPB, crystalloid can be removed from the CPB circuit as bypass is initiated. This can be limited to draining the prime in the venous return line into a collection bag through a side port or Y-connection, or it can be extended to include removal of a majority of the crystalloid prime through the technique of retrograde autologous priming (RAP). According to this technique, immediately prior to the initiation of CPB, blood is drained from the right atrium via the venous line and from the aorta via the arterial line. The crystalloid that is displaced from the circuit is collected in a collection bag off the arterial side of the CPB circuit. Typically 800 to 1000 ml of the original crystalloid circuit prime can be removed using this technique. This removed prime can be returned at any time during CPB when volume is required. Even if the full volume is returned, nothing is lost by having applied the technique. RAP is performed by the perfusionist in conjunction with both the surgeon and anesthesiologist.

Intraoperative Salvage (Cell Saver) (See Chapter 13)

We utilize a Cell Saver centrifugal salvage device for intraoperative salvage prior to heparenization, following protomine reversal of heparin residual and for circuit blood processing. Every attempt is made to salvage as much lost blood as possible from the time of the first incision to the time of chest closure ("skin to skin"). Centrifugation and washing allows us to reclaim pericardial blood and blood from other sources that would also not be appropriately reinfused without washing. After initation of CPB, all "clean" heparenized blood is reclaimed directly into the CPB circuit, using a parallel "cardiotomy" suction circuit. During CPB, any available Cell Saver blood is the first blood product to be infused when the hematocrit drops to 15% or less (17% or less if history of stroke or cerebrovascular disease). The Cell Saver can also be used to concentrate excess reservoir volume (e.g., mitral valve cases), but this should be done only if the hematocrit is low in the setting of this excess volume. Otherwise platelets and coagulation factors are needlessly discarded. When Cell Saver blood is available during CPB, it should only be reinfused if it becomes necessary (i.e., low hematocrit). This is in keeping with the general concept that the CPB pump and apparatus cause red cell damage and hemolysis, and so as many red cells as possible should be kept from exposure to this apparatus for as long as possible. When using the Cell Saver to process residual circuit blood, we first pump as much of the circuit blood as possible into the patient as unprocessed blood. Only the remainder is centrifuged, washed, and returned to the patient as processed Cell Saver blood. In this way loss of additional platelets and factors from the residual circuit volume is minimized. If the last hematocrit on CPB is low and little or no IAD is available for post-CPB reinfusion, it is essential to accelerate processing of the residual CPB circuit volume. In these cases we pump the circuit blood into the Cell Saver and replace this volume with crystalloid so that the circuit remains primed in case the patient must be re-placed on bypass. This rapid processing technique can provide the equivalent of one to two units of packed red cells, eliminating what would otherwise result in a need for homologous red cells during this crucial time.

Hemofiltration (See Chapter 12)

If a large excess of whole autologous blood is left in the CPB circuit and the patient appears euvolemic or hypervolemic and has a low hematocrit, this blood can be processed using an ultrafiltration device. In this setting, use of hemofiltration is theoretically superior to use of the Cell Saver because platelets and coagulation factors are not removed and therefore lost from this large volume of blood. The device is simple to attach postoperatively, and is relatively inexpensive. Because the situation of volume excess/low hematocrit does not commonly occur at our institution, from a cost-effectiveness/resource utilization standpoint we cannot justify including the ultrafiltration device in every circuit setup. We do, however, keep ultrafiltration capability ready for when appropriate circumstances arise.

Optimal Surgical Technical and Maximum Surgical Hemostasis

One of the most important contributions that the surgeon can make to blood conservation efforts is to perform a swift and accurate procedure that incurs minimal intraoperative blood loss and that results in minimum postoperative bleeding. During chest opening and vein graft harvesting all potential bleeding points should be controlled with liberal use of clips, ties, and cautery where appropriate. Lap pads, sponges, and discard sucker should be used sparingly as these result in direct unsalvageable autologous blood loss. All blood should be aspirated/salvaged from the chest before closure, and at any time that the perfusionist indicates that circuit reservoir level is low. Venous cannulae should be adjusted as required to optimize venous return and therefore decrease the amount of crystalloid or blood that must be added to the circuit by the perfusionist to maintain minimum acceptable reservoir levels. Communication between the surgeon and the perfusionist concerning this point is essential. Anastomoses should be checked for leaks prior to chest closure, and all suture lines should be oversewn (aortic, atrial, etc.).

Adequate Patient Warming

Patients should be rewarmed to at least 36°C before separation from CPB to help optimize platelet and coagulation factor function. In addition, the operating room should be warmed to help maintain patient temperature. Upon arrival in the ICU the patient should be placed on a warming blanket. We additionally apply an air convection warming blanket over the patient and strive to rapidly achieve and maintain a temperature of 37°C postoperatively. These efforts should be accelerated and intensified in the setting of clinically significant postoperative bleeding. Adequate patient warming is the job of the perfusionist, anesthesiologist, surgical, and nursing staff. It requires a collaborative team approach.

Shed Mediastinal Blood Reinfusion

The platelets contained in shed mediastinal blood are nonfunctional, and defibrinogenation has occurred. It is useful, therefore, only for the reclamation of red cell mass. This is a very important function, however, which can help to negate the loss in red cell mass that occurs with postoperative bleeding. The fibrin split products, as well as the increased levels of other degradation products found in this blood, at most mildly exacerbate postoperative coagulopathic bleeding, but this is more than offset by the volume of red cells that is restored to the circulation. We reinfuse shed blood intermittently every 3 hours, for a maximum of 12 hours, until the collected volume is less than 100 ml over the preceding 3-hour period. We believe that by waiting 3 hours for the first reinfusion, much of the obligatory coagulopathy of CPB is allowed to resolve, and therefore the negative effects of shed blood with respect to bleeding have less of an exacerbating effect. The argument that the hematocrit of shed blood is low (typically 15–25%, depending on the rate of blood loss and the postoperative time) rendering it useless is fallacious, as the importance of shed blood reinfusion lies in the restoration of red cell mass. For example, if the shed blood hematocrit is 20%, if 400 ml of shed blood are reinfused, this results in the reinfusion of 80 ml of red cell mass. This is the equivalent of between one third and one fourth of a unit of packed red cells. If bleeding is rapid and of larger volumes, significantly more lost red cell mass can be reclaimed. We use the Deknatel Pleurovac ATS shed blood reinfusion system, in which a collection/reinfusion bag is attached proximal and in line to the Pleurovac. Initially only the mediastinal tube (along with any pleural tubes that may be attached to this tube) is attached to a collection bag. We found that it is the mediastinal tube that drains a majority of blood, and this therefore helps to limit waste and control costs. If one of the pleural tubes begins to drain significant volumes of blood, then a collection bag is attached to this tube as well. All blood is reinfused by gravity drainage through a 40-μm Pall blood filter. Our only contraindications to shed blood reinfusion are the presence of gross infection, the use of Betadine irrigation or other toxic substance that might enter into the shed blood, or the intraoperative use of fibrin glue. Such circumstances are rarely encountered in our practice. Under typical circumstances, reinfusion of shed mediastinal blood is primarily the responsibility of the nursing staff.

Occasionally very rapid, clearly surgical bleeding is encountered, and this rapid rate precludes defibrinogenation of the blood prior to its leaving the chest cavity. In this setting, frank clotting of the shed blood can occur, precluding its reinfusion. In this situation heparin must be administered to the collection bag as soon as such clotting is encountered, or if it is anticipated based on the rate of blood loss. We administer enough heparin to anticoagulate for 500 cc of blood, and reinfuse the blood after each 500 cc has been collected. As the patient is brought to the operating room, we place enough heparin for a full 1000-cc bag, and process this blood with the Cell Saver once in the operating room. This is a difficult situation at a time when the major emphasis is, and should be, on return of the patient to the operating room as rapidly as possible. However, careful attention to appropriate collection, treatment (i.e., heparin, if required), and reinfusion of these large volumes of fresh shed blood can markedly reduce concurrent and subsequent allogeneic red cell requirements. While shed mediastinal blood reinfusion is generally performed by the ICU nursing staff, during times of rapid bleeding prior and during return to the operating room, it is helpful to designate a single individual to be in charge of shed blood collection and reinfusion.

Minimum Safe Red Cell Transfusion Triggers (See Chapter 16)
(CPB = 15%, post-CPB = 19%, ICU = 21.9%)

This is one of the key elements of our blood conservation program. The simplest and most cost-effective way to reduce the use of homologous red cells is to transfuse them only when it becomes physiologically necessary. An awareness of the lowest safe level of anemia during each of the perioperative periods is therefore essential. This is discussed in detail in Chapter 16, Indications for Red Cell Transfusion, and Table 27.5 provides a concise summary of what the literature has demonstrated (and what we feel) to work well clinically. Allogeneic red cell use should be safely minimized when given according to these guidelines. An important component of minimum safe transfusion is the need to adjust the transfusion triggers upward or downward depending on the age, disease status, and most importantly clinical symptomatology demonstrated at any given time. Allogeneic red cells should be reinfused at these times only when all available autologous red cell mass has been reinfused (PAD blood, IAD blood, Cell Saver/salvaged blood, shed mediastinal blood).

Postoperative Bleeding Protocol (See Chapter 20)

We feel that it is essential to apply a standard regimen for treatment of the patient with excessive postoperative bleeding. This protocol must provide criteria for identifying the patient with clinically significant bleeding, so that the protocol can be instituted in a timely manner, and it must provide for organized and rapid implementation of all available hemostatic maneuvers. The central themes of our bleeding protocol is the allotment of sufficient time for the obligatory coagulopathy of CPB to resolve with maximum nontransfusion supportive therapy before instituting homologous platelet and coagulation factor therapy. Regardless of the presence of coagulopathic bleeding in the operating room, we virtually never administer homologous platelets and coagulation factors during this immediate post-CPB period. Prophylactic platelet and coagulation factor therapy during this time has never been shown to be of benefit, and our own studies have demonstrated that even the reinfusion of four to five units of fresh IAD blood does not decrease postoperative bleeding (see Chapter 11, Intraoperative Donation Practices).[19] We therefore reserve the use of these homologous blood products for reinfusion in the postoperative care area, and only if the rate of bleeding continues in excess of our guidelines and has not responded to institution of the other technical and pharmacologic treatment modalities. Probably no other single component of our multimodality program has resulted in a larger reduction in the number of total donor exposures than this simple rule of waiting to institute allogeneic blood component therapy. Figure 27.4 is a summary of our approach to the patient with increased postoperative bleeding (as marked by mediastinal drainage).

Minimize Laboratory Blood Sampling Losses (See Chapter 21, Nursing Interventions)

The amount of blood lost through perioperative laboratory testing can be markedly reduced by three basic measures: (1) limiting the number of blood samples obtained during the perioperative period, (2) use of small sample volume (pediatric) blood tubes, and (3) return of arterial line flush volumes.

TABLE 27.5. Guidelines for red blood cell transfusion during the perioperative period.

Perioperative time point	Factors affecting tolerance	Recommended transfusion trigger	Adjustment of trigger upward	Adjustment of trigger downward
Preoperative	Awake Normothermic +Cardiovascular disease	25%	Ongoing ischemia Hemodynamic instability Small body size	Asymptomatic with very large body size
Intraopeative/pre-CPB	Anesthetized Normothermic +Cardiovascular disease	25%	Ongoing ischemia Hemodynamic instability Small body size (calculate hct on CPB)	Asymptomatic with very large body size
Intraoperative/CPB	Anesthetized Hypothermic Cardiopulmonary bypass	(1) 15% or less (2) 17% or less (+ stroke risk)		Profound hypothermia
Postoperative	Anesthetized/awake Normothermic +/−Cardiovascular disease	(1) less than 22% (age 75 or less) (2) less than 24% (age 76 or greater)	Poor revascularization Low cardiac output Pulmonary failure/hypoxia Cardiac/cerebral ischemia	Young, healthy, and asymptomatic

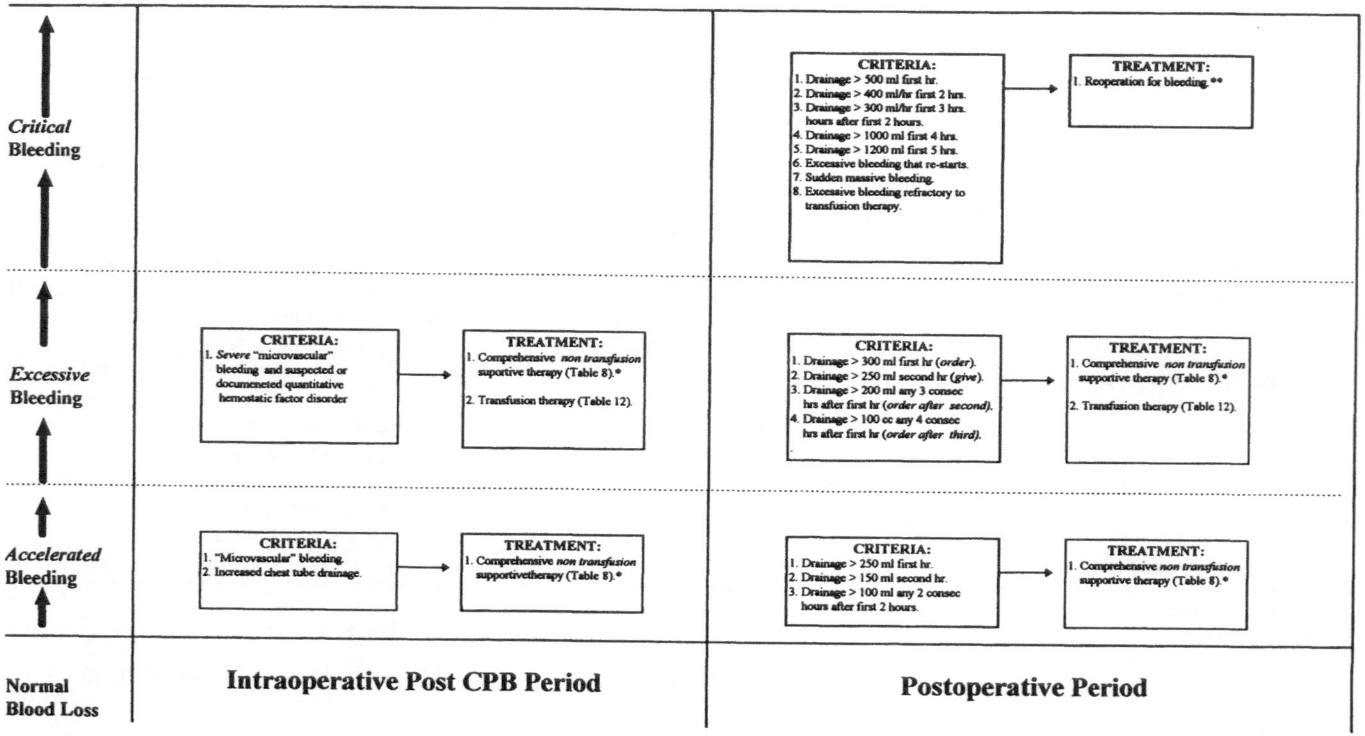

* Non- transfusion supportive therapy includes: (1) adequate and sustained warming, (2) blood pressure control, (3) PEEP increase, (4) pharmacologicRx (protamine, EACA, DDAVP).
** Implied is that the full set of non transfusion modalities has been implemented, and that appropriate blood product support has or is being given.

FIGURE 27.4. Algorithm for the treatment of increased postoperative bleeding.

Remarkably few laboratory tests are required to assess and maintain optimal patient status during the perioperative period. The number of tests performed can be minimized by establishing clinical algorithms or "pathways" based on careful analysis. The initiation of a critical care pathway at our institution reduced the number of laboratory tests by 40%. Pediatric blood tubes reduce sampling volumes by as much as 80%. Finally, return of arterial line flushes during the immediate perioperative period reclaims additional autologous blood mass. This can be done either manually, or with the various closed reinfusion system devices. Together, these three measures can reduce perioperative blood loss by over 60% – decreasing lost volume from 450 cc to 80 cc during a typical CABG patient's hospitalization (see Figure 21.3, Chapter 21).

Pharmacologic Conservation Measures

Erythropoietin (See Chapter 4)

Erythropoietin is administered selectively to those patients at increased risk for requiring red cell transfusion (hematocrit less than 34% *and* red cell mass less than 1600 cc). Begun preoperatively at the time of admission for surgery, the initial (admission) dose is a combined intravenous (300 U/kg IV, in 50-cc D5W administered over 15 minutes) and subcutaneous (500 U/kg SQ) dose designed to achieve the high prolonged initial erythropoietin peak blood levels consistent with the natural maximum erythropoietin response. Erythropoietin is then continued at 500 U/kg every other day until the time of surgery. For obvious reasons of cost containment, we delay surgery only to allow time for an increase in hematocrit in the Jehovah's Witness population. For others, the benefit of this acute erythropoietin therapy is primarily seen during the postoperative period. Erythropoietin therapy is continued postoperatively (500 U/kg) selectively only for those patients with low postoperative hematocrits (less than 25%). Erythropoietin therapy should always be accomplished by the use of oral or intravenous iron therapy to ensure a maximum erythropoietic response. Details related to the clinical application of erythropoietin can be found in Chapter 4.

Aprotinin (See Chapter 15)

Aprotinin is administered intraoperatively selectively to patients at high risk for excessive bleeding (ASA, heparin/thrombolytic agent use within 48 hours, history of bleeding disorder/coagulation factor deficiency). The bleeding prophylaxis protocol that we apply is delineated in Table 27.6. We employ the half-strength Hammersmith regimen for all primary cases: (1) 1 million units intravenous over 15 minutes prior to the first skin incision, (2) 250,000 units per hour until the last of the IAD blood is reinfused, and (3) 1 million units in the CPB circuit prime prior to the initiation of CPB. Reoperative procedures receive the full Hammersmith regimen (each of the three components is doubled). Alternatively, no control costs, intravenous

Amicar (amino caproic acid) can be utilized in place of aprotinin (see below). Recently aprotinin has been used postoperatively to treat increased postoperative bleeding, with promising results.

Amicar

Although Amicar is less effective at preventing the coagulopathy of CPB than aprotinin (it addresses primarily only one component – fibrinolysis), it nevertheless is a useful agent for bleeding prophylaxis. In an effort to contain costs, it can be used in place of aprotinin. It should still be selectively used only for patients at increased risk for postoperative bleeding (ASA <5 days, heparin therapy within 24 hours, thrombolytic therapy within 7 days). Younger patients with a high likelihood of requiring reoperation, and patients with prior aprotinin use or aprotinin sensitivity (on test dose) should also be treated with Amicar (vs aprotinin), if they are at risk for excessive postoperative bleeding (Table 27.6). Amicar can also used postoperatively for patients with excessive bleeding as one component of a comprehensive bleeding protocol. We do not utilize tranexamic acid because its actions are similar to those of Amicar (it differs primarily in half-life and potency), but at a significantly higher cost. Intraoperatively, Amicar is initiated prior to the first skin incision and is administered according to the standard dosing regimen (initial bolus dose of 5 g over 15 minutes, followed by a continuous infusion of 5 g in 250-cc D5W at 1 g per hour for 4 hours or until excessive bleeding has resolved.

Iron

Oral iron therapy (325 mg TID–QID) is initiated at the time of admission and continued to the time of discharge. It is accompanied by the use of vitamin C (500 mg PO BID) to aid in intestinal absorption of iron (it reduces iron to its ferric state, which is the form adsorbed from the ileum and jejunum). The concomitant use of a stool softener such as Colace (300 mg QD) is also helpful to counter the constipating effects of iron. We reserve the use of intravenous iron for Jehovah's Witness patients who require urgent or emergent surgery and are both anemic and iron deficient (for dosing protocol for these patients see Chapter 4). We feel that the small but real incidence of potentially fatal iron anaphylaxis (1:30,000) does not outweigh the risks or costs of the one to two red cell unit transfusions that might be avoided by the use of intravenous iron in the non–Jehovah's Witness population.

DDAVP

Despite initial excitement about reduction in postoperative bleeding with the use of DDAVP, the data indicate that it provides little benefit in routine surgery utilizing cardiopulmonary bypass. Its activity in promoting release of von Willebrand factor from endothelial cells has been shown to provide

TABLE 27.6. Risk factors for postoperative bleeding and suggested prophylaxis.

Increased bleeding risk	Risk factor	Suggested prophylaxis
I. Low	1. Aspirin (<5 days before surgery)[121] 2. Age >70[123]	1. None
II. Moderate	1. Heparin <72 hours prior to surgery[124] 2. Warfarin with PT >15[124] 3. Thrombolytic therapy within 5 days 4. Reopration[123] 5. ETOH abuse, liver dysfunction[124] 6. Anticipated CPB run >90 min[122,123] 7. Procedure type a. Valve-CABG[122] b. Double valve[122] c. Other complex procedure[122] 8. Uremic renal dysfunction[123] 9. Ongoing infection/sepsis[124] 10. Emergency procedure[123] 11. Preoperative bleeding disorder[127]	1. Amicar (full strength regimen) 2. Optional a. DDAVP (if uremic renal dysfunction)
III. High	1. Multiple low or moderate bleeding risk factors[123] 2. Jehovah's Witness	1. Aprotinin (1/2 strength Hammersmith regimen) 2. Optional a. Full Hammersmith regimen aprotinin b. Heparin bonded circuit c. If contraindication to aprotinin give Amicar d. White cell filtration

benefit in the setting of uremic renal failure and in von Willebrand factor deficiency. DDAVP likely provides benefit in patients at high risk for bleeding, or in those with established coagulopathic bleeding. We therefore reserve DDAVP for use in patients who demonstrate clinically significant bleeding, lowering the threshold for use in the setting of renal failure or von Willebrand's disease.

Aspirin

Discontinuing aspirin therapy 5 to 7 days prior to surgery allows time for sufficient platelet turnover by the time of surgery so that platelet thromboxane production and overall platelet function is returned to normal by the time of surgery, decreasing the magnitude of postoperative bleeding

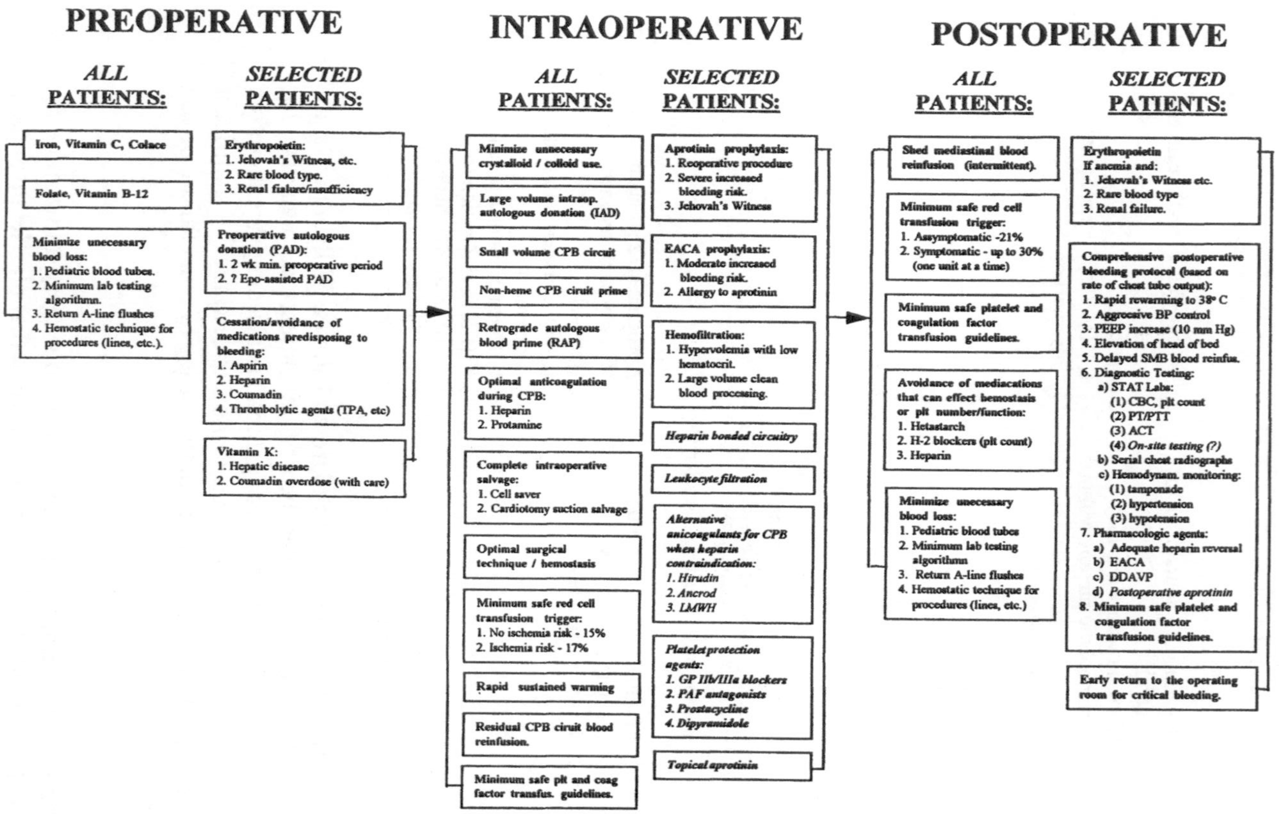
PREOPERATIVE
ALL PATIENTS:
Iron, Vitamin C, Colace
Folate, Vitamin B-12
Minimize unecessary blood loss:
1. Pediatric blood tubes.
2. Minimum lab testing algorithmn.
3. Return A-line flushes
4. Hemostatic technique for procedures (lines, etc.).
SELECTED PATIENTS:
Erythropoietin:
1. Jehovah's Witness, etc.
2. Rare blood type.
3. Renal fialure/insufficiency
Preoperative autologous donation (PAD):
1. 2 wk min. preoperative period
2. ? Epo-assisted PAD
Cessation/avoidance of medications predisposing to bleeding:
1. Aspirin
2. Heparin
3. Coumadin
4. Thrombolytic agents (TPA, etc)
Vitamin K:
1. Hepatic disease
2. Coumadin overdose (with care)
INTRAOPERATIVE
ALL PATIENTS:
Minimize unnecessary crystalloid / colloid use.
Large volume intraop. autologous donation (IAD)
Small volume CPB circuit
Non-heme CPB ciruit prime
Retrograde autologous blood prime (RAP)
Optimal anticoagulation during CPB:
1. Heparin
2. Protamine
Complete intraoperative salvage:
1. Cell saver
2. Cardiotomy suction salvage
Optimal surgical technique / hemostasis
Minimum safe red cell transfusion trigger:
1. No ischemia risk - 15%
2. Ischemia risk - 17%
Rapid sustained warming
Residual CPB ciruit blood reinfusion.
Minimum safe plt and coag factor transfus. guidelines.
SELECTED PATIENTS:
Aprotinin prophylaxis:
1. Reoperative procedure
2. Severe increased bleeding risk.
3. Jehovah's Witness
EACA prophylaxis:
1. Moderate increased bleeding risk.
2. Allergy to aprotinin
Hemofiltration:
1. Hypervolemia with low hematocrit.
2. Large volume clean blood processing.
Heparin bonded circuitry
Leukocyte filtration
Alternative anicoagulants for CPB when heparin contraindication:
1. Hirudin
2. Ancrod
3. LMWH
Platelet protection agents:
1. GP IIb/IIIa blockers
2. PAF antagonists
3. Prostacycline
4. Dipyramidole
Topical aprotinin
POSTOPERATIVE
ALL PATIENTS:
Shed mediastinal blood reinfusion (intermittent).
Minimum safe red cell transfusion trigger:
1. Assymptomatic -21%
2. Symptomatic - up to 30% (one unit at a time)
Minimum safe platelet and coagulation factor transfusion guidelines.
Avoidance of mediacations that can effect hemostasis or plt number/function:
1. Hetastarch
2. H-2 blockers (plt count)
3. Heparin
Minimize unecessary blood loss:
1. Pediatric blood tubes
2. Minimum lab testing algorithmn
3. Return A-line flushes
4. Hemostatic technique for procedures (lines, etc.)
SELECTED PATIENTS:
Erythropoietin
If anemia and:
1. Jehovah's Witness etc.
2. Rare blood type
3. Renal failure.
Comprehensive postoperative bleeding protocol (based on rate of chest tube output):
1. Rapid rewarming to 38° C
2. Aggressive BP control
3. PEEP increase (10 mm Hg)
4. Elevation of head of bed
5. Delayed SMB blood reinfus.
6. Diagnostic Testing:
a) STAT Labs:
(1) CBC, plt count
(2) PT/PTT
(3) ACT
(4) On-site testing (?)
b) Serial chest radiographs
c) Hemodynam. monitoring:
(1) tamponade
(2) hypertension
(3) hypotension
7. Pharmacologic agents:
a) Adequate heparin reversal
b) EACA
c) DDAVP
d) Postoperative aprotinin
8. Minimum safe platelet and coagulation factor transfusion guidelines.
Early return to the operating room for critical bleeding.

FIGURE 27.5. The New York Hospital–Cornell Medical College Multimodality Blood Conservation Program. Techniques and pharmacologic agents are listed under the perioperative period in which they are applied. Newer modalities which have not yet been clearly demonstrated to be of benefit or are investigational are listed in italics. LMWH = low molecular weight heparin; PAF = platelet activating factor; BP = blood pressure; ACT = activated clotting time; EACA = ϵ-aminocaproic acid; DDAVP = D arginine amino vasopressin; PEEP = positive end expiratory pressure; TPA = tissue plasminogen activator.

attributable to this partial platelet defect. However, with the changing nature of the circumstances surrounding cardiac surgery (i.e., a higher proportion of surgeries performed within 7 days of catheterization) and the decision to perform surgery, the ability to discontinue aspirin therapy within 5 to 7 days is becoming less and less common. In addition, the wisdom of discontinuing the use of a drug that has been shown to provide benefit in decreasing the incidence of myocardial infarction prior to the time of repairing lesions that are at risk of causing infarction can be questioned. For these reasons, and because we now have available the means to help counteract other factors contributing to the postoperative coagulopathic state (aprotinin, Amicar, tranexamic acid), we no longer require the discontinuation of aspirin therapy within 5 to 7 days of surgery. In appropriate patients undergoing purely elective surgery, however, we do request that this be done if possible.

Other Drugs

Patients with preoperative anemia should also be given appropriate supplementation of folate (1 mg PO qd) and vitamin B_{12} (1000 μg IM qd) to treat these potential deficiencies.

An Algorithm for Optimal Multimodality Cardiac Surgical Blood Conservation

The preceding section summarized our use of the many available technical and pharmacologic blood conservation modalities. An algorithm demonstrates the way in which these techniques are integrated during the perioperative period (Fig. 27.4). Using a team approach that both optimizes and integrates the use of each of these measures, the use of homologous blood can be markedly reduced in a majority of cardiac surgical patients. This reduction can be achieved both safely and cost-effectively.

References

1. Roche J, Stengle JM. Open-heart surgery and the demand for blood. *JAMA* 1973;225(12):1516–1521.
2. Pekkanen J. America's looming blood shortage. *Reader's Digest* May 1994;1–8.
3. Loussert-Ajaka I, Ly TD, Chaix ML, et al. HIV-1/HIV-2 seronegativity in HIV-1 subtype O infected patients. *Lancet* 1994;343(8910):1393–1394.
4. Dondero TJ, Dale JH, George JR. HIV-1 variants: yet another challenge to public health. *Lancet* 1994;343(8910):1376.
5. Pollack A. Variants of AIDS virus can elude blood tests. *The New York Times* August 8, 1994, p. 5.
6. Cowley G, Springen K, Hager M. In search of safer blood. *Newsweek* August 10, 1992;44–45.
7. Helm RE, Uzzo RG, O'Connor LT, Rosengart TK, Krieger KH, Young G.

Blood conservation techniques in urologic surgery: preliminary experience. *J Urology* 1996;155(5):631A.
8. Rosengart TK, Helm RE, DeBois W, et al. Open heart surgery without transfusion: results of a multimodality strategy in 50 Jehovah's Witness patients. *J Amer Coll Surg* 1997 (in press).
9. Johnson RG, Thurer RL, Kruskall MS, et al. Comparison of two transfusion strategies after elective operations for myocardial revascularization. *J Thorac Cardiovasc Surg* 1992;104:307–314.
10. Watanabe Y, Fuse K, Naruse Y, et al. Subcutaneous use of erythropoietin in heart surgery. *Ann Thorac Surg* 1992;54:479-483.
11. Kulier AH, Gombotz H, Fuchs G, et al. Subcutaneous recombinant erythropoietin and autologous blood donation before coronary artery bypass surgery. *Anesth Analg* 1993;76:102–106.
12. Ovrum E, Holen EA, Abdelnoor M, Oystese R. Conventional blood conservation techniques in 500 consecutive coronary artery bypass operations. *Ann Thorac Surg* 1991;51:500–505.
13. Ovrum E, Holen EA, Lindstein Ringdal MA. Elective coronary artery bypass without homologous blood transfusion. *Scand J Thorac Cardiovasc Surg* 1991;25:13–18.
14. Daily PO, Lamphere JA, Dembitsky WP, et al. Effect of prophylactic epsilon aminocaproic acid on blood loss and transfusion requirements in patients undergoing first time coronary artery bypass grafting. *J Thorac Cardiovasc Surg* 1994;108:99–108.
15. Cosgrove DM, Thurer RL, Lytle BW, et al. Blood conservation during myocardial revascularization. *Ann Thorac Surg* 1979;28(2):184–188.
16. Cosgrove DM, Loop FD, Lytle BW, et al. Determinants of blood utilization during myocardial revascularization. *Ann Thorac Surg* 1985;40(4):381–384.
17. Belcher P, Lennox SC. Reduction of blood use in surgery for coronary artery disease. *J Cardiovasc Surg* 1986;27:657–661.
18. Jones JW, Rawitscher RE, Mclean TR, et al. Benefit from combining blood conservation measures in cardiac operations. *Ann Thorac Surg* 1991; 51:541–546.
19. Owings DV, Kruskall MS, Thurer RL, et al. Autologous blood donations prior to elective cardiac surgery. *JAMA* 1989;262(14):1963–1968.
20. Helm RE, Klemperer JD, Rosengart TK, et al. Intraoperative autologous donation preserves red cell mass but does not decrease postoperative bleeding. *Ann Thorac Surg* 1996;62(5):1431–1441.
21. Karski JM, Teasdale SJ, Norman PH, et al. Prevention of postbypass bleeding with tranexamic acid and epsilon aminocaproic acid. *J Cardiothorac Vasc Anesth* 1993;7(4):431–435.
22. Zubiate P, Kay JH, Mendez AH, et al. Coronary artery surgery. A new technique with use of little blood if any. *J Thorac Cardiovasc Surg* 1974; 68(2):104–109.
23. Hartz RS, Smith JA, Green D. Autotransfusion after cardiac operations. *J Thorac Cardiovasc Surg* 1988;96:178–182.
24. LoCicero J, Massad M, Gandy K, et al. Aggressive blood conservation in coronary artery surgery: Impact on patient care. *J Cardiovasc Surg* 1990; 31:559–563.
25. Paone G, Spencer T, Silverman NA. Blood conservation in coronary artery surgery. *Surgery* 1994;116:672–678.

26. Jones JW, McCoy TA, Rawitscher RE, et al. Effects of intraoperative plasmapheresis on blood loss in cardiac surgery. *Ann Thorac Surg* 1990;49:585–590.
27. Schonberger JP, Bredee JJ, Tijan D, et al. Introaperative predonation contributes to blood saving. *Ann Thorac Surg* 1993;56:893–898.
28. Rousou JA, Engelman RM, Flack JE, et al. Tranexamic acid significantly reduces blood loss associated with coronary revascularization. *Ann Thorac Surg* 1995;59:671–675.
29. Lemmer JH, Stanford, Bonney SL, et al. Aprotinin for coronary bypass operations: Effiacy, safety, and influence on early saphenous vein graft patency. *J Thorac Cardiovasc Surg* 1994;107:543–553.
30. Breyer RH, Engelman RM, Rousou JA, Lemeshow S. Blood conservation for myocardial revascularization. *J Thorac Cardiovasc Surg* 1987;93:512–522.
31. Weisel RD, Charlesworth DC, Mickleborough LL, et al. Limitations of blood conservation. *J Thorac Cardiovasc Surg* 1984;88:26–38.
32. Parrot D, Lancon JP, Merle JP, et al. Blood salvage in cardic surgery. *J Cardiothorac Vasc Anesth* 1991;00:454–456.
33. Petry AF, Jost T, Sievers H. Reduction of homologous blood requirements by blood-pooling at the onset of cardiopulmonary bypass. *J Thorac Cardiovasc Surg* 1994;107:1210–1214.
34. Deitrich W, Barankay A, Dilthey G, et al. Reduction of blood utilization during myocardial revascularization. *J Thorac Cardiovasc Surg* 1989;97:213–219.
35. Tobe CE, Vocelka C, Sepulvada R, et al. Infusion of autologous platelet rich plasma does not reduce blood loss and blood product use after coronary artery bypass. *J Thorac Cardiovasc Surg* 1993;105:1007–1014.
36. Tyson GS, Sladen RN, Spainhour V, et al. Blood conservation in cardiac surgery: Preliminary results with an institutional commitment. *Ann Surg* 1989;209(6):736–742.
37. Yeh T, Shelton L, Yeh TJ. Blood loss and bank blood requirement in coronary bypass surgery. *Ann Thorac Surg* 1978;26(1):11–16.
38. Ward HB, Smith RRA, Landis KP, et al. Prospective, randomized trial of autotransfusion after routine cardiac operations. *Ann Thorac Surg* 1993; 56:137–141.
39. Schaff HV, Hauer J, Gardner TJ, et al. Routine use of autotransfusion following cardiac surgery: Experience in 700 patients. *Ann Thorac Surg* 1979;27(6):493–499.
40. Arom KV, Emery RW. Decreased postoperative drainage with addition of epsilon aminocaproic acid before cardiopulmonary bypass. *Ann Thorac Surg* 1994;57:1108–1113.
41. Davies GG, Wells DG, Mabee TM, et al. Platelet-leukocyte plasmapheresis attenuates the deleterious effects of cardiopulmonary bypass. *Ann Thorac Surg* 1992;53:274–277.
42. Sutton RG, Kratz JM, Spinale FG, Crawford FA. Comparison of three blood processing techniques during and after cardiopulmonary bypass. *Ann Thorac Surg* 1993;56:938–943.
43. Bayer WL, Coenen WM, Jenkins DC, et al. The use of blood and blood components in 1769 patients undergoing open-heart surgery. *Ann Thorac Surg* 1980;29(2):117–122.
44. Rosengart TK, Helm RE, Klemperer JD, et al. Combined aprotinin and erythropoietin use for blood conservation: Results with Jehovah's Witnesses. *Ann Thorac Surg* 1994;58:1397–1403.

45. Beall AC, Yow EM, Bloodwell RD, et al. Open heart surgery without blood transfusion. *Arch Surg* 1967;94:567–570.
46. Sandrelli L, Pardini A, Lorusso R, et al. Impact of autologous blood predonation on a comprehensive blood conservation program. *Ann Thorac Surg* 1995;59:730–735.
47. Helm RE, Klemperer JD, Rosengart T, et al. Intraoperative autologous donation: volume dependent red cell preservation. *Surg Forum* 1994; 45:249–252.
48. Parolari A, Antona C, Rona P, et al. The effect of multiple blood conservation techniques on donor blood exposures in adult coronary and valve surgery performed with a membrane oxygenator: A multivariate analysis on 1310 patients. *J Card Surg* 1995;10:227–235.
49. Wong CA, Franklin ML, Wade LD. Coagulation tests, blood loss, and transfusion requirements in platelet-rich plasmapheresed versus non-pheresed cardiac surgery patients. *Anesth Analg* 1994;78:29–36.
50. Horrow JC, Van Riper DF, Strong MD, et al. Hemostatic effects of tranexamic acid and desmopressin during cardiac surgery. *Circulation* 1991;84:2063–2070.
51. Dzik WH, Fleisher AG, Ciavarella D, et al. Safety and efficacy of autologous blood donation before elective aortic valve operation. *Ann Thorac Surg* 1992;54:1177–1181.
52. Horrow JC, Hlavacek J, Strong MD, et al. Prophylactic tranexamic acid decreases bleeding after cardiac operations. *J Thorac Cardiovasc Surg* 1990;99:70–74.
53. Britton LW, Eastlund T, Dziuban SW, et al. Predonated autologous blood use in elective cardiac surgery. *Ann Thorac Surg* 1989;47:529–532.
54. Johnson RG, Rosenkrantz KR, Preston RA, et al. The efficacy of postoperative autotransfusion in patients undergoing cardiac operations. *Ann Thorac Surg* 1983;36(2):173–179.
55. Love TR, Hendren WG, O'Keefe DD, et al. Transfusion of predonated autologous blood in elective cardiac surgery. *Ann Thorac Surg* 1987; 43:508–512.
56. Shinfeld A, Zippel D, Lavee J, et al. Aprotinin improves hemostasis after cardiopulmonary bypass better than single-donor platelet concentrate. *Ann Thorac Surg* 1995;59:872–876.
57. Carey JS, Cukingnan RA, Carson E. Transfusion therapy in cardiac surgery: Impact of the Paul Gann Blood Safety Act in California. *Am Surg* 1991; 57:830–835.
58. Thurer RL, Lytle BW, Cosgrove DM. Autotransfusion following cardiac operations: A randomized, prospective study. *Ann Thorac Surg* 1979; 27(6):500–507.
59. Schaff HV, Hauer JM, Bell WR, et al. Autotransfusion of shed mediastinal blood after cardiac surgery. *J Thorac Cardiovasc Surg* 1978;75(4):632–641.
60. Del Rossi AJ, Cernaian, Bostros S, et al. Prophylactic treatment of post perfusion bleeding using EACA. *Chest* 1989;96:27–30.
61. Scott WJ, Rode R, Castlemain B, et al. Efficacy, complications, and cost of a comprehensive blood conservation program for cardiac operations. *J Thorac Cardiovasc Surg* 1992;103:1001–1007.
62. Murkin JM, Lux J, Shannon NA, et al. Aprotinin significantly decreases bleeding and transfusion requirements in patients receiving aspirin and undergoing cardiac operations. *J Thorac Cardiovasc Surg* 1994;107:554–561.

63. Axford TC, Dearani JA, Ragno G, et al. Safety and therapeutic effectiveness of reinfused shed blood after open heart surgery. *Ann Thorac Surg* 1994; 57:615–622.
64. Lambert CJ, Marengo-Rowe AJ, Leveson JE, et al. The treatment of post perfusion bleeding using epsilon aminocaproic acid, cryoprecipitate, fresh frozen plasma, and protamine sulfate. *Ann Thorac Surg* 1979;28(5):440–444.
65. Ikeda S, Johnston MFM, Yagi K, et al. Intraoperative autologous blood salvage with cardiac surgery: An analysis of five years' experience in more than 3000 patients. *J Clin Anesth* 1992;4:359–366.
66. Lepore V, Radegram K. Autotransfusion of mediastinal blood in cardiac surgery. *Scand J Thorac Cardiovasc Surg* 1989;23:47–49.
67. Cove H, Matloff J, Sacks JH, et al. Autologous blood transfusion in coronary artery bypass surgery. *Transfusion* 1976;16(3):25–248.
68. Spiess BD, Gillies BSA, Chandler W, et al. Changes in transfusion therapy and reexploration rate after institution of a blood management program in cardiac surgical patients. *J Thor Cardiothorac Vasc Anesth* 1995;9(2):168–173.
69. Page R, Russel GN, Fox MA. Hard-shell cardiotomy reservoir for reinfusion of shed mediastinal blood. *Ann Thorac Surg* 1989;48:514–517.
70. Cohn LH, Fosberg AM, Anderson WP, et al. The effects of phlebotomy, hemodilution, and autologous transfusion on systemic oxygenation and whole blood utilization in open-heart surgery. *Chest* 1975;68(3):283–287.
71. Kaplan JA, Cannarella C, Jones EL, et al. Autologous blood transfusion during cardiac surgery. A re-evaluation of three methods. *J Thorac Cardiovasc Surg* 1977;74(1):4–10.
72. Lilleaasen P. Moderate and extreme hemodilution in open-heart surgery. *Scand J Thorac Cardiovasc Surg* 1977;11:97–103.
73. Giordano GF, Rivers SL, Chung GKT, et al. Autologous platelet-rich plasma in cardiac surgery: Effect on intraoperative and postoperative transfusion requirements. *Ann Thorac Surg* 1988;46:416–419.
74. Giordano GF, Goldman DS, Mammana RB, et al. Intraoperative autotransfusion in cardiac operations: Effect on intraoperative and postoperative transfusion requirements. *J Thorac Cardiovasc Surg* 1988;96:382–386.
75. Cooley DA, Bloodwell RD, Beall AC, et al. Cardiac valve replacement without blood transfusion. *Am J Surg* 1966;112:743–751.
76. Bailey CP, Hirose Teruo, Gollub S, et al. Open heart surgery without blood transfusion. *Vasc Dis* 1968;5(4):179–187.
77. Beall AC, Yow EM, Bloodwell RD, et al. Open heart surgery without blood transfusion. *Arch Surg* 1967;94:567–570
78. Helm RE, Gold JP, Rosengart TK, et al. Erythropoietin in cardiac surgery. *J Cardiovasc Surg* 1993;8(5):579–606.
79. D'Ambra MN, Lynch KE, Boccagno J, et al. The effect of perioperative administration of recombinant human erythropoietin (r-HuEPO) in CABG patients: a double blind, placebo-controlled trial. *Anesthesiology* 1992; 77(3a):A159 (Abstract).
80. Abraham PA, Halstenson CI, Macres MM, et al. Epoetin enhances erythropoiesis in normal men undergoing repeated phlebotomies. *Clin Pharmacol Ther* 1992;52:205–213.
81. Murkin JM, Lux J, Shannon NA, et al. Aprotinin significantly decreases bleeding and transfusion requirements in patients receiving aspirin and undergoing cardiac operations. *J Thorac Cardiovasc Surg* 1994;107:554–561.

82. van Oeveren W, Harder MP, Roozendaal, et al. Aprotinin protects platelets against the initial effects of cardiopulmonary bypass. *J Thorac Cardiovasc Surg* 1990;99:788–797.
83. Horrow JC. Management of the coagulopathy of CPB. In: Gravlee GP, Davis RF, Utley JR, eds. *Cardiopulmonary Bypass: Principles and Practice*. Philadelphia: Williams & Wilkins, 1993.
84. Helm RE, Uzzo RG, O'Conner LT, et al. Blood conservation techniques in urologic surgery: preliminery experience. *J Urology* 1996;155(5):631A.

Index